Handbook of
MEDICAL SURGICAL NURSING

Handbook of
MEDICAL SURGICAL NURSING

BT Basavanthappa MN PhD

Principal
RajaRajeswari College of Nursing
Bengaluru, Karnataka, India

Former Professor and Principal
Government College of Nursing
Bengaluru, Karnataka, India

PhD Guide for Research Work
Ex-Member
Faculty of Nursing, RGUHS, Karnataka, India
Academic Council, RGUHS, Karnataka, India
Examiner
UG, PG and Doctoral Degree Courses on Nursing in various Universities
Ex-Program In-Charge
IGNOU, BSc (N) Course, Karnataka and Goa, India
Life Member
Nursing Research Society of India, New Delhi, India
Trained Nurses Association of India, New Delhi, India
President
RGUHS, Nursing Teachers Association, Karnataka, India
Winner
Bharat Excellence Award and Gold Medal
Vikas Rattan Gold Award
UWA Lifetime Achievement Award
Shree Veeranjaneya 'Shrujanashri' Award

JAYPEE The Health Sciences Publisher
New Delhi | London | Philadelphia | Panama

Jaypee Brothers Medical Publishers (P) Ltd

Headquarters

Jaypee Brothers Medical Publishers (P) Ltd
4838/24, Ansari Road, Daryaganj
New Delhi 110 002, India
Phone: +91-11-43574357
Fax: +91-11-43574314
Email: jaypee@jaypeebrothers.com

Overseas Offices

J.P. Medical Ltd
83 Victoria Street, London
SW1H 0HW (UK)
Phone: +44 20 3170 8910
Fax: +44 (0)20 3008 6180
Email: info@jpmedpub.com

Jaypee-Highlights Medical Publishers Inc
City of Knowledge, Bld. 237, Clayton
Panama City, Panama
Phone: +1 507-301-0496
Fax: +1 507-301-0499
Email: cservice@jphmedical.com

Jaypee Medical Inc
The Bourse
111 South Independence Mall East
Suite 835, Philadelphia, PA 19106, USA
Phone: +1 267-519-9789
Email: jpmed.us@gmail.com

Jaypee Brothers Medical Publishers (P) Ltd
17/1-B Babar Road, Block-B, Shaymali
Mohammadpur, Dhaka-1207
Bangladesh
Mobile: +08801912003485
Email: jaypeedhaka@gmail.com

Jaypee Brothers Medical Publishers (P) Ltd
Bhotahity, Kathmandu, Nepal
Phone +977-9741283608
Email: kathmandu@jaypeebrothers.com

Website: www.jaypeebrothers.com
Website: www.jaypeedigital.com

Inquiries for bulk sales may be solicited at: jaypee@jaypeebrothers.com

Handbook of Medical Surgical Nursing

First Edition: ***2015***

ISBN 978-93-5152-583-7

Printed at Sanat Printers, Kundli

Preface

It gives me immense pleasure and satisfaction to introduce the *Handbook of Medical Surgical Nursing* to our nursing community. In offering this title, I remain grateful to all readers who supported my all titles of nursing.

Actually this book is the handbook for my title *Medical Surgical Nursing*, Third edition. This has been written according to the contents included in the text. This will be the concise, quick reference designed for use by nursing students and members of the nursing profession. This book enables students and readers to gain quick access to key points of information on disease, etiology, pathophysiology, diagnosis and management of diseases. If readers want more information required for the respected diseases, they are requested to refer relevant chapters in Author's Third edition of *Medical Surgical Nursing*.

I am aware that for manifold reasons errors might have crept in and shall feel obliged if such errors are brought to my notice for taking suitable measures. I sincerely welcome constructive criticism from readers.

BT Basavanthappa

Acknowledgments

I owe a great deal of thanks to many people who supported me with their time and encouragement throughout:

- Shri G Basavannappa, Former Minister of Karnataka, for initiating and supporting me to take up this 'Noble Nursing Profession' as my career
- Dr (Mrs) Manjula K Vasundhra, Professor and Head, Department of Community Medicine, Bangalore Medical College, Bengaluru, Karnataka, India, who continuously encouraged me to write textbooks in the field of nursing, a major force in medical and health service
- My father Shri Thukkappa who continues to grace for the progress of my career and all-round development of my personality for welfare of the community
- My mother Smt Hanumanthamma who continues to be bright spot in the lives of all who knew her and whose grace gave me strength to progress in my life
- My wife Smt Lalitha who gives meaning to my life in so many ways; she is the one whose encouragement keeps me motivated, whose support gives me the strength and whose gentleness gives me comfort
- My lovely children BB Mahesh and BB Ganashree, for all the joy they provided me for all the hope that they instill in me and who bear with patience throughout my works of nursing textbook; they keep me young at heart
- Finally my warmest appreciation goes to Shri Jitendar P Vij (Group Chairman), Mr Ankit Vij (Group President) and Mr Tarun Duneja (Director–Publishing) and all the staff of Bengaluru Branch of M/s Jaypee Brothers Medical Publishers (P) Ltd, New Delhi, India, for sharing my vision for this book and giving me the chance to turn vision into reality.

Acknowledgements

Contents

1 Chapter Brief History of Medicine and Nursing in India

MEDICINE IN INDIA

Indian medicine is ancient. Its earliest concepts are set out in the sacred writings called the Vedas, especially in the metrical passages of the Atharvaveda, which may possibly date as far back as the second millennium BC. According to a later writer, the system of medicine called Ayurveda was received by a certain Dhanvantari from Brahma and Dhanvantari was defined as the God of medicine. In later times, his status was gradually reduced, until he was credited with having been an earthly king who died of snakebite. Legends tell of Dhanvantari's relations with snakes and illustrate the skill early Indian practitioners treated snakebites.

The period of Vedic medicine lasted until about 800 BC. The Vedas are rich in magical practices for the treatment of diseases and in charms for the expulsion of the demons traditionally supposed to cause diseases. The chief conditions mentioned are fever, cough, constipation, diarrhea, dropsy, abscesses, seizures, tumors and skin diseases (including leprosy). The herbs recommended for treatment are numerous.

Because, the Hindus were prohibited by their religion from cutting the dead body, their knowledge of anatomy was limited. The Sushruta Samhita recommends that a body be placed in a basket and sunk in a river for 7 days. On its removal, the parts could be easily separated without cutting. As a result of these crude methods, the emphasis in Hindu anatomy was given to the bones and then to the muscles, ligaments and joints. The nerves, blood vessels and internal organs were very imperfectly known.

The Hindus believed that the body contained three elementary substances, microcosmic representatives of the three divine universal forces, which they called spirit (air), phlegm and bile. These were comparable with the humors of the Greeks. Health depends on the normal balance of these three elementary substances. The spirit has its seat below the navel, the phlegm about the heart and the bile between the heart, and the navel. The seven primary constituents of the body are blood, flesh, fat, bone, marrow, chyle and semen are produced by the action of the elementary substances. Semen was supposed to be produced from all parts of the body and not from any individual part or organ.

Both Charaka and Sushruta state the existence of a large number of diseases (Sushruta Samhita contain description of 1,120 illness). Rough classifications of diseases are given. In all texts 'fever' of which numerous types are described, is regarded as important, phthisis (wasting disease, especially pulmonary tuberculosis) was apparently common and the Hindu physicians knew the symptoms of cases likely to terminate fatally. Smallpox was common and it is probable that smallpox inoculation was practiced.

In surgery, ancient Hindu medicine reached its zenith. Detailed instructions about the choice of instruments and the different operations are given in the classical texts. It has been said that the Hindus knew all ancient operations were grouped broadly such as excision of tumors, incision of abscesses punctures of collections of fluid in the abdomen, extraction of foreign bodies (pressing out of the contents of abscesses), probing of fistulas and stitching of wound.

The surgical instruments used by the Hindus have received special attention in modern times. According to Sushruta, the surgeon should be equipped with 20 sharp and 101 blunt instruments. The sharp instruments included knives of various patterns, scissors, trocars (instruments for piercing tissues and draining fluid from them), saws and needles. The blunt instruments included forceps, specula (instruments for inspecting body cavities or passages), tubes, levers, hooks and probes. The Sushruta Samhita does not mention the catheter, but it is referred in later writings. The instruments were largely of steel. Alcohol seems to have been used as a narcotic during operations.

Important Events

A brief description of chronological events related to development of health and medicine in India is given below:

3000 BC: In the Indus Valley Civilization, one finds evidence of well-developed environmental sanitation programs such as underground drains public baths, etc. 'Arogya' or 'Health' was given high priority in daily life and this concept of health included physical, mental, social and spiritual well-being.

2000 BC: Rigveda marks the beginning of the Indian system medicine. Medicine was considered part of Vedas or Scriptures. 'Ayurveda', a 'science of life and art of living' said to be founded by Sage 'Atreya'. Good health implies an ideal balance between tridoshic factors, i.e. wind, bile, phlegm (Vata, Pitta and Kapha) according to Ayurveda. Health promotion and health education were also emphasized by following 'Dinacharya'.

1000 BC: Atharvaveda mentions the twin aims of medical sciences as health and longevity and curative treatment. Hygiene and dietetics are considered important in treatment. Beneficial effects of milk are described in detail.

800 BC: A codification of medical knowledge scattered through Vedas by Bhela called Bhela Samhita.

700 BC: A codification of medical knowledge by Agnivesha said to be desciple of Atreya called Agnivesha Samhita became the basis of later Charaka.

700–600 BC: Atreya was an eminent sage and a pupil of Bharadwaj at Taxila (Taksasila) situated on the banks of the river Sutlej now in Pakistan. He taught medicine and ushered in the age of scientific medicine through his astute observation of symptoms, diseases and their correlation. He is rightly known as the 'Hippocrates of Ancient Indian Medicine' as well as the 'Father of Indian Medicine'. Charaka was one of his students.

600 BC: A treatise by Kashyapa mainly dealing with pediatrics.

600–500 BC: Dhanvantari at Banaras (Varanasi), became a renowned teacher of surgery and later came to be known as the 'Patron Saint of Surgery'.

500 BC: 'Chivaravastu,' a book written by unknown author is found. It mentions prince Jivika, the court physician of Bimbisara, King of Magadha, as a marvelous physician and surgeon. He is credited with such difficult operations as piercing the skull to operate on the brains, surgery of the eyes, etc. and medical treatment of dropsy, internal tumors and varicose veins.

272–236 BC: King Ashoka, convert to Buddhism, built number of hospitals. More emphasis was laid on the preventive aspects. Doctors, nurses and midwives were to be trustworthy and skillful. The nurses were usually men and old women. This period saw famous medical schools at Taxila and Nalanda.

237–201 BC: Buddha instituted a state medical system, appointed doctors for every 10 villages on the main roads of India. Pharmaceutical gardens were also maintained.

200–100 BC: Patanjali explored the yoga system of philosophy of men and physical discipline the starting point of yoga therapy later continued.

100 BC: Charaka Samhita, the first classical exposition of Indian system medicine deals with an almost all the branches of medicine, anatomy, physiology, etiology, prognosis, pathology, treatment procedure and sequence of medication and an extension. Materia medica is a Latin word, which means medical material for more than 600 drugs. This treatise formed the basis of the Atreya School of Medicine in India, in 100 AD. The qualification of attending nurse, enshrined in the Charaka Samhita, i.e. knowledge of preparation and compounding of drugs for administration, cleverness, devotedness to patient under care and purity of both mind and body.

200–300 AD: Sushruta Samhita appears to have been revised by Nagarjuna, laid main emphasis on surgery. This great treatise described more than 300 operations, around 43 different surgical processes and 121 different types of instruments. The materia medica is also extensive covering more than 650 drugs of animals, plant and mineral origin. This treatise forms the basis of Dhanvantari School (300 AD).

Sushruta defines ideal relations of doctor, patient, nurses and medicine as the four upon which a cure must rest.

500–600 AD: Vagbhata wrote Astanga Hridaya (8 limbs and heart) . The eight limbs refer to the eight traditional branches of Ayurvedic knowledge, i.e. therapeutics, surgery, ear, nose and throat (ENT), mental and superstitious diseases, infantile diseases and treatment, toxicology, arresting physical and mental decay and rejuvenation or regaining lost virility potency and procreative ability.

This book is the most concise and scientific exposition of Ayurveda. It is in verse form, making it easy to memorize. It incorporates the teachings of the sages Atreya and Dhanvantari and the Rasayana School of Medicine. It is distinguished, but its knowledge of chemical reactions and laboratory processes are same.

600–800 AD: Sodhala (700 AD) two treatises, Gandanighraha, a medical treatise and Sodhala a medical lexicon. Vrudukunta (750 AD) writes Siddayoga, the earliest treatise on Rasa Chikitsa now existing intact. The Rasa Chikitsa system considers mercury as the king of all medicines. Siddayoga explain the various preparations of mercury and other metals, alloys, metallic compounds, salts and sulfur. This school of medicine is called Siddha school. All of them are made of metals, salts and sulfur. It is supposed to be a continuation of the pre-Aryan medical system in India. It is popular in Eastern and Southern India.

700–800 AD: Siddha Nagarjuna two treatises on the Siddha systems, Rasarathanakara and Arogya Manjari, Madhavacharya wrote Madhava Nidana. This is compilation from the earlier works of Agnivesa, Charaka, Sushruta, Vagbhata. It is specially useful as a chemical guide to preparations. It is famous all over India as the best Ayurvedic work on the diagnosis of diseases.

800–1300 AD: A number of treatises were written in India during this period. Arka Prakasha, a book on tincture extraction, Sarangadhara Samhita, Chikitsa, Sangraha and Yoga Ratnakara are the better known among others.

The period also witnessed a spirit of writing on the Rasa Chikitsa system. Rasha Hridaya by Govind Vagbhata, Rasaratnakara by Siddha Nityananda, Rasara-Tnasammukta by Vagbhata (another), Rasarnava by Sambhu, Rasendrachintamani by Ramachandra and Rasendra Choodamani by Somadeva.

1300–1600 AD: Bhavamisra wrote Bhava Prakasha. This is the most renowned Indian treatise during the period. It contains an exhaustive list of diseases and their symptoms and complete list of drugs including many not mentioned in the earlier works. It includes etiology and treatment of syphilis, a disease brought into India by Portuguese seamen.

Other works of this period are Chikitsaliye by Trisata, a manual on diagnosis; Chintamani by Ballabhendra on etiology and diagnosis and Vaidyamrutha by Moreswara on the treatment of diseases.

Another class of works produced during this period are Medical Lexicons by Madanapala, Nagahari, Bimapala, and Rajavallabha.

1600 AD: East India Company established British Rule in India. Western medicine and surgery started to be practiced and became popular in India.

NURSING IN INDIA

King Ashoka was the first person to improve the medical care in India. He built monasteries and houses for travelers and hospitals for both men and animals. Prevention of disease became the first important thing. Hygienic practices were adopted, i.e. people must wear clean clothes, should keep their nails cut and short. The women after delivery should live in rooms, which are clean and well-ventilated. The nurses usually men or old women.

The past and the progress of nursing in India has been hindered by many difficulties such as, the low status of women, the purdah system among Muslim women, the caste system among Hindus, illiteracy, poverty, political unrest, language differences and the fact that nursing has been looked upon as servants' work. Progress in surgery and medicine during past three centuries increases interest for better nursing service and nurse training.

The era of modern nursing commences with the work of Florence Nightingale in the Crimean War (1854–1856). She was born on May 12, 1820. She was the daughter of wealthy English parents. She felt that God had called her to fulfill 'Mission of Mercy'. She observed the life of poor and tried to relieve the sick. Nursing appeared to her as the field in which she could do the best. The principles relish she adjusted in her school of nursing as St Thomas Hospital were:

- Nurses should have practice training in hospital setup
- Nurses should live in a home to form that moral character and discipline
- Nursing education must be directed by a nurse
- Education is necessary for a nurse because they must know the reason why they have to teach others
- Theory and practice must be correlated
- The school should be economical independent.

She studied sanitary reforms and did considered the nursing done in Kaiser. A war to be a very high standard, but she earned ideas from efficient method of administration when she was 33 years of age she brought charged, which showed her exceptional ability as an organizer and good administrator.

The first influence on nursing in India was that of Florence Nightingale on a request from the Sanitary Commission for Bengal in 1865, Nightingale drew up some details 'suggestion on a system of nursing for hospital in India'. This was the beginning of modern nursing in India. Later, she took up the subject of sanitation in India. Her constant efforts influenced the Indian administration to improve the hygiene conditions, especially in the British Army in India. Nurses were recruited in India for the first time in 1914. Being attached to the Queen Alexandra Military Imperial Nursing Service (QAIMNS), Military Nursing Service was the earliest type of nursing. In 1664, East India Company helped to start a hospital for soldiers at Fort St George, Madras. Later a civilian hospital was built and medical staff appointed by the East India Company. Nurses were brought from England to be in charge and the first such students were those who had previously received their diploma in midwifery. Later, the plan reversed general nursing was taken first followed by course in midwifery.

Important Events

1871: Basic program for combined general nursing and midwifery formulated.

1874–1885:	Christian Mission Hospitals began training of Indian nurses only Christian girls have opted training.
1913:	The first examination was held by South India Board.
1926:	The Mid India Board formed. A nursing council constituted in Madras (now Chennai).
1945:	University education for nurses started at Delhi and Vellore.
1949:	The Indian Nursing Council was constituted.
1951:	Training program of 2 years for Auxillary Nurse Midwife (ANM) program started at Punjab.
1952:	Public Health Nursing started in 10 months course.
1960:	Master of nursing course introduced at Delhi University.
1971:	College of nursing started at Bangalore, Karnataka.

In 1941, first textbooks for nurses in India printed and published by South India Examining Board of Nurses league of Christian Medical Association of India (CMAI). In 1985, textbooks for health workers [female (F)] published. Later, on several authors published manuals textbooks of different topics related to nursing.

Nursing today provides an ever widening scope of opportunity for service. With present trends leading toward greater opportunities, varieties of services and growing social and professional recognition. It should be exciting and challenging for nurses to know that all nurses members of this profession fulfill the criteria of the profession (for further details please read the authors text on 'Nursing Administration').

Medical-surgical nursing is commonly defined as the nursing care of adults with suspected or diagnosed pathology of physiological function. It encompasses such a large scope that the trend is to subdivide medical surgical, oncological (cancer) nursing and only recently have the other specialties been developed.

Currently, all basic nursing programs prepare nurses to practice medical-surgical nursing. Advanced preparation at the master's and doctoral levels is necessary, if the nurse wishes to develop expertise and acquire in-depth knowledge in particular aspects or subdivisions of the specialty. These specialties would include intensive care units and the emergency room.

Medical-surgical nursing is the area of practice concerned with the care of adults with predicted or existing physiologic alterations, trauma or disability. It is the backbone of modern nursing and the practice foundation of virtually all healthcare institutions.

Traditionally, medical-surgical nursing was not considered a specialty area. Rather practices with a focus on a specific type of health problem within the area of medical-surgical nursing were considered specialties. These included cardiovascular, perioperative, neurologic, gynecologic, infection control and emergency nursing and practices limited to problems such as wound care, burns, hypertension and diabetes. Today, this view has changed. Medical-surgical nursing is now formally recognized as a specialty in its own right and the focused practice areas are seen as subspecialties.

Now medical-surgical nursing is a nursing specialty area concerned with the care of adult patients in a broad range of settings. Traditionally, medical-surgical nursing was an entry-level position that most nurses viewed as a stepping stone to specialty areas.

Medical-surgical nursing is the largest group of professionals in the field of nursing. Advances in medicine and nursing have resulted in medical-surgical nursing evolving into its own specialty. Medicine-surgical nursing is the foundation of all nursing practice. Once upon a time and not so very long ago, all nurse practiced the art and science of nursing on wards and everyone was a medical or surgical nurse. Today licensed medical-surgical nurses' work in a variety of positions, inpatient clinics, emergency departments, nursing administration, outpatient surgical centers, home health care, humanitarian relief work, ambulatory surgical care and skilled nursing homes. Some military medical-surgical nurses serve on battlefields.

2 Chapter Nursing Process Application

Nursing is the diagnosis and treatment of human responses to actual or potential problems. Nursing is a dynamic, therapeutic and educative process in meeting the health needs of the individual, family and society.

The term 'nursing process' was introduced by Lydia Hall in 1955. The process is a systemic work of doing things, which includes series of actions. So, nursing process is a set of actions used to determine, plan, implement and evaluate nursing care.

DEFINITION

- Nursing process is defined as deliberate, intellectual activity by which the practice of nursing is approached in an orderly, systematic manner
- Nursing process may be defined as a systematic method of assessing the health status, diagnosing healthcare needs, formulating a plan of care, initiating the implementation of plan and evaluating the effectiveness of the plan.

STEPS

Nursing process involves five steps, which include assessment, nursing diagnosis, planning, implementation and evaluation.

Assessment

Assessment refers to the collection and interpretation of clinical information. If focuses on gathering the data about a client's state of wellness, functional ability, physical status, strength and responses to actual and potential health problems. Hence, data will be collected by observation, interviewing, laboratory date and physical examination. There are four important aspects of assessment:

1. Collection of data in which the data is gathered about clients' health status that includes health history, physical examination, laboratory results and diagnostic tests.
2. Organizing the data, i.e. the collected data is organized systematically.
3. Validating the data: It means cross checking the educated information and making sure that the collected information is factual or true.
4. Recording the data: It should be done systematically.

Nursing Diagnosis

Diagnosis is a summary statement of the cause or basis of the identified problem. It is defined as a deliberate, systematic process of data analysis and synthesis that ends with a clinical judgment about individual, formally or community responses to actual and potential health for life process:

1. Nursing diagnosis is the diagnosis of actual or potential health problems by nurses by virtue of their education and experiences. They are capable and licensed to treat and taking care.
2. Nursing diagnosis is a statement that describes the human reponses (actual or potential) of an individual or group, which the nurse legally identify and for which the nurse can order the definite interventions to maintain the health state or to reduce, eliminate or prevent alterations.

Nursing diagnosis statements includes problem, etiology and defining characterization of problem describes clients responses for which nursing care will be given. Etiology component identifies and/or more causes of health problem and gives directions for nursing interventions. Defining characteristics are the signs and symptoms of problem, which helps in validating the nursing diagnosis (refer NANDA Nursing Diagnosis for more information).

Planning

Planning is a deliberative, systematic phase of the nursing process than involve decision-making and problem solving. It is a category of nursing behavior in which client-centered goal are established and interventions are designed to achieve stated goals and objectives.

The planning phase consists of four steps, which includes setting priorities, determining goals and objectives, selecting the nursing strategies and developing nursing care plans. Planning setting can be ranked according to Maslow's hierarchy of needs:

1. Setting priorities are three types, i.e. high priority, intermediate priority and low priority.
2. Determining goals and objectives: Goals may be long term or short term. The objectives are expected outcome describes the behavior of the patient, which is expected to achieve.

Implementation

Implementation is the action phase in which intimation of the plan, completion and recording of the nursing care is done, which includes nursing intervention for performing, assisting or directing the performance of activities. It is a continuous process and interact with other components of nursing process. In this phase, nurse utilizes their knowledge and skills for giving planned nursing care, which includes reassessment setting priorities, organizing resources, performing nursing interventions and recording actions. In this phase, nurse needs to be competent, cognitive, interpersonal, technical and psychomotor skills.

Evaluation

Evaluation is defined on the judgment of effectiveness of nursing care to meet clients goals. In this process, nurse compares the clients in behavior responses with predetermined client goals and outcome criteria. In other words, evaluation involves checking the outcome of care.

Evaluation is the continuous process in which nurse assesses and reassess the program, patients have made towards reaching the pre-established goals.

The purpose of evaluations includes the following:

- Collect data for making judgments about nursing care provided
- Determine clients behavioral responses to nursing interventions
- Compare the clients response with predetermined outcome criteria
- Appraise/Appreciate the involvement of client in healthcare decision
- Assess the collaboration of client and healthcare team members
- Identify the errors in the plan of care
- Monitor the quality of nursing care.

Evaluation phase of nursing process involves following activities:

- Review client goals and outcome criteria
- Collect data
- Measure goal attainment
- Revise and modify the nursing plan of care
- Review client goals and objectives (outcome criteria).

HEALTH ASSESSMENT

Health assessment is an integral part of holistic nursing. It provides the basis for nursing process. There are two components of health assessment, which includes health history and physical assessment.

Health History

1. Health history is a collection of subjective and objective data that provides a detailed profile of client's health status. The nurse collect the information through interview with client. An interview is a planned communication between nurses and client.
2. The subjective data are the symptoms, which are indications of illness that are perceived by the patient or client. For example, pain, nausea, feeling of nervousness, etc.
3. The objective data are the signs of illness as perceived by the examiner, i.e. doctor or nurse. For example, rashes, altered vital signs, visible drainage, etc.

Phases in Interview

For interview, there are three interrelated phase, which include introductory phase and working phase, termination phase. The purpose of these phases will include:

1. Introductory phase:
   - To establish rapport
   - To ensure a comfort ability sitting
   - To define what both parties expect from interview.
2. Working phase:
   - To collect biographical data
   - To collect data pertaining to client health status
   - To identify and respond to the client needs.
3. Terminate phase:
   - Presummary, summary and follow-up
   - Techniques may be incorporated.

Physical Examination

The physical examination is usually conducted in head-to-toe sequence, but can be adapted to meet the need of the client being examined. It offers objective information about the client.

Preparation for Physical Examination

- Physical examination requires privacy
- An examination room should be soundproof, well-ventilated and should be warm enough to maintain client comfort
- Adequate lighting is needed for proper illumination of body parts
- The equipment or instrument needed for examination should be readily available and arranged in order for easy use
- Physical preparation involves being sure that client is dressed and draped properly
- Emptying full bladder and bowel, if needed
- Psychologically client should be prepared.

Positions Used for Physical Examination

- Sitting position
- Supine position
- Dorsal recumbent position
- Sims' positions
- Prone position
- Knee-chest position
- Lithotomy position
- Standing position.

Technique of Physical Examination

- Observation
- Inspection
- Palpation
- Percussion
- Auscultation.

Instruments, Equipments and Supplies Required for Physical Examination

- Sphygmomanometer
- Stethoscope
- Ophthalmoscope
- Snellen's charts
- Otoscope
- Nasal speculum
- Scale and height measurement
- Vaginal speculum
- Tuning fork
- Percussion hammer
- Thermometer
- Tongue depressor
- Tape measure
- Penlight
- Gloves
- Lubricant
- Flashlight
- Alcohol swabs
- Cotton applicator
- Disposal pad
- Drape or sheet
- Gauze dressing

- Safety pin
- Gown for client
- Paper towels
- Swabs and sponge forceps
- Specimen container
- Wrist watch.

Note: For guidelines on 'head-to-toe' approach to physical examination in details and sample of nursing care plans, please refer Author's book on *'Medical Surgical Nursing'* 3rd edition published by Jaypee Brothers Medical Publishers (P) Ltd, New Delhi, India.

3 Chapter — Common Problems of Adult Patient

STRESS AND ITS MANAGEMENT

Stress is a state produced by change in the environment that is perceived as challenging, threatening or damaging to the persons dynamic balance or equilibrium. It is a state of physiologic and psychological tension that affects the whole person; physically, emotionally, intellectually, socially and spiritually.

Theoretical Models

Theoretical models views stress as—a stimulus, a response and a transaction.

Hans Selye's Model

1. Hans Selye (1976), who identified and defined stress as a non-specific response of the body to any demand made upon to regardless of its nature.
2. Holmes TH et al viewed stress as a stimulus that causes a response.
3. Lazarus and Folkman (1984) focuses on person-environment transaction and defined stress as transaction. They defined psychological stress as a particular relationship between the person and the environment that is appraised by the person as trading his/her resources and endangering his/her well-bieng.

Hans Selye referred stress-inducing demands as 'stressor'. Stressor can be physical or emotional and pleasant or unpleasant as long as they require the individual to adapt. In response to either physical or psychological stressor, a series of physiological changes occur. Selye called these responses as general adaptation syndrome (GAS).

General adaption syndrome has three phases:

1. Stage of alarm reaction: Here, the reactions are those of sympathetic nervous systems stimulate. The signs are increased blood pressure, increased heart rate and respiratory rate, decreased gastrointestinal mobility, pupil dilatations and increased perspiration acidity, nausea, anorexia, etc.
2. Stage of resistance: In this stage, adaptation to anxious stressor occurs involving modification of the external and internal environment. Resistance is light at this time compared with normal state due to increased cortisol activity.
3. Stage of exhaustion: Here, exhaustion sets in and endocrine activity increases producing deleterious effects on the body systems, especially circulation, digestive and immune systems that can lead to death. The physical symptoms of alarm reactions briefly reappear, no final effort by the body to survive.

According to Selye, there is also a local adaption syndrome (LAS). This includes inflammatory response and repair process than occurs at the local site of tissue injury.

Indicators of Stress

1. There are physiological, psychological and cognitive indicators of stress. Physiological indicators are the result of increased activity of the sympathetic and neuroendocrine systems.
2. Common psychological indicators are anxiety, fear, anger and depression. Anxiety, the most common response has four levels, i.e. mild, moderate, severe and panic. Ego defense mechanisms such as denial, rationalization, compensation and sublimation protect individuals from anxiety.
3. Cognitive indicators or thinking responses to stress include problem solving, structuring, self-control (discipline), suppression and fantasy.

Coping Strategies

1. Coping strategies to deal with stress vary significantly among individuals. Strategies may be problem focused or emotion focused, long term or short term and effective or ineffective.
2. The effectiveness of individual coping depends on the number, duration and intensity of the stressors; past experience; support systems available and the personal qualities of the person.
3. Prolonged stress and ineffective coping interfere with the meeting of basic needs and can affect physical and mental health.

Nursing Management

1. Nursing assessment of a client experiencing stress involves a nursing history to identify perceptions of and duration of stressors and coping strategies, and also physical examination for physical indicators of stress.
2. Nursing intervention for clients who are stressed are aimed at encouraging health promotion strategies (exercise, healthy diet, adequate rest and time management), minimizing anxiety, mediating, anger, teaching about specific relaxation techniques and implementing crisis intervention as needed.
3. Because, nursing practice involves many stressors related to both clients and the work environment, nurses are susceptible to anxiety and burnout. Like clients, they need to implement stress reduction measures.

PAIN AND ITS MANAGEMENT

1. Pain is a subjective sensation to which no two people respond in the same way. It can directly impair health and prolong recovery from surgery, disease or trauma.
2. Pain is an unpleasant sensory, emotional experience associated with actual potential tissue damage, it is described in terms of such damage or hurt.

Pain Process

1. Pain threshold is generally similar in all people, but pain tolerance and response vary considerably, for pain to is perceived, nociceptors must be stimulated. Three types of pain stimuli are mechanical, thermal and chemical.
2. Nociception is comprised of the physiologic processes related to pain perception. It involves four processes, i.e. transduction, transmission, perception and modulation.

3. According to the gate control theory, peripheral nerve fibers carrying pain to the spinal cord can have their input modified at the spiral cord level before transmission to the brain. This theory is the basis of many pain intervention strategies.

Factors Influencing Pain

Numerous factors influence a person's perception and reaction to pain, i.e. sex, situation, ethnic and cultural values, development stages, environment and support people earlier pain experience meaning of pain, anxiety and stress.

Types of Pain

- Acute pain, e.g. myocardial infarction (MI) pulmonary infection
- Chronic pain, e.g. nonmalignant and malignant
- Superficial pain, e.g. visceral pain, splanchnic pain (abdominal viscera)
- Deep somatic pain, e.g. rheumatoid (Rh), arthritis, osteomyelitis
- Localized pain, e.g. pain arise from the site
- Referred pain
- Intractable pain
- Headache
- Psychogenic pain.

Nursing Management

1. Pain is subjective and the most reliable indicator of the presence or intensity of pain is the client's self-report.
2. Assessment of a client who is experiencing pain should include a comprehensive pain history.
3. Although, the nursing diagnosis given to clients suffering pain is acute pain or chronic pain, the pain itself may be the etiology of many other nursing diagnoses.
4. Overall client goals include preventing, modifying or eliminating pain so that the client is able to partly or completely resume usual daily activities and to cope more effectively with the pain experience.
5. When planning, nurses need to choose pain relief measures appropriate for the client.
6. Pain management includes two basic types of nursing interventions, i.e. pharmacologic and nonpharmacologic.
7. Scheduling measures to prevent pain is far more supportive to the client than trying to deal with pain once it is established.
8. Major nursing strategies for all clients are to acknowledge and convey belief in the client's pain, assist support people, reduce misconceptions about pain, prevent pain and reduce fear and anxiety associated with the pain.
9. Pharmacological interventions ordered by the physician include the use of opioids, non-opioids/non-steroidal anti-inflammatory drugs (NSAIDs) and adjuvant drugs.
10. The World Health Organization (WHO) recommends a three-step ladder approach to manage chronic cancer pain.
11. Placebos fail to relieve pain for many people. Deceptive use of placebos is unacceptable practice.
12. Analgesic medication can be delivered through a variety of routes and methods to meet the specific needs of the client.

These routes include oral, nasal, rectal, transdermal, topical, subcutaneous or intravenous with a continuous infusion or a bolus dose and intraspinal.

13. Patient-controlled analgesia enables the client to exercise control and treat the pain by self-administering doses of analgesics.
14. Physical non-pharmacological pain interventions include such cutaneous stimulation as hot and cold applications, massage, acupressure and contralateral stimulation such as transcutaneous electrical nerve stimulation, immobilization and acupuncture.
15. Cognitive-behavior interventions are includes the distraction techniques, relaxation techniques, guided imagery, biofeedback, therapeutic touch and hypnosis.
16. Evaluation of the client's pain therapy includes the response of the client, the changes in the pain and the client's perceptions of the effectiveness of the therapy. Ongoing verbal or written feedback from the client and family is integral to this process.

MANAGEMENT OF FLUID, ELECTROLYTE AND ACID-BASE BALANCE

1. A balance of fluids, electrolyte, acids and bases in the body is necessary for health and life. The body fluids is divided into two major compartments such as the intracellular fluid (ICF) inside the cells and extracellular fluid (ECF) outside the cells.
2. Extracellular fluid is subdivided into two compartments, i.e. intravascular (plasma) and interstitial. It constitutes about one fourth or one third of total body fluid. ECF is in constant motion throughout the body. It is the transport system that carries nutrients to and waste products from the cells.

Physiology

1. As the primary body fluid, water is the most important nutrient of life. The following are the primary functions of water in the body:
   - Provide a medium for transporting nutrients to cells and wastes from the cells, and transporting such substances as hormones, enzymes, blood platelets, red blood cells (RBCs) and white blood cells (WBCs)
   - Facilitate cellular metabolism and proper cellular chemical functioning
   - Act as a solvent for electrolytes and nonelectrolytes
   - Helps to maintain normal body temperature
   - Facilitates digestion and promote elimination
   - Act as a tissue lubricant.
2. As water moves through all parts of the body, it is constantly being lost. Fluids leave the body through the kidneys, lungs, skin and gastrointestinal (GI) tract. To maintain homeostasis, the normal daily loss must be met by normal daily intake.

Mechanism of Controlling Fluid and Electrolyte Movement

1. The percentage of total body fluids varies according to the individual's age, body fat and sex. The younger the person, the higher the proportion of water in the body, the less body fat

present, the greater the proportion of body fluid. Postadolescent females have a smaller percentage of fluid in relation to total body weight than do males have.

2. There are two types of body electrolytes (ions), i.e. positively charged ions (cations) and negatively charged ions (anions).
3. The principal ions of ECF are sodium and chloride and the principal ions of ICF are potassium and phosphate.
4. Fluids and electrolytes move among the body compartments by osmosis, diffusion, filtration and active transport.
5. The major fluid pressures exerted as part of the movement of fluid and electrolytes from one compartment to another are osmotic pressure and hydrostatic pressure.

Regulation of Fluids and Electrolytes

1. The three sources of body fluid are fluids taken orally, food ingested and the oxidation of food.
2. Fluid intake is regulated by the thirst mechanism.
3. Fluid output occurs chiefly through excretion of urine, although body fluid is also excreted through sweat, feces and insensible vapor loss.
4. In healthy adults, measurable fluid intake and output should balance (about 1,500 mL per day). The output of urine normally approximates the oral intake of fluids. Water from food and oxidation is balanced by fluid loss through the skin, respiratory process and feces.
5. A number of body systems and organs are involved in regulating the volume and composition of body fluids; the kidneys, the endocrine system, the cardiovascular system, the lungs and the gastrointestinal system. The kidneys are the primary regulator of fluid and electrolyte balance.
6. Substances such as the antidiuretic hormone, the renin-angiotensin-aldosterone system (RAAS) and the atrial natriuretic factor are also involved in maintaining fluid balance.

Fluids Electrolyte, Acid-base Imbalance

1. Fluid imbalances include:
   a. Fluid volume deficit (FVD) also referred to as hypovolemia.
   b. Fluid volume excess (FVE) also referred to as hypervolemia.
   c. Dehydration, a deficit in water only.
   d. Overhydration, an excess of water only.
2. The most common electrolyte imbalances are deficits or excesses in sodium, potassium and calcium.
3. The acid-base balance (pH range) of body fluids is maintained within a precise range of 7.35–7.45.
4. Acid-base balance is regulated by buffers that neutralize excess acids or bases; the lungs, which eliminate or retain carbon dioxide, a potential acid and the kidneys, which excrete or converse bicarbonate and hydrogen ions.
5. Acid-base imbalance occurs when the normal 20:1 ratio of bicarbonate to carbonic acid is upset. Imbalances may be either respiratory or metabolic, both can result in.
6. Factors that influence an individual's fluid, electrolyte and acid-base balance include age, gender and body size, environmental temperature and lifestyle. Illness, trauma, surgery and certain

medications can place individuals at risk for fluid, electrolyte and acid-base imbalances.

7. Fluid, electrolyte and acid-base imbalance is most accurately determined through laboratory examination of blood plasma.

Nursing Management

1. Assessment relative to fluid, electrolyte and acid-base balances includes:
   a. A nursing history.
   b. Physical examination of the skin, oral cavity, eyes, jugular vein, veins of the hand and the neurologic system.
   c. Measurement of body weight, vital signs and fluid intake and output.
   d. Various diagnostic studies of blood and urine.
2. A nursing history includes data about the client's fluid and food intake; fluids output; signs of fluid, electrolyte and acid-base imbalances and medications, therapies or disease processes that may disrupt these balances.
3. North American Nursing Diagnosis Association (NANDA) approved nursing diagnoses that relate specifically to fluid, electrolyte and acid-base imbalances include deficient fluid volume, excess fluid volume, risk for imbalanced fluid volume, risk for deficient fluid volume and impaired gas exchange. Other diagnoses that may be relevant are impaired oral mucous membrane, impaired skin integrity, decreased cardiac output, impaired tissue perfusion, activity intolerance and risk for injury and acute confusion.
4. In many instances, fluids and electrolytes can be provided orally to clients who are experiencing or at risk of developing fluid deficits. The nurse needs to establish with the client 24-hours plan for ingesting the necessary fluids and to respect the client's fluid preferences.
5. For clients with fluid retention, fluids may need to be restricted for a schedule and short-term goals that make the fluid restriction more tolerable need to be developed.
6. For clients experiencing excessive fluid losses, the administration of fluids and electrolytes intravenously is necessary. Meticulous aseptic technique is required when caring for clients with intravenous infusions.
7. Preventing complications such as infiltration, phlebitis, hypervolemia (circulatory overload) and infection are an important aspect of intravenous therapy.
8. The administration of blood transfusions involves accurately matching and identifying the blood for the individual, correctly identifying the recipient and monitoring the client throughout the procedure for transfusion reactions.

4 Chapter Human Genetics and Genomic Nursing

HUMAN GENETICS AND GENOMIC NURSING

Genetics is the science, which deals with heredity and variations. Heredity is the inheritance of characters from parents to offspring. Children resemble their parents because they inherit traits from both parents. Variations are the difference among progeny of same parents as well as among the individuals of the same species.

Human genetic is the study of the human condition as not in influence by inherited factors that affect and determine growth and development, and that can be transmitted from generation to generation. Furthermore gender factors extend beyond the limited view of solely on health, the occurrence of complex disorders, individuals biologic response to illness, potential treatment and medical management appropriate and strategic for prevention and cure.

SCOPE OF GENOMIC NURSING

Nearly, all diseases are now recognized to have a genetic component. The past several years have transformed genetic nursing practice from a nearly hidden entity separately with a visible contribution to the genetic and overall health of individual and family. Genomic nursing will be a challenging for nursing in which nurses studies and recognizes the pattern of inheritance, understand the new technologies of testing and management of gene-based healthcare services and applying genetics principles in respective chemical areas of nursing for assessment, diagnosis, planning and interventions of genetic related health needs of the client. All areas of nursing practice have been influenced by recent advances in genetic knowledge and technology particularly after the completion of the Human Genome Project (HGP). HGP is providing a new and better understanding of the genetic contribution to disease, the development of targeted drug therapy and the development of genetic tests.

Nurses are ideally positioned to incorporate genetics into the care of patients at all ages and stages of life and in all settings. They are in key position to integrate knowledge of genetics influence into health care.

HEREDITY IN HEALTH PROBLEM

There is probably a genetic component in all disease processes. Most of the disorders have a genetic basis to a greater or lesser extent, even conditions such as fractures and infections. A mutant gene can be thought of as an etiological agent to a degree. Genetic disorders can appear at any age, many inherited biochemical disorders have infant, childhood and adult forms. The characteristics age of onset for manifestation of some genetic disorder are as follows:

1. Lethal during prenatal life: Some chromosome aberrations and some gross malformation.
2. Birth: Congenital malformations, i.e. chromosomal aberrations (e.g. Down syndrome), some forms of adrenogenital syndrome and some forms of deafness.

3. Soon after birth: Phenylketonuria, galactosemia, cystic fibrosis (sore bones) and maple syrup urine disease.
4. Infancy: Sickle cell anemia, Tay-Sachs disease and Werdnig-Hoffmann disease.
5. Early childhood: Cystic fibrosis, Duchenne muscular dystrophy.
6. Near puberty: Limb-girdle muscular dystrophy, Turner's syndrome and some forms of adrenagenital syndrome.
7. Young adulthood: Acute intermittent porphyria, hereditary juvenile glaucoma.
8. Variable age of onset: Diabetes mellitus (0–80 year), Huntington's chorea (15–65 year, myotonic dystrophy (birth to old age).

GENES/CHROMOSOMES AND ITS DEFECTS

Gene is defined as a unit of inheritance composed of a segment of deoxyribonucleic acid (DNA) or chromosome situated at a specific locus (gene locus), which carries coded information associated with a specific junction and can undergo crossing over as well as mutation. It is on elementary unit of inheritance, which can be assigned to a particular trait. In other words, gene to be the shortest segment of chromosome, which can be separated through crossing over can undergo mutation and influence expression of one or more traits.

Chromosome is a thread-like structure than in visible during cell division. In the nucleus of each cell, the DNA molecule is packed into thread-like structure called 'chromosome'. Each chromosome made up of DNA, tightly coiled many times around proteins called histones that support its structure. Chromosomes are organized structures of DNA and proteins that are found in cells. Chromosome is a singular piece of DNA, which contain many genes, regulatory elements and other nucleotide sequences. All the hereditary information is located in the genes mutations produced due to change in gene chemistry.

Chromosomal Defects

- Errors in cell division
- Autosomal chromosomal abnormalities
- Sex chromosomal abnormalities
- Single-gene disorders:
  - Autosomal dominant inheritance
  - Autosomal recessive inheritance
  - Linked recessive inheritance
  - X-linked dominant inheritance.
- Multifunctional disorders.

Genetic Testing

Genetic testing is the analysis of human DNA, ribonucleic acid (RNA), chromosomes, protein and certain metabolism in order to detect heritable disease-related genotypes, mutations, phenotypes or karyotypes for clinical purpose. The types or test includes:

- Preimplanting genetic diagnosis
- Prenatal testing
- Newborn screening
- Predictive genetic testing
- Carrier testing
- Diagnosis testing

- Forensic testing
- Research testing.

The length of genetic testing provides for:

- Early screening and preventive measures
- Future planning and life preparation
- Lifestyles adaptations
- Decreased confusion, uncertainty and anxiety
- Psychological stress relief
- Reproduction choice
- Informed extended family member
- Cost medical following reduced.

Genetic Screening

Genetic screening in contrast to genetic testing is a broader concept and applies to testing of population or groups of independent of a positive family history or symptoms manifestation, e.g. newborn are screened for an increasing number of condition, i.e. phenylketonuria (PKU), galactosemia and congenital hypothyroidism.

Management of Genetic Disease

Therapeutic Modification

- Surgical repair: Correction of structural defects
- Diet modification
- Folic acid: To prevent neural tube defect (NTD)
- Product replacement: For some deficiency disorders
- Avoidance of drugs or other substances
- Removal of toxic substances
- Immunological prevents, e.g. rh-negative mother
- Transplantation
- Cofactor administration
- Recombinant DNA
- Gene transfer.

Role of Nurses

Nurses in genetic-related healthcare blend the principles of human genetics with nursing care in collaboration with other professional including genetic specialist, to foster improvement, maintenance and restoration of patient's health, which include health assessment, family history assessment and physical assessment ancestry, cultural, social and spiritual assessment. And also nurses have to play an important role in genetic counseling, i.e. identify persons in need for genetic counseling and assists in genetic screening, testing and research and all take part in genetic services.

5

Chapter Immunological Problems and Nursing

IMMUNITY

Immunity is defined as the activity to destroy pathogens or other foreign material and to prevent cases of certain infectious diseases. Immunity is most often thought the terms of the body's responses to microorganisms such as bacteria, virus and fungi all of which foreign to body. However, immunity also involves process directed toward other cells and/or substances that are identified in the body correctly or incorrectly as foreign ex vivo malignant cells.

The immune system consists of lymphoid organs, tissues lymphocytes and other white blood cells (WBCs) and many chemicals involved in activation of our own cells for the destruction of foreign antigens.

Antigens are chemical markers that identify cells or molecules. Examples of molecular antigen include bacterial toxins, plant pollens or proteins that trigger allergies and the protein products of viral activity in cells. Human cells except red blood cells (RBCs) have their own self-antigens.

These are three types of lymphocytes:

1. Natural killer (NK) cells.
2. Thymus-derived lymphocytes (T cells).
3. Bone marrow-derived lymphocytes (B cells).

Functions of Lymphocytes

1. Natural killer cells are found in the blood, red bone marrow, lymph nodes and spleen, and are to destroy many kinds of infected body cells and tumor cells.
2. T cells and B cells involved in specific immune systems that is each cell is genetically programmed to respond to one kind of foreign antigen.

Antibodies are also called immunoglobulins (Igs) or gamma globulins and are glycoprotein produced by plasma cells in response to foreign antigen. Each antibody is specific for only one antigen and is capable of producing million of different antibodies.

MECHANISM OF IMMUNITY/RESPONSE TO INVASION

When the body is invaded or attacked by bacteria, virus or other pathogens, it has three means of defense, which includes:

1. The phagocytic immune response, which involves WBCs.
2. The humoral response, which involves mainly B cells, but it is assisted by T cells. It is also called antibody immune response. Antibodies may neutralize viruses that is where attach to a virus and render, it unable to enter a cells and antibodies also involved in allergic responses in which the immune system responds to foreign, but harmless antigen, e.g. anaphylactic shock.
3. The cell mediated or cellular immune response involves T cells, but is effective against intracellular pathogens (virus, fungi), malignant cells and grafts of foreign tissue.

TYPES OF IMMUNITY

Passive Immunity

In passive immunity, antibodies are not produced by the person, but are obtained from another source that is:

1. Naturally acquired passive immunity includes placental transmission of antibodies from mother to fetus and transmission of antibodies in breast milk.
2. Artificially acquired passive immunity involves injection of performed antibodies, this may help to prevent disease after exposure to a pathogen such as hepatitis B virus.

Active Immunity

1. In active immunity, the person produces his/her own antibodies. For example, when a person recovers from an infection and then has antibodies and memory cells specific for that pathogen.
2. Artificially acquired active immunity occurs as the result of a vaccine that stimulates product of antibodies and cells. The duration depends on particular disease or vaccine.

CHARACTERISTICS OF IMMUNOGLOBULIN

Immunoglobulin G (IgG): Appears in blood, extracellular fluid and lymph. It crosses the placenta to provide passive immunity in newborns and provides long-term immunity following vaccination or illness to recovery.

Immunoglobulin A (IgA): Appears in external secretions (e.g. tears, saliva) and found in secretions of all mucous membranes. It provides passive immunity for breastfed infants.

Immunoglobulin M (IgM): Appears in blood, lymph and produced first during an infection (IgG production follows).

Immunoglobulin D (IgD): Found in B cells and are antigen-specific receptors on B lymphocytes.

Immunoglobulin E (IgE): Found in mast cells or basophils, which are important in allergic reactions and mast cell release histamine.

PRIMARY IMMUNE ABERRATIONS

Immune response is protective in healthy individuals. However, that protection depends on an intact immune system. There are four primary immune aberrations can lead to disease, which includes:

1. Immunodeficiency: A deficiency of one or more immune components.
2. Gammopathy: An abnormal production of antibodies.
3. Hypersensitivity: An exaggerated or inappropriate immune response.
4. Autoimmunity: An immunologic attack on host cells.

Immunodeficiency

Primary Immunodeficiency

Primary immunodeficiency disorders are characterized by defects of immunologic cell development or function that result in B cell, T cell, complement or phagocytic cell deficiency.

Clinical manifestations: As follows:
- Frequent external and viral injections
- Infection with unusual or opportunistic organisms
- Associated autoimmune disease
- Painful, swollen wrist, elbow, ankle or knee joints
- Digestive problems, nausea and vomiting
- Chronic skin or mucous membrane infections
- Blood disorders.

  Note: Not all patients experience all symptoms.

Secondary Immunodeficiency

Secondary immunodeficiency results from various factors. Generalized immunosuppression is often induced therapeutically to decrease unwanted immune reactions, such as hypersensitivity reactions autoimmune diseases, neoplasia or organ rejection.

Clinical manifestations: The clinical manifestations depend on following factors.

Management

The goal of management of immunodeficiency disorders includes:
- Identify those at risk for the disorders
- Prevent infections or effectively treating existing infections
- Replace missing humoral and cellular immunologic factors.

Diagnostic Evaluation

- History
- Physical examination
- Laboratory findings.

Treatment/Therapy

- Antimicrobial agents to prevent or treat infections
- Immunoglobulin replacement therapy
- Other chemotherapeutic
- Bone marrow transplants.

Nursing Management

1. Assess problems usually associated with immunodeficiency, which includes:
   - Infections
   - Pain and swelling of joints
   - Problems and frequency
   - Chronic skin infections.
2. Assist in diagnostic evaluation.
3. Planning: Patient will:
   - Identify risk for infections
   - Take measures to prevent infections
   - Maintain treatment regimen.

Nursing Interventions

1. Nurse constantly monitors the patient.
2. Take measures to treat infections as per instructions.

3. Teach preventive measures, which includes:
   - Avoid persons with infections
   - Inspect skin daily for lesions or breaks
   - Avoid burping, breaking or tearing skin
   - Eat well-balanced diet
   - Drink at least six glasses of fluid daily
   - Avoid becoming overfatigued
   - Try to get sufficient sleep every night
   - Decrease environmental contamination
   - Take prophylactics before any manipulative or invasive procedures
   - Report signs of infections immediately.

Gammopathies

1. Gammopathies are also known as hypergammaglobulinemia, which refer to elevated levels of serum gamma globulin (antibodies) resulting from overproduction. The blood normally contains a large number of different proteins collectively called plasma proteins.
2. When the majority of protein produced is an identified type of gamma globulin, the abnormally produced proteins are called monoclonal gammopathy or plasma cell dyscrasia. For example, as seen in multiple myeloma and macroglobulinemia. Another form of gammopathies is polyclonal gammopathic, which involves the overproduction of virtual cell classes of immunoglobulin in response to appropriate antigenic stimulation. High levels of dysfunctional immunoglobulins leaving the patient susceptible to infection. Polyclonal gammopathies are associated with chronic bacterial infections and connective tissue diseases such as lupus erythematosus and rheumatoid (Rh) arthritis.

Note: For clinical manifestations, management and nursing management please refer Multiple myeloma, Systemic lupus erythematosus (SLE), RA arthritis.

Hypersensitivities (Anaphylaxis, the Type I)

The immune system is an adaptive system that protects the body. However, sometimes this system can cause injury to the body because of its exaggerated response. One of these occasions is when a hypersensitivity reaction occurs. In 1963, Gell and Coombs developed a system classifying hypersensitivity reactions on types I, II, III and IV according to the way the tissue injured.

Anaphylaxis is a clinical response to an immediate (type I hypersensitivity) immunologic reaction between a specific antigen and an antibody. The reactions results from a rapid release of IgE-mediated chemicals, which can induce a severe life-threatening allergic reaction. Substances that most commonly cause anaphylaxis include foods, medications, insect stings and latex. Foods that are common causes of anaphylaxis include peanuts, tree nuts, shellfish, fish, milk, eggs, soy and wheat. Many medications have been implicated in anaphylaxis. Those that are most frequently reported include antibiotics (e.g. penicillin), radiocontrast agents, intravenous (IV) anesthetics, Aspirin and other non-steroidal anti-inflammatory drugs (NSAIDs) and opioids. Closely related to anaphylaxis is a non-allergic anaphylaxis (anaphylactoid) reaction.

Clinical Manifestations

Anaphylactic reactions produce a clinical syndrome that affects multiple organ systems. Reactions may be categorized as mild, moderate or severe. The severity depends on the degree of allergy and the dose of allergen.

Mild: Symptoms include peripheral tingling, a warm sensation, fullness in the mouth and throat, nasal congestion, periorbital swelling, pruritus, sneezing and tearing eyes. Symptoms begin within 2 hours of exposure.

Moderate: Symptoms include flushing, warmth, anxiety and itching in addition to any of the milder symptoms. More serious reactions include bronchospasm and edema of the airways or larynx with dyspnea, cough and wheezing. The onset of symptoms is the same as for a mild reaction.

Severe: These systemic reactions have an abrupt onset with the same signs and symptoms described previously. Symptoms progress rapidly to bronchospasm, laryngeal edema, severe dyspnea, cyanosis and hypotension. Dysphagia, abdominal cramping, vomiting, diarrhea and seizures can also occur. Cardiac arrest and coma may follow.

Diagnostic Methods

Diagnostic evaluation of the patient with allergic disorders commonly includes blood tests [complete blood count (CBC) with differential, high total serum IgE levels] smears of body secretions, skin tests and the radioallergosorbent test (RAST).

Prevention

Prevention by avoidance of allergens is of utmost importance. If avoidance of exposure to allergens is impossible, the patient should be instructed to carry and administer epinephrine to prevent an anaphylactic reaction in the event of exposure to the allergen. Healthcare providers should always obtain a careful history of any sensitivity before administering medications. Venom immunotherapy may be given to people who are allergic to insect venom. Insulin allergy in patients with diabetes or penicillin-sensitive patients may require desensitization.

Medical Management/Therapeutic Measures

Respiratory and cardiovascular functions are evaluated and cardiopulmonary resuscitation (CPR) is initiated in cases of cardiac arrest. Oxygen is administered in high concentrations during CPR or when the patient is cyanotic, dyspnea or wheezing. Patients with mild reactions need to be educated about the risk for recurrences. Patients with severe reactions need to be observed for 12–14 hours.

Pharmacological Therapy

Epinephrine, antihistamines and corticosteroids may be given to prevent recurrences of the reaction and to relieve urticaria and angioedema. IV fluids (e.g. normal saline solution), volume expanders and vasopressor agents are administered to maintain blood pressure and normal hemodynamic status; glucagon may be administered. Aminophylline and corticosteroids may also be administered to improve airway patency and function.

Nursing Management

1. Explain to the patient who has recovered from anaphylaxis what occurred and instruct about avoiding future exposure to antigens and how to administer emergency medications to treat anaphylaxis.
2. Instruct about antigens that should be avoided and about strategies to prevent recurrence of anaphylaxis.
3. Instruct the patient and family how to use preloaded syringes of epinephrine, if needed and have the patient and family demonstrate correct administration.

Autoimmune Diseases

The cause of autoimmunity or the loss of self-tolerance is not clearly understood. Autoimmune is a condition in which the body does not recognize itself and the immune system attacks normal cells.

Autoimmune diseases occur more frequently in women, especially during childbearing years. Autoimmunity refers to the formation of antibodies against self-cells. Autoimmune disorders are grouped into categories according to the body part or tissue involved. For example, autoimmune hemolytic anemia, idiopathic thrombocytopenic, purpura, rheumatic fever, multiple sclerosis, Gullian-Barré syndrome, myasthenia gravis, Addison's disease, Graves' disease, pernicious anemia, ulcerative colitis, glomerulonephritis, SLE, RA arthritis, etc.

ACQUIRED IMMUNODEFICIENCY SYNDROME

Acquired immunodeficiency syndrome (AIDS) is defined as the most severe form of a continuum of illness associated with human immunodeficiency virus (HIV) infection. HIV belongs to a group of viruses known as retroviruses. These viruses carry their genetic material in the form of ribonucleic acid (RNA) rather than deoxyribonucleic acid (DNA). Infection with HIV occurs when it enters the host CD4 (T) cells and causes this cell to replicate viral RNA and viral proteins, which in turn invade other CD4 cells. The stage of HIV disease is based on clinical history, physical examination, laboratory evidence of immune dysfunction, signs and symptoms and infections and malignancies. The Centers for Disease Control and Prevention (CDC) standard case definition of AIDS categorizes HIV infection and AIDS in adults and adolescents on the basis of clinical conditions associated with HIV infection and CD4+ T cell counts. Four categories of infected states have been denoted:

1. Primary infection (acute/recent HIV infections, acute HIV syndrome; dramatic drops in CD4 T cell counts, which are normally between 500 and 1,500 cell/mm^3).
2. Asymptomatic HIV (CDC category A: More than 500 CD4+ T lymphocytes/mm^3).
3. Symptomatic HIV (CDC category B: 200–499 CD4+ T lymphocytes/mm^3).

4. Acquired immunodeficiency syndrome (CDC category C: Fewer than 200 CD4+ T lymphocytes/mm³).

Risk Factors

The HIV is transmitted through bodily fluids by high-risk behaviors such as heterosexual intercourse with an HIV-infected partner, injection drug use and male homosexual relations. People who received transfusions of blood or blood products contaminated with HIV, children born to mothers with HIV infection, breastfed infants of HIV infected mothers and healthcare workers exposed to needlestick injury associated with an infected patient are also at risk.

Clinical Manifestations

Symptoms are widespread and may affect any organ system. Manifestations range from mild abnormalities in immune response without overt signs and symptoms to profound immunosuppression, life-threatening infection, malignancy and the direct effect of HIV on body tissues.

Respiratory

1. Shortness of breath, dyspnea, cough, chest pain and fever are associated with opportunistic infections such as those caused by *Pneumocystis jiroveci* [pneumocystis pneumonia (PCP), the most common infection], *Mycobacterium avium* (mycobacterium avium-intracellulare infection), cytomegalovirus (CMV) and *Legionella* species.
2. Human immunodeficiency virus associated tuberculosis occurs early in the course of HIV infection, often preceding a diagnosis of AIDS.

Gastrointestine

1. Loss of appetite.
2. Nausea and vomiting.
3. Oral and esophageal candidiasis (white patches, painful swallowing, retrosternal pain and possibly oral lesions).
4. Chronic diarrhea possibly with devastating effects (e.g. profound weight loss, fluid and electrolyte imbalances, perianal skin excoriation, weakness and inability to perform activities of daily living).
5. Wasting syndrome (cachexia):
   a. Multifactorial protein-energy malnutrition.
   b. Profound involuntary weight loss exceeding 10% of baseline body weight.
   c. Either chronic diarrhea (for more than 30 day) or chronic weakness and documented intermittent or constant fever with no concurrent illness.
   d. Anorexia, diarrhea, gastrointestinal (GI) malabsorption, lack of nutrition and for some patients a hypermetabolic state.

Oncologic

Certain types of cancer occur often in people with AIDS and are considered AIDS defining conditions:

1. Kaposi's sarcoma (KS) is the most common HIV-related malignancy and involves the endothelial layer of blood and lymphatic vessels (exhibits a variable and aggressive contour ranging from localized cutaneous lesions to disseminate disease involving multiple organ systems).
2. B-cell lymphomas are the second most malignant that tend to develop outside the lymph nodes, most commonly in the brain, bone marrow and GI tract. These types of lymphomas are characteristically of a higher grade, indicating aggressive growth and resistance to treatment.
3. Invasive cervical cancer.

Neurologic

1. The HIV-associated neurocognitive disorders consist of cognitive impairment that is often accompanied by motor dysfunction and behavioral change.
2. The HIV-related peripheral neuropathy is common across the trajectory of HIV infection and may occur in a variety of pattern with distal sensory polyneuropathy (DSPN) or distal symmetrical polyneuropathy (DSP), the most frequently occurring type. DSPN can lead to significant pain and decreased function.
3. The HIV encephalopathy [formerly referred to as AIDS dementia complex (ADC)] is a clinical syndrome that is characterized by a progressive decline in cognitive behavioral and motor functions. Syndrome includes memory deficits, headache and difficulty in concentrating, progressive confusion, psychomotor slowing, apathy and ataxia and in later stages global cognitive impairments, delayed verbal responses, a vacant stare, spastic paraparesis, hyperreflexia, psychosis, hallucination tremor, incontinence, seizures, mutism and death.
4. *Cryptococcus neoformans,* a fungal infection (fever, headache, malaise, stiff neck, nausea, vomiting, mental status changes and seizures).
5. Progressive multifocal leukoencephalopathy (PML) a central nervous system demyelinating disorder (mental confusion, blindness, aphasia, muscle weakness, paresis and death).
6. Other common infections involving the nervous systems include *Toxoplasma gondii,* CMV and mycobacterium tuberculosis infections.
7. Central and peripheral neuropathies including vascular myelopathy (spastic paraparesis, ataxia and incontinence).

Depressive

1. Causes of depression are multifactorial and may include a history of pre-existing mental illness, neuropsychiatric disturbances, psychosocial factors or response to the physical symptoms.
2. People with HIV/AIDS who are depressed may experience irrational guilt and shame, loss of self-esteem, feelings of helplessness and worthlessness and suicidal ideation.

Integumentary

1. Kaposi's sarcoma, herpes simplex and herpes zoster viruses, and various forms of dermatitis associated with painful vesicles.
2. Folliculitis associated with dry flaking skin or atopic dermatitis (eczema or psoriasis).

Reproductive

1. Persistent recurrent vaginal candidiasis may be the first sign of HIV infection.
2. Ulcerative sexually transmitted diseases (STDs) such as chancroid, syphilis and herpes are more severe in women with HIV.
3. Human papillomavirus causes venerel warts and is a risk factor for cervical intraepithelial neoplasia, a cellular change that is frequently a precursor to cervical cancer.
4. Women with HIV are 10 times more likely to develop cervical intraepithelial neoplasia.
5. Women with HIV have a higher incidence of pelvic inflammatory disease (PID) and menstrual abnormalities (amenorrhea or bleeding between periods).

Diagnostic Methods

Confirmation of HIV antibodies is done using enzyme immunoassay (EIA) formerly enzyme-linked immunosorbent assay (ELISA), Western blot assay and viral load tests such as target amplification methods. In addition to this HIV-1 antibody assay, two additional techniques are now available; the OraSure saliva test and the OraQuick rapid HIV-1 antibody test. In addition, CBC/lymphocyte count CD4+ CD8+ T-lymphocyte count and genotyping.

Medical Management/Therapeutic Measures

Treatment of Opportunistic Infections

Guidelines for the treatment of opportunistic infections should be consulted for the most current recommendations. Immune function should improve with initiation of highly antiretroviral therapy (HAART) resulting in faster resolution of the opportunistic infection:

1. Pneumocystis pneumonia:
   a. Trimethoprim (TMP) and sulfamethoxazole (SMX) is the treatment of choice for PCP; adjunctive corticosteroids should be started as early as possible (certainly within 72 hour).
   b. Alternative therapeutic regimens (moderate-to-severe) include primaquine plus clindamycin or IV pentamidine.
   c. Adverse effects include hypotension, impaired glucose metabolism leading to the development of diabetes mellitus damage to the pancreas, renal damage, hepatic dysfunction and neutropenia.
2. Mycobacterium avium complex (MAC):
   a. The HIV-infected adults and adolescents should receive chemoprophylaxis against disseminated MAC disease, if they have a CD4+ count fewer than 50 cell/μL.
   b. Azithromycin (Zithromax) and clarithromycin (Biaxin) are the preferred prophylactic agents.
   c. Rifabutin is an alternative prophylactic agent, although interactions may make this agent difficult to use.
3. Cryptococcal meningitis:
   a. Current primary therapy for cryptococcal meningitis is amphotericin B with or without oral flucytosine (5-Ancobon) or fluconazole (Diflucan).

b. Serious potential adverse effects of amphotericin B include anaphylaxis, renal and hepatic impairment, electrolyte imbalances, anemia, fever and severe chills.

4. The CMV retinitis:
   a. Oral valganciclovir, IV ganciclovir followed by oral valganciclovir, IV foscarnet, IV cidofovir and the ganciclovir intraocular implant coupled with valganciclovir are all effective treatments for CMV retinitis.
   b. A common adverse reaction to Ganciclovir is severe neutropenia, which limits the concomitant use of zidovudine [azidothymidine (AZT)/compound S, Retrovir].
   c. Common adverse reactions to foscarnet are nephrotoxicity including renal failure and electrolyte imbalances, hypocalcemia, hyperphosphatemia and hypomagnesemia, which can be life-threatening.
   d. Other common adverse effects include seizures, GI tract disturbances, anemia, phlebitis at the infusion site and low back pain.
   e. Possible bone marrow suppression (producing a decrease in WBC and platelet counts), oral candidiasis and liver and renal impairments require close monitoring.
5. Other infections:
   a. Oral acyclovir, famciclovir or valacyclovir may be used to treat infections caused by herpes simplex or herpes zoster.
   b. Esophageal or oral candidiasis is treated topically with clotrimazole (Mycelex) oral troches or nystatin suspension.
   c. Chronic refractory infection with candidiasis (thrush) or esophageal involvement is treated with ketoconazole (Nizoral) or fluconazole (Diflucan).

Prevention of Opportunistic Infections

People with HIV infection who have a T-cell count of lesser than 200 cell/mm^3 should receive chemoprophylaxis with TMP-SMX to prevent PCP.

The PCP prophylaxis can be safely discontinued in patients who are responding to HAART with sustained increase in T lymphocytes.

Antidiarrheal Therapy

1. For diarrhea, antidiarrheal therapy may be initiated with octreotide acetate (Sandostatin).
2. For Kaposi's sarcoma, chemotherapy may be initiated. Treatment goals are to reduce symptoms by decreasing the size of skin lesions, to reduce discomfort associated with edema and ulcerations and to control symptoms associated with mucosal or visceral involvement. Radiation therapy is effective as a palliative measure; alpha-interferon can lead to tumor regression and improved immune system function.
3. For lymphoma, the successful treatment of AIDS-related lymphomas has been limited because of the rapid progression of these malignancies. Combination chemotherapy and radiation therapy regiments may produce an initial response, but it is usually short lived.

Antidepressant Therapy

1. Treatment of depression involves psychotherapy integrated with pharmacotherapy [antidepressants (e.g. imipramine, desipramine and fluoxetine) and possibly a psychostimulant (e.g. methylphenidate)].
2. Electroconvulsive therapy may be an option for patients with severe depression who do not respond to pharmacological interventions.

Nutrition Therapy

1. A healthy diet tailored to meet the nutritional needs of the patient is important.
2. Patients with diarrhea should consume a diet low in fat, lactose, insoluble fiber and caffeine, and high in soluble fiber.
3. Calorie counts should be obtained to evaluate nutritional status and initiate appropriate therapy for patient experiencing unexplained weight loss.
4. Appetite stimulants can be used in patients with AIDS-related anorexia.
5. Oral supplements may be used to supplement diets that are deficient in calories and protein.

Nursing Management

Assessment

Identify potential risk factors including sexual practices and IV injection drug in first history. Assess physical and psychological status. Thoroughly explore factors affecting immune system functioning as mentioned below:

1. Nutritional status:
   - Obtain dietary history
   - Identify factors may interfere with oral intake such as anorexia, nausea, vomiting, oral pain or difficulty swallowing
   - Assess patient's ability to purchase and prepare food
   - Measure nutritional status by weight, anthropometric measurements (triceps, skinfold measurement) and blood urea nitrogen (BUN), serum protein, albumin, and transferring levels.
2. Skin and mucous membranes:
   - Inspect daily for breakdown, ulceration and infection
   - Monitor oral cavity for redness, ulceration and creamy white patches (candidiasis)
   - Assess perianal area for excoriation and infection
   - Obtain wound culture to identify infectious organisms.
3. Respiratory status:
   - Monitor for cough, sputum production, shortness of breath, orthopnea, tachypnea and chest pain; assess breath sounds
   - Assess other parameters of pulmonary function [chest X-rays, arterial blood gases (ABGs), pulse oximetry, pulmonary function tests].
4. Neurologic status:
   - Assess mental status as early as possible to provide a baseline

- Note level of consciousness and orientation to person, place and time, and the occurrence of memory lapses
- Observe for sensory deficits such as visual changes, headache and numbness and tingling in the extremities
- Observe for motor impairments such as altered gait and paresis
- Observe for seizure activity.

5. Fluid and electrolyte status:
   - Examine skin and mucous membranes for turgor and dryness
   - Assess for dehydration by observing for increased thirst, decreased urine output, low blood pressure, weak rapid pulse or urine's specific gravity
   - Monitor electrolyte imbalances (laboratory studies show low serum sodium, potassium, calcium, magnesium, weak rapid pulse or urine specific gravity)
   - Assess for signs and symptoms of electrolyte deficits including altered mental status, muscle twitching muscle cramps, irregular pulse, nausea and vomiting and shallow breathing.
6. Level of knowledge:
   - Evaluate patient's knowledge of disease and transmission
   - Assess level of knowledge of family and friends
   - Explore patient's reaction to the diagnosis of HIV infection or AIDS
   - Explore how patient has dealt with illness and major life suppressors in the past
   - Identify patient's resources for support.
7. Use of alternative therapies:
   - Question patient about the use of alternative therapies
   - Encourage patient to report any use of alternative therapies to primary healthcare provider
   - Become familiar with potential side effects of alternative therapies; if side effect is suspected to result from alternative therapies, discuss with patient and primary and alternative healthcare provider
   - View alternative therapies with an open mind and try to understand the importance of the treatment to patient.

Nursing Diagnoses/Problems

1. Impaired skin integrity related to cutaneous manifestation of HIV infection, excoriation and diarrhea.
2. Diarrhea related to enteric pathogens or HIV infection.
3. Risk for infection related to immunodeficiency.
4. Activity intolerance related to weakness, fatigue, malnutrition, impaired fluid and electrolyte balance and hypoxia associated with pulmonary infections.
5. Disturbed thought process related to shortened attention span, impaired memory, confusion and disorientation associated with HIV encephalopathy.
6. Ineffective airway clearance related to PCP, increased bronchial secretions and decreased ability to cough related to weakness and fatigue.
7. Pain related to impaired perianal skin integrity second to diarrhea, KS and peripheral neuropathy.

8. Imbalanced nutrition less than body requirements related to decreased oral intake.
9. Social isolation related to stigma of the disease, withdrawal of support systems, isolation procedures and fear of infecting others.
10. Anticipatory grieving related to changes in lifestyles and roles, and unfavorable prognosis.
11. Deficient knowledge related to HIV infection means of preventing HIV transmission and self-care.

Potential Complications

- Opportunistic infections
- Impaired breathing or respiratory failure
- Wasting syndrome and fluid and electrolyte imbalance
- Adverse reaction to medications.

Planning and Goals

Goals for the patient may include achievement and maintenance of skin integrity, resumption of usual bowel patterns, absence of infection, improved activity tolerance, improved thought processes, improved airway clearance increased comfort, improved nutritional status, increase socialization, expression of grief, increased knowledge regarding disease prevention and self-care and absence of complications.

Nursing Interventions

Promoting Skin Integrity

1. Assess skin and oral mucosa for changes in appearance, location and size of lesions, and evidence of infection and breakdown; encourage regular oral care.
2. Encourage patient to balance rest and mobility whenever possible; assist immobile patients to change position every 2 hours.
3. Use devices such as alternating pressure mattresses and low-air-loss beds.
4. Encourage patient to avoid scratching to use nonabrasive and non-drying soaps and to use non-perfumed skin moisturizers on dry skin; administer antipruritic agents, antibiotic medications, analgesic agents, medicated lotions, ointments, and dressing as prescribed; avoid excessive use of tape.
5. Keep bed linen free of wrinkles and avoid tight or restrictive cloth to reduce friction to skin.
6. Advise patient with foot lesions to wear white cotton socks and shoes that do not cause feet to perspire.

Maintaining Perianal Skin Integrity

1. Assess perianal region for impaired skin integrity and infection.
2. Instruct patient to keep the area as clean as possible, to cleanse after each bowel movement, to use sitz bath or irrigation and to dry the area thoroughly after cleaning.
3. Assist debilitated patient in maintaining hygiene practices.
4. Promote healing with prescribed topical ointment and lotions.
5. Culture wounds, if infection is suspected.

Promoting Usual Bowel Patterns

1. Assess bowel patterns for diarrhea (frequency and consistency of stool, pain or cramping with bowel movements).
2. Assess factors that increase frequency of diarrhea.
3. Measure and document volume of liquid stool as fluid volume loss; obtain stool cultures.
4. Counsel patient about ways to decrease diarrhea (rest bowel, avoid foods that act as bowel irritants including raw fruits and vegetables); encourage small, frequent meals.
5. Administer prescribed medications such as anticholinergic/ antispasmodic medications or opiates, antibiotic medications and antifungal agents.
6. Assess self-care strategies patient uses to control diarrhea.

Prevention of Infection

1. Instruct patient and caregivers to monitor for signs and symptoms of infections, and the recommended strategies to avoid infection (upper respiratory tract infections).
2. Monitor laboratory values that indicate the presence of infection such as WBC count and differential; assist in obtaining culture specimens as ordered.
3. Strongly urge patients and sexual partners to avoid exposure to body fluids and to use condoms for any sexual activities.
4. Strongly discourage IV injection drug use because of risk of other infections and transmission of HIV infection to the patient.
5. Maintain strict aseptic technique for invasive procedures.
6. Observe universal precautions in all patient care. Teach colleagues and other healthcare workers to apply precautions to blood and all body fluids, secretions and excretions except sweat (e.g. cerebrospinal fluids, synovial, pleural, peritoneal, pericardial, amniotic and vaginal fluids and semen). Consider all body fluids to be potentially hazardous in emergency circumstances when differentiating between fluid types is difficult.

Improving Activity Tolerance

1. Monitor ability to ambulate and perform daily activities.
2. Assist in planning daily routines to maintain balance between activity and rest.
3. Instruct patient in energy conservation techniques (e.g. sitting, while washing or preparing a meal).
4. Decrease anxiety that contributes to weakness and fatigue by using measures such as relaxation and guided imagery.
5. Collaborate with other healthcare team members to uncover and address factors associated with fatigue [e.g. epoetin alfa (Epogen) for fatigue related to anemia].

Maintain Thought Processes

1. Assess for alternations in mental status.
2. Reorient to person, place and time as necessary; maintain and post a regular daily schedule.
3. Give instructions; instruct family to speak to patient in a slow, simple and clear manner.

4. Provide night lights for bedroom and bathroom. Plan safe leisure activities that patient previously enjoyed.
5. Provide around the clock supervision as necessary for patient with HIV encephalopathy.

Improving Airway Clearance

1. At least daily, assess respiratory status, mental status and skin color.
2. Note and document presence of cough and quantity, and characteristics of sputum; send specimen for analysis as ordered.
3. Provide pulmonary therapy such as coughing, deep breathing, postural drainage, percussion and vibration, every 2 hours to prevent stasis of secretions and promote airway clearance.
4. Assist patient into a position (high or semi-Fowler's) that facilitates breathing and airway clearance.
5. Encourage adequate rest to minimize energy expenditure and prevent fatigue.
6. Evaluate fluid volume status; encourage intake of 3 liters daily.
7. Provide humidified oxygen, suctioning, intubation and mechanical ventilation as necessary.

Relieving Pain and Discomfort

1. Assess patient for quality and severity of pain associated with impaired perianal skin integrity, KS lesions and peripheral neuropathy.
2. Explore effects of pain on elimination, nutrition, sleep, affect and communication along with exacerbating and relieving factors.
3. Encourage patient to use soft cushions or foam pads, while sitting and topical anesthetics or ointments as prescribed.
4. Instruct patient to avoid irritating foods and use antispasmodic agents and antidiarrheal preparations, if necessary.
5. Administer NSAIDS and opiates, and use non-pharmacologic approaches such as relaxation techniques.
6. Administer opioids and tricyclic antidepressants, and recommended graduated compression stockings as prescribed to help alleviate neuropathic pain.

Improving Nutritional Status

1. Assess weight, dietary intake, anthropometric measurements and serum albumin, BUN, protein, and transferrin levels.
2. Based on assessment of factors interfering with oral intake and to implement specific measures to facilitate oral intake; consult dietician to determine nutritional requirements.
3. Control nausea and vomiting; encourage patient to eat easy to swallow foods; encourage oral hygiene before and after meals.
4. Encourage rest before meals; do not schedule meals after painful or unpleasant procedures.
5. Instruct patient about ways to supplement nutritional value of meals (e.g. add eggs, butter, milk).
6. Provide enteral or parental feedings to maintain nutritional status as indicated.

Decreasing Sense of Social Isolation

1. Provide atmosphere of acceptance and understanding of AIDS to the patient, their families and partners.
2. Assess patient's usual level of social interaction early to provide a baseline for monitoring changes in behavior.
3. Encourage patient to express feelings to isolation and aloneness; assure patient that these feelings are not unique or abnormal.
4. Assure patients, family and friends that AIDS is not spread through casual contact.

Coping with Grief

1. Help patients explore and identify resources for support and mechanisms for coping.
2. Encourage patient to maintain contact with family, friends and co-workers, and to continue usual activities whenever possible.
3. Encourage patient to use local or national AIDS support groups and hotlines, and to identify losses and deal with them when possible.

Monitoring and Managing Potential Complications

1. Inform patient that signs and symptoms of opportunistic infections include fever, malaise, difficulty breathing, nausea or vomiting, diarrhea, difficulty swallowing and any occurrences of swelling or discharge. These symptoms should be reported to the healthcare provider immediately.
2. Respiratory failure and impaired breathing monitor ABG values, oxygen saturation, respiratory rate and pattern, and breath sounds; provide suctioning and oxygen therapy; assist patient on mechanical ventilation to cope with associated stress.
3. Wasting syndrome and fluid and electrolyte disturbances, monitor weight gain or loss, skin turgor and dryness, ferritin levels, hemoglobin and hematocrit and electrolytes. Assist in selecting foods that replenish electrolytes and initiate measures to control diarrhea. Provide IV fluids and electrolytes as prescribed.
4. Side effects of medications; provide information about purpose, administration, side effects (those reportable to physician) and strategies to manage or prevent side effects of medications. Monitor laboratory test values.

Promoting Home and Community-based Care

1. Teaching patients self-care:
   a. Thoroughly discuss the disease and all fears, and misconceptions; instruct patient, family and friends about the transmission of AIDS.
   b. Discuss precautions to prevent transmission of HIV; use of condoms during vaginal or anal intercourse; using dental dam or avoiding oral contact with penis, vagina or rectum; avoiding sexual practice that might cut or tear the lining of rectum, vagina or penis and avoiding sexual contact with multiple partners those known to be HIV positive, those who use illicit injectable drugs and those who are sexual partners of people who inject drugs.

c. Teach patient and family how to prevent disease transmission including hygiene and methods of safely handling items soiled with bodily fluids.
d. Instruct patient not to denote blood.
e. Emphasize importance of taking medication as prescribed. Assist patient and caregivers in fitting the medication regimen into their lives.
f. Teach medication administration including IV preparations.
g. Teach guidelines about infection, follow-up care, diet, rest and activities.
h. Instruct patient and family how to administer enteral or parental feedings, if applicable.
i. Offer support and guidance in coping with this disease.

2. Continuing care:
   a. Refer patient and family for home care nursing or hospice for physical and emotional support.
   b. Assist family and caregivers in providing supportive care.
   c. Assist in administration of parental antibiotics, chemotherapy, nutrition, complicated wound care and respiratory care.
   d. Provide emotional support to patient and family.
   e. Refer patient to community programs, housekeeping assistance, meals, transportation, shopping, individual and group therapy, support for caregivers, telephone networks for the homebound and legal and financial assistance.
   f. Encourage patient and family to discuss end-of-life decisions.

Evaluation/Expected Patient Outcomes

- Maintains skin integrity
- Experiences no infections
- Maintains adequate level of activity tolerance
- Maintains usual level of thought processes
- Maintains effective airway clearance
- Experiences increase sense of comfort and less pain
- Maintains adequate nutritional status
- Experiences decreased sense of social isolation
- Progresses through grieving process
- Reports increased understanding of AIDS and participate in self-care activities as possible
- Remains free of complications.

KAPOSI'S SARCOMA

Kaposi's sarcoma (KS) is the most common HIV-related malignancy and involves the endothelial layer of blood and lymphatic vessels. In people with AIDS, epidemic KS is most often seen among male, homosexuals and bisexuals. AIDS-related KS exhibits a variable and aggressive course ranging localized cutaneous lesions to disseminated disease involving multiple organ systems.

Clinical Manifestations

1. Cutaneous lesions can occur anywhere on the body and are usually brownish pink to deep purple. They characteristically present as lower extremity skin lesions.

2. Lesions may be flat or raised and surrounded by ecchymosis and edema; they develop rapidly and cause extensive disfigurement.
3. The location and size of the lesions can lead to venous stasis, lymphedema and pain. Common sites of visceral involvement include the lymph nodes, GI tract and lungs.
4. Involvement of internal organs may eventually lead to organ failure, hemorrhage, infection and death.

Diagnostic Findings

1. Diagnosis is confirmed by biopsy of suspected lesions.
2. Prognosis depends on extent of tumor, presence of other symptoms of HIV infection and the CD4+ count.
3. Pathological findings indicate that death occurs from tumor progression, but more often from other complications of HIV infection.

Medical Management/Therapeutic Measures

Treatment goals are to reduce symptoms by decreasing the size of skin lesions, to reduce discomfort associated with edema and ulcerations and to control symptoms associated with mucosal or visceral involvement. No one treatment has been shown to improve survival rates. Radiation therapy is effective in a palliative measure to relieve localized pain due to tumor mass (especially in the legs) and for KS lesions that are in sites such as the oral mucosa, conjunctiva, face and soles of the feet.

Pharmacological Therapy

1. Patients with cutaneous KS treated with alpha-interferon have experienced tumor regression and improved immune system function.
2. Alpha-interferon is administered by the IV, intramuscular (IM) or subcutaneous route. Patients may self-administer interferon at home or receive interferon in an outpatient setting.
3. The NSAIDS and opioids.

Nursing Management

1. Provide thorough and meticulous skin care involving regular turning, cleansing, and application of medicated ointments and dressing.
2. Provide analgesic agents as regular intervals around the clock.
3. Teach patient relaxation and guided imagery, which may be helpful in reducing pain and anxiety.
4. Teach patient to self-administer alpha-interferon at home or arrange for patient to receive it in an outpatient setting.
5. Support patient in coping with disfigurement of the condition; stress that lesions are temporary when applicable (after immunotherapy is discontinued).
6. Provide supportive care and treatment as ordered minimize pain and edema, address complications and promote healing.

6

Chapter Perioperative Nursing

Surgery is the technique by using of instruments during an operation to treat injuries, diseases and deformities. Surgical procedures are named according to the involved body organ, part or location and the suffix that describes, what is done during procedure. Surgery is scheduled based on the urgency required for a successful outcome for the patient. There are three phases in the surgical process, which includes pre-, intra- and post-operative. These phases together referred to as perioperative, which is the time before, during and after surgery.

Surgery, whether elective or emergency, is a stressful, complex event. Surgery may be performed for a variety of reasons. It may be diagnostic (e.g. biopsy specimen, exploratory laparotomy), curative (e.g. excision of tumor mass), reparative (e.g. repair of wounds), reconstructive or cosmetic (e.g. a facelift), palliative (e.g. pain relief). Surgery may also be classified according to the degree of urgency involved (emergency, urgent, required elective and optional).

Whatever its classification, current surgery involves many more ambulatory procedures than ever before and administrative processes that are new to nursing and other healthcare staff. However, perioperative nursing concerns still focus on the patient and his/her well-being. Inpatient or outpatient, all surgical procedures require a comprehensive preoperative nursing assessment and interventions to prepare the patient and family before surgery.

PREOPERATIVE NURSING

Nursing Management

Preoperative care begins with decisions for surgery and ends with patient transfer to the operating room or operation theater.

Informed Consent

1. Reinforce information provided by surgeon.
2. Notify physician if patient needs additional information to make his/her decision.
3. Ascertain that the consent form has been signed before administering psychoactive premedication. Informed consent is required for invasive procedures such as incision biopsy, cystoscopy or paracentesis, procedures require sedation and/or anesthesia and non-surgical procedures that more than slight risk to the patient (arteriography); and procedures involving radiation.
4. Arrange for a responsible family member or legal guardian to be available to give consent when the patient is a minor or is unconscious or incompetent [an emancipated most (married or independently earning own living) may sign his/her own surgical consent form].
5. Place the signed consent form in a prominent place on the patient's chart.

Assessment for Patient Undergoing Surgery

1. Obtain a health history and perform a physical examination to establish vital signs and a database for future comparisons.
2. Determine the existence of allergies, previous allergic reactions, any sensitivities to medications and past adverse reactions to these agents. And report a history of bronchial asthma to the anesthesiologist.
3. During the physical examination, note significant physical findings such as physical abuse, pressure ulcers, edema or abnormal breath sounds that further describe the patient's overall condition.
4. Obtain and document medication history; include dosage and frequency of prescribed and over-the-counter (OTC) preparations, particularly adrenal corticosteroids, diuretics, phenothiazines, antidepressants, tranquilizers, insulin and antibiotics.
5. Assess patient' usual level of functioning and typical daily activities to assist in patient's care and recovery or rehabilitation plans.
6. Determine nutritional needs on the basis of patient's height and weight. Body mass index (BMI), triceps skinfold thickness, upper arm circumference, serum protein levels or nitrogen balance. Nutrition deficiencies should be corrected before surgery.
7. Assess mouth for dental caries, dentures and partial plates. Decayed teeth or dental prostheses may become dislodged during intubation for anesthetic delivery and occlude the airway.
8. Assess cardiovascular status to meet oxygen and circulatory demands.
9. Determine the value and reliability of patient's support systems; determine role of patient's family and friends.
10. Elicit patient concerns that can have a bearing on the surgical experience.
11. Identify the ethnic group to which the patient belongs and the customs, and beliefs that the patient holds about illness and healthcare providers.
12. Monitor patients who are obese for abdominal distension, phlebitis; and cardiovascular, endocrine, hepatic and biliary diseases, which occur more readily in the obese.
13. Be alert for a history of drug or alcohol abuse when obtaining the patient's history; remain patient, ask questions frankly and maintain a non-judgmental attitude.
14. Investigate the mildest symptoms or slightest temperature elevation in patients with disorders affecting the immune system [e.g. acquired immunodeficiency syndrome (AIDS), leukemia]; use strict asepsis.

Assessment of Ambulatory Surgery

1. Obtain the health history of the ambulatory or same-day surgical patient by telephone interview or at preadmission testing. Ask about recent and past health history, allergies, medications, preoperative preparation, and psychosocial and demographic factors.
2. Complete the physical assessment on the day of surgery.
3. Monitor the older person undergoing surgery for subtle clues that indicate underlying problems because elderly patients have

less physiologic reserve [cardiac, renal and hepatic function, and gastrointestinal (GI) activity] than younger patients. Also monitor elderly patients for dehydration, hypovolemia and electrolyte imbalances, which can be a significant problem in the elderly population.

Nursing Diagnosis/Problems

1. Anxiety related to the surgical experience (anesthesia, pain) and the outcome of surgery.
2. Risk for ineffective therapeutic management regimen related to deficient knowledge of preoperative procedures and protocols, and postoperative expectations.
3. Fear related to perceived threat of the surgical procedure and separation from support system.
4. Deficient knowledge related to the surgical process.

Planning and Goals

The surgical patient's major goals may include relief of preoperative anxiety, adequate nutrition and fluids, optimal respiratory and cardiovascular status, optimal hepatic and renal function, mobility and active body movement, spiritual comfort, and knowledge of pre- and post-operative expectations.

Nursing Interventions

Providing Psychosocial Support to Reduce Anxiety and Fear

1. Be a good listener, be empathetic and provide information that helps alleviate concerns.
2. During preliminary contacts, give the patient opportunities to ask questions and to become acquainted with those who might be providing care during and after surgery.
3. Acknowledge patient concerns or worries about impending surgery by listening and communicating therapeutically.
4. Explore any fears of patient and arrange for the assistance of other health professionals if required.
5. Teach patient cognitive strategies that may be useful for relieving tension, overcoming anxiety and achieving relaxation including imagery, distractions or optimistic affirmations.

Managing Nutrition and Fluids

1. Provide nutritional support as ordered to correct any nutrient deficiency before surgery to provide enough protein for tissue repair.
2. Instruct patient that, oral intake of food or water should be withheld 8–10 hours before the operation (most common), unless physician allows clear fluids up to 3–4 hours before surgery.
3. Inform patient that a light meal may be permitted on the preceding evening when surgery is scheduled in the morning or provide a soft breakfast, if prescribed, when surgery is scheduled to take place afternoon and does not involve any part of the GI tract.
4. In dehydrated patients especially older patient, encourage fluids by mouth as ordered, before surgery and administer fluids intravenously as ordered.

5. Monitor the patient with a history of chronic alcoholism for malnutrition and other systemic problems that increase the surgical risk as well as for alcohol withdrawal (delirium tremens up to 72 hours after alcohol withdrawal).

Promoting Optimal Respiratory and Cardiovascular Status

1. Urge patient to stop smoking 2 months before surgery (or at least 24 hours).
2. Teach patient breathing exercises and how to use an incentive, spirometer if indicated.
3. Assess patient with underlying respiratory disease [e.g. asthma, chronic obstructive pulmonary disease (COPD)] carefully for current threats to pulmonary status; assess patient's use of medications that may affect postoperative recovery.
4. In the patient with cardiovascular disease, avoid sudden changes of position, prolonged immobilization, hypotension or hypoxia and overloading of the circulatory system with fluids or blood.

Supporting Hepatic and Renal Function

1. If patient has a disorder of the liver, carefully assess various liver function tests and acid-base status.
2. Frequently monitor blood glucose levels of the patient with diabetes—before, during and after surgery.
3. Report the use of steroid medications for any purpose by the patient during the preceding year to the anesthesiologist and surgeon.
4. Monitor the patient for signs of adrenal insufficiency.
5. Assess the patients with uncontrolled thyroid disorders for history of thyrotoxicosis (with hyperthyroid disorders) or respiratory failure (with hypothyroid disorders).

Promoting Active Body Movement and Exercise

1. Explain the rationale for frequent position changes after surgery (to improve circulation, prevent venous stasis and promote optimal respiratory function) and show patient, how to turn from side to side, and assume the lateral position without causing pain or disrupting intravenous (IV) lines, drainage tubes or other apparatus.
2. Discuss any special position, which will need to maintain after surgery by the patient (e.g. adduction or elevation of an extremity) and the importance of maintaining mobility as much as possible, despite restrictions.
3. Instruct patient in exercise of the extremities including extension, and flexion of the knee and hip joints (similar to bicycle riding, while lying on the side); foot rotation (tracing the largest possible circle with great toe); and range of motion of the elbow and shoulder.
4. Use proper body mechanics and instruct patient to do the same. Maintain patient's body in proper alignment when patient is placed in any position.

Respecting Spiritual and Cultural Beliefs

1. Help the patient obtain to spiritual help if he/she requests it; respect and support the beliefs of each patient.

2. When assessing pain, remember that some cultural groups are unaccustomed to expressing feelings openly. Individuals from some cultural groups may not make direct eye contact with other; this lack of eye contact is not avoidance or a lack of interest, but a sign of respect.
3. Listen carefully to patient, especially when obtaining the history. Correct use of communication and interviewing skills can help the nurse acquire invaluable information and insight. Remain unhurried, understanding and caring.

Providing Preoperative Patient Education

1. Teach each patient as an individual with consideration for any unique concerns or learning needs.
2. Begin teaching as soon as possible from starting in the physician's office and continuing during the preadmission visit, when diagnostic tests are being performed through arrival in the operating room.
3. Space instruction over a period of time to allow patient to assimilate information and ask questions.
4. Combine teaching sessions with various preparation procedures to allow for an easy flow of information. Include descriptions of the procedures and explanation of the sensations that the patient will experience.
5. During the preadmission visit, arrange for the patient to meet and ask questions of the perianesthesia nurse, view audiovisuals, and review written materials. Provide a telephone number for patient to call, if questions arise closer to the date of surgery.
6. Reinforce information about the possible need for ventilator and the presence of drainage tubes or other types of equipment to help the patient adjust during the postoperative period.
7. Inform the patient, when family and friends will be able to visit after surgery and that a spiritual advisor will be available, if desired.

Teaching the ambulatory surgical patient

1. For the 'same-day' or 'ambulatory' surgical patient, teach about discharge and follow-up home care. Education can be provided by a videotape, over the telephone or during a group meeting, night classes, preadmission testing, or the preoperative interview.
2. Answer questions and describe what to expect.
3. Inform the patient when and where to report, what to bring (insurance care, list of medications and allergies), what to leave at home (jewelry, watch, medications and contact lenses) and what to wear (loose-fitting, comfortable clothes and flat shoes).
4. During the last preoperative phone call, remind the patient not to eat or drink as directed; brushing teeth is permitted, but no fluids should be swallowed.

Teaching deep breathing and coughing exercises

1. Teach the patient, how to promote optimal lung expansion and consequent blood oxygenation after anesthesia by assuming sitting positions, taking deep and slow breath (maximal sustained inspiration), and exhaling slowly.
2. Demonstrate, how patient can splint the incision, how to minimize pressure and control pain (if there will be a thoracic or abdominal incision).

3. Inform the patient that medications are available to relax pain and that they should be taken regularly for pain relief to enable effective deep breathing and coughing exercises.

Explaining pain management

1. Instruct patient to take medications as frequently as prescribed during the initial postoperative period for pain relief.
2. Discuss the use of oral analgesic agents with patient before surgery and assess patient's interest, and willingness to participate in pain relief methods.
3. Instruct the patient in the use of pain rating scale to promote postoperative pain management.

Preparing the bowel for surgery

1. If ordered preoperatively, administer or instruct the patient to take the antibiotic and a cleansing enema or laxative at the evening before the surgery and repeat it at the morning of surgery.
2. Have the patient use the toilet or bedside commode rather than bedpan for evacuation of the enema, unless the patient's condition presents some contraindication.

Preparing patient for surgery

1. Instruct patient to use detergent germicide for several days at home (if the surgery is not an emergency).
2. If hair is to be removed, remove it immediately before the operation using electric clippers.
3. Dress patient with hospital gown that is left untied and open in the back.
4. Cover patient's hair completely with a disposable paper cap; if patient has long hair, it may be braided; hairpins are removed.
5. Inspect patient's mouth and remove dentures or plates.
6. Remove jewelry including wedding rings (if patient objects, securely fasten the ring with tape).
7. Handover the valuable articles including dentures and prosthetic devices to family members, or if needed label articles clearly with patient's name and store in a safe place according to agency policy.
8. Assist patients (except those with urologic disorders) to void immediately before going to the operating room.
9. Administer preanesthetic medication as ordered and keep the patient in bed with the side rails raised. Observe patient for any untoward reaction to the medications. Keep the immediate surroundings quiet to promote relaxation.

Transporting Patient to Operating Room

1. Send the completed chart with patient to operating room; attach surgical consent form and all laboratory reports, and nurses records, noting any unusual last-minute observations that may have a bearing on the anesthesia or surgery at the front of the chart in a prominent place.
2. Take the patient to preoperative holding area and keep the area quiet, avoiding unpleasant sounds or conversation.
3. Someone should be there with the preoperative patient at all times to ensure safety and provide reassurance (verbally as well as nonverbally by facial expressions, manner or the warm grasp of a hand).

Attending the Special Needs of Older Patients

1. Assess the older patient for dehydration, constipation and malnutrition, report if present.
2. Maintain a safe environment for the older patient with sensory limitations such as impaired vision or hearing and reduced tactile sensitivity.
3. Initiate protective measures for the older patient with arthritis, which may affect mobility and comfort. Use adequate padding for tender areas. Move patient slowly and protect bony prominences from prolonged pressure. Provide gentle massage to promote circulation.
4. Take added precautions when moving elderly patient because decreased perspiration leads to dry, itchy, fragile skin, i.e. easily abraded.
5. Apply a lightweighted cotton blankets as a cover when the elderly patient is moved to and from the operating room because decreased subcutaneous fat makes older people more susceptible to temperature changes.
6. Provide the elderly patient with an opportunity to express fears; this enables patient to gain some peace of mind and a sense of being understood.

Attending to the Family's Needs

1. Assist the family to the surgical waiting room, where the surgeon may meet the family after surgery.
2. Reassure the family that they should not judge the seriousness of an operation by the length of time the patient is in the operating room.
3. Inform the people, those who waiting to see the patient after surgery that, the patient may have certain equipment or devices in a place (i.e. IV lines, indwelling urinary catheter, nasogastric tube, suction bottles, oxygen lines, monitoring equipment and blood transfusion lines).
4. When the patient returns to the room, provide explanations regarding the frequent postoperative observations.

Evaluation/Expected Patient Outcomes

- Reports decreased fear and anxiety
- Voices understanding of surgical intervention.

INTRAOPERTAIVE NURSING

Intraoperative nursing begins with transfer of patient to operating room and ends with admission to postanesthesia care unit (PACU). Here, nurses assist the surgeon depending upon the nature of surgical process.

POSTOPERATIVE NURSING

Nursing Management

The postoperative period extends from the time, the patient leaves the operating room until the last follow-up visit with the surgeon (as short as a day or two, or as long as several months). During the postoperative period, nursing care is directed at re-establishing the patient's physiologic equilibrium, alleviating pain, preventing complications and teaching the patient's self-care. Careful assessment and immediate intervention assist the patient in returning to optimal function quickly, safely and as comfortable as possible. Ongoing care in the community through home care, telephone follow-up and clinic or office visits promotes an uncomplicated recovery.

Postanesthesia care in some hospitals and ambulatory surgical centers is divided into three phases. Phase I is the immediate recovery phase, requires intensive nursing care. In phase II, the patient is prepared for self-care or care in the hospital, or an extended care setting. In phase III, the patient is prepared for discharge.

In the Postanesthesia Care Unit

Patients still under anesthesia or recovering from it, are placed in the PACU, formerly called the postanesthesia recovery room, which is located adjacent to the operating rooms. Patients may be in the PACU for as long as 4–6 hours or little as 1–2 hours. In some cases, the patient is discharged to home directly from this unit. Documentation of information and events germane to PACU care includes the following:

- Medical diagnosis and type of surgery performed
- Patient's age and general condition, airway patency, vital signs, etc.
- Anesthetic and other medications used (e.g. opioids and other analgesics, muscle relaxant, antibiotics, etc.)
- Any problems that occurred in the operating room that might influence postoperative care (e.g. extensive hemorrhage, shock and cardiac arrest)
- Amount of fluid administered, estimated blood loss and replacement
- Any tubing, drains, catheters or other supportive aids
- Specific information, which the surgeon, anesthesiologist or anesthetist wishes to be notified
- Pathology encountered (if malignancy, whether to the patient or family has been informed).

The nursing management objectives for the patient in the PACU are to provide care until the patient has recovered from the effects of anesthesia (i.e. until return of motor and sensory functions), is oriented, has stable vital signs and shows no evidence of hemorrhage.

Role of PACU Nurse

The PACU nurse obtain frequent assessments of the patient's oxygen saturation, pulse volume and regularity, depth and nature of respirations, skin color, level of consciousness, and ability to respond to commands. In some cases, end-tidal carbon dioxide ($ETCO_2$) levels are monitored as well. The nurse also performs a baseline assessment followed by checking the surgical site for drainage or hemorrhage and connecting the drainage tubes, and monitoring lines. After the initial assessment, the nurse monitors vital signs and assesses the patient general physical status at every 15 minutes including assessment of cardiovascular function with the above assessments. The nurse maintains airway patency and supplemented oxygen; maintains cardiovascular stability with prevention, and prompt recognition and treatment of hemorrhage, hypertension, dysrhythmias, hypotension and shock; relieves pain and anxiety; and controls nausea and vomiting. The nurse also notes any pertinent information from the patient history that may be significant (e.g. hard of hearing, blind and history of seizures, diabetes, allergies to certain medications or other substances).

Usually, the following measures are used to determine the patient's readiness for discharge from the PACU:

- Uncompromised pulmonary function
- Pulse oximetry readings of adequate oxygen saturation
- Stable vital signs
- Orientation to place, events and time
- Urine output not less than 30 milliliter per hour
- Nausea and vomiting under control
- Minimal pain.

Patients being discharged directly to home are given teaching, written instructions and information about follow-up care. Usually, the nurse makes sure that they are transported home safely by responsible person.

Management of Same-day Surgery Patient

1. Inform the patient and caregiver (i.e. family member or friend) about expected outcomes and immediate postoperative changes anticipated in the patient's capacity for self-care.
2. Provide written instructions about wound care, activity and dietary recommendations, medications and follow-up visits to the same-day surgery unit or the surgeon. Provide caregiver with verbal and written instructions about, what to observe the patient for and about the actions to take, if complications occur.
3. Give prescriptions to patient, provide the nurse's or surgeon's telephone number, and encourage patient and caregiver to call, if questions arise. Follow-up telephone calls from the nurse or surgeon may be used to assess patient's progress and to answer any questions.
4. Instruct patient limit activity for 24–48 hours (avoid driving a vehicle, drinking alcoholic beverages or performing tasks that require energy or skill); to consume fluids as desired; and to consume smaller amounts of food than normal.
5. Caution the patient not to make important decisions at this time because the medications, anesthesia and surgery may affect thinking ability.
6. Refer patient form home care as indicated (aged or frail patients, those who live alone and patients with other healthcare problems that may interfere with self-care or resumption of usual activities).

In Home Care

1. The home care nurse assesses the patient's physical status (e.g. respiratory and cardiovascular status, adequacy of pain management and surgical incision), and the patient's and family's ability to adhere to the recommendations given at the time of discharge. Previous teaching is reinforced as needed.
2. The home care nurse may change surgical dressings and catheters, or teach the patient or family how to do so, monitor the patency of a drainage system, administer medications or teach the patient and family to do so and assess for surgical complications.

3. The home care nurse determines if any additional services are needed and assists the patient and family to arrange for them (needed supplies, resources or support groups the patient may want to contact).
4. The home care nurse reinforces previous teaching and reminds the patient to keep follow-up appointments. The patient and family are instructed about signs and symptoms to report to the surgeon.
5. Prepare the patient's unit by assembling the necessary equipment and supplies; IV pole, drainage receptacle holder, basin, tissues, disposable pads (Chux), blankets and postoperative charting forms.
6. Receive report form the PACU nurse containing baseline data including demographic data, medical diagnosis, procedure performed, comorbid conditions, unexpected intraoperative events, estimated blood loss, type and amount of fluids received, about patient's condition, and specific information about which the surgeon, anesthesiologist, wishes to be notified.
7. Review the postoperative orders, admit patient to unit, perform an initial assessment and attend to patient's immediate needs.
8. During the 1st hour after surgery, interventions focus on helping the patient recover from the effects of anesthesia, performing frequent assessments, monitoring for complications, managing pain and implementing measures to promote self-care, successful management of the therapeutics regimen, discharge to home and full recovery.
9. In the initial hours after admission to the clinical unit, adequate ventilation, hemodynamic stability, incisional pain, surgical site integrity, nausea and vomiting, neurologic status, and spontaneous voiding are primary concerns.
10. Unless indicated more frequently, record the pulse, blood pressure and respirations every 15 minutes for the 1st hour and every 30 minutes for the next 2 hours. Thereafter, they are measured less frequently, if they remain stable. Monitor the patient's temperature every 4 hours for the first 24 hours.

Nursing Interventions

Maintaining Patient Airway

1. Check the orders for and apply supplement oxygen. Assess respiratory rate and depth, ease of respirations, oxygen saturation and breath sounds.
2. Monitor patient for airway obstruction in which the tongue falls backward, and the patient has choking, noisy and irregular respirations, and within minutes, a blue, dusky color (cyanosis) of the skin. Maintain hard rubber or plastic airway in patient's mouth or nose until gag reflex resumes.
3. Encourage patient to turn frequently and take deep breaths, and cough at least every 2 hours.
4. Carefully assist patient to splint an abdominal or thoracic incision site to help patient overcome the fear that the exertion of coughing might open the incision.
5. Administer pain medications to permit more effective coughing, suction the patient as needed.
6. Assist and encourage the patient to use incentive spirometer hourly, while awake (10 breaths per hour).

7. Coughing is contraindicated in patients have head injuries or who have undergone intracranial surgery, eye surgery or plastic surgery.

Maintain Cardiovascular Stability

1. Monitor cardiovascular stability by assessing patient's mental status, vital signs, cardiac rhythm, skin temperature, color and moisture, and urine output.
2. Assess patency of all IV lines.
3. On patient's arrival in the clinical unit, observe the surgical site for bleeding, type and integrity of dressing, and drains (e.g. Penrose, Hemovac and Jackson-Pratt).
4. Assess output from wound drainage systems and amount of bloody drainage on the surgical dressing frequently. Mark and time spots of drainage on dressings; report excess drainage or fresh blood to surgeon immediately.
5. Reinforce dressing with sterile gauze bandages and record the time. Do not change initial dressings; surgeon will normally wish to be present.
6. A systolic blood pressure is less than 90 mm Hg is usually considered reportable at once. However, the patient's preoperative or baseline blood pressure is used to make informed postoperative comparisons. A previously stable blood pressure that shows a downward trend of 5 mm Hg, at each 15 minute reading should also be reported.

Assessing and Managing Pain

1. Assess pain level using a verbal or visual analog scale and assess the characteristics of the pain.
2. Discuss option in pain relief measures with patient to determine the best medication. Assess effectiveness of medication periodically beginning 30 minutes after administration (sooner, if given intravenously).
3. Administer medication at prescribed intervals or if ordered as needed, before pain becomes severe or unbearable. Risk of addiction is negligible with use of opioids for short-term pain control.
4. Provide other pain relief measures (changing patient's position, using distraction, applying cool washcloths to the face and rubbing the back with a soothing lotion) to relieve general discomfort temporarily.

Maintaining Normal Body Temperature

1. Monitor body systems function and vital signs with temperature at every 4 hours for the first 24 hours and every shift thereafter.
2. Report signs of hypothermia to physician. This is a particular risk in old age patients and those with long surgeries.
3. Maintain the room at a comfortable temperature and provide blankets to prevent chilling.
4. Monitor patient for cardiac dysrhythmias.
5. Take efforts to identify malignant hyperthermia and to treat it early.

Assessing Mental Status

1. Assess mental status (level of consciousness, speech and orientation) and compare to preoperative baseline; change may be related to anxiety, pain, medications, oxygen deficit or hemorrhage.
2. Assess for possible causes of discomfort such as tight, drainage-soaked bandages or distended bladder.
3. Address sources of discomfort and report signs of complications to surgeon for immediate treatment.
4. Assess neurovascular status (have patient move the hand or foot distal to the surgical site through a full range of motion, ensuring that all surfaces have intact sensation and assessing peripheral pulses).

Assessing and Managing Gastrointestinal Function and Promoting Nutrition

1. Maintain nesogastric tube in place, and monitor patency and drainage.
2. Provide symptomatic therapy including antiemetic medications for nausea and vomiting.
3. Administer phenothiazine medications as prescribed for severe, persistent hiccups.
4. Assist patient to return to normal dietary intake gradually at a pace set by patient (liquids first, then soft foods such as gelatin, junket, custard, milk and creamed soups are added gradually, then solid food).
5. Remember that paralytic ileus and intestinal obstruction are potential postoperative complications that occur more frequently in patients undergoing intestinal or abdominal surgery. Check specific GI disorder for discussion of treatment.
6. Arrange for patient to consult with the dietitian to plan for appealing high-protein meals, which provide sufficient fiber, calories and vitamins. Nutritional supplements such as Ensure or Sustacal, etc. may be recommended.
7. Instruct patient to take multivitamins, iron and vitamin C supplements postoperatively, if prescribed.
8. At the slightest indication of nausea, turn patient completely on one side to promote mouth drainage and prevent aspiration of vomitus, which can cause asphyxiation and death.

Assessing and Managing Voluntary Voiding

1. Assess for bladder distension and urge to avoid on patient's arrival in the unit and frequently thereafter (patient should void within 8 hours of surgery).
2. Obtain order for catheterization before the end of the 8-hour time limit if patient has an urge to void and cannot or if the bladder is distended and no urge is felt, or patient cannot void.
3. Initiate methods to encourage the patient to void (e.g. letting water run, applying heat to perineum).
4. Warm the bedpan to reduce discomfort and automatic tightening of muscles, and urethral sphincter.
5. Assist the patient who complains of not being able to use the bedpan to use a commode, or stand or sit to void (males), unless contraindicated.

6. Take safeguards to prevent the patient, from falling or fainting due to loss of coordination from medications or orthostatic hypotension.
7. Note the amount of urine voided (report less than 30 mL/h) and palpate the suprapubic area for distension or tenderness or use a portable ultrasound device to assess residual volume.
8. Continue intermittent catheterization at every 4–6 hours until patient can void spontaneously and postvoid residual is less than 100 mL.

Encouraging Early Ambulation

1. Encourage most surgical patients to ambulate as soon as possible.
2. Remind of the importance of early mobility in preventing complications (helps overcome fears) to the patients.
3. Anticipate and avoid orthostatic hypotension (postural hypotension is 20 mm Hg fall in systolic blood pressure or 10 mm Hg fall in diastolic blood pressure, weakness, dizziness and fainting).
4. Assess patient's feeling of dizziness and his/her blood pressure first in the supine position, after patient sits up, again after patient stands, and 2–3 minutes later.
5. When patient gets out of bed, remain at patient's side to give physical support and encouragement.
6. Take care not to tire patient.
7. Initiate and encourage patient to perform bed exercises to improve circulation (range of motion to arms, hands and fingers; feet and legs; leg flexion and leg lifting; abdominal and gluteal contraction).
8. Encourage frequent position changes early in the postoperative period to stimulate circulation. Avoid positions that compromise venous return (raising the knee gatch or placing a pillow under the knees, sitting for long periods and dangling the legs with pressure at the back of the knees).
9. Apply antiembolism stockings and assist patient in early ambulation. Check postoperative activity orders before getting patient out of bed. Then have patient sit on the edge of bed for a few minutes initially, advance ambulation as tolerated.

Promoting Fluid Balance and its Maintenance

1. Monitor patient closely to detect and correct conditions such as fluid volume deficit, altered tissue perfusion and decreased cardiac output.
2. Assess patency of IV lines, ensuring that appropriate fluids are administered at prescribed rate (up to 24 hours or until patient is tolerating oral fluids).
3. Record intake and output including emesis and output from wound drainage systems, separately and add them to determine fluid balance (with indwelling urinary catheter, monitor outputs hourly and report rates of less than 30 mL/h; if the patient is voiding, report output of less than 240 milliliter per shift).
4. Monitor electrolyte levels and hemoglobin and hematocrit levels.

Promoting Self-care

1. Encourge patient to perform as much routine hygiene care as possible on first postoperative day (setting up patient to bath with a bedside wash basin or, if possible, assisting patient to bathroom to sit at a chair near the sink).
2. Assist patient to build up ambulating a functional distance (length of house or apartment), get in and out of bed unassisted and be independent with toileting, to prepare for discharge at home.
3. Ask patient to perform daily activity as much as possible and then look for assistance. Collaborate with patient for progressive activity and assess vital signs before, during and after a scheduled activity.
4. Provide physical support to maintain patient's safety and provide a positive attitude about patient's ability to perform the activity, promoting confidence.
5. While changing the dressing, teach patient, how to care for incision and change dressings at home. Observe for indicators that patient is ready to learn such as looking at the incision, expressing interest or assisting in the dressing change.

Maintaining a Safe Environment

1. Keep side rails up and keep the cot or bed in the low position.
2. Assess level of consciousness and orientation.
3. Determine whether patient needs his/her eyeglasses or hearing aid and provide them as soon as possible.
4. Place all objects, which patient may need within reach including of course, the call bell.
5. Implement any immediate postoperative orders concerning special positioning, equipment or intervention.
6. Ask patient to seek assistance with any activity.
7. Use restrains only if needed (disordered patient) and assess neurovascular status frequently.

Providing Emotional Support to Patient and Family

1. Help patient and family work through their anxieties by providing reassurance and information, and by spending time to listening to and addressing concerns.
2. Describe hospital routines and what to expect in the hours and days until discharge.
3. Explain the purpose of nursing management and interventions.
4. Inform patients when they can take fluids or eat; when they will be getting out of bed; when tubes and drains will be removed and so forth, to help them to gain a sense of control and participation in recovery.
5. Acknowledge family's concerns and accept, and encourage their participation in patient's care.
6. Manipulate the environment to enhance rest and relaxation; provide privacy, reduce noise, adjust lightning, provide enough seating for family members and perform any other supportive measures.

Monitoring and Preventing Postoperative Complications

Deep vein thrombosis

1. Monitor for symptoms of deep vein thrombosis (DVT), which may include a pain or a cramp in the calf elicited on ankle dorsiflexion (Homan's gin); pain and tenderness may be followed by a painful swelling of the entire leg and may be accompanied by slight fever and sometimes chills, and perspiration.
2. Administer prophylactic treatment for postoperative patients at risk (low-dose subcutaneous heparin and then warfarin, external pneumatic compression, and thigh-high elastic pressure stockings).
3. Avoid using blanket rolls, pillow rolls or any form of elevation that can constrict vessels under the knees. Even prolonged 'dangling' (having the patient sit on the edge of the bed with legs hanging over the side) can be dangerous and is not recommended in susceptible patients.
4. Encourage adequate hydration (offer juice and water throughout the day).

Monitoring and treating hypotension and shock

1. Monitor closely for signs of shock (a fall in venous pressure, a rise in peripheral resistance and tachycardia or a fall in blood pressure). If the amount of blood loss exceeds 500 mL (especially if the loss is rapid), replacement is usually indicated.
2. Monitor for the classic signs of shock such as pallor, cool, moist skin, rapid breathing, cyanosis of the lips, gum and tongue; a rapid, weak, thready pulse; decreasing pulse pressure; low blood pressure; and concentrated urine.
3. Prevent hypovolemic shock by timely administration of IV fluids, blood and medications that elevate blood pressure.
4. Control pain by making patient as comfortable as possible and by using opioids judiciously. Avoid exposure and maintain normothermia to prevent vasodilation.
5. Administer volume replacement as ordered (lactated Ringer's solution or blood component therapy).
6. Administer oxygen by nasal cannula, facemask or medical ventilation.
7. Administer cardiotonics, vasodilators or steroids to improve cardiac function and reduce peripheral vascular resistances. Keep the patient warm; however, avoid overheating to prevent dilation.
8. Place patient flat in bed with legs elevated.
9. Monitor respiratory and pulse rate, blood pressure, oxygen concentration, urinary output, level of consciousness, central venous pressure (CVP); pulmonary artery pressure, pulmonary capillary wedge pressure and cardiac output to provide information about respiratory and cardiovascular status.
10. Monitor vital signs continuously until condition has stabilized.

Directing and minimizing hemorrhage

1. Note signs of extreme blood loss (apprehensiveness, restlessness and thirst; cold, moist, pale skin; increased pulse rate; decreasing temperature; and rapid and deep respirations, often of the gasping type spoken of as 'air hunger').
2. If the hemorrhage progresses untreated, cardiac output decreases, arterial and venous blood pressure, and hemoglobin level fall rapidly, the lips and the conjunctive become pallid, spots appear

before the eyes, a ringing is heard in the ears and the patient grows weaker, but remains conscious until near death.

3. Administer blood or blood produce transfusion and determine the cause of hemorrhage.
4. Inspect the surgical site and incision for bleeding. If bleeding is evident, apply a sterile gauze pad and a pressure dressing, and elevate the site of the bleeding to the level of the heart. If possible, place patient in the shock position (lying flat on back with legs elevated at 20° angle, while knees are kept straight). If indicated, prepare patient for return to surgery.
5. Give special considerations to patients who decline blood transfusions such as Jehovah's Witness and to those who identify specific requests on their advance directives or living wall.
6. Giving a too large quantity of IV fluid or administering it too rapidly may raise the blood pressure enough to start the bleeding again.

Managing wound complications

1. Hematoma: Monitor for bleeding beneath the skin at the surgical site, which may result in clot formation (hematoma) within the wound (if clot is large, the wound may bulge and healing is delayed unless the clot is removed). Prepare patient for removal of several sutures by the physician, evacuation of the clot and light wound packing with gauze. Healing occurs usually by granulation or a secondary closure may be performed.
2. Infection (wound sepsis): Monitor for (or instruct patient and family to monitor) wound infection, which may not present until postoperative day 5. Risk factors for wound sepsis include wound contamination, foreign body, faulty suturing, devitalized tissue, hematoma, debilitation, dehydration, malnutrition, anemia, advanced age, extreme obesity, shock, length of postoperative hospitalization and duration of surgery, and associated disorders (e.g. diabetes mellitus, immunosuppression). Signs and symptoms of infection include elevated pulse and temperature; increased white blood cells (WBC) count; wound swelling, warmth, tenderness or discharge; and incisional pain. Local signs may be absent, if the infection is deep.
3. If wound infection results from beta-hemolytic streptococci or *Clostridium* species, take care not to spread infection to others; provide intensive nursing care and care for open incision and drainage, if present. If needed, prepare patient for incision and drainage, if the infection is deep.
4. Administer antimicrobial therapy and initiate wounds to regimen.
5. Wound dehiscence and evisceration: Monitor for wound dehiscence (disruption of surgical incision or wound) and evisceration (protrusion of wound contents), which are serious complications, especially when they involve abdominal incisions or wounds. The earliest signs may be a gush of bloody (sersanguineous) peritoneal fluid from the wound coils of intestine may push out of the abdomen, pain and vomiting may be noted, and frequently the patient will say that 'something gave way.' Monitor patient with risk factors particularly and closely (patients with infection, marked distension and the presence of pulmonary or cardiovascular disease in patients, and the presence of cardiovascular disease in patients who undergo abdominal surgery). If wound disruption occurs, place patient

in low Fowler's position and instruct him/her to lie quietly to minimize protrusion of body tissues. Cover the protruding tissue or coils of intestine with sterile dressings moistened with sterile saline and notify the surgeon at once. Apply the abdominal binder as a prophylactic measure against an abdominal incision evisection.

Promoting Family and Community-based Care

Although certain needs are germane to individual patients and the specific procedures they have undergone. Patient education needs for postoperative care include the following:

1. Provide the detailed discharge instructions to assist patient to becoming proficient in self-care needs after surgery.
2. Arrange for care by community-based services such as home care nurse, if necessary (older patients, patients who live alone, or patients without family support).
3. Arrange for necessary services early in the acute care hospitalization.
4. Wound care, drain management, catheter care, infusion therapy and physical or occupational therapy are some of the needs addressed by community healthcare providers.
5. Instruct patient to continue to perform bed exercise, wet pressure stockings when in bed and rest as needed. Spray silicone over the adhesive used to hold dressings in place; the silicone waterproofs the dressing, so that the patient can bathe or swim and it isolates the area from contamination.
6. Elderly patient continue to be at increased risk for postoperative complications. Age-related physiologic changes in respiratory, cardiovascular and renal function, and the increased incidence of comorbid conditions demand skilled assessment to detect early signs of deterioration. Anesthetics and opioids can cause confusion in older adult and altered pharmacokinetics results in delayed excretion and prolonged respiratory depressive effects. Careful monitoring of electrolyte, hemoglobin and hematocrit levels, and urine output is essential because the older adult is less able to correct and compensate for fluid and electrolyte balance. Elderly patients may need frequent reminders and demonstrations to participate in care effectively.
7. Maintain physical activity when patient is confused. Physical deterioration can worsen delirium and place patient at increased risk for other complications.
8. Avoid restraints, because they can also worsen confusion. If possible, family or staff member is asked to sit with patient instead.
9. Administer haloperidol (Haldol) or lorazepam (Ativan) as ordered during episodes of acute confusion; discontinue these medications as soon as possible to avoid side effects.
10. Assist the older postoperative patient in early and progressive ambulation to prevent the development of problems such as pneumonia, altered bowel function, deep vein thrombosis (DVT), weakness and functional decline; avoid sitting positions that promote venous stasis in the lower extremities.
11. Provide assistance to keep patient from bumping into objects and falling. A physical therapy referral may be indicated to promote safe, regular exercise for the older adult.

12. Provide easy access to call bell and commode; prompt voiding to prevent urinary incontinence.
13. Provide extensive discharge planning to coordinate both professional and family care providers; the nurse, social worker or Nurse Case Manager may institute the plan for continuing care.

Evaluation/Expected Patient Outcomes

The total postoperative evaluation is based on the objective, i.e. expected patient outcomes as given below:

- Experiences decreased pain
- Maintains optimal respiratory function
- Does not develop DVT
- Exercises and ambulates as prescribed
- Wound heals without complication
- Resumes oral intake and normal bowel function
- Acquires knowledge and skills necessary to manage therapeutic regimen
- Experiences no complications and has normal vital signs.

7

Chapter Oncological Nursing

Oncology is the branch of medicine dealing with tumors. Oncological nursing is also called cancer nursing. It is an important component in medical-surgical nursing. Cancer is a group of cells that grow out of control, taking over the junction of the affected organ. Cancer cells are described as poorly constructed, loosely formed and without organization. Cancer is a disease process that begins when an abnormal cell is transformed by the genetic mutation of the cellular deoxyribonucleic acid (DNA). An organ with a cancerous tumor eventually ceases to function. Cancer is the second leading cause of death in United States, with most cancer occurring in men and in people older than 65 years. Cancer also has a higher incidence in industrialized sectors and nations.

CANCER

Cancer is a disease process that begins when an abnormal cell is transformed by the genetic mutation of the cellular DNA.

Pathophysiology

The normal cell forms a clone and begins to proliferate abnormally, ignoring growth-regulating signals in the environment surrounding the cell. The cells acquire invasive characteristics and changes occur in surrounding tissues. The cells infiltrate these tissues, and gain access to lymph and blood vessels, which carry the cells to other areas of the body. This phenomenon is called metastasis (cancer spread to other parts of the body).

Cancerous cells are described as malignant neoplasm, and are classified and named by tissue of origin. The failure of the immune system to promptly destroy abnormal cells permits these cells to grow too large, to be managed by normal immune mechanisms. Certain categories of agents or factors implicated in carcinogenesis (malignant transformation) include viruses and bacteria, physical agents, chemical agents, genetic or familial factors, dietary factors and hormonal agents.

Clinical Manifestations

1. Cancerous cells spread from one organ or body part to another by invasion and metastasis; therefore, manifestations are related to the system affected and degree of disruption (refer the specific type of cancer for clinical manifestation accordingly in this book).
2. Generally cancer causes anemia, weakness, weight loss (dysphagia, anorexia and blockage) and pain (often in late stages).
3. Symptoms are from tissue destruction and replacement with non-functional cancer or overproductive cancer (e.g. bone marrow disruption and anemia or excess adrenal steroid production); pressure on surrounding structures increased metabolic demands and disruption of producing of blood cells.

Diagnostic Findings

Screening to detect early cancer usually focuses on cancer with the highest incidence or those that have improved survival rates, if diagnosed early. For example, of these cancers include breast, colorectal, cervical, endometrial, testicular skin and oropharyngeal cancers. Patients with suspected cancer undergo extensive testing to:

- Determine the presence and extent of tumor
- Identify possible spread (metastasis) of disease or invasion of other body tissues
- Evaluate the function of involved and uninvolved body systems and organs
- Obtain tissue and cells for analysis, including evaluation of tumor stage and grade.

Diagnostic tests may include tumor marker identification, genetic profiling, imaging studies [mammography, magnetic resonance imaging (MRI), computed tomography (CT), fluoroscopy, ultrasonography, endoscopy, nuclear medicine imaging, positron emission tomography (PET), PET fusion and radioimmunoconjugates] and biopsy.

Staging and Grading

Staging determines the size of the tumor and existence of local invasion and distant metastasis. Several systems exist for classifying the anatomic extent of disease. The TNM system frequently used (T refers to extent of the primary tumor, N refers to lymph node involvement and M refers to the extent of metastasis). A variety of other staging systems are used to describe the extent of cancers, such as central nervous system (CNS) cancers, hematological cancers.

Stages of Tumors

Stage I: Tumor less than 2 cm, negative lymph node involvement, no detectable metastases.

Stage II: Tumor greater than 2 cm, but less than 5 cm, negative or positive unfixed lymph node involvement, no detectable metastases.

Stage III: Large tumor greater than 5 cm or a tumor of any size with invasion of the skin or chest wall, or positive fixed lymph node involvement, distant metastases and malignant melanoma that are not well-described by the TNM system.

Grading

Grading refers to the classification of the tumor cells. Grading systems seek to define the type of tissue from which the tumor originated and the degree to which the tumor cells retain the functional and histological characteristics of the tissue of origin (differentiation). Samples of cells to be used to establish the grade of a tumor may be obtained from tissue scrapings, body fluids, secretions or washings, biopsy, or surgical excision. This information helps the healthcare team to predict the behavior and prognosis of various tumors. The tumor is assigned a numeric value ranging from one (well-differentiated) to four (poorly differentiated or undifferentiated).

Medical Management/Therapeutic Measures

The range of possible treatment goals may include complete eradication of malignant disease (cure), prolonged survival and containment of cancer cell, growth (control) or relief of symptoms associated with the disease (palliation). A variety of therapies may be used, including the following:

1. Surgery (e.g. excisions, video-assisted endoscopic surgery, salvage surgery, electrosurgery, cryosurgery, chemosurgery or laser surgery). Surgery may be the primary method of treatment or it may be prophylactic, palliative or reconstructive. The goal of surgery is to remove the tumor or as much as is feasible.
2. Radiation therapy and chemopathy (may be used individually or in combination).
3. Bone marrow transplantation (BMT).
4. Hyperthermia.
5. Other targeted therapies, e.g. biological response modified (BRM), gene therapy, complementary and alternative medicine (CAM).

Nursing Management

Maintaining Tissue Integrity

Some of the most frequently encountered disturbances of tissues integrity include stomatitis, skin and tissue reactions to radiation therapy, alopecia, and malignant skin lesions.

Managing Stomatitis

1. Assess oral cavity daily.
2. Instruct patient to report oral burning, pain, areas of redness, open lesions on the lips, pain associated with swallowing or decreased tolerance to temperature extremes of food.
3. Encourage and assist oral hygiene (brush with soft toothbrush, use non-abrasive toothpaste after meals and bedtime, floss every 24 hours unless painful or platelet count below 40,000/ mm^3); advise patient to avoid irritants such as commercial mouthwashes, alcoholic beverages and tobacco.
4. For mild stomatitis, use normal saline mouth rinses and a soft toothbrush or Toothette, remove dentures except for meals (make sure dentures fit properly), apply water-soluble lip lubricant, and avoid foods that are spicy or hard to chew and those with extremes of temperature.
5. For severe stomatitis, obtain tissue sample for culture and sensitivity tests, assess gap reflex, and ability to chew and swallow, use oral rinses as prescribed or position patient on side and irrigate mouth with suction available, remove dentures, use Toothette or gauze soaked with solution for cleansing, use water-soluble lip lubricant, provide liquid or pureed diet and monitor for dehydration.
6. Help patient minimize discomfort by using prescribed topical anesthetic, administering prescribed systemic analgesics and performing appropriate mouth care.

Managing radiation-associated skin impairments

1. Provide careful skin care by avoiding the use of soaps, cosmetics, perfumes, powders, lotions and ointment, and deodorants. Use

only lukewarm water to bathe the area, and avoid applying hot water bottles, heating pads, ice and adhesive tape to the area. Do not shave the area.

2. Instruct the patient to avoid rubbing or scratching the area, exposing the area to sunlight or cold weather, or wearing tight clothing over the area.
3. If wet desquamation occurs, do not disrupt any blisters that have formed, report blistering and use prescribed ointments. If the area weeps, apply a non-adhesive absorbent dressing. If the area is without drainage, use moisture and vapor permeable dressings, such as hydrocolloids and hydrogels on non-infected areas.

Addressing alopecia

1. Discuss potential hair loss and regrowth with patient and family; advise that hair loss may occur on body parts other than the head.
2. Explore potential impact on hair loss on self-image, interpersonal relationships and sexuality.
3. Prevent or minimize hair loss (use scalp hypothermia and scalp tourniquets, if appropriate, cut long hair before treatment, avoid excessive shampooing and any hair processing, avoid excessive combing or brushing).
4. Suggest ways to assist in coping with hair loss (e.g. purchase wig or hairpiece before hair loss; wear head coverings).
5. Explain that hair growth usually begins again once therapy is completed.

Managing malignant skin lesions

1. Carefully assess and cleanse the skin, reducing superficial bacteria, controlling bleeding, reducing odor, protecting from pain and trauma, and relieving pain.
2. Assist and guide to the patient and family regarding care of these skin lesions at home; refer for home care as indicated.

Promoting Nutrition

1. Most patient with cancer experience weight loss due to their illness. Anorexia, malabsorption and cachexia are common examples of nutritional problems.
2. Teach the patient to avoid unpleasant sights, odors and sounds in the environment during mealtime.
3. Suggest food that are preferred and well-tolerated by patient, preferably high calorie and high protein foods. Respect ethnic and cultural food preferences.
4. Encourage adequate fluids, fluid intake, but limit fluids at mealtime.
5. Suggest smaller, more frequent meals.
6. Promote relaxed, quiet environment during mealtime, increased social interactions as desired.
7. Encourage frequent oral hygiene and provide pain relief measures to make meals more pleasant.
8. Provide control of nausea and vomiting.
9. Decrease anxiety by encouraging verbalization of fears concerns, use of relaxation techniques and imagery mealtime.
10. For collaborative management, provide enteral tube feed of commercial liquids diets, elemental diets or blended foods as prescribed.
11. Administer appetite stimulants as prescribed by physician.

12. Encourage family and friends not to nag or cajole patient about eating.
13. Assess and address other contributing factors to nausea, vomiting and anorexia, such as other symptoms, constriction, gastrointestinal (GI) irritation, electrolyte imbalance radiation therapy, medications and CNS metastasis.

Relieving Pain

1. Use a multidisciplinary team approach to determine the management of pain for optimal quality of life.
2. Assure patient that you know that pain is real and will aid him/her in reducing it.
3. Help patient and family play an active role in managing pain.
4. Provide education and support to correct fears, and misconceptions about opioid use.
5. Encourage strategies of pain relief that patient has used successfully in previous pain experience.
6. Teach patient new strategies to relieve pain and discomfort, distraction, imagery, relaxation, cutaneous stimulation, etc.

Decrease Fatigue

1. Help patient and family to understand that fatigue is usually an expected and temporary side effect of the cancer process and treatment.
2. Help patient to rearrange daily schedule and organize activities to conserve energy expenditures; encourage patient to alternate periods of rest and activity.
3. Encourage patient and family to plan, and reallocate responsibilities such as child care, cleaning and preparing meals. A patient who is employed full time may need to reduce the number of hours worked each week.
4. Encourage adequate intake of protein and calorie; assess for fluid and electrolyte disturbances.
5. Encourage use of relaxation techniques and mental imagery.
6. Address factors that contribute to fatigue and implement pharmacological and non-pharmacological strategies to manage pain.
7. Administer blood products as prescribed.

Promote Body Image and Self-esteem

1. A creative and positive approach is essential when caring for the patient with altered body image. It is also important to individualize care for each patient.
2. Assess patient's feelings about body image and level of self-esteem. Encourage patient to verbalize concerns.
3. Identify potential threats to patient's self-esteem (e.g. altered appearance, decreased sexual function, hair loss, decreased energy and role changes). Validate concerns with patient.
4. Encourage continued participation in activities and decision-making.
5. Assist patient in self-care when fatigue, lethargy, nausea, vomiting and other symptoms prevent independence.
6. Assist patient in selecting and using cosmetics, scarves, hair pieces and clothing that increase his/her sense of attractiveness.

7. Encourage patient and partner to share concerns about altered sexuality and sexual function, and to explore alternatives to their usual experiences.
8. Refer patient to collaborating specialist as needed.

Assisting in Grieving

1. Encourage verbalization of fears, concerns, negative feelings, and question regarding disease, treatment and future implications. Explore previous successful coping strategies.
2. Encourage active participation of patient and family in care and treatment decisions.
3. Visit family frequently to establish and maintain relationships, and physical closeness.
4. Involve spiritual advisor as desired by the patient and family.
5. Allow for progression though the grieving process at the individual pace of the patient and family.
6. Advise professional counseling as indicated for patient or family to alleviate pathological grieving.
7. If patient enters the terminal phase of disease, assist patient and family to acknowledge and cope with their reactions and feelings.
8. Maintain contact with the surviving family members after death of the patient. This may help them to work through their feelings of loss and grief.

Monitoring and Managing Potential Complications

Managing infection

1. Assess patient for evidence of infection: Check vital signs every 4 hours, monitor white blood cell (WBC) count a differential each day and inspect all sites that may sever entry ports for pathogens [e.g. intravenous (IV) sties, wound skin folds, bony prominences, perineum, and oral cavity].
2. Report fever [≥ 38.3°C (101°F) or ≥ 38°C (100.4°F) ≥1 hour], chills, diaphoresis, swelling, heat, erythema and exudate on body surfaces. Also report chart in respiratory or mental status, urinary frequency or burning, malaise, arthralgias, rash or diarrhea.
3. Discuss with patient and family about placing patient in private room if absolute WBC count is less than 1,000/n and the importance of patient avoiding contact with person who have known or recent infection or recent vaccination.
4. Instruct all personnel in careful, hand hygiene before and after entering room.
5. Avoid rectal or vaginal procedures (rectal temperature, examinations, suppositories and vaginal tampons) and in muscular injections. Avoid insertion of urinary catheter. Catheters are necessary, use strict aseptic technique.

Managing septic shock

1. Assess frequently for infection and inflammation through the course of the disease.
2. Prevent septicemia and septic shock or detect, and record for prompt treatment.
3. Monitor for signs and symptoms of septic shock [alter mental status, either abnormal or elevated temperature, cool and clammy skin, decreased urine output, hypotension, tachycardia,

other dysrhythmias, electrolyte imbalance, tachypnea, and abnormal arterial blood gas (ABC) value].

4. Instruct the patient and family about signs of septicemia, nodes for preventing infection, and actions take if inferior septicemia occurs.

Managing bleeding and hemorrhage

1. Monitor platelet count and assess for bleeding (e.g. petechiae or ecchymosis; decrease in hemoglobin or hematocrit; longed bleeding from invasive procedures, venipuncture minor cuts or scratches; frank or occult blood in any excretion, emesis or sputum; bleeding from anybody orifice; altered mental status).
2. Instruct the patient and family about the ways to minimize bleeding (e.g. use soft toothbrush or Toothette for mouth care, electric razor for shaving and avoid foods that are difficult to chew).
3. Initiate measures to minimize bleeding (e.g. draw blood, all laboratory work with one daily venipuncture; avoiding temperature rectally or administering suppositories/enemas; avoid intramuscular injections, use as smallest as possible, if necessary; maintain the fluid intake at least 3 L/24 h unless contraindicated; avoid the medication that will interfere with clotting such as, Aspirin, recommend use of water-based lubricant before sexual intercourse).
4. When platelet count is less than 20,000/mm^3, institute bedrest with padded side rails, avoidance of strenuous activity and platelet transfusions as prescribed.

Promoting Family- and Community-based Care

Teaching patient self-care

1. Provide information needed by patient and family to address the most immediate care needs likely to be encountered at home.
2. Verbally review, and reinforce with written information, the side effects of treatments and changes in the patient's status that should be reported.
3. Discuss strategies to deal with side effects of treatment with patient and family.
4. Identify learning needs on the basis of the priorities identified by patient and family as well as on the complexity of home care.
5. Instruct patient and family, and provide care and support for patients receiving advanced technical care.
6. Provide follow-up visits and phone calls to patient and family, and evaluate patient progress and ongoing needs.

Continuing care

1. Refer patient for home care (assessment of the home environment, suggestions for modifications to assist patient and family in addressing patient's physical needs and physical care, and ongoing assessment of the psychological and emotional effects of the illness on patient and the family).
2. Assess changes in the patient's physical status and report relevant changes to the physician.
3. Assess adequacy of pain management and the effectiveness of other strategies to prevent or manage side effects of treatment.
4. Help coordinate patient care by maintaining close communication with all health care providers involved in the patient's care.

5. Make referrals and coordinate available community resources (e.g. local office of the American Cancer Society, home aides, church groups and support groups) to assist patients and caregivers.

Nursing Management Related to Treatment of Cancer

Cancer surgery

1. Complete a thorough preoperative assessment for all factors that may affect patients undergoing surgery.
2. Assist patient and family in dealing with the possible changes and outcomes resulting from surgery; provide education and emotional support by assessing patient and family needs, and exploring with them their fears and coping mechanisms. Encourage them to take an active role in decision-making when possible.
3. Explain and clarify the information that the physician has provided about the results of diagnostic testing and surgical procedures, if asked.
4. Communicate frequently with the physician and other healthcare team members to ensure that the information provided is consistent.
5. After surgery, assess patient's responses to the surgery and monitor for complications such as infection, bleeding, thrombophlebitis, wound dehiscence, fluid and electrolyte imbalance, and organ dysfunction.
6. Provide for patient comfort.
7. Provide postoperative teaching that address wound care, activity, nutrition and medications.
8. Initiate plans for discharge, follow-up care and treatment as early as possible to ensure continuity of care.
9. Encourage patient and family to use community resources such as the American Cancer Society for support and information.

Radiation therapy

1. Answer questions and allay fears of patient and family about the effects of radiation on others, on the tumor, and on normal tissues and organs.
2. Explain the procedure for delivering radiation. Describe the equipment; the duration of the procedure (often minutes); the possible need for immobilizing the patient during the procedure; and the absence of new sensations, including pain, during the procedure.
3. Assess patient's skin and oropharyngeal mucosa, nutritional status, and general feeling of well-being.
4. Reassure the patient that systemic symptoms (e.g. weakness and fatigue) are a result of the treatment and do not represent deterioration or progression of disease.
5. If a radioactive implant is used, inform patient about the restrictions placed on visitors and healthcare personnel and other radiation precautions as well as the patient's own role before, during and after procedure.
6. Maintain bedrest for patient with an intracavitary delivery device. Use the log-roll maneuver, when positioning patient to prevent displacing the intracavitary device. Provide a low-residue diet and antidiarrheal agents to prevent bowel movements during therapy to prevent the radioisotopes from

being displaced. Maintain an indwelling urinary catheter to ensure that the bladder empties.

7. Assist the weak or fatigued patient with activities of daily living and personal hygiene, including gentle oral hygiene to remove debris, prevent irritation and promote healing.
8. Follow the instructions provided by the radiation safety officer from the radiology department, which identify the maximum time a healthcare provider can spend safely in the patient's room, the shielding equipment to be used, and special precautions and actions to be taken if the implant is dislodged. Explain the rationale for these precautions to patient.
9. For safety in brachytherapy, assign the patient to a private room and post appropriate notices about radiation safety precautions. Have staff members wear dosimeter badges. Make sure that pregnant staff members are not assigned to this patient's care. Prohibit visits by children or pregnant women and limit visits from others to 30 minutes daily. Instruct and monitor visitors to ensure they maintain a 6 feet distance from the radiation source.

Chemotherapy

1. Assess patient's nutritional and fluid, and electrolyte status frequently. Use creative ways to encourage adequate fluid and dietary intake.
2. Decrease the risk of anemia, infection and bleeding disorders, focus nursing assessment, and care on identifying and modifying factors that further increase the risk.
3. Use aseptic technique and gentle handling to prevent infection and trauma.
4. Closely monitor laboratory test results (blood cell counts), and promptly report untoward changes and signs of infection or bleeding.
5. Carefully select peripheral veins and perform venipuncture, and carefully administer drugs. Monitor for indications of extravasation during drug administration (e.g. absence of blood return from the IV catheter, resistance to flow of IV fluid; or swelling, pain, or redness at the site).
6. If extravasation is suspected, stop the drug administration immediately and apply ice to the site (unless the extravasated vesicant is a vinca alkaloid).
7. Assist patient with delayed nausea and vomiting (occurring later than 48–72 hour after chemotherapy) by teaching the patient to take antiemetic medications as necessary for the 1st week at home after chemotherapy and by teaching relaxation techniques, and imagery, which can help to decrease stimuli contributing to symptoms.
8. Monitor blood cells counts frequently, note and report neutropenia, and protect the patient from infection and injury, particularly when blood cell count is depressed.
9. Monitor blood urea nitrogen (BUN), serum creatinine, creatinine clearance and serum electrolyte levels, and report any findings that indicate decreasing renal function.
10. Provide adequate hydration, dieresis and alkalinization of the urine to prevent formation of uric acid crystals; administer allopurinol to prevent these side effects.
11. Monitor closely for signs of heart failure, cardiac ejection fraction (volume of blood ejected from the heart with each beat) and pulmonary fibrosis (e.g. pulmonary function test results).

12. Inform patient that the taxanes and plant alkaloids, especially vincristine, can cause peripheral neurologic damage with sensory alterations in the feet and hands; these side effects are usually reversible after completion of chemotherapy, but they may take months to resolve.
13. Help patient and family to plan strategies to combat fatigue.
14. Use precautions developed by the healthcare agencies to protect healthcare personnel who handle chemotherapeutic agents.

Bone marrow transplantation

1. Before BMT, perform nutritional assessments and extensive physical examinations, and ensure that organ function tests as well as psychological evaluations, are completed as ordered.
2. Ensure that patient's social support system and financial, and insurance resources are evaluated.
3. Reinforce information for informed consent.
4. Provide patient teaching about the procedure and pretransplantation and post-transplantation care.
5. During the treatment phase, closely monitor for signs of acute toxicities (e.g. nausea, diarrhea, mucositis and hemorrhagic cystitis) and give constant attention to patient.
6. During the bone marrow infusions or stem cell reinfusions, monitor vital signs, and blood oxygen saturation, assess for adverse effects (e.g. fever, chills, shortness of breath, chest pain, cutaneous reactions, nausea, vomiting, hypotension or hypertension, tachycardia, anxiety and taste changes), provide ongoing support and patient teaching.
7. Because of the high risk for dying from sepsis and bleeding, support patient with blood products and hematopoietic growth factors and protect from infection.
8. Assess for early graft-versus-host disease (GVHD) effects on the skin, liver and encephalopathy). Monitor for pulmonary complications, such as pulmonary edema, and interstitial and other pneumonias, which often complicate recovery after BMT.
9. Provide for ongoing nursing assessment in follow-up visits to detect late effects (100 day or later) after BMT, such as infections (e.g. varicella zoster), restrictive pulmonary abnormalities and recurrent pneumonias as well as chronic GVHD involving skin, liver, intestine, esophagus, eye, lungs, joints and vaginal mucosa. Cataracts may develop after total body irradiation.
10. Provide ongoing psychological patient assessment, including the stressors affecting patients at each phase of the transplantation experience.
11. Assess and address the psychosocial needs of marrow donors and family members. Educate and support donor and family members to reduce anxiety and promote coping. Assist family members to maintain realistic expectations of themselves as well as of the patients.

Hyperthermia

1. Explain the patient and family about the procedure, its goals and its effect.
2. Assess the patient for adverse effects, and make efforts to reduce their occurrence and severity.
3. Provide local skin care at the site of the implanted hyperthermic probes.

Biological response modifiers

1. Assess the need for education and guidance for both patient and family (often the same needs as patients having other treatment approaches, but BRMs may be perceived as a last-chance effort by patients who have no responded to standard treatments).
2. Monitor therapeutic and adverse effects (e.g. fever, myalgia, nausea and vomiting, as seen with interferon therapy) and life-threatening side effects (e.g. capillary leak syndrome pulmonary edema and hypotension).
3. Teaches self-care and assist in providing for continuing care.
4. Teach patients and families, as needed, how to administer BRM agents through subcutaneous injections.
5. Provides instructions about side effects, and help the patient and family to identify strategies to manage many of the common side effects of BRM therapy (e.g. fatigue, anorexia and flu-like symptoms).
6. Arrange for home care nurses to monitor patient's responses to treatment, and provide teaching and continued care.

8

Chapter Respiratory Nursing

DEVIATED SEPTUM

The septum dividing the nasal passages is slightly deviated in most adults. This may result from nasal trauma, but often has no cause. Some septa may be so deviated that they lock sinus drainage or interfere with breathing.

Clinical Manifestations

The client may report any of these:
- A chronically stuffy
- Discomfort from blocked sinus drainage
- Headaches and nosebleed.

Therapeutic Measures

1. Symptomatic treatment with decongestant, antihistamines or intranasal corticosteroid sprays to reduce inflammation.
2. When it causes deviated septum (DS) chronic discomfort nasoseptoplasty or submucous resection needed, i.e. making incision through the mucous membrane.
3. Covering the septum and reviving or removing the deviated portion.

Nursing Management

1. Administer decongestants and antihistamines sprays as prescribed.
2. After nasoseptoplasty, nurse has to:
   - Monitor vital signs and bleeding up to patient unstable
   - Check for blood running down back of throat (excessing swallowing)
   - Teach the patient should maintain semi-Fowler's position to avoid anything that might increase pressure and cause bleeding, i.e. sneezing, coughing or straining to move bowels
   - Administer stool softeners and cough depressant, if ordered
   - Avoid Aspirin and such medications to avoid increase risk of bleeding
   - Administer antibiotics or anticoagulants, if instructed.
3. Advice patient with precautions:
   - Change the mustache dressing as often needs
   - Donor blow nose and sneeze with mouth open
   - Drink plenty of fluid unless any special instruction by doctor
   - Use cool mist vaporizer to humidify air and prevent nose drying
   - Keep the patient head elevated on a two pillow or sleep in recliner
   - Take medication as prescribed
   - Report any high fever.

EPISTAXIS (NOSEBLEED)

Epistaxis is hemorrhage from the nose caused by the rupture of tiny, distended vessels in the mucous membrane of any area of the nasal passage. The anterior septum is the most common site. Risk factors include infections, low humidity and nasal inhalation of illicit drugs, trauma (including vigorous nose blowing and nose picking), arteriosclerosis, hypertension, nasal tumors, thrombocytopenia, Aspirin use, liver disease and hemorrhagic syndromes.

Medical Management/Therapeutic Measures

A nasal speculum, penlight or headlight may be used to identify the site of bleeding in the nasal cavity. The patient sits upright with the head tilted forward to prevent swallowing and aspiration of blood, and is directed to pinch the soft outer portion of the nose against the midline septum for 5 or 10 minutes continuously. Alternatively, a attempt is made by using cotton tampon to stop the bleeding. Suction may be used to remove excess blood and clots from the field of inspection. Application of anesthetics and nasal decongestants (phenylephrine, one or two sprays), which act as vasoconstrictors may be necessary. Visible bleeding cannot to identified, the nose may be packed with gauze impregnated with petroleum jelly or antibiotic ointment. The packing may remain in place for 48 hours or up to 5 or 6 days, if necessary to control bleeding. Antibiotics may be prescribed to prevent and manage infection.

Nursing Management

1. Monitor vital signs, airway and breathing, and assist in control of bleeding.
2. Provide tissues and an emesis basin for expectoration of blood.
3. Reassure patient in a calm and efficient manner that bleeding can be controlled.
4. Once bleeding is controlled, instruct the patient to avoid vigorous exercise for several days and to avoid hot or spicy foods and tobacco.
5. Teach the patient to provide self-care by reviewing ways to prevent epistaxis, avoid forceful nose blowing, straining, high altitudes and nasal trauma (including nose picking).
6. Provide adequate humidification to prevent drying of nasal passages.
7. Instruct patient how to apply pressure to nose with thumb and index finger for 15 minutes, if nosebleed recurs.
8. Instruct the patient to seek medical attention, if recurrent bleeding cannot be stopped.

INFLUENZA

Influenza is an acute viral disease that causes worldwide epidemics every 2–3 years with a highly variable degree of severity. The virus is easily spread from host to host through droplet exposure. Previous infection with influenza does not guarantee protection from future exposure. Mortality is probably attributable to accompanying pneumonia (viral or superimposed bacterial pneumonia) and other chronic cardiopulmonary sequelae. Transmission is most likely to occur in the first 3 days of illness.

Management

Goals of medical and nursing management include relieving symptoms, treating complications and preventing transmission (refer 'Nursing and Medical Management' under 'Pharyngitis' and 'Pneumonia' for additional information).

Prevention

Annual influenza vaccinations are recommended for those at high risk for complications of influenza. These include people older than 50 years, children 6–59 months of age, pregnant women, residents of extended care facilities and those with chronic medical diseases or disabilities. In addition, healthcare providers and household members of those in high-risk groups should receive the vaccine to reduce the risk of transmission to people vulnerable to influenza sequelae.

RHINITIS (COMMON COLD)

Rhinitis is inflammation of the nasal mucous membrane, the release of histamine and other substances cause vasodilation and edema. It may occur in reaction to allergens like pollen dust, molds or some foods. It may be caused by bacteria or viruses.

Clinical Manifestations

- Nasal congestion
- Localized itching
- Sneezing, sore throat
- Nasal discharge
- Viral rhinitis may accompanied by fever and malaise
- Sometimes difficult to differentiate.

Diagnostic Methods

- Skin test to determine offending allergens
- Blood test for immunoglobulin E (IgE) antibodies.

Therapeutic Measures

- Antihistamines to carotid allergen
- Desensitization (allergy shorts)
- Symptomatic treatment for viral rhinitis
- Antibiotic are not effective in viral type
- Acetaminophen can be used for generalized discomfort
- Decongestants cause vasoconstriction, which reduces swelling and congestion, but may increase blood pressure, so use with caution
- Cough syrups and cold medicine may be used into caution.

Nursing Management

- Administer prescribed drugs by monitor adverse effect
- Teach the patient that rest and fluids are the most effective treatment.

SINUSITIS

Sinusitis is inflammation of the mucosa of one or more sinuses, the maxillary and ethmoid sinuses are most commonly affected. Inflammation is often the result of bacterial infection and may follow viral illness. The common infectious organisms are *Streptococcus pneumonia* and *Haemophilus influenzae*. Sinusitis may be cause by allergies, nasal polyps, fungal infection or intubations.

Clinical Manifestations

- Pain over the region of the affected sinus
- Purulent nasal discharge
- Fever may be present in acute infection with or without generalized fatigue and foul breathe
- If not treated properly, risk for complications such as infection may spread to surrounding areas causing osteomyelitis, cellulitis of the orbit and abscess or meningitis.

Diagnostic Measures

- Uncomplicated sinusitis diagnosed on the basis of symptoms
- If episodes are repeated then X-ray, nasal endoscopy, computed tomography (CT) and magnetic resonance image (MRI) needed.

Therapeutic Measures

- Treatment aims at relieving pain and promoting sinus drainage
- Nasal irrigation with normal saline for chronic sinusitis
- Corticosteroid via nasal spray as ordered to reduce inflammation
- Adrenergic nasal spray for constricted blood vessels and reduce swelling
- Sprays may be used for up to 3 days, longer use may rebound congestion
- Acetaminophen or ibuprofen may be used for pain and fever
- Expectorant or antihistamine may be used, if instructed.

Nursing Management

- Uncomplicated ones can be taken care at their home
- Instruct the patient to increase water intake of 8–10 glass per day
- Patient with cardiovascular or kidney disease, intake to be restricted accordingly
- Pressure may be relieved by semi-Fowler's position
- Explain the use of hot moist packs, analgesics and prescribed medication
- Instruct the patient not to take antibiotics as prescribed duration, even if symptom relieve.

ACUTE PHARYNGITIS

Acute pharyngitis commonly referred to as a 'sore throat,' is sudden painful inflammation of the pharynx caused mostly by viral infections with bacterial infections accounting for the remainder of cases. When group A streptococci cause acute pharyngitis, the condition is known as strep throat. The inflammatory response results in pain, fever, vasodilation edema and tissue damage, which is manifested by redness and swelling in the tonsillar pillars, uvula and soft palate.

Uncomplicated viral infections usually subside within 3–10 days. Pharyngitis caused by more virulent bacteria is more severe illness because of dangerous complications (e.g. sinusitis, otitis, media, peritonsillar abscess, mastoiditis and cervical adenitis). In rare cases, the infection may lead to bacteremia, pneumonia, meningitis, rheumatic fever and nephritis.

Clinical Manifestations

- Fiery red pharyngeal membrane and tonsils
- Lymphoid follicles swollen and freckled with white-purple exudates
- Cervical lymph nodes enlarged and tender
- Fever, malaise and sore throat
- Hoarseness.

Diagnostic Tests

- Swab specimens obtained from posterior pharynx and tonsils (tongue not included)
- Rapid strept test (RST) used with professional clinical evaluation
- Backup culture of negative RST.

Medical Management/Therapeutic Measures

Viral pharyngitis is treated with supportive measures, whereas antibiotic agents are used to treat pharyngitis caused by bacteria; penicillin (5 day) for group A streptococci, cephalosporins and macrolides (from 3 to 10 day) for patients with penicillin allergies is erythromycin resistance. In addition, liquid or soft diet is recommended during the acute stage. In severe instances, intravenous (IV) fluids are administered if the patient cannot swallow. If the patient can swallow, he\she is encouraged to drink at least 2–3 liter of fluid daily.

Analgesic medications [e.g. Aspirin or acetaminophen (Tylenol)] can be given at 4–6 hours intervals, if required acetaminophen with codeine can be taken three or four times daily.

Nursing Management

- Encourage bedrest during febrile stage of illness; instruct frequent rest periods once patient is up and about
- Instruct patient about secretion precautions (e.g. disposing of used tissue properly) to prevent spread of infection
- Examine skin once or twice daily for possible rash because acute pharyngitis may precede some other communicable disease (e.g. rubella)
- Administer warm saline gargles or irrigations [40.6°C–43.3°C (105°F–110°F)] to ease pain, and also instruct patient regarding purpose and technique for warm gargles (as warm as patient can tolerate) to promote maximum effectiveness
- Apply an ice collar for symptomatic relief
- Perform mouth care to prevent fissures of lips and inflammation in the mouth
- Permit gradual resumption of activity
- Advise patient about the importance of taking the full course of antibiotic therapy

- Inform patient and family to watch for symptoms that may indicate development of complications including nephritis and rheumatic fever.

CHRONIC PHARYNGITIS

Chronic pharyngitis is common in adults who work or live in dusty surroundings, use their voice to excess, suffer from chronic cough, and habitually use alcohol and tobacco. Three types are recognized such as hypertrophic, a general thickening and congestion of the pharyngeal mucous membranes; atrophic, a late stage of type; 1 and chronic granular marked by numerous swollen lymph follicles of the pharyngeal wall.

Clinical Manifestations

- Constant sense of irritation or fullness in the throat
- Mucus that collects in the throat and is expelled by coughing
- Difficulty in swallowing.

Medical Management

Treatment is based on symptom relief, avoidance of exposure to irritants and correction of any upper respiratory, pulmonary or cardiac condition that might be responsible for chronic cough. Nasal sprays or medications containing ephedrine sulfate or phenylephrine hydrochloride are used to relieve nasal congestion. Aspirin (for patients older than 20 year) or acetaminophen may be recommended to control inflammation and relieve discomfort. Tonsillectomy may be an effective option, if consideration is given to morbidity and complications relating to the surgery.

Nursing Management

1. Advise patient to avoid contact with others until fever has subsided completely to prevent infection from spreading.
2. Instruct patient to avoid alcohol, tobacco, secondhand smoke, exposure to cold, and environmental and occupational pollutants. Suggest wearing a disposable mask for protection.
3. Encourage patient to drink plenty of fluids and encourage gargling with warm salt water to relieve throat discomfort. Using lozenges may help to keep the throat moist.

TONSILITIS/ADENOIDITIS

The tonsils are masses of lymph tissue that lie on each side of the oropharynx. They filter microorganisms to prevent the lungs from infections. The adenoids and mass of lymphoid tissue located at the back of the nasopharynx. Infection of these occurs when filtering function becomes overwhelmed with a virus or bacteria. Tonsillitis in viral, but bacteria that is commonly associated with it include *Staphylococcus aureus, H. influenza* and pneumococcus species. It is common in children than adults.

Clinical Manifestations

- Onset with sore throat, fever, chills and pain or swelling
- General symptoms—headache, malaise and myalgia

- Tonsils appear red and swollen, and may have yellow or white exudates
- Patient voice like hot potato in his/her mouth
- Adenoids involves—snoring, nasal obstruction and nasal tone.

Diagnostic Tests

- Throat culture to determine causative organisms
- White blood cell (WBC) count
- Chest X-ray (if respiratory symptom positive).

Therapeutic Measures

- Antibodies for bacterial infection
- Acetaminophen, lozenges and saline gargle for comfort
- Tonsillitis becomes chronic—tonsillectomy/adenoidectomy.

Nursing Management

- Nursing care plan for patient with upper respiratory tract infections (URTS)
- Care of patient undergoing tonsillectomy
- Patient should maintain semi-Fowler's position to reduce swelling and drainage
- Monitor the patient for bleeding and airway potency
- Provide comfort measures
- Encourage fluids for hydration
- Cold fluids may help reduce pain and bleeding
- Red-colored drinks should be avoided
- Room humidified to prevent drying
- Keep suction equipment for emergencies.

LARYNGITIS

Laryngitis is an inflammation of the mucous membrane lining the larynx. It can be caused by irritation from smoking, alcohol, chemical exposure, gastroesophageal reflux disease (GERD) or a viral, fungal or bacterial infection. It often follows upper respiratory infection.

Clinical Manifestations

- Hoarseness (most common)
- Cough, dysphagia and fever may be present.

Therapeutic Measures

- Rest, fluids, humidified air
- Aspirin in adults or acetaminophen
- Antibiotics (if bacterial infection)
- Medication to control acid reflux 'GERD'
- Encourage patient to avoid speaking (to rest voice)
- Obtain paper and pen for communication
- Use throat lozenges, which help to increase comfort.

Nursing Management

- Help the patient to identify and avoid causative factors
- Use nursing care plan with URTI.

CANCER OF LARYNX

Cancer of larynx accounts for approximately 50% of all the head and neck cancers. Almost all malignant tumors of the larynx arise from the surface epithelium and are classified as squamous cell carcinoma. Risk factors include male gender, age 60–70 years, tobacco use (including smokeless), alcohol use, vocal straining, chronic laryngitis, occupational exposure to carcinogens, nutritional deficiencies (riboflavin) and family predisposition.

Clinical Manifestations

- Hoarseness, noted early with cancer in glottic area; harsh, raspy and low-pitched voice
- Persistent cough, pain and burning in the throat when drinking hot liquids and citrus juices
- Lump felt in the neck
- Late symptoms—dysphagia, dyspnea, unilateral nasal obstruction or discharge, persistent hoarseness or ulceration and foul breath
- Enlarged cervical nodes, weight loss, general debility and pain radiating to the ear may occur with metastasis.

Diagnostic Methods

- Physical examination of the head and neck
- Indirect laryngoscopy
- Endoscopy, virtual endoscopy, optical imaging, CT, MRI, and position emission tomography (PET) scanning (to detect recurrence of tumor after treatment)
- Direct laryngoscopic examination under local or general anesthesia
- Biopsy of suspicious tissue.

Medical Management/Therapeutic Measures

1. The goals of treatment of laryngeal cancer include care, preservation of safe effective swallowing and useful voice, and avoidance of permanent tracheostomy.
2. Treatment options include surgery, radiation therapy and chemotherapy or combinations.
3. Before treatment begins, a complete dental examination is performed to rule out oral disease. Dental problems should be resolved before surgery and after radiotherapy.
4. Radiation therapy provides excellent results in early-stage glottic tumors, when only one cord is affected and mobile and may be used preoperatively to reduce tumor size combined with surgery in advanced laryngeal cancer (stages 3 and 4) or as a palliative measure.
5. Surgical procedures for early-stage tumors may include transoral endoscopic laser resection, classic open vertical hemilaryngectomy for glottic tumors or classic horizontal supraglottic laryngectomy.
6. Other surgical option includes the following:
   a. Vocal cord stripping—used to treat dysplasia, hyperkeratosis and leukoplakia, and is often curative for these lesions.
   b. Cordectomy—for lesions limited to the middle third of the vocal cord.
   c. Laser surgery for treatment of early glottic cancers.

d. Partial laryngectomy is recommended in early stages of glottic cancer with only one vocal cord involved high cure rate.
e. Total laryngectomy can provide the desire cure in most advanced stage four laryngeal cancers, when the tumor extends beyond the vocal cords or for cancer that recurs or persists after radiation therapy.
f. Speech therapy when indicated; esophageal speech, artificial larynx (electrolarynx) or tracheoesophageal puncture.

Nursing Management

Nursing Assessment

1. Obtain a health history and assesses the patient's physical psychosocial and spiritual domains.
2. Assess for hoarseness, sore throat, dyspnea, dysphagia or pain and burning in the throat.
3. Perform a thorough head and neck examination; palpate the neck and thyroid for swelling, nodularity or adenopathy.
4. Assess patient's ability to hear, see, read and write; evaluation by speech therapist, if indicated.
5. Determine nature of surgery, assess patient psychological status, evaluate patient's and family's coping methods preoperatively and postoperatively and give effective support.

Nursing Diagnoses/Problems

Based on all the assessment data, major nursing diagnoses may include the following:

1. Deficient knowledge about the surgical procedure and postoperative course.
2. Anxiety and depression related to the diagnosis of cancer and impending surgery.
3. Ineffective airway clearance related to excess mucus production secondary to surgical.
4. Alternations in the airway.
5. Impaired verbal communication related to anatomic deficit secondary to removal of larynx and to edema.
6. Imbalanced nutrition less than body requirements related to inability to ingest food secondary to swallowing difficulties.
7. Disturbed body image and low self-esteem secondary to major neck surgery change in appearance and altered structure and function.
8. Self-care deficit related to pain, weakness and fatigue; musculoskeletal impairment related to surgical procedure and postoperative course.

Based on assessment data, potential complications that may develop include the following:

- Respiratory distress (hypoxia, airway obstruction and tracheal edema)
- Hemorrhage, infection and wound breakdown
- Aspiration
- Tracheostomal stenosis.

Planning and Goals/Objectives

Major goals for the patient may include knowledge about treatment, reduced anxiety, maintenance of a patent airway, effective use of alternative means of communication, optimal levels of nutrition and hydration, improvement in body image and self-esteem, improved self-care management and absence of complications. The objectives include the following:

- Demonstrate an adequate level of knowledge, verbalizing an understanding of the surgical procedure and performing self-care adequately
- Demonstrate less anxiety and depression
- Maintains clear airway and handles own secretions
- Demonstrates practical, safe and correct technique for cleaning, and changing the tracheostomy or laryngectomy tube
- Acquires effective communication techniques
- Maintains adequate nutrition and fluid intake
- Exhibits improved body image, self-esteem and self-concept
- Exhibits no complications
- Adheres to rehabilitation and home care program.

Nursing Interventions

Preoperative Teaching

1. Clarify any misconceptions and for provide educational materials about surgery patient and family (written and audiovisual) for review and reinforcement.
2. Explain to patient that natural voice will be lost if complete laryngectomy is planned.
3. Assure patient that much can be done through training in a rehabilitation program.
4. Review equipment and treatments that will be a part of postoperative care.
5. Teach coughing and deep breathing exercise; provide for return demonstration.

Reducing Anxiety and Depression

1. Assess patient's psychological preparation; give patient and family opportunity to verbalize feelings; and share perceptions. Give patient and family complete and concise answers to questions.
2. Arrange a visit from a postlaryngectomy patient; help patient cope with situation; and know that rehabilitation is possible.
3. Surgical site, purulent drainage, odor and increase in wound drainage.
4. Observe stoma area for wound breakdown, hematoma and bleeding, and report significant changes to the surgeon.
5. Monitor patient carefully, particularly for carotid hemorrhage.
6. Monitor for possible reflux and aspiration, keep suction equipment available.
7. Perform tracheostomy care routinely.
8. Postoperatively be alert for the possible serious complications of rupture of the carotid artery, if this occur, apply direct pressure over the artery, summon assistance and provide psychological support until the vessel can be ligated.

Promoting Family- and Community-based Care

Teaching patient self-care

1. Provide discharge instructions as soon as patient is able to participate and assess readiness to learn.

2. Assess knowledge about self-care management; reassure patient and family that strategies can be mastered.
3. Give specific information about tracheostomy and stomal care, wound care, and oral hygiene including suctioning and emergency measures. Instruct the patient about the need for adequate dietary intake, safe hygiene and recreational activities.
4. Instruct patient to provide adequate humidification of the environment, minimize air conditioning and drink fluids.
5. Teach patient to take precautions when showering to prevent vent water from getting into the stoma.
6. Discourage swimming because the patient with laryngectomy can drown.
7. Recommend that patient avoid getting hairspray, loose hair and powder into stoma.
8. Teach the patient and caregiver about the signs and symptoms of infection; identify indications that require contacting the physician after discharge.
9. Stress that activity should be undertaken in moderation; when tired, the patient has more difficulty speaking with low voice.
10. Instruct patient to wear or carry medical identification such as bracelet or card to alert medical personnel to the special requirements for resuscitation when the need arise.

Continuing care

1. Refer to home care agency for patient and family assistance, follow-up assessment and teaching.
2. Encourage patient to visit physician regularly for physical examinations and advice.
3. Remind the patient to participate in health promotion activities and health screening.

Evaluation

Evaluation will be on the basis of expected patient outcomes/ objectivities as mentioned in planning:

- Demonstrate an adequate level of knowledge, verbalizing an understanding of the surgical procedure and performing self-care adequately
- Demonstrate less anxiety and depression
- Maintains clear airway and handles own secretions
- Demonstrates practical, safe and correct technique for cleaning and changing the tracheostomy or laryngectomy tube
- Acquires effective communication techniques
- Maintains adequate nutrition and fluid intake
- Exhibits improved body image, self-esteem and self-concept
- Exhibits no complications
- Adheres to rehabilitation and home care program.

PNEUMONIA

Pneumonia is an inflammation of the lung parenchyma caused by various microorganisms including bacteria, mycobacteria, fungi and viruses. Pneumonias are classified as community-acquired pneumonia (CAP), hospital-acquired (nosocomial) pneumonia (HAP), pneumonia in the immunocompromised host and aspiration pneumonia. There is overlap in how specific pneumonias are classified because they may occur in different settings. Those at risk for pneumonia often have chronic underlying disorders, severe acute illness, a suppressed immune system from disease or medication, immobility and other factors that interfere with normal lung protective mechanisms. The elderly are also at high risk.

Pathophysiology

An inflammatory reaction can occur in the alveoli, producing an exudate that interferes with diffusion of oxygen and carbon dioxide; bronchospasm may also occur if the patient has reactive airway disease. Bronchopneumonia, the most common form, is distributed in a patchy fashion extending from the bronchi to surrounding lung parenchyma. Lobar pneumonia is the term used if a substantial part of one or more lobes is involved. Pneumonia is caused by a variety of microbial agents in the various settings. Common organisms include *Pseudomonas aeruginosa* and *Klebsiella* species, *Staphylococcus aureus, H. influenza, Streptococcus pneumoniae;* and enteric gram-negative bacilli, fungi and viruses (most common in children).

Clinical Manifestations

Clinical features vary depending on the causative organism and the patient's disease:

1. Sudden chills and rapidly rising fever [38.5°C–40.5°C (101°F–105°F)].
2. Pleuritic chest pain aggravated by respiration and coughing.
3. Severely ill patient has marked tachypnea (25–45 breaths per minute) and dyspnea; orthopnea when not propped up.
4. Pulse rapid and bounding, may increase 10 beats per minute per degree of temperature elevation (Celsius).
5. A relative bradycardia for the amount of fever suggests viral infection, mycoplasma infection or infection with a *Legionella* organism.
6. Other signs are upper respiratory tract infection, headache, low-grade fever, pleuritic pain, myalgia, rash and pharyngitis; after a few days, mucoid or mucopurulent sputum is expectorated.
7. Severe pneumonia: Flushed cheeks, lips and nail beds demonstrating central cyanosis.
8. Sputum purulent, rusty, blood tinged, viscous or green depending on etiological agent.
9. Appetite is poor and the patient is diaphoretic.

Signs and symptoms of pneumonia may also depend on a patient's underlying condition (e.g. different signs occur in patients with condition such as cancer and in those who are undergoing treatment with immunosuppressant, which decrease the resistance to infection).

Diagnostic Methods

- Primary history, physical examination
- Chest X-rays, blood and sputum cultures, Gram stain.

Pneumonia in elderly patient may occur as a primary stenosis or as a complication of a chronic disease. Pulmonary infections in older people frequently difficult to treat result in a higher mortality rate than in younger people. Early deterioration, weakness, abdominal symptoms, anorexia confusion, tachycardia and tachypnea may signal the onset of pneumonia. The diagnosis of pneumonia may be mild, because the classic symptoms of cough, chest pain, sputum production and fever may be absent or masked in elderly patients. Also, the presence of some signs may be misleading. For example, abnormal breath sounds may cause microatelectasis that occurs as a result of decreased mobility, decreased lung volumes or other respiratory function change. Chest X-rays may be needed to differentiate chronic heart failure (HF) and pneumonia as the cause of clinical signs and symptoms.

Supportive treatment includes hydration (caution with frequent assessment because of the risk of fluid in the elderly), supplemental oxygen therapy, and assistance with deep breathing, coughing, frequent position changes and early ambulation. To reduce or prevent serious complication of pneumonia in the elderly, vaccination against pneumococcal and influenza infections is recommended.

Medical Management/Therapeutic Measures

1. Antibiotics are prescribed on the basis of Gram stain result and antibiotic guidelines (resistance patterns risk factor etiology must be considered). Combination therapy may also be used.
2. Supportive treatment includes hydration, antipyretics, antitussive medications, antihistamines or nasal decongestant.
3. Bedrest is recommended until infection shows signs clearing.
4. Oxygen therapy is given for hypoxemia.
5. Respiratory support includes high-inspired oxygen concentrations, endotracheal intubation and mechanical ventilation.
6. Treatment of atelectasis, pleural effusion, shock, respiratory failure or superinfection is instituted, if needed.
7. For groups at high risk for CAP, pneumococcal vaccination is advised.

Nursing Management

Nursing Assessment

1. Assess for fever, chills, night sweats, pleuritic type pain, fatigue, tachypnea, use of accessory muscles for breathing, bradycardia or relative bradycardia, coughing and purulent sputum.
2. Monitor the patient for the following; changes in temperature and pulse; amount, odor and color of secretions; frequency and severity of cough; degree of tachypnea or shortness of breath; changes in physical assessment findings (primarily assessed by inspecting and auscultation the chest); and changes in the chest X-ray findings.
3. Assess the elderly patient for unusual behavior, altered mental status, dehydration, excessive fatigue and concomitant HF.

Nursing Diagnoses

- Ineffective airway clearance related to copious tracheobronchial secretions
- Activity intolerance related to impaired respiratory function
- Risk for deficient fluid volume related to fever and a rapid respiratory rate
- Imbalanced nutrition, less than body requirements
- Deficient knowledge about treatment regimen and preventive health measures

- Continuing symptoms after initiation of therapy
- Shock
- Respiratory failure
- Atelectasis
- Pleural effusion
- Confusion.

Planning and Goals/Objectives

The major goals of the patient may include improved airway patency, rest to conserve energy, maintenance of proper fluid volume, maintenance of adequate nutrition, an understanding of treatment protocol, preventive measures and absence of complications.

Nursing Interventions

Improving Airway Patency

- Encourage hydration and fluid intake (2–3 L/day) to loosen secretions
- Provide humidified air using high-humidity face mask
- Encourage patient to cough effectively and provide correct positioning, chest physiotherapy, and incentive spirometry
- Provide nasotracheal suctioning, if necessary
- Provide appropriate method of oxygen therapy
- Monitor effectiveness of oxygen therapy.

Promoting Rest and Conserving Energy

1. Encourage the debilitated patient to rest, avoid overexertion and possible exacerbation of symptoms.
2. Patient should assume a comfortable position to promote rest and breathing (e.g. semi-Fowler's position), and should change positions frequently to enhance secretion clearance, pulmonary ventilation and perfusion.
3. Instruct outpatients not to overexert themselves and to engage in only moderate activity during the initial phases of treatment.

Promoting Fluid Intake and Maintaining Nutrition

- Encourage fluids (2 L/day minimum with electrolytes and calories)
- Administer IV fluids and nutrients, if necessary.

Promoting Patient's Knowledge

1. Instruct on cause of pneumonia, management of symptoms, signs and symptoms that should be reported to the physician or nurse, and the need for follow-up.
2. Explain treatments in simpler manner and using appropriate language; provide written instructions and information, and alternative formats of patients with hearing or vision loss.
3. Repeat instructions and exploration as needed.

Monitoring and Preventing Potential Complications

1. Monitoring for continuing symptoms of pneumonia (patients usually begin to respond to treatment within 24–48 hours after antibiotic therapy is initiated).

2. Assess for signs and symptoms of shock, multisystem organ failure and respiratory failure (e.g. evaluate vital signs, pulse oximetry and hemodynamic monitoring parameters).
3. Assess for atelectasis and pleural effusion.
4. Assist with thoracentesis and monitor for patient for pneumothorax after procedure.
5. Assess for confusion or cognitive changes; assess underlying factors.

Promoting Family- and Community-based Care

Teaching patients about self-care

1. Instruct patient to continue taking full course of antibiotics as prescribed. Teach the patient about their proper administration and potential side effects.
2. Instruct patient about symptoms that require contacting the healthcare provider; difficulty breathing, worsening cough, recurrent/increasing fever and medication intolerance.
3. Advise patient that fatigue and weakness may linger.
4. Encourage breathing exercise to promote lung expansion and clearing.

Continuing care

1. Encourage follow-up chest X-rays.
2. Encourage patient to stop smoking.
3. Instruct patient to avoid stress, fatigue, sudden changes in temperature and excessive alcohol intake, all of which lower resistance to pneumonia.
4. Review principles of adequate nutrition and rest.
5. Recommended influenza vaccine (Pneumovax) to all patients at risk.
6. Refer patient for home care to facilitate adherence to therapeutic regimen as indicated.

PULMONARY TUBERCULOSIS

Tuberculosis (TB), an infectious disease primarily affecting the lung parenchyma, is most often caused by *Mycobacterium tuberculosis*. It may spread to almost any part of the body including the meninges, kidney, bones and lymph nodes. The initial infection usually occurs 2–10 weeks after exposure. The patient may then develop active disease because of comprised or inadequate immune system response. The active process may be prolonged and characterized by long remissions when the disease is arrested, only to be followed by period of renewed activity. Tuberculosis is a worldwide public health problem that is closely associated with poverty, malnutrition, overcrowding, substandard housing and inadequate health care. Mortality and morbidity rates continue to rise.

Tuberculosis is transmitted when a person with active pulmonary disease expels the organisms. A susceptible person inhales the droplets and becomes infected. Bacteria are transmitted to the alveoli and multiply. An inflammatory reaction results in exudate in the alveoli and bronchopneumonia, granulomas and fibrous tissue. Onset is usually insidious.

Risk Factors

- Close contact with someone who has active TB
- Immunocompromised status [e.g. elderly, cancer, corticosteroid therapy and human immunodeficiency virus (HIV)]

- Injection drug use and alcoholism
- People lacking adequate health care (e.g. homeless or impoverished, minorities, children and young adults)
- Pre-existing medical conditions including diabetes, chronic renal failure, silicosis and malnourishment
- Immigrants from countries with a high incidence of TB (e.g. Haiti, Southeast Asia)
- Institutionalization (e.g. long-term care facilities, prisons)
- Living in overcrowded, substandard housing
- Occupation (e.g. healthcare workers, particularly those performing high-risk activities).

Clinical Manifestations

- Low-grade fever, cough, night sweats, fatigue and weight loss
- Non-productive cough, which may progress to mucopurulent sputum with hemoptysis.

Diagnostic Methods

- The TB skin test (Mantoux test), QuantiFERON-TB Gold (QFT-G) test
- Chest X-ray
- Acid-fast bacillus smear
- Sputum culture.

Elderly patients may have atypical manifestations such as unusual behavior or disturbed mental status, fever, anorexia and weight loss. TB is increasingly encountered in the nursing home population. In many elderly people, the TB skin test produces no reaction.

Medical Management/Therapeutic Measures

Pulmonary TB is treated primarily with antituberculosis agents for 6–12 months. Prolonged treatment duration is necessary to ensure eradication of the organisms and to prevent relapse.

Pharmacologic Therapy

1. First-line medications: Isoniazid or INH (Nydrazid), rifampin (Rifadin), pyrazinamide and ethambutol (Myambutol) daily for 8 weeks and continuing for up to 4–7 months.
2. Second-line medications: Capreomycin (Capastat), ethionamide (Trecator), para-aminosalicylate sodium and cycloserine (Seromycin).
3. Vitamin B (pyridoxine) usually administered with INH.

Nursing Management

Promoting Airway Clearance

- Encourage increased fluid intake
- Instruct about best position to facilitate drainage.

Advocating Adherence to Treatment Regimen

1. Explain that TB is a communicable disease and that taking medications is the most effective way of preventing transmission.

2. Instruct about medications, schedule and side effects; monitor for side effects of anti-TB medications.
3. Instruct about risk of drug resistance if the medications regimen is not strictly and continuously followed.
4. Carefully monitor vital signs and observe for spikes in temperature or changes in the patient's clinical status.
5. Teach caregivers of patients who are not hospitalized, so monitor the patient's temperature and respiratory status; report any changes in the patient's respiratory status to the primary healthcare provider.

Promoting Activity and Adequate Nutrition

1. Plan a progressive activity schedule with the patient or increase activity tolerance and muscle strength.
2. Devise a complementary plan to encourage adequate nutrition. A nutritional regimen of small, frequent meals and nutritional supplements may be helpful in meeting daily caloric requirements.
3. Identify facilities (e.g. shelters, soup kitchen and meal on wheels) that provide meals in the patient's neighborhood and increase the likelihood that the patient with limited resource and energy will have access to more nutritious intake.

Preventing Spreading of Tuberculosis Infection

1. Carefully instruct the patient about important hygiene measures including mouth care, covering the mouth and nose when coughing and sneezing, proper disposal of tissue and handwashing.
2. Report any cases of TB to the health department to other parts of the body (spread or dissemination of TB infection to non-pulmonary sites of the body in known as military TB).
3. Carefully monitor patient for military TB: Monitor vital signs and observe for spikes in temperature as well as changes in renal and cognitive functions, few physical signs may be elicited on physical examination of the chest, but at this stage, the patient has a severe cough and dyspnea. Treatment of military TB is the same as for pulmonary TB.

BRONCHIECTASIS

Bronchiectasis is a chronic, irreversible dilation of the bronchi and bronchioles, and is considered a disease process separate from chronic obstructive pulmonary disease (COPD). The result is retention of secretions, obstructions and eventual alveolar collapse. Bronchiectasis may be caused by a variety of conditions including airway obstruction, diffuse airway injury, pulmonary infection and obstruction of the bronchus or complications of long-term pulmonary infections, genetic disorders (e.g. cystic fibrosis), abnormal host defense (e.g. ciliary dyskinesia or humoral immunodeficiency) and idiopathic causes. Bronchiectasis is usually localized, affecting a segment or lobe of a lung most frequently the lower lobes. People may be predisposed to bronchiectasis as a result of recurrent respiratory infection in early childhood, measles and influenza, tuberculosis or immunodeficiency disorders.

Clinical Manifestations

- Chronic cough and production of copious purulent sputum
- Hemoptysis, clubbing of the fingers and repeated episodes of pulmonary infection.

Diagnostic Findings

- Definite diagnostic clue is prolonged history of productive cough with sputum consistently negative for tubercle bacilli
- Diagnosis is established on the basis of CT scan.

Medical Management/Therapeutic Measures

- Treatment objectives are to promote bronchial drainage to clear excessive secretions from the affected portion of the lung and to prevent or control infection
- Chest physiotherapy with percussion, postural drainage, expectorants or bronchoscopy to remove bronchial secretions
- Antimicrobial therapy guided by sputum sensitivity studies
- Year-round regimen of antibiotics and alternating types of drugs at required intervals
- Vaccination against influenza and pneumococcal pneumonia
- Bronchodilators
- Smoking cessation
- Surgical intervention (segmental resection of lobe or lung removal), used infrequently
- During preparation for surgery employ vigorous postural drainage, suction through bronchoscope and antibacterial therapy.

Nursing Management

Please refer Nursing Management of COPD.

CHRONIC BRONCHITIS

Chronic bronchitis is a disease of the airways, is defined as the presence of cough and sputum production for at least 3 months in each of two consecutive years. Although chronic bronchitis is clinically and epidemiologically useful, it does not reflect the major impact of airflow limitation in morbidity and mortality in COPD. In many cases, smoke or other environmental pollutants irritate the airways resulting in inflammation and hypersecretion of mucus. Constant irritation causes the mucus secretion of glands and goblet cells to increase in number, leading to increase mucus production. Mucus plugging of the airways reduce ciliary function. Bronchial walls also become thickened further narrowing the bronchial lumen. Alveoli adjustment in altered function of the alveolar macrophage, this is significant because the macrophages play an important role in destroying foreign particles including bacteria. As a result, the patient becomes more susceptible to respiratory infection. A wide range of viral, bacterial and mycoplasmal infections can produce acute episodes bronchitis. Exacerbations of chronic bronchitis are most likely to occur during the winter when viral and bacterial infections are more prevalent (refer Nursing Management of COPD).

EMPYEMA

Empyema is a collection of thick, purulent (infected) fluid in the pleural space. At first, the pleural fluid is thin with a low-leukocyte count, but it frequently progresses to a fibropurulent stage and then to a stage at which it encloses the lung with a thick exudative membrane (loculated empyema).

Clinical Manifestations

1. Patient is acutely ill with signs and symptoms similar to those of an acute respiratory infection or pneumonia (fever, night sweats, pleural pain, cough, dyspnea, anorexia and weight loss).
2. Symptoms may be vague, if the patient is immunocompromised; symptoms may be less obvious, if patient has received antimicrobial therapy.

Assessment and Diagnostic Methods

1. Chest auscultation, which demonstrates decreased or absent breath sounds over the affected area, dullness on chest percussion, decreased fremitus.
2. Chest CT and thoracentesis (under ultrasound guidance).

Medical Management/Therapeutic Measures

The objectives of treatment are to drain pleural cavity and to achieve complete expansion of the lung. The fluid is drained and appropriate antibiotics, in large dose are prescribed on the basis of the causative organism. Drainage of the pleural fluid depends on the stage of the disease and accomplished by one of the following methods:

1. Needle aspiration (thoracentesis), if volume is good and fluid is not too thick.
2. Tube thoracostomy with fibrinolytic agents instilled through chest tube and when indicated.
3. Open chest drainage via thoracotomy to remove thickened pleura, pus and debris and to remove the underlying diseased pulmonary tissue.
4. Decortication and surgical removal, if inflammation has been long standings.
5. Provide care specific to method of drainage of pleural and fluid.
6. Help patient cope with condition, instruct in lung expansions breathing exercises to restore normal respiratory function.
7. Instruct patient and family about care of drainage system and drain site and measurement and observation of drainage.
8. Teach patient and family, signs and symptoms of infection, and how and when to contact healthcare provider.

LUNG ABSCESS

Lung abscess is necrosis of the pulmonary parenchyma caused by microbial infection; the lesion collapses and forms a cavity. It is generally caused by aspiration of anaerobic bacteria. Most lung abscess is a complication of bacterial pneumonia or is caused by aspiration of oral anaerobes into the lung. Abscesses also may occur secondary to mechanical or functional obstruction of the bronchi. At risk patients include with impaired cough reflexes, loss of glottal closures or swallowing difficulties, which may cause aspiration of foreign material. Other at risk patient include those with central nervous system disorders (e.g. seizure, stroke, drug addiction, alcoholism, esophageal disease or comprised immune function); patients without teeth and those receiving nasogastric tube feedings; and patients with an altered state of consciousness due to anesthesia. The site of lung abscess is related to gravity and is determined by the patient's position. For patients in a recumbent position, the posterior segment of upper lobe and the superior segment of the lower lobe are the most common areas. The organisms frequently associated with lung abscesses are *S. aureus, Klebsiella pneumoniae* and other gram-negative species.

Clinical Manifestations

1. The clinical features vary from a mild productive cough to acute illness.
2. Fever is accompanied by a productive cough of moderate to copious amounts of foul-smelling sputum, often bloody.
3. Leukocytosis may be present.
4. Pleurisy or dull chest pain, dyspnea, weakness, anorexia and weight loss are common.
5. Chest dullness on percussion and decreased or absent breath sounds are found with an intermittent pleural friction rub and possibly crackles on auscultation.

Diagnostic Methods

Chest radiography, sputum culture and fiberoptic bronchoscopy are performed, and CT of the chest may be required.

Medical Management/Therapeutic Measures

1. To reduce the risk for lung abscesses, give appropriate antibiotic therapy before dental procedures and maintain adequate dental and oral hygiene. Give appropriate antimicrobial therapy for pneumonia.
2. Findings of the history, physical examination, chest X-ray and sputum culture indicate type of organism and treatment.
3. Coughing, postural drainage (chest physiotherapy) and possibly percutaneous catheter placement or infrequently bronchoscopy for abscess drainage is used.
4. The patient is advised to eat high-protein and high-calorie diet.
5. Surgical intervention is rare. Pulmonary resection (lobectomy) is performed when there is massive hemoptysis or no response to medical management.

Pharmacological Therapy

1. The IV antimicrobial therapy: Clindamycin (Cleocin) is the medication of choice. Large IV doses are required because the antibiotic must penetrate necrotic tissue and abscess fluid.
2. Antibiotics are administered orally instead of intravenously after signs of improvement [normal temperature, lowered WBC count and improvement on chest X-ray (reduction in size of cavity)]. Antibiotic therapy may last 4–8 weeks.
3. Administer antibiotic and IV therapy as prescribed and monitor for any adverse effects.

Nursing Management

1. Initiate chest physiotherapy as prescribed to drain abscess.
2. Teach patient deep breathing and coughing exercises.
3. Encourage diet high in protein and calories.
4. Provide emotional support; abscess may take a long time to resolve.
5. Teach patient or caregiver how to change the dressings to prevent skin excoriation and odor, how to monitor for signs and symptoms of infection and how to care for and maintain the drain or tube.
6. Remind patient to perform deep breathing and coughing exercises every 2 hours during the day.
7. Teach postural counseling for attaining and maintaining an optimal state of nutrition.
8. Emphasize importance of completing antibiotic regimen, rest and appropriate activity levels to prevent relapse.
9. Arrange home health nursing and visits by an IV therapy nurse to administer IV antibiotic therapy.

CHEST TRAUMA

The term pneumothorax literally means air in the chest and is used to describe conditions in which air has entered the pleural space outside the lungs. Common types are:

1. Pneumothorax occurs without an associate injury is called 'spontaneous pneumothorax': This mostly occurs in tall, thin persons and in smokers. There is risk for recurrence patient with underlying lung disease (empysema) may have blister; like defects in lungs (blebs), than can rupture.
2. In traumatic pneumothorax, penetrating trauma to the chest wall and parietal pleura allows air to enter the pleural space. This can occur as a result of knife or gunshot wounds or from protruding broken ribs.
3. In open pneumothorax, air can enter and escape through the opening in the pleural space.
4. In closed pneumothorax, air collects in the space and is unable to escape.
5. In tension pneumothorax, if a pneumothorax is closed, air and tension, increases, pressure is applied in the heart and great vessels, pushing away from the affected side of the chest. This is called mediastinal shift, when the heart and vessels are compress. Venous return to the heart is impaired resulting in reduced cardiac output and symptoms of shock.
6. Hemothorax refers to the presence of blood in the pleural space, this can occur with or without pneumothorax and often the result of traumatic injury. Other causes are lung cancer, pulmonary embolism and anticoagulant use.

Clinical Manifestations

- Sudden dyspnea, chest pain, tachypnea, tachycardia, restlessness and anxiety
- Asymmetric chest expansion on inspiration (on edema)
- Breath sounds are absent or diminished on affected side
- In a sucking chest, wound air can be heard
- In tension pneumothorax:

- Patient becomes hypoxemia and hypotensive
- Heart sounds may be muffed
- Brachycardia and shock occurs.

Diagnostic Measures

- History, physical examinations
- Chest X-ray, CT scan
- Bedside ultrasound, if available
- Monitoring arterial blood gas (ABG) and oxygen saturation.

Therapeutic Measures/Medical Management

- Rest or high-flow oxygen for small pneumothorax or trapped air can be removed with small needlenose inserts into pleural space
- Chest tubes connected to water-seal drainage system to remove up large amount of air or blood
- For a recurrent pneumothorax, pleurodesis needed
- Pleurodesis is painful. Prepare patient with analgesic prior to procedure.

Nursing Management

- Close monitoring of the condition
- Frequent and through assessment, which includes:
  - Level of conciousness, skin and mucous membrane color
  - Vital signs, oxygen saturation, respiratory rate and depth
  - Presence of dyspnea, chest pain, restlessness and anxiety, and care of patient with chest tube and water drainage system (refer Management of Pneumothorax and Hemothorax).

RIB FRACTURE

Chest trauma is often accompanied by fractured ribs.

Clinical Manifestations

- Uncontrolled coughing
- Cause of broken ribs usually falls in older patients
- Broken ribs are very painful
- May result in atelectasis or pneumonia
- Displaced ribs lead to damage of abdominal organs or lung tissue, causing pneumothorax.

Therapeutic Measures

- Pain control: Non-steroidal anti-inflammatory drug (NSAID) or opioids, or intercostal nerve block
- Keeping patient in comfortable position allows coughing and deep breathing, which can prevent complications.

FLAIL CHEST

Flail chest is a condition of the chest wall caused by two or more fractures on each affected rib, resulting in a segment of rib that is not attached on either end's the flail portion moves paradoxically in with inspiration and out with expiration.

Clinical Manifestations

- Paradoxical respiration: As a result of affected part of the chest collapse with the negative pressure of inspiration and bulges with expiration
- Paradoxical respiration may be ineffective in ventilating the lungs and result in hypoxia
- Patient exhibits chest movements that is opposite to usual seen with respiration
- Patient in dyspnea, anxious, tachypenia or tachycardia.

Therapeutic Measures

- Supplemental oxygen and analgesics
- Intubation and mechanical ventilation may be needed (but to be avoided for risk of infection)
- If lung damage, treatment of pneumothorax
- Surgical stabilization of the ribs, if required.

PNEUMOTHORAX AND HEMOTHORAX

Pneumothorax occurs when the parietal or visceral pleura are breached and the pleural space is exposed to positive atmospheric pressure. Normally, the pressure in the pleural space is negative or subatmospheric; the negative pressure is required to maintain lung inflation. When pleura are breached, air enters the pleural space and the lung or a portion of it collapses. Hemothorax is the collection of the blood in the chest cavity because of torn intercostal vessels or laceration of the lungs injured through trauma. Often both blood and air are found in the chest cavity (hemopneumothorax).

Types of Pneumothorax

Simple Pneumothorax

A simple or spontaneous, pneumothorax occurs when air enters the pleura space through a breach of either the parietal or visceral pleural. Most commonly this occurs as air enters the pleural space through the rupture of a bleb or a bronchopleural fistula. A spontaneous pneumothorax may occur in an apparently healthy person in the absence of trauma due to rupture of air-filled bleb or blister, on the surface of the lung, allowing air from the airways to enter the pleural cavity. It may be associated with diffuse interstitial lung disease and severe emphysema.

Traumatic Pneumothorax

A traumatic pneumothorax occurs, when air escapes from a laceration in the lung itself and enters the pleural space or from a wound in the chest wall. It may result from blunt trauma (e.g. rib fractures), penetrating chest or abdominal trauma (e.g. stab wounds or gunshot wounds), or diaphragmatic tears. Traumatic pneumothorax may occur during invasive thoracic procedures (i.e. thoracocentesis, transbronchial lung biopsy, insertion of a subclavian line) in which the pleural is inadvertently punctured or with barotraumas from mechanical ventilation. A traumatic pneumothorax resulting from major injury to the chest is often is accompanied by hemothorax. Open pneumothorax is one form of traumatic pneumothorax. It occurs when a wound in the chest wall is large enough to allow air to pass freely in and out of the thoracic cavity with each attempted respiration.

Traumatic open pneumothorax calls for emergency interventions. Stopping the flow of air through the opening in the chest wall is a life saving measure.

Tension Pneumothorax

A tension pneumothorax occurs when air is drawn into the pleural space and is trapped with each breath. Tension builds up in the pleural space, causing lung collapse. Mediastinal shift (shift of the heart and great vessels and trachea towards the unaffected side of the chest) is a life-threatening medical emergency. Both respiratory and circulatory functions are compromised.

Clinical Manifestations

Signs and symptoms associated with pneumothorax depend on its size and cause:

1. Pleuritic pain of chest onset.
2. Minimal respiratory distress with small pneumothorax; acute respiratory distress, if large.
3. Anxiety, dyspnea, air hunger, use of accessory muscles and central cyanosis (with severe hypoxemia).
4. In simple pneumothorax, the trachea is midline, expansion of the chest is decreased, breath sounds may be diminished and percussion of the chest may reveal normal sounds or hyper-resonance depending on the size of the pneumothorax.
5. In a tension pneumothorax, the trachea is shifted away from the affected side, chest expansion may be decreased or fixed in a hyperexpansion state, breath sounds are diminished or absent and percussion to the affected side is hyper-resonant. The clinical picture is one of air hunger, agitation, increasing hypoxemia, central cyanosis, hypotension, tachycardia and profuse diaphoresis.

Medical Management/Therapeutic Measures

The goal is evacuation of air or blood from the pleural space:

1. A small chest tube is inserted near the second intercostal space for a pneumothorax.
2. A large diameter chest tube is inserted, usually in the fourth or fifth intercostal space for hemothorax.
3. Autotransfusion has begun, if excessive bleeding from chest tube occurs.
4. Traumatic open pneumothorax is plugged (petroleum gauze); patient is asked to inhale and strain against a closed glottis to eject air from the thorax until the chest tube is inserted, with water-seal drainage.
5. Antibiotics are usually prescribed to combat infection from contamination.
6. The chest wall is opened surgically (thoracotomy) if more than 1,500 mL of blood is aspirated initially by thoracentesis (or is the initial chest tube output) or if chest tube output continues at greater than 200 mL/h. Urgency is determined by the degree of respiratory compromise.
7. An emergency thoracotomy may also be performed in the emergency department, if a cardiovascular injury secondary to chest or penetrating trauma is suspected.

8. The patient with a possible tension pneumothorax should immediately be given a high concentration of supplemental oxygen to treat the hypoxemia and pulse oximetry should be used to monitor oxygen saturation.
9. In an emergency situation, a tension pneumothorax can be decompressed or quickly converted to a simple pneumothorax by inserting a large-bore needle (14 gauge) at the second intercostal space, midclavicular line on the affected side. A chest tube is then inserted and connected to suction to remove the remaining air and fluid, re-establish the negative pressure, and re-expand the lung.

Nursing Management

1. Promote early detection through assessment and identification of high-risk population; report symptoms.
2. Assist chest tube insertion; maintain chest drainage or water seal.
3. Monitor respiratory status and re-expansion of lung, with interventions (pulmonary support) performed in collaboration with other healthcare professionals (e.g. physician, respiratory therapist and physical therapist).
4. Provide information and emotional support to patient and family.

PLEURISY

Pleurisy refers to inflammation of both the visceral and parietal pleurae. When inflamed, pleural membranes rub together, the result is severe, sharp, knife-like pain with breathing, i.e. intensified on inspiration. Pleurisy may develop in conjunction with pneumonia or an URTI, tuberculosis, or collagen disease; after trauma to the chest, pulmonary infarction, or pulmonary embolism (PE) in patients with primary or metastatic cancer and after thoracotomy.

Clinical Manifestations

1. Pain is usually occurs on the side and worsens with deep breaths, coughing and sneezing.
2. Pain is decreased when the breath is held. Pain is localized or radiates to the shoulder or abdomen.
3. As pleural fluid develops, pain lessens. A friction rub can be auscultated, but disappears as fluid accumulates.

Diagnostic Measures

- Auscultation for pleural friction rubs
- Chest X-rays
- Sputum culture
- Thoracentesis for pleural fluid examination, pleural biopsy (less common).

Management/Therapeutic Measures

1. Objectives of management are to discover the underlying condition causing pleurisy and to relieve pain.
2. Patient is monitored for signs and symptoms of pleural effusion; shortness of breath, pain assumption of a position that decreases pain, and decreased chest wall excursion.

3. Prescribed analgesics, such as NSAIDs, are given to relieve pain and allow effective coughing.
4. Applications of heat or cold are provided for symptomatic relief.
5. An intercostal nerve block is done for severe pain.

Nursing Management

1. Enhance comfort by turning patient frequently on affected side to splint chest wall.
2. Teach patient to use hands or pillow to splint rib care while coughing.

PLEURAL EFFUSION

Pleural effusion, a collection of fluid in the pleural space, is usually secondary to other diseases (e.g. pneumonia, pulmonary infections, nephritic syndrome, connective tissue decrease neoplastic tumors and congestive heart failure). The effusion can be relatively clear fluid (a transudate or an exudate), or it can be blood or pus. Pleural fluid accumulates due to an imbalance in hydrostatic or oncotic pressures (transudate), or as a result of inflammation by bacterial products or tumors (excudated).

Clinical Manifestations

Some symptoms are caused by the underlying disease. Pneumonia causes fever, chills and pleuritic chest pain. Malignant effusion may result in dyspnea and coughing. The size of the effusion, the speed of its formation and the underlying long disease determine the severity of symptoms:

1. Large effusion; shortness of breath to acute respiratory distress.
2. Small to moderate effusion; dyspnea may not be present.
3. Dullness or flatness to percussion over areas of fluid, minimal or absence of breath sounds, decreased fremitus and tracheal deviation away from the affected side.

Diagnostic Measures

- Physical examination
- Chest X-rays (lateral decubitus)
- Chest computed tomography scan
- Thoracentesis
- Pleural fluid analysis (culture, chemistry and cytology)
- Pleural biopsy.

Management/Therapeutic Measures

Objectives of treatment are to discover the underlying cause to prevent reaccumulation of fluid; and to relieve discomfort, dyspnea and respiratory compromise. Specific treatment is directed at the underlying cause:

1. Thoracentesis is performed to remove fluid, collect specimen for analysis and relieve dyspnea.
2. Chest tube and water-seal drainage may be necessary for drainage and lung re-expansion.
3. Chemical pleurodesis: Adhesion formation is promoted when drugs are instilled into the pleural space to obliterate the space and prevent further accumulation of fluid.

4. Other treatment modalities include surgical pleurectomy (insertion of a small catheter attached to a drainage bottle) or implantation of a pleuroperitoneal shunt.

Nursing Management

1. Implement medical regimen; prepare and position patient for thoracentesis and offer support throughout the procedure.
2. Monitor chest tube drainage and water-seal drainage and water-seal system; record amount of drainage at prescribed intervals.
3. Administer nursing care related to the underlying cause of the pleural effusion.
4. Assist patient in pain relief. Assist patient to assume positions that are painful. Administer pain medication as prescribed and needed to continue frequent turning and ambulation.
5. If the patient is to be managed as an outpatient with a pleural catheter for drainage, educate the patient and family about management and care of the catheter and drainage system.

PULMONARY EMBOLISM

Pulmonary embolism refers to the obstruction of the pulmonary artery or one of its branches by a thrombus (or thrombi) that originate somewhere in the venous system or in the right side of the heart. Gas exchange is impaired in the lung mass supplied by the obstructed vessel. Massive PE is a life-threatening emergency, death commonly occurs within 1 hour after the onset of the symptoms. It is a common disorder associated with trauma, surgery (orthopedic, major abdominal, pelvic and gynecologic), pregnancy, HF, age group more than 50 years, hypercoagulable stress and prolonged immobility. It also may occur in apparently healthy people. Most thrombi originate in the deep veins of the legs.

Clinical Manifestations

1. Symptoms depend on the size of the thrombus and the area of the pulmonary artery occlusion.
2. Dyspnea is the most common symptom. Tachypnea is the most frequent sign.
3. Chest pain is common, usually sudden in onset and pleuritic in nature; it can be substernal and may mimic angina pectoris or a myocardial infarction.
4. Anxiety, fever, tachycardia, apprehension, cough, diaphoresis, hemoptysis, syncope, shock and sudden death may occur.
5. Clinical picture may mimic that of bronchopneumonia or HF.
6. In atypical instances, PE causes few signs and symptoms, whereas in other instances it mimics various other cardiopulmonary disorders.
7. Because the symptoms of PE can vary from few to severe, a diagnostic workup is performed to rule out other diseases.
8. The initial diagnostic workup may include chest X-ray, electrodiography (ECG), ABG analysis and ventilation-perfusion scan.
9. Pulmonary angiography is considered the best method to diagnose PF; however, it may not be feasible, cost-effective or easily performed, especially with critical ill patients.
10. Spiral CT of the lung, D-dimer assay (blood test for evidence of blood clots) and pulmonary arteriogram may be warranted.

Medical Management/Therapeutic Measures

1. Ambulation of leg exercise in patients on bedrest.
2. Applications of sequential compression devices.
3. Anticoagulant therapy for patients whose hemostasis is adequate and who are undergoing major elective abdominal or thoracic surgery.

Pharmacological Measures

1. Immediate objective is to stabilize the cardiopulmonary system.
2. Nasal oxygen is administered immediately to relieve hypoxemia, respiratory distress and central cyanosis.
3. The IV infusion lines are inserted to establish routes for medications or fluids that will be needed.
4. A perfusion scan, hemodynamic measurements, and ABG determinations are performed. Spiral (helical) CT or pulmonary angiography maybe performed.
5. Hypotension is treated by a slow infusion of dobutamine (Dobutrex), which has a dilating effect on the pulmonary vessels and bronchi or dopamine (Intropin).
6. The ECG is monitored continuously for dysrhythmia and right ventricular failure, which may occur suddenly.
7. Digitalis glycosides, IV diuretics and antiarrhythmic agents are administered when appropriate.
8. Blood is drawn for serum electrolytes, complete blood cell count and hematocrit.
9. If clinical assessment and ABG analysis indicate the need, the patient is intubated and placed on a mechanical ventilator.
10. If the patient has suffered massive embolism and is hypotensive, an indwelling urinary catheter is inserted to monitor urinary output.
11. Small doses of IV morphine or sedatives are administered to relieve patient anxiety, to alleviate chest discomfort to improve tolerance of the endotracheal tube and to ease adaptation to the mechanical ventilator.
12. Anticoagulant therapy (heparin, warfarin sodium) has traditionally been the primary method for managing acute deep venous thrombosis (DVT) and PE (numerous specific options for treatment are available.
13. Patients must continue to take some form of anticoagulation for at least 3–6 months after embolic event.
14. Major side effects are bleeding anywhere in the body and anaphylactic reaction resulting in shock or death. Other side effects include fever, abnormal liver function and allergic skin reaction.
15. Thrombolytic therapy may include urokinase, streptokinase and alteplase. It is reserved for PE affecting a significant area and causing hemodynamic instability.
16. Bleeding is significant side effect; non-essential invasive procedures are avoided.
17. A surgical embolectomy is rarely performed, but may be indicated if the patient has a massive PE or hemodynamic instability, or if there are contraindications to thrombolytic therapy.
18. Transvenous catheter embolectomy with or without insertion of an inferior vena caval filter (e.g. Greenfield).

Nursing Management

The nurse must have a high degree of suspicious for PE in all patients, but particularly in those with conditions, predisposing to a slowing of venous return by taking following measures.

Preventing Thrombus Formation

- Encourage early ambulation, active and passive leg exercises
- Instruct patient to move legs in a 'pumping' exercise
- Advise patient to avoid prolonged sitting, immobility and constructive clothing
- Do not permit dangling of legs and feet in a dependent position
- Instruct patient to place feet on the floor or chair and to avoid crossing legs
- Do not leave IV catheters in veins for prolonged periods.

Monitoring Anticoagulant and Thrombolytic Therapy

- Advise bedrest, monitor vital signs every 2 hours and limit invasive procedures
- Measure international normalized ratio (INR) or activated partial thromboplastin time (PTT) every 3–4 hours after thrombolytic infusion is started to confirm activation of fibrinolytic systems
- Perform only essential ABG studies on upper extremities, with manual compression of puncture site for atleast 30 minutes.

Minimizing Chest Pain Pleuritic

- Place patient in semi-Fowler's position; turn and reposition frequently
- Administer analgesics as prescribed for severe pain.

Managing Oxygen Therapy

- Assess the patient frequently for signs of hypoxemia and monitors the pulse oximetry values
- Assist patient with deep breathing and incentive spirometer
- Nebulizer therapy or percussion and postural drainage may be necessary for management of secretions.

Alleviating Anxiety

- Encourage patient to express feelings and concerns
- Answer questions concisely and accurately
- Explain therapy and describe how to recognize untoward effects early.

Monitoring Complications

Be alert for potential complications of cardiogenic shock or right ventricular failure subsequent to the effect of PE on the cardiovascular system.

Providing Postoperative Care

- Measure pulmonary arterial pressure and urinary output
- Assess insertion site of arterial catheter for hematoma formation and infection

- Maintain blood pressure to ensure perfusion of vital organs
- Encourage isometric exercises, antiembolism stockings and walking when permitted out of bed; elevate foot of bed when patient is resting
- Discourage sitting/Hip flexion compresses large veins in the legs.

Promoting Family-based Care

1. Before discharge and at follow-up clinic or home visits, teach patient how to prevent recurrence and which signs and symptoms should alert patient to seek medical attention.
2. Teach patient to look for bruising and bleeding when taking anticoagulants, and to avoid bumping into objects.
3. Advise patient to use a toothbrush with soft bristles to prevent gingival bleeding.
4. Instruct patient not to take aspirin (an anticoagulant) or and histamine drugs while taking warfarin sodium (Coumadin).
5. Advise patient to check with physician before taking any medication, including over-the-counter (OTC) drugs.
6. Advise patient to continue wearing antiembolism stockings as long as directed.
7. Instruct patient to avoid laxatives, which effect vitamin K absorption (vitamin K promotes coagulation).
8. Teach patient to avoid sitting legs crossed for prolonged periods.
9. Recommend that patient change position regularly when traveling, walking occasionally and do active exercises of legs and ankles.
10. Advise patient to take plenty of liquids.
11. Teach patient to report dark, tarry stools immediately.
12. Recommend that patient wear identification stating that he/she is taking anticoagulants.

PULMONARY HYPERTENSION

Pulmonary hypertension occurs when the arteries that carry deoxygenated blood from the heart to the lungs become narrowed as a result of changes in the lining and smooth muscle of the vessels. The result is elevated pressure in the pulmonary arteries causing right ventricles to work harder to push blood into them, which leads to failure of right ventricle (cor pulmonales).

Secondary pulmonary hypertension occurs as a result of other disorders like coronary artery disease or mitral valve disease both which increase pressure in left side of the heart. Liver diseases, systemic lupus erythematosus (SLE) and scleroderma associated with pulmonary hypotension and not also caused by appetite suppressants (fen-phen) and dexfenfluramine.

Clinical Manifestations

- Dyspnea, weakness and syncope
- If heart failure—peripheral edema and distended jugular veins
- Angina may result from right ventricular ischemia.

Diagnostic Measures

- Arterial blood gas show hypoxemia and hypocapnia
- Cardiac catheterization will determine high pulmonary pressures

- Electrocardiography may show right ventricle hypotrophy
- Chest X-ray, spirometry, lung scan, pulmonary angiogram in secondary pulmonary hypertension.

Therapeutic Measures

- No treatment available except lung or heart-lung transplant
- In secondary pulmonary hypertension, supportive care needed, which includes:
  - Low-sodium diet and diuretics to reduce blood volume
  - Oxygen administration
  - Cardiac monitoring
  - Use of vasodilators (calcium-channel blockers)
  - Warfarin to prevent clotting.

Nursing Management

- Administer prescribed medication
- Provide Fowler's position or high-Fowler's position to relieve dyspnea and discomfort
- Bedrest and comfort measures to treat fatigue and anxiety.

PULMONARY ARTERIAL HYPERTENSION

Pulmonary arterial hypertension is a condition that is not clinically evident until late in the disease. Pulmonary arterial hypertension exists when the mean pulmonary artery pressure exceeds 25 mm Hg with a pulmonary capillary wedge pressure of less than 15 mm Hg. There are two forms: Idiopathic (or primary) pulmonary artery hypertension and pulmonary arterial hypertension. Pulmonary hypertension is due to a known cause. Primary pulmonary hypotension occurs most often in women aged 20–40 years, either sporadically or in patients with a family history and is usually fatal within 5 years of diagnosis. There are several possible causes, but the exact cause is unknown. The clinical presentation may occur with no evidence of pulmonary or cardiac disease. Secondary pulmonary hypertension is more common and results from existing cardiac or pulmonary disease. The prognosis depends on the severity of the underlying disorder and the changes in the pulmonary vascular bed. A common cause of pulmonary arterial hypertension is pulmonary artery constriction due to hypoxemia from COPD (cor pulmonale). When the pulmonary vascular bed is destroyed or obstructed its ability to handle the blood volume received is impaired. The increase blood flow increases the pulmonary artery pressure, pulmonary vascular resistance and hypertension.

Clinical Manifestations

- Dyspnea, the main symptom is noticed first with exertion and then at rest
- Substernal chest pain is common
- Weakness, fatigability, syncope and occasional hemotype may occur
- Signs of right-sided HF (peripheral edema, ascites, distended neck veins, liver engorgement, crackles and heart murmur) as noted
- Anorexia and abdominal pain may also occur in the right upper quadrant

- Partial pressure of oxygen (PaO_2) is decreased (hypoxemia)
- In ECG changes (right ventricular hypertrophy) are seen, with right axis deviation and tall peaked P waves in inferior leads and tall anterior R waves and ST segment depression of T-wave inversion anteriorly.

Diagnostic Methods

Complete diagnostic evaluation includes a history, physical examination, chest X-ray, pulmonary function studies, ECG, echocardiogram, ventilation-perfusion scan, sleep studies, autoantibody tests (to identify diseases of collagen vascular origin), HIV tests, liver functioning tests and cardiac catheterization.

Management/Therapeutic Measures

The goal of treatment is to manage the underlying condition related to pulmonary hypertension of known cause:

1. Most patients with pulmonary hypertension do not have hypoxemia at rest, but require supplemental oxygen with exercise.
2. Anticoagulation should be considered for patients with pulmonary hypertension and patients with an indwelling catheter for administration of medications.
3. Different classes of medications are used to treat pulmonary hypertension. These include calcium-channel blockers, phosphodiesterase 5 inhibitors [e.g. sildenafil (Revatio, Viagra)], endothelin antagonists [e.g. bosentan (Tracleer)], and prostanoids [e.g. epoprostenol (Flolan), treprostinil (Remodulin) and iloprost (Ventavis)]. The choice of therapeutic agents is based on the severity of the disease.
4. A small number of patients with pulmonary hypertension respond favorably to acute vasodilation and do well with a calcium-channel blocking agent.
5. Lung transplantation remains an option for all eligible patients who shows severe disease and symptoms after 3 months of receiving epoprostenol; atrial septostomy may be considered for selected patients.

Nursing Management

- Be alert for signs and symptoms
- Administer prescribed oxygen therapy appropriately
- Inform and instruct patient and family about home oxygen supplementation
- Identify patients at high risk for developing pulmonary hypertension, i.e. those with COPD, pulmonary emboli, congenital heart disease and mitral valve disease.

PULMONARY EMPHYSEMA

In emphysema, impaired oxygen and carbon dioxide exchange results from destruction of the walls of overdistended alveoli. Emphysema is a pathological term that describes detention of the air spaces beyond the terminal and destruction of the walls of the alveoli. This is the end of process that progresses slowly for many years. The wall of the alveoli are destroyed (process accelerated by infections), the alveolar surface area in direct contact with pulmonary capillaries continually decreases. The increase in dead space (lung area where no gas exchange occur) and impaired oxygen diffusion, which leads to emphysema. In the later stages of disease, carbon dioxide is impaired, resulting in increased carbon dioxide arterial blood (hypercapnia) leading to respiratory acidosis. The alveolar walls continue to breakdown, the pulmonary capillary bed is reduced in size. Consequently, resistance of pulmonary blood flow is increased, forcing the right ventricle to maintain a higher blood pressure in the pulmonary vein. Hypoxemia may further increase pulmonary artery. For this reason, right-sided heart failure (cor pulmonale) of the complications of emphysema, congestion-depended edema, distended neck veins or pain in the region of the suggested development of cardiac failure.

There are two main types of emphysema, based on the changes taking place in the lung. Both types may occur in the same patient. In the panlobular (panacinar) type of emphysema, there is destruction of the respiratory bronchiole, alveolar duct and alveolus. All air spaces within the lobules are essentially enlarged, but there is little inflammatory disease. A hyperinflated (hyperexpanded) chest, marked dyspnea on exertion and weight loss typically occur. To move air in and out of the lungs, negative pressure is required during expansion an adequate level of positive pressure must be and maintained during expiration. Instead of being voluntary passive act, expiration becomes active and muscular effort.

In the centrilobular (centroacinar) form, action take place mainly in the center of the secondary lobular persevering the peripheral portions of the acinus. Frequently, there is a derangement of ventilation-perfusion producing chronic hypoxemia, hypercapnia, polypsis and episodes of right-sided heart failure. This leads to cyanosis and respiratory failure. The patient also develops peripheral edema, which is treated with diuretic therapy.

Nursing Management

Refer 'Nursing Management' under COPD for additional information.

ASTHMA

Asthma is a chronic inflammatory disease of the airways characterized by hyper-responsives, mucosal edema and mucus production. This inflammation ultimately leads to recurrent episodes of asthma symptoms such as cough, chest tightness, wheezing and dyspnea. Patients with asthma may experience symptom-free periods alternating with acute exacerbations that last from minutes to hours or days.

Asthma, the most common chronic disease of childhood, can begin at any age. Risk factors for asthma include family history, allergy (strongest factor) and chronic exposure to airway irritant or allergens (e.g. grass, weed, pollens, mold, dust or animals). Common triggers for asthma symptoms and exacerbations include airway irritants (e.g. pollutants, cold, heat, strong odors, smoke and perfumes), exercise, stress or emotional upset, rhinosinusitis with postnasal drip, medications, viral respiratory tract infections and gastroesophageal reflux.

Clinical Manifestations

1. Most common symptoms of asthma are cough (with or without mucus production), dyspnea and wheezing (first on expiration, then possibly during inspiration as well).
2. Asthma attacks frequently occur at night or in the early morning.
3. An asthma exacerbation is frequently preceded by increasing symptoms over days, but it may begin abruptly.
4. Chest tightness and dyspnea occur.
5. Expiration requires effort and becomes prolonged.
6. As exacerbation progresses, central cyanosis secondary severe hypoxia may occur.
7. Additional symptoms, such as diaphoresis, tachycardia and a widened pulse pressure, may occur.
8. Exercise-induced asthma included maximum symptoms during exercise, absence of nocturnal symptoms and sometimes only a description of a 'choking' sensation during exercise.
9. In severe, continuous reaction and status asthmaticus may occur. It is life-threatening.
10. Edema, rashes and temporary edema are allergic reactions that may be noted with asthma.

Diagnose Methods

Present environment and occupational history is essential. During acute episodes, sputum and blood test, pulse oximetry, ABGs hypocapnia and respiratory alkalosis, and pulmonary function [forced expiratory volume (FEV) and forced vital capacity (FVC) decreased] tests are performed.

Therapeutic Measures/Management

The two classes of medications include long-acting and quick-relief medications, as well as there are combination products:

- Short acting beta 2-adrenergic agonists
- Anticholinergic
- Corticosteroids: Metered dose inhaler (MDI)
- Leukotrene: Modifier inhibitors
- Methylxanthines.

Nursing Management

1. The immediate nursing care of patients with asthma depends on the severity of symptoms. The patient and family are often frightened and anxious because of patient's dyspnea. A calm approach is an important aspect of care.
2. Assess the patient's respiratory status by monitoring the severity of symptoms, breath sounds, peak flow, pulse oximetry and vital signs.
3. Observe a history of allergic reactions to medications before administering medications.
4. Identify medications the patient is currently taking.
5. Diagnose medications as prescribed and monitor the patient responses to those medications; medications may include an antibiotic, if the patient has an underlying respiratory infection.
6. Administer fluids if the patient is dehydrated.
7. Assist with intubation procedure, if required.

Promoting Family- and Community-based Care

Teaching patient about self-care

1. Teach patient and family about asthma (chronic inflammatory) purpose and action of medications, triggers to avoid and how to do so, and proper inhalation technique.
2. Instruct patient and family about peak-flow monitoring.
3. Teach patient how to implement an action plan and how and when to seek assistance.
4. Obtain current educational materials for the patients based on the patient's diagnosis, causative factors, education level and cultural background.

Continuing care

1. Emphasize adherence to prescribed therapy, preventive measures and need for follow-up appointments.
2. Refer for home health nurse as indicated.
3. Home visit to assess for allergens may be indicated (with recurrent exacerbations).
4. Refer patient to community support groups.
5. Remind patients and families about the importance of health promotion strategies and recommended health screening.

STATUS ASTHMATICUS

Status asthmaticus is severe and persistent asthma that does not respond to conventional therapy; attacks can occur with little or no warning and can progress rapidly to asphyxiation. Infection anxiety, nebulizer abuse, dehydration, increased adrenergic blockage and non-specific irritants may contribute to these episodes. An acute episode may be precipitated by hypersensitivity to Aspirin. Two predominant problems occur; a decrease bronchial diameter and a ventilation-perfusion abnormality.

Clinical Manifestations

- Same as those in severe asthma
- To correlate between severity of attack and number of wheezes; with greater obstruct, wheezing may disappear, possibly signaling impending respiratory failure.

Diagnostic Measures

- Primarily pulmonary function studies and ABG analysis
- Respiratory alkalosis most common finding
- Partial pressure of carbon dioxide ($PaCO_2$) to normal or higher is a danger sign, which signaling respiratory failure.

Medical Management/Therapeutic Measures

1. Initial treatment includes β_2-adrenergic agonists, corticosteroids, supplemental oxygen and IV fluids to hydrate patient. Sedatives are contraindicated.
2. High-flow supplemental oxygen is best delivered using partial or complete non-rebreather mask (PaO_2 at a minimum of 92 mm Hg or O_2 saturation greater than 95%).
3. Magnesium sulfate, a calcium antagonist, may be administered to induce smooth muscle relaxation.

4. Hospitalization, if no response to repeated treatments or if blood gas levels deteriorate, or pulmonary function scores are low.
5. Mechanical ventilation, if patient is tiring or in respiratory failure or if condition does not respond to treatment.

Nursing Management

The main focus of nursing management is to actively assess the airway and the patient's response to treatment. The nurse should be prepared for the next intervention, if the patient does not respond to treatment:

1. Constantly monitor the patient for the first 12–24 hours or until status asthmaticus is under control. Blood pressure and cardiac rhythm should be monitored continuously during the acute phase and until the patient stabilizes and responds to therapy.
2. Assess the patient skin turgor for signs of dehydration; fluid intake is essential to combat dehydration, to loosen secretions and to facilitate expectoration.
3. Administer IV fluids as prescribed, up to 3–4 L/day, unless contraindicated.
4. Encourage the patient to conserve energy.
5. Ensure patient's room is quite and free of respiratory irritants (e.g. flowers, tobacco, smoke, perfumes or odors of cleaning agents); non-allergic pillows should be used.

CHRONIC OBSTRUCTIVE PULMONARY DISEASE

Chronic obstructive pulmonary disease is a disease characterized by airflow limitation that is fully reversible. The airflow limitation is usually progressive and associated with an abnormal inflammatory response of the lung to noxious particles or gases, resulting in narrowing of airways, hypersecretion of mucus, and changes in the pulmonary vasculature. Other disease such as cystic fibrosis, bronchiectasis and asthma that were previously classified as types of COPD are now classified as chronic pulmonary disorders, although symptoms may overlap with those of COPD. Cigarette smoking, air pollution, to occupational exposure and cotton dusts grain are important risk factors that contribute to COPD development, which may occur over a 20–30 year span. Complications of COPD vary, but include respiratory insufficiency and failure (major complications) as well as pneumonia, atelectasis and pneumothorax.

Clinical Manifestations

1. Chronic obstructive pulmonary disease is characterized by chronic cough, sputum production and dyspnea on exertion; often worsen overtime.
2. Weight loss is common.
3. Symptoms are specific to the disease. Refer 'Clinical Manifestations' under 'Asthma,' 'Bronchiectasis,' 'Bronchitis' and 'Emphysema.'
4. It accentuates many of the physiologic changes associated with aging and is manifested in airway obstruction (in bronchitis) and excessive loss of elastic lung recoil (in emphysema). Additional changes in ventilation-perfusion ratios occur.

Management/Therapeutic Measures

1. Smoking cessation, if appropriate.
2. Bronchodilators, corticosteroids and other drugs of α antitrypsin augmentation therapy, antibiotic agents, mucolytic agents, antitussive agents, vasodilators and narcotics. Vaccines may also be effective.
3. Oxygen therapy, including nighttime oxygen.
4. Varied treatment specific to disease. Refer 'Medical Management' under 'Asthma', 'Bronchiectasis,' 'Bronchitis' and 'Emphysema.'
5. Surgery: Bullectomy to reduce dyspnea; lung volume reduction to improve lobar elasticity; and function and lung transplantation.

Nursing Management

Obtain information about current symptoms as well as previous disease manifestations. In addition to the history, nurse review the results of available diagnostic tests.

Airway Clearance

1. Monitor the patient for dyspnea and hypoxemia.
2. If bronchodilators or corticosteroids are prescribed, administer the medications properly and be alert for potential side effects.
3. Confirm relief of bronchospasm by measuring improvement in expiratory flow rates and volumes (the force of expiration, how long it takes to exhale and the amount of air exhaled) as well as by assessing the dyspnea and making sure that it has lessened.
4. Encourage patient to eliminate or reduce all pulmonary irritants, particularly cigarette smoking.
5. Instruct the patient in directed or controlled coughing.
6. Chest physiotherapy with postural drainage, intermittent positive-pressure breathing, increased fluid intake and bland aerosol mists (with normal saline solution or water) may be useful for some patients with COPD.
7. Inspiratory muscle training and breathing retraining may help to improve breathing patterns.
8. Training in diaphragmatic breathing reduces the respiratory rate, increases alveolar ventilation and sometimes helps to expel as much air as possible during expiration.
9. Pursed-lip breathing helps in slow expiration, prevent collapse of small airway, and control the rate and depth of respiration; it also promotes relaxation.

Improving Activity Tolerance

1. Evaluate the patient's activity tolerance and limitations, and use teaching strategies to promote independent activities of daily living.
2. Determine, if patient is a candidate for exercise training to strengthen the muscles of the upper and lower extremities and to improve exercise tolerance and endurance.
3. Recommend use of walking aids, if appropriate to improve activity levels and ambulation.
4. Consult with other healthcare professionals (rehabilitation therapist, occupational therapist and physical therapist), as needed.

Monitoring and Managing Complications

1. Assess patient from complications (respiratory insufficiency and failure, respiratory infection and atelectasis).
2. Monitor pulse oximetry values and administer oxygen as prescribed.
3. Instruct patient and family about signs and symptoms of infection or other complication and to report changes in physical or cognitive status.
4. Encourage patient to be immunized against influenza and *Streptococcus pneumoniae.*
5. Caution patient to avoid going outdoors, if the pollen count is high or if there is significant air pollution and to avoid exposure to high outdoor temperatures with high humidity.
6. If a rapid onset of shortness of breath occurs, quickly evaluate the patient for potential pneumothorax by assessing the symmetry of chest movement, differences in breath sounds and pulse oximetry.
7. Provide instructions about self-management; assess the knowledge of patients and family members about self-care and the therapeutic regimen.
8. Teach patients and family members about early signs and symptoms of infection, and other complications, so that they send appropriate healthcare promptly.
9. Instruct patient to avoid extremes of heat, cold and air pollutants (e.g. fumes, smoke, dust, talcum, lint and aerosol sprays). High altitudes aggravate hypoxemia.
10. Encourage patient to adopt a lifestyle of modern activity ideally in a climate with minimal shifts in temperature and humidity. Patient should avoid emotional disturbances and stressful situations; patient should be encouraged to stop smoking.
11. Review educational information and to demonstrate patient correct metered dose inhaler (MDI) use before discharge, during follow-up visits and during home visits.

Promoting Family-based Care

1. Refer patient for home care is necessary.
2. Direct the patient to community resources (e.g. pulmonary rehabilitation programs and smoking cessation programs); remind the patient and family about the importance of participating in general health promotion activities and health screening.
3. Address quality of life and issues surrounding the end of life in patients with end-stage COPD (e.g. symptom management quality of life, satisfaction with care, information/communication, use of care professionals, use of care facilities, hospital admission and place of death).

CYSTIC FIBROSIS

Cystic fibrosis is a disorder of the exocrine glands that affects primarily the lungs, GI tract and sweat glands. Abnormal sodium and chloride transport across cell membranes, causing these tenacious secretions, is responsible for many of the characteristics symptoms. Thick sticky respiratory secretions those are difficult to remove the causes of airway obstruction, resulting in air trapping and frequent respiratory infections. It is a genetic disorder. First symptoms appear in infancy or childhood.

Clinical Manifestations

1. Respiratory symptoms of chronic sinusitis to production of thick, tenacious sputum.
2. Risk for frequent respiratory infections with cough and purulent sputum.
3. Clubbing of fingers.
4. Hemoptysis (later) due to damaged blood vessels within lungs.
5. Frequent foul smelling stools for lack of enzymes in intestine.
6. Inability to absorb fat-soluble vitamins, poor appetite malnutrition.
7. Bowel obstructions, cirrhosis, cholecystitis and cholelithiasis may occur.
8. Chronicity cause delayed sexual maturity and infertility.
9. Complications: Bronchiectasis, pneumothorax, cor pulmonale and respiratory failure.

Diagnostic Measures

- Genetic testing
- Sweat chloride test
- Chest X-ray, spirometry.

Therapeutic Measures/Nursing Management

- No cure for cystic fibrosis
- Controlling infections and relieving symptoms
- Removal of thick sputum in promoting with hydration use of vibratory positive expiratory pressure (PEP) device
- Chest physiotherapy or high frequency chest wall oscillation
- Regular exercise to mobilize secretions
- Nebulizations.

CANCER OF THE LUNG (BRONCHOGENIC CARCINOMA)

Lung cancers arise from a single transformed epithelial cell in the tracheobronchial airways. A carcinogen (cigarette smoke, radon gas, other occupational and environmental agents) damages the cell, causing abnormal growth and development into a malignant tumor. Most lung cancer are classified into one of two major categories; small cell lung cancer (15%–20% of tumors) and non-small cell lung cancer (NSCLC) approximately 80% of tumors. NSCLC cell types include squamous cell carcinoma (20%–30%), which is usually more centrally located; large cell carcinoma (15%), which is fast growing and tends to arise peripherally and adenocarcinoma (40%), which presents as peripheral masses often metastasizes and includes bronchoalveolar carcinoma. Most small cell cancer arises in the major bronchi and spread by infiltration along the bronchial wall.

Risk factor include tobacco smoke, second-hand (passive) smoke, environmental and occupational exposures, gender, genetics, and dietary deficits. Other factors that have been associated with lung cancer include genetic predisposition and underlying respiratory diseases, such as COPD and TB.

Clinical Manifestations

1. Lung cancer often develops insidiously and is asymptomatic until late in its course.
2. Signs and symptoms depend on location, tumor size, degree of obstruction, and existence of metastases to regional or distant sites.
3. Most common symptoms is cough or change in a chronic cough.
4. Dyspnea may occur early in the disease.
5. Hemoptysis or blood tinged-sputum may be expectorated.
6. Chest pain or shoulder pain may indicate chest wall or pleural involvement. Pain is a late symptom and may be related to bone metastasis.
7. Recurring fever may be an early symptom.
8. Chest pain, tightness, hoarseness, dysphagia, head and neck edema, and symptoms of pleural or pericardial infusion exist if the tumor spreads to adjacent structures and lymph nodes.
9. Common sites of metastases are lymph nodes, bone, brain, contralateral lung, adrenal glands and liver.
10. Weakness, anorexia and weight loss may appear.
11. A cough that changes in character should arouse suspicion of lung cancer.

Diagnostic Measures

1. Chest X-ray, CT, bone scans, abdominal scans, PET scans, liver ultrasound and MRI.
2. Sputum examinations, fiberoptic bronchoscopy, transthoracic fine-needle aspiration, endoscopy with esophageal ultrasound, mediastinoscopy or mediastinotomy and biopsy.
3. Pulmonary function tests, ABG analysis scans and exercise testing.
4. Staging of the tumor refers to the size of the tumor its location, whether lymph nodes are involved and whether the cancer has spread (refer 'Tumor Staging and Grading' under 'Cancer' for additional information).

Therapeutic Measures/Management

Refer 'Medical Management' under 'Cancer' for additional information.

The objective of management is to provide a cure if possible. Treatment depends on cell type, stage of the disease and physiologic status.

Treatment may involve surgery (preferred), radiation therapy or chemotherapy or else a combination of these. Newer and more specific therapies to modulate the immune system (gene therapy, with defined tumor antigens) are under study and show promise.

Nursing Management

Refer 'Nursing management' under 'Cancer' for additional information other than the following.

Managing Symptoms

Instruct patient and family about the side effects of specific treatments and strategies to manage them.

Relieving Breathing Problems

1. Maintain airway patency. Remove secretions through deep breathing exercises, chest physiotherapy, directed cough, suctioning and in some instances bronchoscopy.
2. Administer bronchodilator medications; supplemental oxygen will probably be necessary.
3. Encourage patient to assume positions that promote lung expansion and to perform breathing exercise.
4. Teach energy conservation and airway clearance techniques. Refer to pulmonary rehabilitation as indicated.

Reducing Fatigue

1. Assess level of fatigue; identify potentially treatable causes.
2. Educate patient in energy conservation techniques and guided exercise as appropriate.

Refer to physical or occupational therapist as indicated.

Providing Psychological Support

- Help patient and family deal with poor prognosis and progression of the disease (when indicated)
- Assist patient and family with informed decision-making regarding treatment options
- Suggest methods to maintain the patient quality of life during the course of this disease
- Support patient and family in end-of-life decisions and treatment options
- Help identify potential resources for the patient and family.

ACUTE RESPIRATORY DISTRESS SYNDROME

Acute respiratory distress syndrome (ARDS) is a severe form of acute lung injury characterized by sudden and progressive pulmonary edema, increasing bilateral infiltrates, hypoxemia unresponsive to oxygen supplementation, and the absence of an left atrial pressure. ARDS occurs when inflammatory triggers initiate the release of cellular and chemical mediators, causing injury to the alveolar capillary membrane in addition to other structural damage to the lungs. Factors associated with the development of ARDS include direct injury to the lungs (e.g. smoke inhalation) or indirect insult to the lungs (e.g. shock). ARDS has been associated with a mortality rate ranging from 25% to 58% with the major cause of death in ARDS being non-pulmonary multiple-system organ failure, often with sepsis.

Clinical Manifestations

- Rapid onset of severe dyspnea, usually 12–48 hours after an initiating event
- Intercostal retraction and crackles may be present
- Arterial hypoxemia not responsive to oxygen supplementation
- Lung injury then progresses to fibrosing alveolitis with persistent, severe hypoxemia
- Increased alveolar dead space and decreased pulmonary compliance.

Diagnostic Findings

- Plasma brain natriuretic peptide (BNP) levels
- Echocardiography
- Pulmonary artery catheterization.

Medical Management/Therapeutic Measures

1. Identify and treat the underlying condition, provide aggressive, supportive care (intubation and mechanical ventilation; circulatory support, adequate fluid volume, and nutritional support).
2. Use supplement oxygen as patient begins the initial spiral of hypoxemia.
3. Monitor ABG values, pulse oximetry, and pulmonary functioning testing.
4. As disease progresses, use positive end-expiratory pressure (PEEP).
5. Treat hypovolemia carefully; avoid overload (inotropic or vasopressor agents may be required).
6. There is no specific pharmacological treatment for ARDS except supportive care. Numerous pharmacological treatments are under investigation to stop the cascade events leading to ARDS (e.g. surfactant replacement therapy, pulmonary antihypertensive agents and antiagents).
7. Provide nutritional support (35–45 kcal/kg/daily).

Nursing Management

1. Closely monitor the patient, frequently assess effectiveness treatment (e.g. oxygen administration, nebulizer therapy, chest physiotherapy, endotracheal intubation or tracheostomal mechanical ventilation, suctioning and bronchoscopy).
2. Consider other needs of the patient (e.g. positioning and rest).
3. Identify any problems with ventilation that may cause anxiety reaction; tube blockage, other acute respiratory problems (e.g. pneumothorax, pain), a sudden decrease in the oxygen level, the level of dyspnea or ventilator function.
4. Sedation may be required to decrease the patient's oxygen consumption, allow the ventilator to provide full support ventilation, and decrease the patient's anxiety.
5. If sedatives do not work, paralytic agents (used for the shortest time possible) may be administered (with adequate sedation and pain management); reassure the patient that paralysis is a result of the medication and is temporary; describe the purpose and effects of the paralytic agents to the patient's family.
6. Closely monitor patients on paralytic agents; ensure that the patient is not disconnected from ventilator and that all ventilator and patient alarms are ON at all times, provide every care, minimize complications related to neuromuscular blockade, anticipate the patient's needs regarding pain and comfort.

ACUTE PULMONARY EDEMA

Pulmonary edema is the abnormal accumulation of fluid in the interstitial spaces of the lungs that diffuses into the alveoli. Pulmonary edema is an acute event that results from left ventricular failure. With increased resistance to left ventricular filling, blood backup into the pulmonary edema, sometimes called 'flash pulmonary edema' from the blood volume overload in the lungs. Pulmonary edema can also be caused by non-cardiac disorders, such as renal failure and other conditions that affect the body to retain fluid. The pathophysiology is similar to that seen in HF, in that the left ventricle cannot handle the volume overload and blood volume and pressure buildup in the left atrium. The rapid increase in atrial pressure, which produces an increase in hydrostatic pressure that forces fluid out of the pulmonary capillaries into the interstitial space and alveoli lymphatic drainage of the excess fluid, is ineffective.

Clinical Manifestations

1. As a result of decreased cerebral oxygenation, the patient becomes increasingly restless and anxious.
2. Along with a sudden onset of breathlessness and sense of suffocation, the patient's hands become cold and moist, the nail beds become cyanotic (bluish), and the skin turns ashes (gray).
3. The pulse is weak and rapid, and the neck veins are distended.
4. Incessant coughing may occur, producing increasing quantities of foamy sputum.
5. As pulmonary edema progresses, the patient's anxiety and restlessness increases the patient becomes confused then stuporous.
6. Breathing is rapid, noisy and moist sounding; the patient's oxygen saturation is significantly decreased.
7. The patient, nearly suffocated by blood-tinged frothy fluid filling the alveoli, is literally drowning in secretions. The situation demands action.

Diagnostic Methods

1. Diagnosis is made by evaluating the clinical manifestations resulting from pulmonary congestion.
2. Abrupt onset signs of left-sided HF (e.g. crackles on auscultation of the lungs) may occur without evidence of right-sided HF) [e.g. no jugular venous distention (JVD), no dependent edema].
3. Chest X-ray reveals increased interstitial markings.
4. Pulse oximetry to assess ABG levels.

Management/Therapeutic Measures

Goals of medical management are to reduce overload, improve ventricular function and increase respiratory exchange using a combination of oxygen, and medication therapies, which includes the following.

Oxygenation

1. Oxygen concentrations adequate to relieve hypoxia and dyspnea.
2. Oxygen by intermittent or continuous positive pressure, if signs of hypoxemia persist.
3. Endotracheal intubation and mechanical ventilation, if respiratory failure occurs.
4. Positive end-expiratory pressure.
5. Monitoring of pulse oximetry and ABGs.

Medications

1. Morphine given intravenously in small doses to reduce anxiety and dyspnea; contraindicated in cerebral vascular accident, chronic pulmonary disease, or cardiogenic shock; have naloxone hydrochloride (Narcan) available for excessive respiratory depression.
2. Diuretics (e.g. furosemide) to produce a rapid diuretic effect.
3. Vasodilators such as IV nitroglycerin or nitroprusside (Nipride) may enhance symptom relief.

Nursing Management

1. Assist with administration of oxygen, intubation and mechanical ventilation.
2. Position patient upright (in bed if necessary) or with legs and feet down to promote circulation. Preferably position patient with legs dangling over the side of bed.
3. Provide psychological support by reassuring patient that touch to convey a sense of concrete reality. Maximize time at the bedside.
4. Give frequent, simple and concise information about what is being done to treat the condition, and what the response to treatment mean.
5. Monitor the effects of medications. Observe patient for excessive respiratory depression, hypotension and vomiting. Keep a morphine antagonist available (e.g. naloxone hydrochloride). Insert and maintain an indwelling catheter, if ordered or provide beside commode.
6. The patient receiving continuous IV infusions of vasoactive medication requires ECG monitoring and frequent measurement of vital signs.

9

Chapter Gastrointestinal Nursing

CANCER OF ORAL CAVITY AND PHARYNX

Cancer of oral cavity and pharynx can occur in any part of the mouth (lips, lateral tongue, floor of mouth most common) or throat and is curable if discovered early. Risk factors for cancer of the oral cavity and pharynx include cigarette, cigar and pipe smoking; use of smokeless tobacco; and excessive use of alcohol. Oral cancers are often associated with the combined use of alcohol and tobacco. Other factors include gender (male), age (older than 50 year), and African American descent. Malignancies of the oral cavity are usually squamous cell cancers.

Clinical Manifestations

1. Few or no symptoms; most commonly a painless sore or mass that will not heal.
2. Typical lesion is a painful indurated ulcer with raised edges.
3. As the cancer progresses, patient may complain of tenderness; difficulty in chewing, swallowing or speaking, coughing if blood-tinged sputum; or enlarged cervical lymph nodes.

Diagnostic Methods

Oral examination, assessment of cervical lymph nodes and biopsies of suspicious lesions (not healed within 2 week).

Medical Management/Therapeutic Measures

1. Management varies with the nature of lesions preference of the physician and patient choice. Resectional surgery, radiation therapy, chemotherapy or a combination may be effective.
2. Lip cancer: Small lesions are excised liberally; larger lesions may be treated by radiation therapy.
3. Tongue cancer: Treated aggressively, recurrence rate is high. Radiation and surgery (total resection or hemiglossectomy) are performed.
4. Radical neck dissection for metastases of oral cancer to lymphatic channel in the neck region with reconstructive surgery.

Nursing Management

Preoperative

1. Assess the patient's nutritional status preoperatively; a dietary consultation may be necessary.
2. Implement enteral [through the gastrointestinal (GI) tract or parenteral intravenous (IV)] feedings as needed to maintain adequate nutrition.
3. If a radial graft is to be performed, perform an Allen test on the donor arm must to ensure that the ulnar artery is patent and can provide blood flow to the hand after removal of the radial artery.

4. Assess the patient's ability to communicate in writing as verbal communication may be impaired by radical surgery for oral cancer (provide a pen and paper after surgery to patients who can use them to communicate).
5. Obtain a communication board with commonly used words or pictures (give after surgery to patients who cannot write so that they may point to needed items).
6. Consult a speech therapist.

Postoperative

1. Assess for patent airway.
2. Perform suctioning if the patient is unable to manage oral secretions; if grafting was part of the surgery, suctioning must be performed with care to prevent damage to the graft.
3. Assess the graft for viability, assess color (white may indicate arterial occlusion and blue mottling may indicate venous congestion) although it can be difficult to assess the graft by looking into the mouth.
4. A Doppler ultrasound device may be used to locate the radial pulse at the graft site and to assess graft perfusion.

NAUSEA AND VOMITING

Nausea is the subjective feeling of the urge to vomit. Vomiting is the act of expelling stomach content from the body through the esophagus and mouth. Vomiting is a protective function to rid the body of harmful substance from GI tract. Many stimuli and conditions that are directly related to the GI tract or independent of it can trigger nausea and vomiting. Viral GI infections, other infections, motion sickness, stress, pregnancy, medications (narcotics) uremia and other conditions may cause nausea and vomiting.

Clinical Manifestations

1. If dehydrated electrolytes imbalance treat rehydrate and maintain metabolic alkalosis due to hydrochloride loss.
2. Emis looks like coffee ground color, bleeding from stomach.

Therapeutic Measures/Management

1. Usually nausea and vomiting may be self-limited require no interventions.
2. If prolonged, needs measures like:
   - Protection of the airway during vomiting to prevent aspiration
   - Place patient (unconscious) on this side, when begin to vomit
   - Allow the gastric contents to be expelled from the mouth.
3. If cause is known, administer prescribed medications, e.g. diphenhydramine, metaloperamide, promethazine, antimetics, etc.
4. For severe prolonged, give IV fluids.
5. Occasionally nasogastric suction needed to decompress stomach.
6. After vomiting resolved, clear liquids are started.

GASTROESOPHAGEAL REFLUX DISEASE

Gastroesophageal reflux disease (GERD) is a condition in which gastric secretion reflux into esophagus. The esophagus can be damaged by acidic gastric secretions and exposure to digestive enzymes. It can be caused by primarily by conditions that affect the ability of the lower esophagus sphincter to close tightly, such as hiatal hernia.

Clinical Manifestations

- Heartburn, regurgitation, dysphagia and bleeding
- Aspiration is a concern
- Scar tissue can develop from the inflammation.

Complications: Esophagitis, Barrett's syndrome, respiratory symptoms.

Diagnostic Measures

- X-ray studies
- Endoscopy
- Fluoroscopy.

Therapeutic Measures/Management

- Medications to decrease acid, improve gastric emptying and function of lower esophageal sphincter
- Antacids, histamine receptor antagonists
- Proton pumps inhibitors, cytoprotective agents
- Cholinergic drugs
- Controlling symptoms
- Low-fat high protein diet
- Avoiding triggers
- Raising head of bed on 4–6 inch blocks
- Instructing patient to drink fluids between meals rather than with meals.

Nursing Management

- Identify factors that increase pain to develop teaching plan
- Monitor pain level using pain rating scale to identify pain level
- Instruct patient regarding factors that aggravate pain
- Instruct patient to sleep with head of bed elevated 4–6 inches, eat small meals and avoid lying down for 2 hours after eating to prevent reflux
- Instruct patient to avoid smoking and alcohol, and avoid food cause discomfort
- Review medications schedule and teach patient take medications of pain reduction
- Provide pain medications on routine schedule.

HIATAL HERNIA

Hiatal (hiatus) hernia is the opening in the diaphragm through which the esophagus passes becomes enlarged and part of the upper stomach tends to move up into the lower portion of the thorax. There are two types of hernias—sliding and paraesophageal. Sliding or type I, hiatal hernia occurs when the upper stomach and the gastroesophageal junction are displaced upward and slide in and out of the thorax; this occurs in about 90% of patients with esophageal hiatal hernias. The less frequent paraesophageal hernias are classified extent of herniation (type II, III or IV) and occur when all or part of the stomach pushes through the diaphragm beside the esophagus. Hiatal hernia occurs more often in women than men.

Clinical Manifestations

Sliding Hernia

- Heartburn, regurgitation and dysphagia; at least half of cases are asymptomatic
- Often implicated in reflux.

Paraesophageal Hernia

- Sense of fullness or chest pain after eating or may be asymptomatic
- Reflux does not usually occur
- Complications of hemorrhage, obstruction and strangulation possible.

Diagnostic Methods

Diagnostic is confirmed by X-ray studies, barium swallow and fluoroscopy.

Medical Management/Therapeutic Measures

1. Frequent, small feedings that easily pass through the esophagus are given.
2. Advise patient not to recline for 1 hour after eating (prevents reflux or hernia movement).
3. Elevate the head of bed on 4–8 in blocks to prevent hernia from sliding upward.
4. Surgery is indicated in about 15% of patients; paraesophageal hernias may require emergency surgery.
5. Medical and surgical management of paraesophageal hernias is similar to that for gastroesophageal reflux; antacids, histamine blockers, gastric acid pump inhibitors or prokinetic agents [metoclopramide (Reglan), cisapride (Propulsid)].

Nursing Management

Assessment

- Take a complete health history, including pain assessment and nutrition assessment
- Determine if patient appears emaciated
- Auscultate chest to determine presence of pulmonary complications.

Nursing Diagnoses/Problems

- Imbalanced nutrition; less than body requirements related to difficulty in swallowing
- Risk for aspiration due to difficulty in swallowing or tube feeding
- Acute pain related to difficulty in swallowing, ingestion of abrasive agent, a tumor or reflux
- Deficit knowledge about the esophageal disorder, diagnostic studies, treatments and rehabilitation.

Planning and Goals

Major goals may include adequate nutritional intake, avoidance of respiratory compromise from aspiration, relief of pain and increased knowledge level. The objective will be that patient:

- Achieves an adequate nutritional intake
- Does not aspirate or develop pneumonia
- Is free of pain or able to control pain within a tolerable level
- Increase knowledge level of esophageal condition and treatment.

Nursing Interventions

Encouraging Adequate Nutritional Intake

1. Encourage patient to eat slowly and chew all food thoroughly.
2. Recommend small frequent feedings of non-irritating foods; sometimes drinking liquids with food helps to passage.
3. Prepare food in an appealing manner to help stimulate appetite; avoid irritants (tobacco, alcohol).
4. Obtain a baseline weight and record daily weights, and assess nutrient intake.

Decreasing Risk of Aspiration

1. If patient has difficulty in swallowing or handling secretions, keep him or her in at least a semi-Fowler's position.
2. Instruct patient in the use of oral suction to decrease risk of aspiration.

Relieving Pain

1. Teach patient to eat small meals frequently (i.e. 6–8 meals daily).
2. Advise patient to avoid any activities that increase pain and to remain upright for 1–4 hours after each meal to prevent reflux.
3. Elevate the head on 4–8 in blocks; discourage eating before going to bed.
4. Advise patient not use over-the-counter antacids because of possible rebound acidity.
5. Instruct in use of prescribed antacids or histamine antagonists.

Promoting Family- and Community-based Care

Teaching patients about self-care

1. Help patient plan for needed physical and psychological adjustments and follow-up care if condition is chronic. Teach patient and family to use special equipment (enteral or parenteral feeding devices and suction).
2. Help in planning meals, using medications as prescribed and resuming activity.
3. Educate about nutritional requirements and how to measure the adequacy of nutrition (particularly in elderly and debilitated patients). Refer 'Nursing Management' under the 'Preoperative and Postoperative Patient' for additional information.

Continuing care

1. Arrange for home healthcare nursing support and assessment when indicated.
2. Teach patient to prepare blenderized or soft food if indicated.
3. Assist patient to adjust medication schedule to daily activities when possible.
4. Arrange for nutritionist, social worker or hospice care when indicated.

CANCER OF ESOPHAGUS

Carcinoma of the esophagus is usually the squamous cell epidermoid type; the incidence, of adenocarcinoma of the esophagus is increasing in the United States. Tumor cells may involve the esophageal mucosa and muscle layers, and can spread to the lymphatics; in later stages, they may obstruct the esophagus, perforate the mediastinum or erode into the great vessels.

Risk Factors

- Gender (male)
- Race (African American)
- Age (greater risk fifth decade of life)
- Geographic locale (much higher incidence in China and Northern Iran)
- Chronic esophageal irritation
- Use of alcohol and tobacco
- Gastroesophageal reflux disease.

Other factors may include chronic ingestion of hot liquids or foods, nutritional deficiencies, poor oral hygiene and exposure to nitrosamines in the environment or food.

Clinical Manifestations

1. Patient usually presents with an advanced ulcerated lesion of the esophagus.
2. Dysphagia, first with solid foods and eventually liquids.
3. Feeling of a lump in the throat and painful swallowing.
4. Substernal pain or fullness; regurgitation of undigested food with foul breath and hiccups later.
5. Hemorrhage; progressive loss of weight and strength from inadequate nutrition.

Diagnostic Methods

Esophagogastroduodenoscopy (EGD) with biopsy and brushings confirms the diagnosis most often. Other studies include computed tomography (CT), positron emission tomography (PET), endoscopic ultrasound (EUS) and exploratory laparoscopy.

Management/Therapeutic Measures

1. Treatment of esophageal cancer is directed toward cure if cancer is in early stage; in late stages, palliation is the goal or therapy. Each patient is approached in a way that appears best for him or her.
2. Surgery (e.g. esophagectomy), radiation chemotherapy or a combination of these modalities, depending on extent of disease.
3. Palliative treatment to maintain esophageal patency; dilation of the esophagus, laser therapy, placement of an endoprosthesis (stent), radiation and chemotherapy.

Nursing Management

Refer 'Nursing management of the patient with Cancer' under 'Cancer' for additional information. Intervention for esophageal cancer is directed toward improving the patient's nutritional and physical status in preparation for surgery, radiation therapy or chemotherapy:

1. Implement program to promote weight gain based on a high-calorie and high-protein diet, in liquid or soft form, if adequate food can be taken by mouth. If this is not possible initiate parenteral or enteral nutrition.
2. Monitor nutritional status throughout treatment.
3. Inform patient about the nature of the postoperative equipment that will be used, including that required for closed chest drainage, nasogastric suction, parenteral fluid therapy and gastric intubation.
4. Immediate postoperative care is similar to that provided for patients undergoing thoracic surgery. Place patient in a low Fowler's position after recovery from anesthesia and later in a Fowler's position.
5. Observe patient carefully for regurgitation and dyspnea.
6. Implement vigorous pulmonary plan of care that includes incentive spirometry, sitting up in a chair and, if necessary, nebulizer treatments; avoid chest physiotherapy due to the risk of aspiration.
7. Monitor the patient's temperature to detect any elevation that may indicate an esophageal leak.
8. Monitor for and treat complications.
9. Once feeding begins, encourage the patient to swallow small sips of water. Eventually, the diet is advanced as tolerated to a soft, mechanical diet; discontinue parenteral fluids when appropriate.
10. Have patient remain upright for at least 2 hours after eating to allow the food to move through the GI tract.
11. Family involvement and home-cooked favorite food may help the patient to eat; antacids may help patients with gastric distress; metoclopramide (reglan) is useful in promoting gastric motility.
12. If esophagitis occurs liquid supplements may be more easily tolerated (avoid supplements such as Boost and ensure because they promote vagotomy syndrome (dumping syndrome).
13. Provide oral suction if the patient cannot handle oral secretions, or place a wick-type gauze at the corner of the mouth to direct secretions to a dressing or emesis basin.
14. When the patient is ready to go home, instruct the family about how to promote nutrition, what observations to make, what measure to take if complications occur, how to keep the patient comfortable, and how to obtain needed physical and emotional support.

ESOPHAGEAL VARICES AND BLEEDING

Bleeding or hemorrhage from esophageal varices is one of the major causes of death in patients with cirrhosis. Esophageal varices are dilated tortuous veins usually found in the submucosa of the lower esophagus; they may develop higher in the esophagus or extent into the stomach. The condition is nearly always caused by portal hypertension. Risk factors for hemorrhage include muscular strain from heavy lifting; straining at stool; sneezing, coughing or vomiting, esophagitis or irritation of vessels (rough food or irritating fluids); reflux of stomach contents (especially alcohol) and salicylates or any drug that erodes the esophageal mucosa.

Clinical Manifestations

1. Hematemesis, melena, or general deterioration in mental or physical status; often a history of alcohol abuse.

2. Signs and symptoms of shock (cool clammy skin, hypertension and tachycardia) may be present.
3. Bleeding esophageal varies can quickly lead to hemorrhagic shock and should be considered an emergency.

Diagnostic Methods

1. Endoscopy, barium swallow, ultrasonography, angiography and CT.
2. Neurologic and portal hypertension assessment.
3. Liver function tests (serum aminotransferases, bilirubin alkaline phosphate and serum proteins).
4. Splenoportography, hepatoportography and celiac angiography.

Provide support before and during examination by endoscopy to relieve stress. Monitor carefully to detect early signs of cardiac dysrhythmias, perforation and hemorrhage. Do not allow to the patient to drink fluids after the examination until the gag reflex returns. Offer lozenges and gargles to relieve throat discomfort, but withhold any oral intake if patient is actively bleeding. Provide support and explanations regarding care and procedures.

Medical Management/Therapeutic Measures

1. Aggressive medical care includes evaluation of extent of bleeding and continuous monitoring of vital signs when hematemesis and melena are present.
2. Signs of potential hypovolemia are noted; blood volume is monitored with a central venous catheter or pulmonary artery catheter.
3. Oxygen is administered to prevent hypoxia and to maintain adequate blood oxygenation, and IV fluids and volume expanders are administered to restore fluid volume and replace electrolytes.
4. Transfusion of blood components may also be required.

Non-surgical Treatment

Surgical management is preferred because of high mortality associated with emergency surgery to control bleeding from esophageal varices and because of the poor physical condition of most of these patients. Non-surgical measures include:

1. Pharmacological therapy; vasopressin (Pitressin), vasopressin with nitroglycerin, somatostatin and octreotide (Sandostatin), β-blocking agents and nitrates, balloon tamponade, saline lavage and endoscopic sclerotherapy.
2. Esophageal banding therapy and variceal band ligation.
3. Transjugular intrahepatic portosystemic shunt (TIPS).

Surgical Management

If necessary surgery may involve the following:

- Direct surgical ligation of varices
- Splenorenal, mesocaval and portacaval venous shunts
- Esophageal transaction with devascularization.

Nursing Management

1. Provide postoperative care similar to that of any thoracic or abdominal operation. Refer 'Preoperative and Postoperative Nursing Management' for additional information.

2. The risk for postsurgical complications (hypovolemic or hemorrhagic shock, hepatic encephalopathy, electrolyte imbalances, metabolic and respiratory alkalosis, alcohol withdrawal syndrome and seizures) is high. In addition, bleeding may present as new collateral vessels develop.
3. Monitor patient's physical condition and evaluate emotional responses, and cognitive status.
4. Monitor and record vital signs. Assess nutritional status.
5. Perform a neurologic assessment, monitoring for signs of hepatic encephalopathy and coma).
6. Treat bleeding by complete rest of the esophagus. Initiate parenteral nutrition (PN) as ordered.
7. Assist patient to avoid straining and vomiting. Maintain gastric suction to keep the stomach empty as possible.
8. Provide frequent oral hygiene and moist sponges to the lips to relieve thirst.
9. Closely monitor blood pressure.
10. Provide vitamin K therapy and multiple blood transfusions as ordered for blood loss.
11. Provide a quiet environment and calm reassurance to reduce anxiety and agitation. Provide emotional support and performed explanations regarding medical and nursing interventions.
12. Monitor closely to detect and manage complications including hypovolemic or hemorrhagic shock, hepatic encephalopathy, electrolyte imbalance, metabolic and respiratory alkalosis, alcohol withdrawal syndrome and seizures.

GASTRITIS

Gastritis is an inflammation of the stomach mucosa and can be acute or chronic. The cause of gastritis may be diet (alcohol, spicy foods), microorganisms [(*Helicobacter pylori*), *Salmonella*]. Medications [Aspirin, non-steroidal anti-inflammatory drugs (NSAIDs), corticosteroids, digitalis, chemotherapy)] stress (physiologic and psychological), trauma and other factors (reflux of bile, smoking, radiations, nasogastric suction and endoscopic).

Acute gastritis lasts several hours to few days and is often caused by dietary indiscretion (eating irritating food that is highly seasoned or food that is infected). Other causes include excessive use of Aspirin, and other NSAIDs, excessive alcohol intake, bile reflux and radiation therapy. A more severe form of acute gastritis is caused by strong acids or alkali, which may cause the mucosa to become gangrenous or to perforate. Gastritis may also be the first sign of acute systemic infection.

Chronic gastritis is a prolonged inflammation of stomach that may be caused either by benign or malignant ulcers of the stomach or by bacteria such as *H. pylori*. Chronic gastritis may be associated with autoimmune diseases such as pernicious anemia, dietary factors such as caffeine, the use of medications such as NSAIDs or bisphosphonates [e.g. alendronate (Fosamax), risedronate (Actonel), ibandronate (Boniva)], alcohol smoking or chronic reflux of pancreatic secretions and bile into the stomach. Superficial ulceration may occur and can lead to hemorrhage.

Clinical Manifestations

Acute Gastritis

1. Abdominal pain accompanied by nausea and anorexia.
2. Patient experience abdominal tenderness a feeling of fullness reflux, belching and hematemesis, diarrhea (due to

contaminated food): In chronic poor appetite, heartburn, belching and sour taste in mouth.
3. May have rapid onset of symptoms; abdominal discomfort, headache, lassitude, nausea, anorexia, vomiting and hiccupping.

Chronic Gastritis

1. May be asymptomatic.
2. Complaints of anorexia, heartburn after eating, belching, a sour taste in the mouth, or nausea and vomiting.
3. Patients with chronic gastritis from vitamin deficiency usually have evidence of malabsorption of vitamin B_{12}.

Diagnostic Measures

Acute Gastritis

1. Gastritis is sometimes associated with achlorhydria and hypochlorhydria (absence or low levels of hydrochloric acid or with high acid levels).
2. Upper GI X-ray series and endoscopy.
3. Biopsy with histologic examination is performed.
4. Serologic testing for antibodies to the *H. pylori* antigen and a breath test may be performed.

Chronic Gastritis

- Endoscopy
- Upper GI X-ray
- Gastric aspiration analysis.

Medical Management/Therapeutic Measures

Acute Gastritis

1. The gastric mucosa is capable of repairing itself after an episode of gastritis. As a rule, the patient recovers in about 1 day although the appetite may be diminished for an additional 2 or 3 days. The patient should refrain from alcohol and eating until symptoms subside. Then the patient can progress to a non-irritating diet. If symptoms persist, intravenous fluids may be necessary. If bleeding is present, management is similar to that of upper GI tract hemorrhage.
2. If gastric is due to ingestion of strong acids or alkali, dilute and neutralize the acid with common antacids (e.g. aluminum hydroxide); neutralize alkali with diluted lemon juice or dilute vinegar. If corrosion is extensive or severe, avoid emetics and lavage because of danger of perforation.
3. Supportive therapy may include nasogastric intubation, analgesic agents and sedatives, antacids and IV fluids.
4. Fiberoptic endoscopy may be necessary; emergency surgery may be required to remove gangrenous or perforated tissue; gastric resection (gastrojejunostomy) may be necessary to treat pyloric obstruction.

Chronic Gastritis

Diet modification, rest, stress reduction, avoidance of alcohol and NSAIDs, and pharmacotherapy are key treatment measures. Gastritis related to *H. pylori* infection is treated with selected drug combinations.

Nursing Management

Reducing Anxiety

1. Carry out emergency measures for ingestion of acids or alkalis.
2. Offer supportive therapy to patient and family during treatment and after the ingested acid or alkali has been neutralized or diluted.
3. Prepare patient for additional diagnostic studies (endoscopy) or surgery.
4. Calmly listen and answer question as completely as possible; explain all procedures and treatments.

Promoting Optimal Nutrition

1. Provide physical and emotional support for patient with acute gastritis.
2. Help patient manage symptoms (e.g. nausea, vomiting, heartburn and fatigue).
3. Avoid foods and fluids by mouth for hours or days until acute symptoms subside.
4. Offer ice chips and clear liquids when symptoms subside.
5. Encourage patient to report any symptoms suggesting a repeat episode of gastritis as food is introduced.
6. Discourage caffeinated beverages (caffeine increases gastric activity and pepsin secretion), alcohol and cigarette smoking (nicotine inhibits neutralization of gastric acid in the duodenum).
7. Refer patient for alcohol counseling and smoking cessation when appropriate.

Promoting Fluid Balance

1. Monitor daily intake and output for dehydration (minimal intake of 1.5 L/day and urine output of 30 mL/h); infuse intravenous fluids if prescribed.
2. Assess electrolyte values every 24 hours for fluid imbalance.
3. Be alert for indicators of hemorrhagic gastritis (hematemesis, tachycardia and hypotension) and notify physician.

Relieving Pain

1. Instruct patient to avoid foods and beverages that may irritating to the gastric mucosa.
2. Instruct patient in the correct use of medications to relieve chronic gastritis.
3. Assess pain and attainment of comfort through use of medications and avoidance of irritating substances.

Educating About Self-care

1. Assess knowledge about gastritis and develop an individualized teaching plan that incorporates patient's pattern of caring, daily caloric needs and food preferences.

2. Provide a list of substances to avoid (caffeine, nicotine, spicy foods, irritating highly seasoned food and alcohol); consult with nutritionist if indicated.
3. Educate about antibiotic agents, antacids, bismuth slats, sedative medications or anticholinergic agents that may be prescribed.
4. When necessary, reinforce the importance of completing the medication regimen as prescribed to eradicate H. pylori infection.

GASTRIC BLEEDING

Gastric bleeding may be caused by ulcer perforation, tumors, gastric surgery or other conditions and bleeding peptic ulcer leads to blood loss into the stomach or intestine. Blood loss can be hidden blood in the stools, observable vomited blood or black tarry stools. When blood mixes with hydrochloric acid and enzymes in the stomach a dark, granular maternal resembling coffee grounds produced.

Clinical Manifestations

- With mild bleeding, slight weakness or diaphoresis
- Severe blood loss (>1 L × 24 h) result in hypovolemic shock hypotension, weak thready pulse, chills, palpitation and diaphoresis
- Occult blood stools
- Hematemesis.

Diagnostic Measures

- Endoscopy
- Low Hb and hematocrit.

Therapeutic Measures

- Treat hypovolemic shock, nasopharyngeal oxygen (NPO), IV fluids, O_2 therapy, nasogastric (NG) tube
- Removal or ligation of bleeding area
- Medication to decrease gastric aux.

Nursing Management

- Monitor color, amount, frequency of fluid loss for changes in fluid balance
- Monitor vital signs and report abnormal findings for proper treatment
- Monitor levels of consciousness, mucus membrane and skin turgor
- Obtain daily weight, to detect change in fluid volume
- Offer oral fluids to ensure adequate intake
- Monitor intravenous infusion as order to prevent hypovolemic
- Monitor hemoglobin and hematocrit levels as ordered.

PEPTIC ULCER

A peptic ulcer is an excavation formed in the mucosal wall of the stomach, pylorus, duodenum or esophagus. It is frequently referred to as a gastric, duodenal or esophageal ulcer, depending on its location. It is caused by the erosion of a circumscribed area of mucous membrane. Peptic ulcers are more likely to be in the duodenum than in the stomach. They tend to occur singly, but there may be several present at one time. Chronic ulcers usually occur in the lesser curvature of the stomach, near the pylorus. Peptic ulcer has been associated with bacterial infection, such as *H. pylori.* The greatest, frequency is noted in people between ages of 40 and 60 years. After menopause, the incidence among women is almost equal to that in men. Predisposing factors including family history of peptic ulcer, blood type O, chronic use of NSAIDs, alcohol ingestion, excessive smoking and possibly high stress. Esophageal ulcer results from the backward flow of hydrochloric acid from the stomach into the esophagus.

Zollinger-Ellison syndrome (gastrinoma) is suspected when a patient has several peptic ulcer or an ulcer that is resistant to standard medical therapy. This syndrome involves extreme gastric hyperacidity (hypersecretion of gastric juice), duodenal ulcer and gastrinomas (islet cell tumors). About 90% of tumors are found in the gastric triangle. About one third of gastrinomas are malignant. Diarrhea and steatorrhea (unabsorbed fat in the stool) may be evident. These patients may have coexistent parathyroid adenomas or hyperplasia and exhibit signs of hypercalcemia. The most frequent complaint is epigastric pain. The presence of *H. pylori* is not a risk factor.

Stress ulcer (not be confused with Cushing's or Curling's ulcers) is a term given to acute mucosal ulceration of the duodenal or gastric area that occurs after physiologically stressful events, such as burns, shock, severe sepsis and multiple organ trauma. Fiberoptic endoscopy within 24 hours of trauma of injury shows shallow erosions of the stomach wall; by 72 hours multiple gastric erosions are observed and the stressful condition continues, the ulcer spread. When the patient recovers the lesions is reversed; this pattern is typical of stress ulceration.

Clinical Manifestations

1. Symptoms of an ulcer may last days, weeks or months and may subside only to reappear without cause. Many patients have asymptomatic ulcers.
2. Dull, gnawing pain and a burning sensation in the midepigastrium or in the back are characteristics.
3. Pain is relieved by eating or taking alkali; once the stomach has emptied or the alkali wears off, the pain returns.
4. Sharply localized tenderness is elicited by gentle pressure on the epigastrium or slightly right of the midline.
5. Other symptoms include pyrosis (heartburn) and a burning sensation in the esophagus and stomach, which moves up to the mouth, occasionally with sour eructation (burping).
6. Vomiting is rare in uncomplicated duodenal ulcer; it may or may not be preceded by nauseas and usually follows about of severe pain and bloating; it is relieved by ejection of the acid gastric contents.
7. Constipation or diarrhea may result from diet and medications.
8. Bleeding (15% of patients with gastric ulcers) and tarry stools may occur; a small portion of patients who bleed from an acute ulcer have only very mild symptoms or none at all.

Medical Management/Therapeutic Measures

The goals of treatment are to eradicate *H. pylori* and manage gastric acidity.

Pharmacological Therapy

1. Antibiotics combined with proton pump inhibitors and bismuth salts to suppress *H. pylori.*
2. Administer histamine 2 (H_2) receptor antagonists (in high doses in patient with Zollinger-Ellison syndrome) to decrease stomach acid secretion; maintenance does of H_2 receptor antagonists are usually recommended for 1 year. Proton pump inhibitors may also be prescribed.
3. Cytoprotective agents (protect mucosal cells from acid or NSAIDs).
4. Antacids in combination with cimetidine (Tagamet) or ranitidine (Zantac) for treatment of stress ulcer and for prophylactic use.

Lifestyle Changes

1. Stress reduction and rest are priority interventions. The patient needs to identify situations that are stressful or exhausting (e.g. rushed lifestyle and irregular schedules) and implement changes, such as establishing regular rest periods during the day in the acute phase of the disease. Biofeedback, hypnosis, behavior modification, massage or acupuncture may also be useful.
2. Smoking cessation is strongly encouraged because smoking raises duodenal acidity and significantly inhibits ulcer repair. Support groups may be helpful.
3. Dietary modification may be helpful; patient should eat whatever aggresses with them; small, frequent meals are not necessary if antacids or histamine blockers are part of therapy. Over secretion and hypermotlity of the GI tract can be minimized by avoiding extremes of temperature and over stimulation by meat extracts. Alcohol and caffeinated beverages such as coffee (including decaffeinated coffee, which stimulates acid secretion) should be avoided. Diets rich in milk and cream should be avoided also because they are potent acid stimulators. The patient is encouraged to eat three regular meals a day.

Diagnostic Methods

1. Physical examination (epigastric tenderness, abdominal distention).
2. Endoscopy (preferred, but upper GI barium study may be done).
3. Diagnostic test include analysis of stool specimens for occult blood, gastric secretory studies, and biopsy and histology with culture to detect *H. pylori* (serologic testing, stool antigen tests, or breath test may also detect *H. pylori*).
4. With the advent of H_2 receptor antagonists, surgical intervention is less common.
5. If recommended, surgery is usually for intractable ulcer (particularly with Zollinger-Ellison syndrome), life-threatening hemorrhage, perforation or obstruction. Surgical procedures include vagotomy, or vagotomy with pyloroplasty or Billroth I or II.

Nursing Management

Assessment

1. Assess pain and methods used to relieve it; take a thorough history, including a 72-hour food intake history. If patient has vomited, determine whether emesis is bright red or coffee ground in appearance. This helps to identify source of blood.

2. Ask patient about usual food habits, alcohol, smoking and medication use NSAIDs, and level of tension or nervousness.
3. Ask how patient expresses anger (especially at work and with family, and determine whether patient is experiencing occupational stress or family problems.
4. Obtain family history of ulcer disease.
5. Assess vital signs for indicators of anemia (tachycardia, hypotension).
6. Assess for blood in the stools with an occult blood test.
7. Palpate abdomen for localized tenderness.

Nursing Diagnoses/Problems

1. Acute pain related to the effect of gastric acid secretions on damaged tissue.
2. Anxiety related to coping with an acute disease.
3. Imbalanced nutrition related to changes in diet.
4. Deficient knowledge about preventing symptoms and managing the condition.

Potential Complications

- Hemorrhage upper GI
- Perforation
- Penetration
- Pyloric obstruction (gastric outlet obstruction).

Planning and Goals

The major goals of the patient may include relief of pain, reduced anxiety, maintenance of nutritional requirements, knowledge about the management and prevention of ulcer recurrence, and absence of complications. The objective will be that patient:

- Remains free of pain between meals
- Experiences less anxiety
- Complies with therapeutic regimen
- Maintains weight
- Experiences no complications.

Nursing Interventions

Relieving Pain and Improving Nutrition

1. Administer prescribed medications.
2. Avoid Aspirin, which is anticoagulant, and foods and beverages that contain acid-enhancing caffeine (colas, tea, coffee and chocolate), along with decaffeinated coffee.
3. Encourage patient to eat regularly spaced meals in a relaxed atmosphere; obtain regular weights and encourage dietary modifications.
4. Encourage relaxation techniques.

Reducing Anxiety

1. Assess what patient wants to know about the disease, and evaluate level of anxiety, encourage patient to express fears openly and without criticism.

2. Explain diagnostic tests and administering medications on schedule.
3. Interact in a relaxing manner, help in identifying stressors and explain effective coping techniques, and relaxation methods.
4. Encourage family to participate in care and give emotional support.

Monitoring and Managing Complications

1. If hemorrhage is a concern:
   a. Assess for faintness or dizziness and nausea, before or with bleeding; test stool for occult or gross blood; monitor vital signs frequently (tachycardia, hypotension and tachypnea).
   b. Insert an indwelling urinary catheter and monitor intake and output; insert and maintain an IV line for infusing fluid, and blood.
   c. Monitor laboratory values (hemoglobin and hematocrit).
   d. Insert and maintain a nasogastric tube and monitor drainage; provide a lavage as ordered.
   e. Monitor oxygen saturation and administering oxygen therapy.
   f. Place the patient in the recumbent position with the legs elevated to prevent hypotension, or place the patient on the left side to prevent aspiration from vomiting. Treat hypovolemic shock as indicated.
2. If perforation and penetration are concerns:
   a. Note and report symptoms of penetration (back and gastric pain not relieved by medications that were effective in the past).
   b. Note and report symptoms of perforation (sudden abdominal pain, referred pain to shoulders, vomiting and collapse, extremely tender and rigid abdomen, hypotension and tachycardia or other signs of shock).
   c. Refer 'Preoperative Nursing Management' under 'Clinical Manifestation' for additional information.

Promoting Family- and Community-based Care

Teaching patient self-care

1. Assist the patient in understanding the condition and doctor that help or aggravate it.
2. Teach patient about prescribed medications, including name, dosage, frequency and possible side effects. Also identify medications such as Aspirin that patient should avoid.
3. Instruct patient about particular foods that will upset the gastric mucosa, such as coffee, tea, colas and alcohol, which have acid-producing potential.
4. Encourage patient to eat regular meals in a relaxed setting and to avoid overeating.
5. Explain that smoking may interfere with ulcer healing; refer patient to programs to assist smoking cessation.
6. Alter patient to signs and symptoms of complications to be reported. These complications include hemorrhage (cool skin, confusion, increased heart rate, labored breathing and blood in the stool), penetration and perforation (severe abdominal pain, rigid and tender abdomen, vomiting, elevated temperature and increase heart rate) and pyloric obstruction (nausea, vomiting, distended abdomen and abdominal pain). To identify

obstruction, insert and monitor nasogastric tube; more than 400 mL residual suggest obstruction.

Continuing care

1. Teach patient that follow-up supervision is necessary for about 1 year.
2. Tell patient that the ulcer could recur; advise patient to seek medical assistance if symptoms recur.
3. Inform patient and family that surgery is no guarantee of cure. Discuss possible postoperative sequelae, such as intolerance to dairy products and sweet foods.

Evaluation/Expected Patient Outcomes

- Remains free of pain between meals
- Experiences less anxiety
- Complies with therapeutic regimen
- Maintains weight
- Experiences no complications.

GASTRIC CANCER

Most gastric cancers are adenocarcinomas; they can occur anywhere in the stomach. The tumor infiltrates the surrounding mucosa, penetrating the wall of the stomach and adjacent organs, and structures. It typically occurs in males and people older than 40 years (occasionally in younger people). The incidence of gastric cancer is greater in Japan. Diet appears to be a significant factor (i.e. high in smoked foods and lacking in fruits and vegetables). Other factors related to the incidence of stomach cancer include chronic inflammation of the stomach, H. pylori infection, pernicious anemia, smoking, achlorhydria, gastric ulcers, previous subtotal gastrectomy (more than 20 years ago) and genetics. Prognosis is poor because most patients have metastases (liver, pancreas and esophagus or duodenum) at the time of diagnosis.

Clinical Manifestations

1. Early stages; symptoms may be absent or may resemble those of patients with benign ulcers (e.g. pain relieved with antacids).
2. Progressive disease; symptoms include dyspepsia (indigestion), early satiety, weight loss, abdominal pain just above the umbilicus, loss or decrease in appetite, bloating after meals, nausea and vomiting, and symptoms similar to those of peptic ulcer disease.
3. Advanced gastric cancer may be palpable as a mass.

Diagnostic Methods

- The EGD for biopsy and cytologic washings is the diagnostic study of choice
- Barium X-ray examination of the upper GI tract, endoscopic ultrasound (EUS) and CT may be used.

Medical Management/Therapeutic Measures

1. Removal of gastric carcinoma; curative if tumor can be removed, while still localized to the stomach.

2. Effective palliation (to prevent symptoms such as obstruction) by resection of the tumor; total gastrectomy; radical subtotal gastrectomy; proximal subtotal gastrectomy; esophagogastrectomy.
3. Chemotherapy for further disease control or for palliation (fluorouracil, cisplatin, Doxorubicin, Etoposide and Mitomycin-C).
4. Radiation for palliation.
5. Tumor marker assessment to determine treatment effectiveness.

Nursing Management

Assessment

1. Elicit history of dietary intake.
2. Identify weight loss, including time frame and amount; assess appetite and eating habits; include pain assessment.
3. Obtain smoking and alcohol history, and family history (e.g. any first or second-degree relatives with gastric or other cancer).
4. Assess psychological support (marital status, coping skills, emotional and financial resources).
5. Performa complete physical examination (palpate and percuss abdomen for tenderness, masses or ascites).

Nursing Diagnoses/Problems

- Anxiety related to disease and anticipated treatment
- Imbalanced nutrition, less than body requirements, related to early satiety or anorexia
- Pain related to tumor mass
- Anticipatory grieving related to diagnosis of cancer
- Deficient knowledge regarding self-care activities.

Planning and Goals

The major goals for the patient may include reduced anxiety, optimal nutrition, relief of pain, and adjustment to the diagnosis and anticipated lifestyle changes.

Nursing Interventions

Reducing Anxiety

1. Provide a relaxed, non-threatening atmosphere (helps patients, express fears, concerns and anger).
2. Encourage family in efforts to support the patient, offering assurance and supporting positive coping measures.
3. Advise about any procedures and treatments.

Promoting Optimal Nutrition

1. Encourage small, frequent feedings or non-irritating foods to decrease gastric irritation.
2. Facilitate tissue repair by ensuring food supplements are high in calories and vitamins A and C, and iron.
3. Administer parenteral vitamin B_{12} indefinitely if a total gastrectomy is performed.

4. Monitor rate and frequency of IV therapy.
5. Record intake, output and daily weights.
6. Assess signs of dehydration (thirst, dry mucous membranes, poor skin turgor, tachycardia and decreased urine output).
7. Review results of daily laboratory studies to note any metabolic abnormalities [sodium, potassium, glucose, blood urea nitrogen (BUN)].
8. Administer antiemetic agents as prescribed.

Relieving Pain

1. Administered analgesic agents as prescribed (continuous infusion of an opioid).
2. Assess frequency, intensity and duration of pain to determine effectiveness of analgesic agent.
3. Work with patient to help manage pain by suggesting non-pharmacological methods for pain relief, such as position changes, imagery, distraction, relaxation exercises (using relaxation audiotapes), back rubs, massage, and periods of rest and relaxation.

Providing Psychosocial Support

1. Help patient express fear, concerns and grief about diagnosis.
2. Answer patients' questions honestly.
3. Encourage patient to participate in treatment decisions.
4. Support patient's disbelief and time needed to accept diagnosis.
5. Offer emotional support and involve family members, and significant others whenever possible; reassure that emotional responses are normal and expected.
6. Beware of mood swings and defense mechanisms (denial, rationalization, displacement and regression).
7. Provide professional services as necessary (e.g. clergy, psychiatric clinical nurse specialists, psychologists, social workers and psychiatrists).
8. Assist with decisions regarding end-of-life care and make referrals as warranted.

Promoting Family- and Community-based Care

Teaching patients about self-care

1. Teach self-care activities specific to treatment regimen.
2. Include information about diet and nutrition, treatment regimens, activity and lifestyles changes, pain management and complications.
3. Explain that the possibility of dumping syndrome exists with any enteral feeding and teach ways to manage it.
4. Explain need for daily rest periods and frequent visits to physician after discharge.
5. Refer home care; nurse for supervise any enteral or parenteral feeding and teach patient and family members how to use equipment, and formulas as well as how to detect complications.
6. Teach patient to record daily intake and output, and weight.
7. Teach patient how to cope with pain, nausea, vomiting and bloating.
8. Teach patient to recognize and report complications that require medical attention, such as bleeding (overt or covert

hematemesis, melena), obstruction, perforation or any symptoms that become consistently worse.

9. Explain chemotherapy or radiation regimen and the care needed during and after treatment.

Refer 'Nursing Management' under 'Cancer' for additional information.

IRRITABLE BOWEL SYNDROME

Irritable bowel syndrome (IBS) is a disorder of altered intestinal motility in which the color does not contract in normal pattern. Instead it contracts in a disorderly way that can be violent and last for long time or at times, it may not contract at all. The abnormal contractions lead to changes in bowel pattern: diarrhea and constipation or both, abdominal discomfort. There is a hereditary tendency for IBS. It is more common in females than males. Flare-ups can be caused by other illness, infections or the menstrual cycle.

Clinical Manifestations

- There will be reports of gas, bloating, constipation and diarrhea
- Alternating constipation and diarrhea
- Feeling of abdominal bloating, with or without abdominal distention
- Rectal passage of mucus, feeling of incomplete evacuation
- Abdominal pain, depression, anxiety and palpitations.

Diagnostic Measures

- History, physical examination and stool examination
- Colonoscopy and sigmoidoscopy
- Lactose intolerance test for anxiety milk producing test.

Therapeutic Measures/Medical Management

1. Usually, symptoms controlled by lifestyle modification, diet, stress management and medication.
2. Higher fiber and high-bran diet.
3. Avoid food causing distress and gas formation, i.e. fresh fruits or vegetables, spices, milk, coffee, carbonated drinks, alcohol.
4. Eat smaller frequent meals, to reduce bowel contraction.
5. Stress management, behavioral therapy (biofeedback, hypnosis, physiotherapy and exercise.
6. Maintain diary of food eaten, stressors and symptoms.
7. Administer medications as give below.
8. Antidepressant to block brain perception of abdominal pain.
9. Serotonin reuptake inhibitors (e.g. paxil).
10. Antispasmodies (e.g. hyoscyamine).
11. Lubiprostone for women with constipation.
12. Antidiarrheal medications.
13. Intravenous fluids if required as prescribed.

DIARRHEA

Diarrhea is a condition defined by an increased frequency of bowel movements (more than three per day), increased amount of stool (more than 200 g/day) and altered consistency (liquid stool). It is usually associated with urgency, perianal discomfort, incontinence or a combination of these factors. Diarrhea can result from any condition that causes increased intestinal secretions, decreased mucosal absorption or altered (increased) motility.

Types of diarrhea include secretory, osmotic, malabsorptive, infectious and exudative. It can be acute (self-limiting and often associated with infection) or chronic (persists for a long period and may return sporadically). It can be caused by certain medications, tube feed formulas, metabolic and endocrine disorders, and viral and bacterial infections. Other causes are nutritional and malabsorptive disorders, anal sphincter deficit, Zollinger-Ellison syndrome, paralytic ileus, acquired immunodeficiency syndrome (AIDS) and intestinal obstruction.

Clinical Manifestations

1. Increased frequency and fluid content of stool.
2. Abdominal cramps, distention, intestinal rumbling, anorexia and thirst.
3. Painful spasmodic contractions of the anus and stiff straining (tenesmus) with each defecation.
4. Other symptoms, depending on the cause and severity, and related to dehydration and fluid and electrolyte imbalance include the following:
   - Watery stools, which may indicate small bowel disease
   - Loose, semisolid stools, which are associated with disorders of the large bowel
   - Voluminous greasy stools, which suggest intestinal malabsorption
   - Blood, mucus and pus in the stools, which denote inflammatory enteritis or colitis
   - Oil droplets on the toilet water, which are diagnostic of pancreatic insufficiency
   - Nocturnal diarrhea, which may be a manifestation of the diabetic neuropathy.

Complications

Complications of diarrhea include cardiac dysrhythmias due to fluid and electrolyte (potassium) imbalance, urinary output less than 30 mL/h, muscle weakness, paresthesia, hypotension, anorexia, drowsiness [report if potassium level is less than mEq/L (3.5 mmol/L)], skin care issues related to irritant dermatitis and death if imbalance become severe.

Diagnostic Findings

When the cause is not obvious; complete blood cell count, serum chemistries, urinalysis; routine stool examination and stool examinations for infectious or parasitic organisms, bacterial toxins, blood, fat, electrolytes and white blood cells. Endoscopy or barium enema may assist identifying the cause.

Medical Management/Therapeutic Measures

1. Primary medical management is directed at controlling symptoms, preventing complications and eliminating or treating the underlying disease.

2. Certain medications (e.g. antibiotics, anti-inflammatory agents) and antidiarrheals, e.g. loperamide (Imodium), diphenoxylate (Lomotil); may reduce the severity of diarrhea and the disease.
3. Increase oral fluids, oral glucose and electrolyte solution may be prescribed.
4. Antimicrobials are prescribed when the infectious agent has been identified or diarrhea is severe.
5. Intravenous (IV) therapy is used for rapid hydration in very young or elderly patients.

Nursing Management

1. Elicit a complete health history to identify character and pattern of diarrhea, and the following; any related signs and symptoms, current medication therapy, daily dietary patterns and intake, past related medical and surgical history, and recent exposure to an acute illness or travel to another geographic area.
2. Perform a complete physical assessment, paying special attention to auscultation (characteristic bowel sounds), palpation for abdominal tenderness and inspection of stool (obtain a sample for testing).
3. Inspect mucous membranes and skin to determine hydration status, and assess perianal area.
4. Encourage bed rest, liquids and foods low in bulk until acute period subsides.
5. Recommended bland diet (semisolids to solids), when food intake is tolerated.
6. Encourage patient to limit intake of caffeine and carbonated beverages, and avoid very hot and cold foods, because these increase intestinal motility.
7. Advise patient to restrict intake of milk products, fat, whole grain products, fresh fruits and vegetables for several days.
8. Administer antidiarrheal drugs as prescribed.
9. Monitor serum electrolyte levels closely.
10. Report evidence of dysrhythmias or change in level of consciousness immediately.
11. Encourage patient to follow a perianal skin care routine decrease irritation and excoriation.
12. Skin in elderly patients is sensitive to rapid perianal excoriation because of decreased turgor and reduced subcutaneous fat layers.

CONSTIPATION

Constipation refers to abnormal infrequency or irregularly of defecation, abnormal hardening of stools that make their passage difficult and sometimes painful, decrease in stool volume or prolonged retention of stool in the rectum. It can be caused by certain medications; rectal or anal disorders; obstruction; metabolic, neurologic and neuromuscular conditions endocrine disorders; lead poisoning; connective tissue disorders, and a variety of disease conditions. Other causes may include weakness, immobility, debility, fatigue and inability to increase intra-abdominal pressure to pass stools. Constipation develops when people do not take the time or ignore the urge to defecate or as the result of dietary habits (low consumption of fiber and inadequate fluid intake), lack of regular exercise and a stress-filled life. Perceived constipation is a subjective problem that occurs when an individual's bowel elimination pattern is not constituent with what he/she perceives as normal. Chronic laxative use contributes to this problem.

Clinical Manifestations

1. Fewer than three bowel movements per week, abdominal distention, and pain and pressure.
2. Decreased appetite, headache, fatigue, indigestion and sensation of incomplete emptying.
3. Straining at stool; elimination of small volume of hard and dry stool.
4. Complications such as hypotension, hemorrhoids, fissures, fecal impaction and magacolon.

Diagnostic Methods

Diagnosis is based on history, physical examination, possible a barium enema or sigmoidoscopy, stool for occult blood, anorectal manometry (pressure studies), defecography and colonic transit studies. Newer tests such as pelvic floor magnetic resonance imaging (MRI) may identify occult pelvic floor defects.

Medical Management/Therapeutic Measures

1. Treatment should target underlying cause of constipation and aim to prevent recurrence, including education, bowel habit training, increased fiber and fluid intake, and judicious use of laxatives.
2. Discontinue laxative abuse; increase fluid intake; include fiber in diet; try biofeedback and exercise routine to strengthen abdominal muscles.
3. If laxative is necessary, then use bulk-forming agents, saline and osmotic agents, lubricants, stimulants or fecal softeners.
4. Specific medication therapy to increase intrinsic motor function (e.g. cholinergic, cholinesterase inhibitors or prokinetic agents).

Nursing Management

Use tact and respect with patient when talking about bowel habits and obtaining health history. Note the following:

1. Onset and duration of constipation, current and past elimination patterns, patient's expectation of normal bowel elimination, and lifestyle information (e.g. exercise and activity level, occupation, food and fluid intake, and stress level).
2. Past medical and surgical history, current medications, history of laxative or enema use.
3. Report of any of the following; rectal pressure or fullness, abdominal pain, straining at defecation and flatulence.
4. Sets specific goals for teaching; goals for the patient include restoring or maintaining a regular pattern of elimination by responding to the urge to defecate ensuring about bowel eliminations patterns and avoiding complications.

APPENDICITIS

The appendix is a small, finger-like appendage attached to the cecum just below the ileocecal valve. Because it empties into the colon inefficiently and its lumen is small, it is prone to becoming obstructed and is vulnerable to infection appendicitis. The obstructed appendix becomes inflamed and edematous and eventually fills with pus. It is the most common cause of acute inflammation in the right lower quadrant of the abdominal cavity and the most common cause of emergency abdominal surgery. Although, it can occur at any age, it more commonly occurs between the ages of 10 and 30 years.

Clinical Manifestations

1. Lower right quadrant pain usually accompanied by low-grade fever, nausea and sometimes vomiting, loss of appetite is common; constipation can occur.
2. At McBurney's point (located halfway between the umbilicus and the anterior spine of the ilium), local tenderness with pressure and some rigidity of the lower portion of the right rectus muscles.
3. Rebound tenderness may be present; location of appendix dictates amount of tenderness, muscle spasm and occurrence of constipation or diarrhea.
4. Bowsing's sign (elicited by palpating left lower quadrant, which paradoxically causes pain in right lower quadrant).
5. If appendix ruptures, pain becomes more diffuse; abdominal distention develops from paralytic ileus and condition worsens.

Diagnostic Findings

1. Diagnosis is based on a complete physical examination and imaging tests.
2. Elevated white blood cell (WBC) count with an elevation of the neutrophils; abdominal radiographs, ultrasound studies and CT scans, may reveal right lower quadrant density or localized distention of the bowel.
3. In the elderly, signs and symptoms of appendicitis may vary greatly. Signs may be very vague and suggestive of bowel obstruction or another process; some patients may experience no symptoms until the appendix ruptures. The incidence of perforated appendix is higher in the elderly, because many of these people do not seek health care quickly as younger people.

Medical Management/Therapeutic Measures

1. Surgery (conventional or laparoscopic) is indicated, if appendicitis is diagnosed and should be performed as soon as possible to decrease risk of perforation.
2. Administer antibiotics and IV fluids, until surgery is performed.
3. Analgesic agents can be given after diagnosis is made.

Complications of Appendectomy

1. The major complication is perforation of the appendix, which can lead to peritonitis, abscess formation (collection of purulent material) or portal pylephlebitis.
2. Perforation generally occurs 24 hours after the onset of pain. Symptoms include a fever of 37.7°C (100°F) or greater, a toxic appearance and continued abdominal pain or tenderness.

Nursing Management

1. Nursing goals include relieving pain, preventing fluid volume deficit, reducing anxiety, eliminating infection due to the potential or actual disruption of the gastrointestinal (GI) tract, maintaining skin integrity and attaining optimal nutrition.
2. Preoperatively prepare patient for surgery, start IV line, administer antibiotic and insert nasogastric tube (if evidence of paralytic ileus). Do not administer an enema or laxative (could cause perforation).
3. Postoperatively place patient in high Fowler's position, give narcotic analgesic as ordered, administer oral fluids when tolerated and give food as desired on day of surgery (if tolerated). If dehydrated before surgery, administer IV fluids.
4. If a drain is left in place at the area of the incision; monitor carefully for signs of intestinal obstruction, secondary hemorrhage or secondary abscesses (e.g. fever, tachycardia and increased leukocyte count).

Promoting Family- and Community-based Care

1. Teaching patient self-care.
2. Teach patient and family to care for the wound and perform dressing changes and irrigations as prescribed.
3. Reinforce need for follow-up appointment with surgeon.
4. Discuss incision care and activity guidelines.
5. Refer for home care nursing, as indicated to assist with care, and continued monitoring of complications and wound healing.

PERITONITIS

Peritonitis, inflammation of the peritoneum, is usually the result of bacterial infection, with the organisms coming from disease of the GI tract. It can also result from external sources, such as injury or trauma or inflammation from an extraperitoneal organ, such as the kidney.

Pathophysiology

Peritonitis is cause by leakage of contents from abdominal organs into the abdominal cavity, usually as a result of inflammation, infection, ischemia, trauma or tumor perforation. The most common bacteria implicated are *Escherichia coli, Klebsiella, Proteus,* and *Pseudo monas* species. Other common causes are appendicitis, perforated ulcer, diverticulitis and bowel perforation. Peritonitis may also be associated with abdominal surgical procedures and peritoneal dialysis. Sepsis is the major cause of death from peritonitis (shock, from sepsis or hypovolemia). Intestinal obstruction from bowel adhesion may develop.

Clinical Manifestations

1. Clinical features depend on the location and extent of inflammation.
2. Diffuse pain becomes constant, localized and more intense near site of the process.
3. Pain is aggravated by movement.

4. Affected area of the abdomen becomes extremely tender and distended, and the muscles become rigid.
5. Rebound tenderness and paralytic ileus may be present.
6. Anorexia, nausea and vomiting occur, and peristalsis is diminished.
7. Temperature and pulse increase; hypotension may develop.

Diagnostic Methods

1. Leukocytes (elevated) and serum electrolytes (altered potassium, sodium and chloride).
2. Abdominal X-rays, ultrasound, CT scan, MRI and peritoneal aspiration with culture and sensitivity studies.

Medical Management/Therapeutic Measures

1. Fluid, colloid and electrolyte replacement with an isotonic solution is major focus of medical management.
2. Analgesics are administered for pain; antiemetics are administered for nausea and vomiting.
3. Intestinal intubation and suction are used to relieve abdominal distention.
4. Oxygen therapy by nasal cannula or mask is instituted to improve ventilatory function.
5. Occasionally airway intubation and ventilatory assessment are required.
6. Massive antibiotic therapy may be instituted (sepsis to the major cause of death).
7. Surgical objectives include removal of infected material; surgery is directed toward excision (appendix), resection (intestine), repair (perforation) or drainage (abscess).

Nursing Management

1. Monitor the patient's blood pressure by arterial line, if shock is present.
2. Monitor central venous or pulmonary artery pressure and urine output frequently.
3. Provide ongoing assessment of pain, GI function, and fluid and electrolyte balance.
4. Assess nature of pain, location in the abdomen, and shift of pain and location.
5. Administer analgesic medication and position for comfort (e.g. on side with knees flexed to decrease tension on abdominal organs).
6. Record intake and output central venous pressure (CVP) and/or pulmonary artery pressures.
7. Administer and monitor IV fluids closely; nasogastric and intubation may be necessary.
8. Observe for decrease in temperature and pulse rate, softening of abdomen, return of peristaltic sounds, and passage of flatus and bowel movements; which indicate increase food and oral fluids gradually, and decrease parenteral fluid intake when peritonitis subsides.
9. Observe and record character of drainage from postoperative wound drains if inserted; take care to avoid dislodging drains.
10. Postoperatively, prepare patient and family for discharge; teach care of incision and drains, if still in place at discharge.
11. Refer for home care, if necessary.

DIVERTICULAR DISEASE

A diverticular is a sac-like herniation of the lining of the bowel that extends through a defect in the muscle layer. Diverticular may occur anywhere in the small intestine or colon, but most commonly occur in the sigmoid colon. Diverticulosis exists when multiple diverticula are present without inflammation symptoms. It is most common in people older than 80 years. A low intake of dietary fiber is considered a major disposing factor. Diverticulitis results when food and bacteria retained in the diverticulum produce infection and inflammation that can impede draining and lead to perforation in abscess. It may occur in acute attacks or persist as a chronic, smoldering infection. A congenital predisposition is likely to when the disorder is present in those younger than 40 years. Complications of diverticulitis include abscess, fistula (abnormal tract) formation, obstruction, perforation, peritonitis and hemorrhage.

Clinical Manifestations

1. Frequently no problematic symptoms are noted; chronic constipation often precedes development.
2. Bowel irregularity with intervals of diarrhea, nausea and anorexia, and bloating or abdominal distention.
3. Cramps, narrow stools and increased constipation at times during intestinal obstruction.
4. Weakness, fatigue and anorexia.

Symptoms of Diverticulitis

- Acute onset of mild to severe pain, in the left lower quadrant
- Nausea, vomiting, fever, chills and leukocytosis
- If untreated, peritonitis and septicemia.

The incidence of diverticular disease increases with age because of degeneration and structural changes in the circular muscle layers of the colon and cellular hypertrophy. Symptoms are less pronounced among elderly patients, who may not experience abdominal pain until infection occurs. They may delay reporting symptoms, because they fear surgery or cancer. Blood in stools may frequently be overlooked because of failure to examine stool or inability to notice changes due to impaired vision.

Diagnostic Findings

- Colonoscopy and possibly barium enema studies
- Computed tomography scan with contrast agent
- Abdominal X-ray
- Laboratory tests; complete blood cell count, revealing an elevated WBC count and elevated erythrocyte sedimentation rate (ESR).

Medical Management/Therapeutic Measures

Dietary and Pharmacological

1. Diverticulitis can usually be treated on an outpatient basis with diet and medication; symptoms treated with rest, analgesics and antispasmodics.
2. The patient is instructed to ingest clear liquids until inflammation subsides, then a high-fiber, low-fat diet. Antibiotics are

prescribed for 7–10 days and a bulk forming laxative is also prescribed.
3. Patient with significant symptoms and often those who are elderly, immunocompromised or taking corticosteroids are hospitalized. The bowel is rested by withholding oral intake, administering IV fluids and instituting nasogastric suctioning.
4. Broad-spectrum antibiotics and analgesics are prescribed and an opioid is prescribed for pain relief. Oral intake is increased as symptoms subside. A low-fiber diet may be necessary.
5. Antispasmodics such as propantheline bromide and oxyphencyclimine (Daricon) may be prescribed.
6. Normal stools can be achieved by administering bulk preparation of psyllium, stool softeners, warm oil enemas and evacuant suppositories.

Surgical Management

Surgery (resection) is usually necessary only if complications (e.g. perforation peritonitis, hemorrhage and obstruction) occur. Type of surgery performed varies according to the extent of complications (one-stage resection or multistaged procedures). In some cases fecal diversion (colostomy) may be performed.

Nursing Management

Assessment

1. Assess health, including onset and duration of pain, dietary habits (fiber intake), and past and present elimination patterns [straining at stool, constipation with diarrhea, tenesmus (spasm of the anal sphincter with pain and persistent urge to defecate), abdominal bloating and distention].
2. Auscultate for presence and character of bowel sounds; palpate for tenderness, pain or firm mass over left lower quadrant; inspect stool for pus, mucus or blood.
3. Monitor blood pressure, temperature and pulse for abnormal variations.

Nursing Diagnoses/Problems

Constipation related to narrowing of the colon secondary to thickening muscular segments and strictures. Acute pain related to inflammation and infections.

Potential complications: Peritonitis, abscess formation and bleeding.

Planning and Goals

The major goals of the patient may include attainment and maintenance of normal elimination patterns, pain related and absence of complications.

Nursing Interventions/Implementation

Maintain Normal Elimination Patterns

1. Increase fluid intake to 2 L/day within limits of patient's cardiac and renal reserve.
2. Promote foods that are soft, but that have increased fiber content.

3. Encourage individualized exercise program to improve abdominal muscle tone.
4. Review patient's routine to establish a set time for meals and defecation.
5. Encourage daily intake of bulk laxatives, e.g. psyllium (Metamucil), stool softeners or oil retention enemas.
6. Administer stool softeners or oil retention enemas as prescribed.
7. Urge patient's to identify food triggers (e.g. nut and popcorn) that may bring on an attack of diverticulitis and avoid them.

Relieve Pain

1. Administer analgesic agents (usually opioid analgesics) for pain and antispasmodic medications.
2. Record and monitor intensity, duration and location of pain.

Maintain and Managing Potential Complications

1. Identify patients at risk and manage their symptoms as needed.
2. Ask for indicators of perforation; increased abdominal pain and tenderness accompanied by abdominal rigidity, elevated WBC count, elevated ESR, increased temperature, tachycardia and hypotension.
3. Perforation is a surgical emergency; monitor vital signs and urine output, and administer IV fluids as prescribed.

Evaluation/Expected Patient Outcomes

- Attains a normal pattern of elimination
- Reports decreased pain
- Recovers without complications.

ULCERATIVE COLITIS

Ulcerative colitis is a recurrent ulcerative and inflammatory disease of the mucosal and submucosal layers of the colon and rectum. It is a serious disease, accompanied by as systemic complications and a high mortality rate; approximately 5% of patients with ulcerative colitis develop colon cancer. It is characterized by multiple ulcerations, diffuse inflammation and desquamation or shedding of the colon epithelium of the colonic epithelium, with alternating periods of exacerbation and remission. Bleeding occurs from the ulceration and the mucosa becomes edematous and inflamed, with continuous lesions and abscesses. Ulcerative colitis most commonly affects people of Caucasian and Jewish heritage.

Clinical Manifestations

1. Predominant symptoms; diarrhea, passage of mucus and pus, left lower quadrant abdominal pain, intermittent tenesmus, and rectal bleeding.
2. Bleeding may be mild or severe; pallor, anemia and fatigue result.
3. Anorexia, weight loss, fever, vomiting, dehydration, cramping and feeling an urgent need to defecate (may report passing 10–20 liquid stools daily).
4. Hypocalcemia may occur.

5. Rebound tenderness in right lower quadrant.
6. Skin lesions, eye lesions (uveitis), joint abnormalities and liver disease.

Diagnostic Methods

1. Assess for tachypnea, tachycardia, hypotension, fever and pallor.
2. Abdomen is examined for bowel sounds, distention and tenderness.
3. Stool examination to rule out dysentery, occult blood test.
4. Abdominal X-rays, CT scans and MRI.
5. Sigmoidoscopy or colonoscopy and barium enema.
6. Blood studies (low hematocrit and hemoglobin, WBC cell count, decreased albumin level and electrolyte imbalance).

Medical Management/Therapeutic Measures

Medical treatment for both Crohn's disease and ulcerative colitis is aimed at reducing inflammation, suppressing inappropriate immune responses, providing rest for a diseased bowel so that healing may take place, improving quality of life and preventing or minimizing complications.

Nutritional Therapy

Initial therapy consists of diet and fluid management with oral fluids; low-residue, high-protein, high-calorie diets; supplemental vitamin therapy; and iron replacement. Fluid and electrolyte balance may be corrected by IV therapy. Additional treatment measures including smoking cessation and avoiding foods that exacerbate symptoms, such as milk and cold foods. Parenteral nutrition (PN) may be provided as indicated.

Pharmacological Therapy

- Sedative, antidiarrheal and antiperistaltic medications
- Aminosalicylates; sulfasalazine (Azulfidine); effective for mild or moderate inflammation
- Corticosteroids [e.g. oral; prednisone (Deltasone); parenteral—hydrocortisone (Solu-Cortef); topical—budesonide (Entocort)]
- Immunomodulator agents [e.g. azathioprine (Imuran)]
- Biologic agents [e.g. infliximab (Remicadel)].

Surgical Management

When non-surgical measures fail to relieve the severe symptoms of inflammatory bowel disease, surgery may be recommended. A common procedure performed for strictures of the small intestines is laparoscope-guided strictureplasty. In some cases, a small bowel resection is performed. In case of severe Crohn's disease of the colon, a total colectomy and ileostomy may be the procedure of choice. A new option may be intestinal transplantation, especially for children and young adults who have lost intestinal function because of the disease. At least 25% of patients with ulcerative colitis eventually have total colectomies. Proctocolectomy with ileostomy (i.e. complete excision of colon, rectum and anus) is recommended when the rectum is severely diseased. If the rectum can be preserved, restorative protocolectomy with ileal pouch anal anastomosis (IPAA) is the procedure of choice. Fecal diversions may be needed.

Nursing Management

Both regional enteritis (Crohn's disease) and ulcerative colitis are categorized as inflammatory bowel disease.

Assessment

1. Determine the onset, duration and characteristics of abdominal pain; the presence of diarrhea or fecal urgency straining at stool (tenesmus), nausea, anorexia or weight loss; and family history.
2. Nursing assessment findings in ulcerative colitis and regional enteritis are:
   a. Ulcerative colitis:
      - Dominant sign is rectal bleeding
      - Distended abdomen with rebound tenderness may be present.

   b. Regional enteritis:
      - Most prominent symptom is intermittent pain associated with diarrhea that does not decrease with defecation
      - Pain usually localized in the right lower quadrant
      - Abdominal tenderness noted on palpation
      - Periumbilical region pain suggests involvement of ileum
      - Explore dietary pattern, including amounts of alcohol, caffeine and nicotine used daily or weekly
      - Determine bowel elimination patterns, including character, frequency and presence of blood, pus, fat or mucus
      - Inquire about allergies, especially to milk (lactose)
      - Ask about sleep pattern disturbances, if diarrhea or pain occurs at night.

Nursing Diagnosis/Problems

- Diarrhea related to inflammatory process
- Acute pain related to increased peristalsis and gastrointestinal inflammation
- Deficient fluid volume related to anorexia, nausea and diarrhea
- Imbalanced nutrition, nausea and malabsorption
- Activity intolerance related to generalized weakness
- Anxiety related to impending surgery
- Ineffective individual coping related to repeated episodes of diarrhea
- Risk for impaired skin integrity related to malnutrition and diarrhea
- Risk for ineffective management of therapeutic regimen related to insufficient knowledge concerning process and management of disease.

Potential complications: Electrolyte imbalance, cardiac dysrhythmias related to electrolyte imbalances, gastrointestinal bleeding with fluid volume loss, perforation of bowel, etc.

Planning and Goals

Major goals may include attainment of normal bowel elimination patterns, relief of abdominal pain and cramping, prevention of fluid volume deficit, maintenance of optimal nutrition and weight, avoidance of fatigue, reduction of anxiety, promotion of effective coping, absence of skin breakdown, increased knowledge about the disease process of therapeutic regimen and avoidance of complications.

Nursing Interventions/Implementation

Maintaining Normal Elimination Patterns

1. Provide ready access to bathroom, commode or bedpan; keep environment clean and odor free.
2. Administer antidiarrheal agents as prescribed and record frequency and consistency of stools after therapy has started.
3. Encourage bedrest to decrease peristalsis.

Relieving Pain

1. Describe character of pain (dull, burning or cramplike) and its onset, pattern, and medication relief.
2. Administer anticholinergic medications 30 minutes before a meal to decrease intestinal motility.
3. Give analgesic agents as prescribed; reduce pain by position changes, local application of heat (as prescribed), diversional activities and prevention of fatigue.

Maintaining Fluid Intake

1. Record intake and output, including wound or fistula drainage.
2. Monitor weight daily.
3. Assess for signs of fluid volume deficit, dry skin and mucous membranes, decreased skin turgor, oliguria, fatigue, decreased temperature, increased hematocrit, elevated urine specific gravity and hypotension.
4. Encourage oral intake; monitor IV flow rate.
5. Initiate measures to decrease diarrhea; dietary restrictions, stress reduction and antidiarrheal agents.

Maintain Optimal Nutrition

1. Use PN when symptoms are severe.
2. Record fluid intake and output daily weights during PN therapy; test for glucose every 6 hours.
3. Give feedings high in protein and low in fat and residues after PN therapy; note intolerance (e.g. vomiting, diarrhea and distention).
4. Provide small frequent, low-residue feedings if oral foods are tolerated.
5. Restrict activities to conserve energy, reduce peristalsis and reduce calorie requirements.

Promoting Rest

1. Recommend intermittent rest periods during the day; schedule or restrict activities to conserve energy and reduce metabolic rate.
2. Encourage activity within limits; advise bedrest with active or passive exercise for a patient who is febrile, has frequent stools or is bleeding.
3. If the patient cannot perform active exercises, perform passive exercises and joint range of motion for the patient.

Reducing Anxiety

Tailor information about impending surgery to patient's level of understanding and desire for detail; pictures and illustrations help to explain the surgical procedure and help the patient to visualize what a stoma looks like.

Enhancing Coping Measures

1. Develop a relationship with the patient that supports all attempts to cope with stressors of anxiety, discouragement and depression.
2. Implement stress reduction measures such as relaxation techniques, visualization, breathing exercises and biofeedback.
3. Refer to professional counseling, if needed.

Preventing Skin Breakdown

- Examine skin, especially perianal skin
- Provide perianal care after each bowel movement
- Give immediate care to reddened or irritated areas over bony prominences
- Use pressure relieving devices to avoid skin breakdown
- Consult with a wound, ostomy and continence nurse as indicated.

Monitoring and Managing Potential Complications

1. Monitor serum electrolyte levels; administer replacements.
2. Report dysrhythmias or change in level of consciousness (LOC).
3. Monitor rectal bleeding and give blood volume expanders.
4. Monitor blood pressure; obtain laboratory blood studies; administer vitamin K as prescribed.
5. Monitor for indications of perforation; acute increase in abdominal pain, rigid abdomen, vomiting or hypotension.
6. Monitor for signs of obstruction and toxic megacolon, i.e. abdominal distention, decreased or absent bowel sounds, changes in mental status, fever, tachycardia, hypotension, dehydration and electrolyte imbalances.

Promoting Family- and Community-based Care

Teaching patients about self-care

1. Assess need for additional information about medical management (medications, diet) and surgical interventions.
2. Provide information about nutritional management (bland, low-residue, high-protein, high-calorie and high-vitamin diet).
3. Give rationale for using corticosteroids and anti-inflammatory, antibacterial antidiarrheal and antispasmodic medications.
4. Emphasize importance of taking medications as prescribed and not abruptly discounting regimen.
5. Review ileostomy care as necessary. Obtain education information from reliable resources.

Continuing care

1. Refer for home care nurse, if nutritional status is compromised and patient is receiving PN.
2. Explain that disease can be controlled and patient can lead a healthy life between exacerbations.

3. Instruct about medications and the need to take them on schedule, while at home. Recommend use of medication reminders (containers that separate pills according to day and time).
4. Encourage patient to rest as needed and modify activities according to energy levels during a flare-up. Advise patient to limit take that impose strain on the lower abdominal muscles and to sleep close to bathroom because of frequent diarrhea. Suggest room deodorizers for odor control.
5. Recommend low-residue, high-protein, high-calorie diet during an acute phase. Encourage patient to keep a record of foods that irritate bowel and to eliminate them from diet. Recommend intake of eight glass of water per day.
6. Provide support for prolonged nature of disease because it is a strain on family life and financial resources. Arrange for individual and family counseling as indicated.
7. Provide time for patient to express fears and frustrations.

Evaluation/Expected Patient Outcomes

- Reports decrease in frequency of diarrheal stools
- Experiences less pain
- Maintains fluid volume balance
- Attains optimal nutrition
- Avoids fatigue
- Experiences less anxiety
- Copes successfully with diagnosis
- Maintain skin integrity
- Acquires an understanding of the disease process
- Recovers with complications.

REGIONAL ENTERITIS (CROHN'S DISEASE)

Regional enteritis is a subacute and chronic inflammation of the GI tact wall that extends through all layers. Crohn's disease is usually first diagnosed in adolescents or younger adults, but can appear at any time of life. Although, the most areas in which it is found are the distal ileum and colon; it can occur anywhere along with the GI tract. Fistula, fissures and abscesses form as the inflammation extends into the peritoneum. In advanced cases, the intestinal mucosa has a cobblestone-like appearance. As the disease advances, the bowel wall thickens and becomes fibrotic and the intestinal lumen narrows. The clinical course and symptoms vary. In some patients, periods of remission and exacerbation occur, but in others the disease follows a fulminating course.

Clinical Manifestations

1. Onset of symptoms is usually insidious, with prominent right lower quadrant abdominal pain and diarrhea unrelieved by defecation.
2. Abdominal tenderness and spasm.
3. Crampy pain occurs after meals; the patient tends to limit intake, causing weight loss, malnutrition and secondary anemia.
4. Chronic diarrhea may occur, resulting in patient who is uncomfortable and is thin and emaciated from inadequate fold intake and constant fluid loss. The inflamed intestine may perforate and form intra-abdominal and anal abscesses.

5. Fever and leukocytosis occur.
6. Abscesses, fistulas, and fissures are common.
7. Symptoms extend beyond the GI tact to include joint disorders (e.g. arthritis), skin lesions (e.g. erythema nodosum), ocular disorders (e.g. conjunctivitis) and oral ulcers.

Diagnostic Methods

1. Barium study of the upper GI tract is the most conclusive diagnostic aid; shows the classic 'string sign' of the terminal ileum (constriction of a segment of intestine) as well as cobblestone appearance, fistula and fissures.
2. Endoscopy, colonoscopy and intestinal biopsies may be used to confirm the diagnosis.
3. Proctosigmoidoscopic examination, CT scan.
4. Stool examination for occult blood and steatorrhea.
5. Complete blood cell count [decreased mercury (Hg) and hematocrit], sedimentation rate (elevated), albumin and protein levels (usually decreased due to malnutrition).

Medical Management

Refer nursing process for the patient with 'Inflammatory Bowel Disease' and 'Ulcerative Colitis' for additional information.

LARGE BOWEL OBSTRUCTION

Intestinal obstruction (mechanical or functional) occurs when blockage prevents the flow of contents through the intestinal tract. Large bowel obstruction results in an accumulation of intestinal contents, fluid and gas proximal to the obstruction. Obstruction in the colon can lead to severe distention and perforation unless gas and fluid can flow back through the ileal valve. Dehydration occurs more slowly than in small bowel obstruction. If the blood supply is cut off, intestinal strangulation and necrosis occur; this condition is life-threatening.

Clinical Manifestations

1. Symptoms develop and progress relatively slowly.
2. Constipation may be the only symptom for months (obstruction in sigmoid colon or rectum).
3. Blood loss in the stool, which may result in iron-deficiency anemia.
4. The patient may experience weakness, weight loss and anorexia.
5. Abdomen eventually becomes markedly distended, loops of large bowel become visibly outlined through the abdominal wall and patient has crampy lower abdominal pain.
6. Fecal vomiting develops; symptoms of shock may occur.

Diagnostic Methods

Symptoms plus imaging studies (abdominal X-ray and abdominal CT scan or MRI; barium studies are contraindicated).

Medical Management/Therapeutic Measures

1. Restoration of intravascular volume, correction of electrolyte abnormalities and nasogastric aspiration and decompression are instituted immediately.

2. Colonoscopy to untwist and decompress the bowel, if obstruction is high in the colon.
3. Cecostomy may be performed for patients who are poor surgical risks and urgently need relief from the obstruction.
4. Rectal tube to decompress an area that is lower in the bowel.
5. Usual treatment is surgical resection to remove the obstructing lesion; a temporary or permanent colostomy may be necessary; an ileoanal anastomosis may be performed if entire large bowel must be removed.

Nursing Management

1. Monitor symptoms indicating worsening intestinal obstruction.
2. Provide emotional support and comfort.
3. Administer IV fluids and electrolyte replacement.
4. Prepare patient for surgery if no response to medical treatment.
5. Provide preoperative teaching patient's condition indicates.
6. After surgery, provide general abdominal wound care and routine postoperative nursing care.

SMALL BOWEL OBSTRUCTION

Most bowel obstruction occurs in the small intestine. Intestinal contents, fluids and gas accumulate above the intestinal obstruction. The abdominal distention and retention of fluid reduce the absorption of fluids and stimulate more gastric secretion. With increasing distention, pressure within the intestinal lumen increases, causing a decrease in venous and capillary pressure. This causes edema, congestion, necrosis and eventual rupture or perforation of the intestinal wall, with resultant peritonitis. Reflux vomiting may be caused in abdominal distention. Vomiting results in loss of hydrogen gas and potassium in the blood and leading to metabolic alkalosis. Dehydration and acidosis develop from loss of water and sodium. With acute fluid losses, hypovolemic shock may occur.

Clinical Manifestations

1. General symptoms are usually crampy pain, i.e. wave like and anxiety. Patient may pass blood and mucus, but no fecal matter or latus. Vomiting occurs, if the obstruction is complete, peristaltic waves become extremely vigorous and assume a reverse direction, propelling intestinal contents toward the mouth.
2. If the obstruction is in the ileum, fecal vomiting takes place.
3. Dehydration results in intense thirst, drowsiness, generalized malaise, aching and a parched tongue and mucous membranes.
4. Abdomen becomes distended (the lower the obstruction) the gastrointestinal tract, the more marked the distention.
5. If uncorrected, hypovolemic shock occurs due to dehydration and loss of plasma volume.

Diagnostic Findings

Symptoms plus imaging studies (abnormal quantities of gas and/or fluid in intestines) and laboratory studies (electrolytes and complete blood count show dehydration and possible infection).

Medical Management/Therapeutic Measures

Decompression of the bowel may be achieved through nasogastric or small bowel tube. However, when the bowel is completely obstructed, the possibility of strangulation warrants surgical interventions. Surgical treatment depends on the cause of obstruction (e.g. hernia, repair). Before surgery, IV therapy is instituted to replace water, sodium, chloride and potassium.

Nursing Management

1. For the non-surgical patient, maintain the function of the nasogastric tube; assess and measure nasogastric output assess for fluid and electrolyte imbalance; monitor nutritional status; and assess improvement (e.g. return of normal bowel sounds, decreased abdominal distention, subjective improvement in abdominal pain and tenderness, and passage of flatus or stool).
2. Report discrepancies in intake and output, worsening pain or abdominal distention and increased nasogastric output.
3. If patient's condition does not improve, prepare him/her for surgery.
4. Provide postoperative nursing care similar to that for other abdominal surgeries (refer 'Preoperative and Postoperative Nursing Management' in chapter for additional information).

CANCER OF THE COLON AND RECTUM (COLORECTAL CANCER)

Colorectal cancer is predominantly (95%) adenocarcinoma, with colon cancer affecting more than twice as many people as rectal cancer. It may start as a benign polyp, but may become malignant, invade and destroy normal tissues, and extend into surrounding structures. Cancer cells may migrate away from the primary tumor and spread to other parts of the body (most often to the liver, peritoneum and lungs). Incidence increases with age (the incidence is highest in people older than 85 years) and is higher in people with family history of colon cancer and those with inflammatory bowel disease (IBD) or polyps. If the disease is detected and treated at an early stage before the disease spreads, the 5-year survival rate is 90%; however, only 39% of colorectal cancers are detected in early stage. Survival rates late diagnosis is very low.

Clinical Manifestations

1. Changes in bowel habits (most common presenting symptom), passage of blood in or on the stools (second most common symptom).
2. Unexplained anemia, anorexia, weight loss and fatigue.
3. Right-sided lesions are possibly accompanied by dull abdominal pain and melena (black tarry stools).
4. Left-sided lesions are associated with obstruction (abdominal pain and cramping, narrowing stools, constipation and distention) and bright red blood in stool.
5. Rectal lesions are associated with tenessmus (ineffective painful straining at stool), rectal pain, feeling of incomplete evacuation after a bowel movement, alternating constipation and diarrhea, and bloody stool.
6. Signs of complications partial or complete bowel obstruction, tumor extension and ulceration into the surrounding blood vessels (perforation, abscess formation, peritonitis, sepsis or shock).

7. In many instances, symptom, do not develop until colorectal cancer is at an advanced stage.

The incidence of carcinoma of the colon and rectum increases with age. These cancers are considered common malignancies in advanced age. In men, only the incidence of prostate cancer and lung cancer exceeds that of colorectal cancer. In women, only the incidence of breast cancer exceeds that of colorectal cancer. Symptoms are often insidious. Patients with colorectal cancer usually report fatigue, which is caused primarily by iron-deficiency anemia. In early stages, minor changes in bowel patterns and occasional bleeding may occur. The later symptoms most commonly reported by the elderly are abdominal pain, obstruction, tenesmus and rectal bleeding.

Colon cancer in the elderly has been closely associated with dietary carcinogens. Lack of fiber is a major causative factor, because the passage of feces through the intestinal tract is prolonged, which extends to possible carcinogens. Excess dietary fat, high alcohol consumption and smoking increase the incidence of colorectal tumors. Physical activity and dietary folate have protective effects.

Diagnostic Measures

1. Abdominal and rectal examination; fecal occult blood testing; barium enema; proctosigmoidoscopy; and colonoscopy, biopsy or cytology smears.
2. Carcinoembrionic antigen (CEA) studies should return to normal within 48 hours of tumor excisions (reliable in predicting prognosis and recurrence).

Medical Management/Therapeutic Measures

Treatment of cancer depends on the stage of disease and related complications. Obstruction is treated with IV fluids and nasogastric suction and with blood therapy, if bleeding is significant. Supportive therapy and adjuvant therapy (e.g. chemotherapy, radiation therapy and immunotherapy) are included.

Surgical Management

1. Surgery is the primary treatment for most colon and rectal cancers; the type of surgery depends upon the location and size of tumor and it may be curative or palliative.
2. Cancers limited to one site can be removed through colonoscopy.
3. Laparoscopic colostomy with polypectomy minimizes the extent of surgery needed in some cases.
4. Neodymium: Yttrium aluminum garnet (Nd:YAG) laser effective with some lesions.
5. Bowel resection with anastomosis and possible temporary or permanent colostomy or ileostomy (less than one third of patient) or coloanal reservoir (colonic pouch).

Nursing Management

Assessment

1. Obtain a health history about the presence of fatigue abdominal or rectal pain, past and present elimination patterns and characteristics of stool.

2. Obtain a history of IBD or colorectal polyps, a family history of colorectal disease and current medication therapy.
3. Assess dietary patterns, including fat and fiber intake, amounts of alcohol consumed and history of smoking; describe and document a history of weight loss and feelings of weakness and fatigue.
4. Auscultate abdomen for bowel sounds; palpate for areas tenderness, distention and solid masses; inspect stool for blood.

Nursing Diagnoses/Problems

1. Imbalanced nutrition; less than body requirements related to nausea and anorexia.
2. Risk for deficient fluid volume related to vomiting and dehydration.
3. Anxiety related to impending surgery and diagnosis of cancer.
4. Risk for ineffective therapeutic regimens management related to deficient knowledge concerning the diagnosis, surgical procedure and self-care after discharge.
5. Impaired skin integrity related to surgical incisions, stomal and fecal contamination of peristomal skin.
6. Ineffective sexuality patterns related to ostomy and self-concept.

Potential complications: Intraperitoneal infection, complete large bowel obstruction, gastrointestinal bleeding and hemorrhage, bowel perforation, peritonitis, abscess and sepsis.

Planning and Goals

The major goals may include attainment of optimal level of nutrition; maintenance of fluid and electrolyte balance; reduction of anxiety, learning about the diagnosis, surgical procedure, and self-care after discharge; maintenance of optimal tissue healing, protection of peristomal skin; learning how to irrigate the colostomy (sigmoid colostomies) and change the appliance; expressing feelings and concerns about the colostomy and the impact on self; and avoidance of complications. The objectives of the care will be:

- Consumes a healthy diet and maintains fluid balance
- Experiences reduced anxiety
- Learns about diagnosis, surgical procedure, postoperative preparation and self-care after discharge
- Maintain clean incision, stoma and perineal wound
- Verbalizes feelings and concerns about self
- Recovers without complications.

Nursing Interventions/Implementation

Preparing Patient for Surgery

1. Physically prepare patient for surgery (diet high in calories, protein and carbohydrates and low in residue; full liquid diet 24–48 hours before surgery or PN is prescribed).
2. Administer antibiotics, laxatives, enemas or colonic irrigations as prescribed.
3. Perform intake and output measurements of hospitalized patient (including vomitus); nasogastric tube, and IV fluid and electrolytic management.

4. Observe for signs of hypovolemia (e.g. tachycardia, hypotension, decreased pulse volume); monitor hydration status (e.g. skin turgor, mucous membranes).
5. Monitor for signs of obstruction or perforation (increased abdominal distention, loss of bowel sounds and pain or rigidity).
6. Reinforce and supplement patient's knowledge about diagnosis, prognosis, surgical procedure, and expected level of function postoperatively. Include information about postoperative wound and ostomy care, dietary restrictions, pain control and medical management.
7. Refer 'Nursing Management' under 'Cancer' in Chapter 7 'Respiratory Nursing' for additional information.

Providing Emotional Support

1. Assess patient's level of anxiety and coping mechanisms and suggest methods for reducing anxiety, such as deep breathing exercises and visualizing a successful recovery from surgery and cancer.
2. Arrange meetings with a spiritual advisor, if desired.
3. Provide meeting for patient and family with physician and nurses to discuss treatment and prognosis; a meeting with an enterostomal therapist may be useful.
4. Help to reduce fear by presenting facts about the surgical procedure and the creation and management of the ostomy.

Maintaining Optimal Nutrition

1. Teach about the health benefits of a healthy diet; diet is individualized as long as it is nutritionally sound and does not cause diarrhea or constipation.
2. Advise patient to avoid foods that cause excessive odor and gas, including food in the cabbage family, eggs, asparagus, fish, bean and high cellulose products such as peanuts, non-irritating foods are substituted for those that are restricted so that deficiencies are corrected.
3. Suggest fluid intake of at least 2 L/day.

Maintaining Fluid and Electrolyte Balance

1. Administer antiemetics and restrict fluids and food to prevent vomiting; monitor abdomen for distention, loss of bowel sounds or pain or rigidity (signs of obstruction or perforation).
2. Record intake and output, and restrict fluids and oral food to prevent vomiting.
3. Monitor serum electrolytes to detect hypokalemia and hyponatremia.
4. Assess vital signs to detect sings of hypovolemia; tachycardia, hypotension, and decreased pulse volume.
5. Assess hydration status and report decreased skin turgor, dry mucous membranes and concentrated urine.

Supporting a Positive Body Image

1. Encourage patient to verbalize feelings and concerns.
2. Provide a supportive environment and attitude to promote adaptation to lifestyle changes related to stoma care.

3. Listen to patient's concerns about sexuality and function (e.g. mutilation, fear of impotence and leakage during sex). Offer support and if appropriate refer to an enterostomal therapist sex counselor or therapist, or advanced practice nurse.

Monitoring and Managing Complications

1. Before and after surgery, observe for symptoms of complications; report; and institute necessary care.
2. Administer antibiotics as prescribed to reduce intestinal bacteria in preparation for bowel surgery.
3. Postoperatively examine wound dressing frequently during first 24 hours, checking for infection, dehiscence, hemorrhage and excessive edema.

Promoting Family- and Community-based Care

Teaching patient about self-care

1. Assess patient's need and desire for information, and provide information to patient and family (refer 'Providing Emotional support' under 'Nursing Interventions' of cancer).
2. Provide patients been discharged with specific information relevant to their needs.
3. If patient has an ostomy, include information about ostomy care and complications to observe for, including obstruction, infection, stoma stenosis, retraction or prolapse and peristomal skin irritation.
4. Provide dietary instructions to help patient identify and eliminate foods that can cause diarrhea or constipation.
5. Provide patient with a list of prescribed medications, with information on action, purpose and possible side effects.
6. Demonstrate and review treatments and dressing changes, stoma care, ostomy irrigations, and encourage family to participate.
7. Provide patient with specific directions about when to call the physician and what complications require prompt attention (e.g. bleeding, abdominal distention and rigidity, diarrhea, fever, wound drainage and disruption of suture line).
8. Review side effects of radiation therapy (anorexia, vomiting, diarrhea and exhaustion), if necessary.
9. Refer patient for home nursing care as indicated.

Evaluation/Expected Patient Outcomes

- Consumes a healthy diet and maintains fluid balance
- Experiences reduced anxiety
- Learns about diagnosis, surgical procedure, preoperative preparation and self-care after discharge
- Maintains clean incision, stoma and perineal wound
- Verbalizes feelings and concerns about self
- Recovers without complications.

ANORECTAL PROBLEMS

1. Hemorrhoids are enlarged veins within the anal tissue. They are caused by an increase in pressure in the veins, often from increased intra-abdominal pressure.
2. Internal hemorrhoids occur above the internal sphincter.

3. External hemorrhoids occur below the external sphincter.
4. Most hemorrhoids caused by straining during bowel movements.
5. Common during pregnancy. Prolonged sitting or standing, obesity or chronic constipation are also contributes to it.

Clinical Manifestations

1. Internal hemorrhoids usually not painful unless they prolapse may bleed during bowel movement.
2. External hemorrhoids cause itching and pain when inflamed and filled with blood (thrombosis).
3. Inflammation and edema occur with thrombosis cause severe pain.
4. Possible infarction of the skin and mucosa over hemorrhage.

Medical Management/Therapeutic Measures

1. The goal is to prevent constipation; avoiding straining during defecation; maintain good personal hygiene; and making lifestyle changes to relieve discomfort and symptoms.
2. Increase fluid intake and stool softeners reduce straining.
3. Avoid prolonged sitting and standing.
4. Daily sit bath to increase circulation around and for healing comfort.
5. Astringents (hazel) to relieve symptoms.
6. Anti-inflammatory medications may be tried, e.g. steroid creams or suppositories.
7. Rubber band or ligation around hemorrhoid, if posted for or surgery.
8. Care of patient undergoing surgery:
   - Analgesic for severe pain
   - Comfort measures; side lying position, measures, to relieve pain
   - Stool softeners may be used
   - Dressing and/or package changes
   - Sit bath used to keep area clean and promote healing after bowel movements
   - Patient are instructed to importance of clean and dry of area
   - Other usual postoperative measures.

VIRAL HEPATITIS (TYPES A, B, C, D, E AND G)

Hepatitis A

Hepatitis A is caused by a ribonucleic acid (RNA) virus of the genus *Enterovirus*. This form of hepatitis is transmitted primarily through the fecal-oral route, by the ingestion of food or liquids infected by the virus. The virus is found in the stool of infected patient before the onset of symptoms and during the 1st few days of illness. The incubation period is estimated to be 2–6 weeks, with a mean of approximately 4 weeks. The course of illness may last 4–8 weeks. The virus is present only briefly in the serum; by the time jaundice appears, the patients are likely to be noninfectious. A person who is immune to hepatitis A may contract other forms of hepatitis. Recovery from hepatitis A is usual; it rarely progresses to acute liver necrosis and fulminant hepatitis. No carrier state exists and no chronic hepatitis is associated with hepatitis A.

Clinical Manifestations

1. Many patients are anicteric (without jaundice) and symptomless.
2. When symptoms appear, they are of a mild, flu-like upper respiratory infection, with low-grade fever.
3. Anorexia is an early symptom and is often severe.
4. Later, jaundice and dark urine may be apparent.
5. Indigestion is present in varying degrees.
6. Liver and spleen are often moderately enlarged for a few days after onset.
7. Patient may have an aversion to cigarette smoke and strong odor; symptoms tend to clear when jaundice reaches its peak.
8. Symptoms may be mild in children; in adults, they may be more severe and the course of the disease prolonged.

Diagnostic Methods

- Stool analysis for hepatitis A antigen
- Serum hepatitis A virus antibodies, immunoglobulin.

Prevention

1. Scrupulous handwashing, safe water supply and proper control of sewage disposal.
2. Hepatitis vaccine.
3. Administration of immune globulin, if not previously vaccinated; to prevent hepatitis A, if given within 2 weeks of exposure.
4. Immune globulin is recommended for household members and for those who are in sexual contact with people with hepatitis A.
5. Pre-exposure prophylaxis is recommended for those traveling to developing countries or setting with poor or uncertain sanitation conditions who do not have sufficient time to acquire protection by administration of hepatitis A vaccine.

Medical Management/Therapeutic Measures

1. Bedrest during acute stage; encourage a nutritious diet.
2. Give small, frequent feedings supplemented by IV glucose if necessary during period of anorexia.
3. Promote gradual, but progressive ambulation to hasten recovery. Patient is usually managed at home unless symptoms are severe.
4. Assist patient and family to cope with the temporary disability and fatigue that are common problems in hepatitis.
5. Teach patient and family the indications to seek additions health care, if the symptoms persist or worsen.
6. Instruct patient and family regarding diet, rest and follow-up blood work, avoidance of alcohol, and sanitation and hygiene measures (handwashing) to prevent spread of disease to other family members.
7. Teach patient and family about reducing risk for contracting hepatitis A; good personal hygiene with careful handwashing; environmental sanitation with safe food and water supply, and sewage disposal.

Hepatitis B

Hepatitis B virus (HBV) is a deoxyribonucleic (DNA) virus transmitted primarily through blood. The virus has found in saliva, semen and vaginal secretions and can be transmitted through mucous membranes and breaks in the skin. Hepatitis B has a long incubation period (1–6 month). It replicates in the liver and remains in the serum for long periods, allowing transmission of the virus. Those at risk include all healthcare workers, patients in hemodialysis and oncology units, sexually active homosexual and bisexual men, and IV drug users. About 10% of patients progress to a carrier state or develop chronic hepatitis. Hepatitis B remains a major worldwide cause of cirrhosis and hepatocellular carcinoma.

Clinical Manifestations

1. Symptoms may be insidious and variable; subclinical episodes frequently occur, fever and respiratory symptoms are rare; some patient have arthralgias and rashes.
2. Loss of appetite, dyspepsia, abdominal pain, general aching, malaise and weakness may occur.
3. Jaundice may or may not be evident. With jaundice, there are light-colored stools and dark urine.
4. Liver may be tender and enlarged; spleen is enlarged and palpable in a few patients. Posterior cervical lymph nodes may also be enlarged.

Diagnostic Findings

1. Hepatitis B surface antigen appears in blood of up to 90% of patients. Additional antigens help to confirm diagnosis.
2. Elderly patients who contract hepatitis B have a serious risk for severe liver cell necrosis or fulminant hepatic failure. Because the patient is seriously ill and the prognosis is poor, efforts should be undertaken to eliminate other factors (e.g. medications, alcohol) that may affect liver function.

Prevention

- Screening of blood donors
- Good personal hygiene
- Education
- Hepatitis B vaccine.

Medical Management/Therapeutic Measures

1. Alpha interferon has shown promising results.
2. Lamivudine (Epivir) and adefovir (Hepsera).
3. Bedrest and restriction of activities until hepatic enlargement and elevation of serum bilirubin and liver enzymes have disappeared.
4. Maintain adequate nutrition; restrict proteins when the ability of the liver to metabolize protein byproducts is impaired.
5. Administer antacids and antiemetics for dyspepsia and general malaise; avoid all medications, if patient is vomiting.
6. Provide hospitalization and fluid therapy, if vomiting persists.

Nursing Management

1. Convalescence may be prolonged and recovery may take 3–4 months; encourage gradual activity after complete clearing of jaundice.
2. Identifies psychological issues and concerns, particularly the effects of separation from family and friends if the patient is hospitalized; if not hospitalized, the patient will be unable to work and must avoid sexual contact.
3. Include family in planning to help reduce their fears and anxieties about the spread of the disease.
4. Educate patient and family in home care and convalescence.
5. Instruct patient and family to provide adequate rest and nutrition.
6. Inform family and intimate friends about risks of contracting hepatitis B.
7. Arrange family and intimate friends to receive hepatitis B vaccine or hepatitis B immune globulin as prescribed.
8. Caution patient to avoid drinking alcohol and eating raw shellfish.
9. Inform family that follow-up home visits by home care nurse are indicated to assess progress and understanding; reinforce teaching and answer questions.
10. Encourage patient to use strategies to prevent exchange of body fluids, such as avoiding sexual intercourse or using condoms.
11. Emphasize importance of keeping follow-up appointments and participating in other health promotion activities and recommended health screenings.

Hepatitis C

A significant portion of cases of viral hepatitis are not, A, B or D, they are classified as hepatitis C. It is the primary form of hepatitis associated with parenteral means (sharing contaminated needles, needle sticks or injuries to healthcare workers and blood transfusions) or sexual contact. The incubation period is variable and may range from 15 to 160 days. The clinical course of hepatitis C is similar to that of hepatitis B; symptoms are usually mild. A chronic carrier state occurs frequently. There is an increased risk for cirrhosis and liver cancer after hepatitis C. A combination therapy using ribavirin (Rebetol) and interferon (Intron-A) is effective for treating patients with hepatitis C and in treating relapses.

Hepatitis D

Hepatitis D (delta agent) occurs in some cases of hepatitis B, because the virus requires hepatitis with hepatitis B surface antigen for its replication, so only patients B are at risk. It is common in IV drug users, hemodialysis patients and recipient of multiple blood transfusions. Sexual contact is an important mode of transmission of hepatitis B and D; incubation varies between 30 and 150 days. The symptoms are similar to those of hepatitis B except that patients are more likely to have fulminant hepatitis and progress to chronic hepatitis and cirrhosis. Treatment is similar to that for other forms of hepatitis.

Hepatitis E

The hepatitis E virus is transmitted by the fecal-oral rout, principally through contaminated water and poor sanitation. Incubation is variable and is estimated to range between 15 and 65 days. In general, hepatitis E resembles hepatitis A has a self-limited course with an abrupt onset. Jaundice almost always present. Chronic forms do not develop. The major method of prevention is avoiding contact with the virus through hygiene (handwashing). The effectiveness of immune globulin in protecting against hepatitis E virus is uncertain.

Hepatitis G

Hepatitis G (the latest form) is a post-transfusion hepatitis with an incubation period of 14–145 days. Autoantibodies are absent. The risk factors are similar to those for hepatitis C.

HEPATITIS ENCEPHALOPATHY AND HEPATIC COMA

Hepatic encephalopathy or portosystemic encephalopathy (PSE), is a life-threatening complication so liver disease occurs with profound liver failure. Ammonia is considered the major etiological factor in the development of encephalopathy. Patient have no over signs, but do have abnormalities on neuropsychological testing. Hepatic encephalopathy is the neuropsychiatric manifestations of hepatic failure associated with portal hypotension and shunting of blood from the portal venous system into the systemic circulation. Circumstances that increase serum ammonia levels precipitate or aggravate hepatic encephalopathy, such as digestion of dietary and blood proteins, and ingestion of ammonia salts. Other factors that may cause hepatic encephalopathy include excessive diuresis, dehydration, infections, fever, surgery, some medications, and additionally elevated levels of serum manganese and changes in the types of circulating amino acids, mercaptans, and levels of dopamine and other neurotransmitters in the central nervous system.

Clinical Manifestations

1. Earliest symptoms of hepatic encephalopathy include minor mental changes and motor disturbances. Slight confusion and alterations in mood occur; the patient becomes unkempt, experiences disturbed sleep patterns, and tends to sleep during the day and to experience restlessness and insomnia at night.
2. With progression, patient may be difficult to awaken and be completely disoriented with respect to time and place; with further progression, at the patient lapses into frank coma and may have seizures.
3. Asterixis (flapping tremor of the hands) may occur. Simple tasks, such as handwriting become difficult.
4. In early stages, patient's reflexes are hyperactive; with worsening encephalopathy, reflexes disappear and extremities become flaccid.
5. Occasionally, fetor hepaticus, a characteristic breath odor like freshly mowed grass, acetone or old wine, may be noticed.

Diagnostic Findings

1. Electroencephalogram (EEG) shows generalized slowing, an increase in the amplitude of brain waves and characteristic triphasic waves.

2. Serum ammonia measurements are evaluated.
3. Assess symptoms in a susceptible patient; daily handwriting or drawing sample; constructional apraxia reveals progression.

Medical Management/Therapeutic Measures

1. Administer lactulose (Cephulac) to reduce serum ammonia level. Observe for watery diarrheal stools, which indicate lactulose overdose; monitor for hypokalemia and dehydration.
2. Administer IV glucose to minimize protein breakdown and vitamins to correct deficiencies, correct electrolyte imbalances (especially potassium) and administer antibiotics if needed.
3. Assess neurologic and mental status.
4. Record fluid intake and output, and body weight daily; vital signs every 4 hours.
5. Assess potential sites of infections; report abnormal findings promptly.
6. Monitor serum ammonia level daily.
7. Moderately restrict protein intake in patients who are comatose or who have encephalopathy that is refractory to lactulose and antibiotic therapy.
8. Give enema as prescribed to reduce ammonia absorption from the gastrointestinal tract.
9. Discontinue medications that may precipitate encephalopathy (e.g. sedative medications, tranquilizers and analgesic agents).
10. Administer benzodiazepine antagonists (flumazenil).

Nursing Management

1. Maintain a safe environment to prevent bleeding, injury and infection.
2. Administer the prescribed treatments and monitor the patient for the numerous potential complications.
3. Encourage deep breathing and position changes to prevent the development of atelectasis, pneumonia and other respiratory complications.
4. Communicate with the patient's family to inform them about the patient's status and supports them by explaining the procedures and treatment that are part of the patient's care.
5. Instruct family to observe patient for subtle signs of recurrent encephalopathy. Explain that rehabilitation after recovery is likely to be prolonged.
6. Instruct in maintenance of moderate-protein and high-calorie diet. Protein may then be added (10 g increments every 3–5 day). Reduce, if relapse noted.
7. Teach how to administer lactulose and monitor for side effects.
8. Refer for home care nurse visits to assess patient's physical and mental status and compliance with prescribed therapeutic regimen.
9. Emphasize importance of periodic follow-up.

HEPATIC CIRRHOSIS

Cirrhosis is a chronic disease characterized by replacement of normal liver tissue with diffuse fibrosis that disrupts the structure and function of the liver. Cirrhosis, or scarring of the liver is divided into three types; alcoholism (the most common type of cirrhosis), postnecrotic a late result of a previous acute viral hepatitis and biliary, (a result of chronic biliary obstruction and infection, i.e. least common type of cirrhosis).

Clinical Manifestations

1. Compensated cirrhosis, usually found secondary to routine physical examination vague and symptoms.
2. Decompensated cirrhosis; symptoms of decreased proteins, clotting factors and other substances, and manifestations of portal hypertension.
3. Liver enlargement early in the course (fatty liver); later in course, liver size decreases from scar tissue.
4. Portal obstruction and ascites; organs become the seat of chronic passive congestion; indigestion and altered bowel function result.
5. Infection and peritonitis; clinical signs may be absent, necessitating paracentesis for diagnosis.
6. Gastrointestinal varices; prominent, distended abdominal blood vessels; distended blood vessels throughout the GI tract; varices or hemorrhoids, hemorrhage from the stomach.
7. Edema.
8. Vitamin deficiency (A, C and K) and anemia.
9. Mental deterioration with impending hepatic encephalopathy and hepatic coma.

Diagnostic Methods

- Ultrasound scanning
- Computed tomography scan
- Magnetic resonance imaging
- Radioisotopic liver scans
- Liver function tests [e.g. serum alkaline phosphatase, aspartate aminotransferase (AST), serum glutamic oxaloacetic transaminase (SGOT), alanine aminotransferase (ALT) serum glutamic pyruvic transaminase (SGPT), gamma-glutamyl transferase (GGT), serum cholinesterase and bilirubin], prothrombin time, arterial blood gases (ABGs) biopsy.

Medical Management/Therapeutic Measures

1. Medical management is based on presenting symptoms.
2. Treatment includes antacids, vitamins and nutritional supplements, balanced diet; potassium-sparing diuretics for ascites; avoidance of alcohol.
3. Colchicine may increase the length of survival in patient with mild to moderate cirrhosis.

Nursing Management

Promoting Rest

1. Positioning bed for maximal respiratory efficiency; provide oxygen, if needed.
2. Initiate efforts to prevent respiratory, circulatory and vascular disturbances.

3. Encourage patient to increase activity gradually and plan rest with activity and mild exercise.
4. Improving nutritious status.
5. Provide a nutritious, high-protein diet supplemented by complex vitamins and others, including A, C and K.
6. Encourage patient to eat; provide small, frequent meals. Consider patient preferences and provide protein supplements, if needed.
7. Provide nutrients by feeding tube or total PN, if needed.
8. Provide patient who have fatty stools (steatorrhea) with water-soluble forms of fat-soluble forms vitamins A, D and E, and give folic acid and iron to prevent anemia.
9. Provide a low-protein diet temporarily, if patient shows signs of impending or advancing coma; restrict sodium, if needed.

Providing Skin Care

1. Change patient's position frequently.
2. Avoid using irritating soaps and adhesive tape.
3. Provide lotion to soothe irritated skin; take measures to prevent patient from scratching the skin.

Reducing Risk Injury

1. Use padded side rails, if patient becomes agitated or restless.
2. Orient to time, place and procedures to minimize agitation.
3. Instruct patient to ask for assistance to get out of bed.
4. Carefully evaluate any injury because of the possibility of internal bleeding.
5. Provide safety measures to prevent injury or cuts (electric razor, soft toothbrush).
6. Apply pressure to venipuncture sites to minimize bleeding.

Monitoring and Managing Complications

1. Monitor for bleeding and hemorrhage.
2. Monitor the patient's mental status closely and report changes, so that treatment of encephalopathy can be initiated promptly.
3. Carefully monitor serum electrolyte levels and correct, if abnormal.
4. Administer oxygen, if oxygen desaturation occurs; monitor for fever or abdominal pain, which may signal the onset of bacterial peritonitis or other infection.
5. Assess cardiovascular and respiratory status; administer diuretics, implement fluid restrictions and enhance patient positioning, if needed.
6. Monitor intake and output, daily weight changes, in abdominal girth and edema formation.
7. Monitor for nocturia and later for oliguria, because these states indicate increasing severity of liver dysfunction.

Refer 'Nursing Management' under 'Hepatic Encephalopathy' for additional information.

Promoting Family- and Community-based Care

1. Prepare for discharge by providing dietary instruction, including exclusion of alcohol.

2. Refer to alcoholic anonymous, psychiatric care, counseling or spiritual advisor, if indicated.
3. Continue sodium restriction; stress avoidance of raw shellfish.
4. Provide written instruction, teaching, support and reinforcement to patient and family.
5. Encourage rest and probably a change in lifestyle (adequate, well-balanced diet and elimination of alcohol).
6. Instruct family about symptoms of impending encephalopathy and possibility of bleeding tendencies and infection.
7. Offer support and encouragement to the patient and provide positive feedback when the patient experiences success.
8. Refer patient to home care nurse and assist in transport from hospital to home.

CHOLELITHIASIS AND CHOLECYSTITIS

In cholelithiasis, calculi (gallstones) usually form in the gallbladder from solid constituents of bile and vary greatly in size, shape and composition. There are two major type of gallstones, i.e. pigment stones, which contain an excess of unconjugated pigments in the bile and cholesterol stones (the more common form), which result from bile supersaturated with cholesterol due to increased synthesis of cholesterol and decreased synthesis of bile acids that dissolve cholesterol. Risk factors for pigment stones include cirrhosis, hemolysis and infections of the biliary tract. These stones cannot be dissolved and must be removed surgically. Risk factors for cholesterol stones include gender (women are two to three times more likely to develop cholesterol stones); use of oral contraceptives, estrogens and clofibrate; age (usually older than 40 year); multiparous status; and obesity. There is also an increased risk related to diabetes, GI tract disease, T-tube fistula and ileal resection or bypass.

Cholecystitis, an acute complication of cholelithiasis, is an acute infection of the gallbladder. Most patients with cholecystitis have gallstones (acalculous cholecystitis). A gallstone obstructs bile outflow and bile in the gallbladder initiates a chemical reaction, resulting in edema, compromise of the vascular therapy, and gangrene. In the absence of gallstones, cholecystitis (acalculous) may occur after surgery, severe trauma or burns, or with torsion, cystic duct obstruction, multiple blood transfusion and primary bacterial infections of the gallbladder. Infection causes pain, tenderness and rigidity of the upper right abdomen; is associated with nausea and vomiting, and the usual signs of inflammation. Purulent fluid inside the gallbladder indicates an empyema of the gallbladder. Refer 'Nursing Process' for additional information.

Clinical Manifestations

1. May be silent, producing no pain and only GI symptoms.
2. May be acute or chronic with epigastric distress (fullness abdominal distention, and vague upper right quadrant pain may follow a meal rich in fried of fatty foods).
3. If the cystic duct is obstructed, the gallbladder becomes distended, inflamed and eventually infected; fever and palpable abdominal pain, radiating to back or right shoulder with nausea and vomiting several hours after a heavy meal, restlessness and constant or colicky pain.
4. Jaundice, accompanied by marked itching, with obstruction of the common bile duct, in a small percentage of patients.

5. Very dark urine; grayish or clay-colored stool.
6. Deficiencies of vitamins A, D, E and K (fat-soluble vitamins).

Diagnostic Findings

- Cholecystogram, cholangiogram; celiac axis arteriography
- Laparoscopy
- Endoscopic ultrasound (EUS)
- Helical CT, MRI, endoscopic retrograde cholangiopancreatography (ERCP), etc.
- Serum alkaline phosphate; GGT, gamma-glutamyl transpeptidase (GGTP) and lactate dehydrogenase (LDH)
- Cholesterol levels.

Medical Management/Therapeutic Measures

Major objectives of medical therapy are to reduce the incidence of acute episodes of gallbladder pain and cholecystitis by supportive and dietary management and, if possible, to remove the cause by pharmacotherapy, endoscope procedures or surgical intervention:

1. Surgical intervention for disease of the biliary tract is the most common operation performed in the elderly.
2. Dietary disease may be accompanied or preceded by symptoms of septic shock; oliguria, hypotension, mental changes, tachycardia and tachypnea.
3. Cholecystectomy is usually well-tolerated and carries a low risk, if expert assessment and care are provided before, during and after surgery.
4. Mortality from serious complications is high. Risk of complications and shorter hospital stays make it essential that older patients and their family members receive specific information about signs and symptoms of complications and measures to prevent them.

Nutritional and Supportive Therapy

1. Achieve remission with rest, IV fluids, nasogastric suction, analgesia and antibiotics.
2. Diet immediately after an episode is usually low-fat liquids with high protein and carbohydrates followed by soft solid foods as tolerated, avoiding eggs, cream, pork, fried foods, cheese, rich dressings, gas-forming vegetables and alcohol.

Pharmacological Therapy

1. Ursodeoxycholic acid [UDCA (Urso, Actigall)] and chenodeoxycholic acid or chenodiol (CDCA)/(Chenix) are effective in dissolving primarily cholesterol stones.
2. Patients with significant frequent symptoms; cystic duct occlusion; or pigment stones are not candidates for therapy with UDCA.

Non-surgical Removal of Gallstones

In addition to dissolving gallstones, they can be removed by other instrumentation (e.g. catheter and instrument with a basket attached are threaded through the T-tube tract or fistula formed at the time of T-tube insertion, ERCP endoscope), intracorporeal lithotripsy (laser pulse) or extracorporeal shock wave therapy, i.e. lithotripsy or extracorporeal shock wave lithotripsy (ESWL).

Surgical Management

1. Goal of surgery is to relieve persistent symptoms, to remove the cause of biliary colic and to treat acute cholecystitis.
2. Laparoscopic cholecystectomy; performed through and incision or puncture made through the abdominal with the umbilicus.
3. Cholecystectomy; gallbladder is removed through the abdominal incision (usually right subcostal) after the cystic duct and artery are ligated.
4. Minicholecystectomy: Gallbladder is removed through small incision.
5. Choledochostomy; incision into the common duct for removal.
6. Cholecystostomy (surgical or percutaneous); gallbladder if opened; the stone, bile or purulent drainage is removed.

Nursing Management

Assessment

1. Assessment health history; note history of smoking or respiratory problems.
2. Assess respiratory status; note shallow respirations, persistent cough or ineffective or adventitious breath sounds.
3. Evaluate nutritional status (dietary history, general examination and laboratory study results).

Nursing Diagnoses/Problems

1. Acute pain and discomfort related to surgical incision.
2. Impaired gas exchange related to high abdominal surgical incision.
3. Impaired skin integrity related to altered biliary drainage after surgical incision.
4. Imbalanced nutrition; less than body requirements, related to inadequate bile secretions.
5. Deficient knowledge about self-care activities related to incisional care, dietary modifications (if needed), medications and reportable signs or symptoms such as fever.

Potential complications: Bleeding and gastrointestinal symptoms.

Planning and Goals

Goals include relief of pain, adequate ventilation, intact skin and improved biliary drainage, optimal nutritional intake, absence of complications and understanding of self-care routines.

Nursing Interventions

Postoperative

- Place patient in lower Fowler's position
- Provide IV fluid and nasogastric suction
- Provide water and other fluids, and soft diet, after bowel sounds return.

Relieving Pain

- Administer analgesic agents as ordered
- Help patient turn, cough, breathe deeply and ambulate as indicated
- Instruct patient to use a pillow or binder to splint incision.

Improving Respiratory Status

1. Remind patient to take deep breath and cough every hour, to expand the lungs fully and prevent atelectasis; promote early ambulation.
2. Monitor elderly and obese patients and those with pre-existing pulmonary disease most closely for respiratory problems.

Maintaining Skin Integrity and Promoting Biliary Drainage

1. Connect tubes to drainage receptacle and secure tubing to avoid kinking (elevated abdomen).
2. Place drainage bag in patient's pocket when ambulating.
3. Observe for indication of infections, leakage of\ bile and obstruction of bile drainage.
4. Observe for jaundice (check the sclera).
5. Note and report right upper quadrant abdominal pain, nausea and vomiting, bile drainage around any drainage tube, clay-colored stools and a change in vital signs.
6. Change dressing frequently using ointment to protect skin from irritation.
7. Measure bile collected every 24 hours; document amount, color and character of drainage.
8. Keep careful record of intake and output.

Improving Nutritional Status

1. Encourage the patient to eat a diet that is low in fat, and high in carbohydrate and proteins.
2. Immediately after surgery. At the time of discharge, advice patient to maintain diet and avoid excessive fats; fat restriction is usually lifted in 4–6 weeks.

Monitoring and Managing Complications

1. Bleeding; assess periodically for increased tenderness and rigidity of abdomen and report; instruct patient and family to report change in color of stools. Monitor vital signs closely. Inspect incision for bleeding.
2. Gastrointestinal symptoms; assess for loss of appetite, vomiting, pain, distention of abdomen and temperature elevation; report promptly and instruct patient and family to report symptoms promptly, provide written reinforcement of verbal instructions.

Promoting Family- and Community-based Care

1. Teach about medications and their actions.
2. Instruct patient to report to physician symptoms of jaundice, dark urine, pale stools, pruritus or signs of inflammation and infection (e.g. pain and fever).

3. Instruct patient verbally and in writing, about care of drainage tubes and to report to physician promptly changes in amount or characteristics of drainage.
4. Refer to home care, if necessary.
5. Emphasize importance of keeping follow-up appointment.

Evaluation/Expected Patient Outcomes

- Reports decrease in pain
- Demonstrates appropriate respiratory function
- Exhibits normal skin integrity around biliary drainage sites
- Obtains relief from dietary intolerance
- Absence of complications.

ACUTE PANCREATITIS

Pancreatitis (inflammation of the pancreas) is a serious disorder that can range in severity from a relatively mild, self-limiting disorder to a rapidly fatal disease that does not respond to any treatment.

Acute pancreatitis is commonly described as an autodigestion of the pancreas by the exocrine enzymes it produces, principally trypsin. About 80% of patients with acute pancreatitis have biliary tract disease or a history of long-term alcohol abuse. Other less common causes of pancreatitis include bacterial or viral infection; with pancreatitis occasionally developing as a complication of mumps virus. Many disease process and condition have been associated with an increased incidence of pancreatitis including surgery on or near the pancreas, medications, hypercalcemia and hyperlipidemia. Up to 10% of cases are idiopathic and there is a small incidence of hereditary pancreatitis.

Mortality rate is high because of shock, anoxia, hypotension or fluid and electrolyte imbalances. Attacks of acute pancreatitis may result in complete recovery, may recur without permanent damage or may progress to chronic pancreatitis.

Clinical Manifestations

1. Severe abdominal pain is the major symptoms.
2. Pain in the midepigastrium may be accompanied by abdominal distention, poorly defined, palpable abdominal mass; decreased peristalsis; and vomiting that fails to relieve the pain or nausea.
3. Pain is frequently acute, in onset (24–48 hours after a heavy meal or alcohol ingestion); may be more severe after meals and unrelieved by antacids.
4. Patient appears acutely ill.
5. Abdominal guarding; rigid or board-like abdomen (generally an ominous sign, usually indicating peritonitis).
6. Ecchymosis in the flank or around the umbilicus, which may indicate severe hemorrhagic pancreatitis.
7. Nausea and vomiting, fever, jaundice and mental condition agitation.
8. Hypotension related to hypovolemia and shock.
9. May develop tachycardia, cyanosis, cold and clammy skin.
10. Acute renal failure common.
11. Respiratory distress and hypoxia.
12. May develop diffuse pulmonary infiltrates, dyspnea, tachypnea and abdominal blood gas values.

13. Myocardial depression, hypocalcemia hyperglycemia, and disseminated intravascular coagulation (DIC).

Diagnostic Measures

Diagnosis is based on history of abdominal pain, the presence of known risk factor, physical examination findings and diagnostic findings (increased urine amylase level and WBC count; hypocalcemia; transient hyperglycemia; glucosamine and increased serum bilirubin levels in some patients). X-rays of abdomen and chest, ultrasound, and contrast enhanced CT scan may be performed. Hematocrit and hemoglobin levels are used to monitor the patient for bleeding.

Serum amylase and lipase levels are most indicative (elevated within 24 hours; amylase may returns to normal within 48–72 hours; lipase remains elevated for longer period). Peritoneal fluid is elevated for increase in pancreatic enzymes.

The mortality from acute pancreatitis increases with advancing age. Patterns of complications change with age (e.g. the incidence of multiple organ failure increases with age). Close monitoring of major organ function (lungs and kidneys) is essential and aggressive treatment is necessary to reduce mortality in the elderly.

Medical Management/Therapeutic Measures

Acute Phase

During the acute phase, management is symptomatic and directed toward preventing or treating complications:

1. Oral intake is withheld to inhibit pancreatic stimulation and secretion of pancreatic enzymes.
2. Parenteral nutrition is administered to the debilitated patient.
3. Nasogastric suction is used to relieve nausea and vomiting, and to decrease painful abdominal distention and paralytic ileus.
4. Histamine 2 receptor antagonists (cimetidine, ranitidine) or sometimes, proton pump inhibitors are given to decrease hydrochloric acid secretion.
5. Adequate pain medication, such as morphine is administered.
6. Antiemetic agents may be prescribed to prevent vomiting.
7. Correction of fluid, blood loss and low albumin levels is necessary.
8. Antibiotics are administered, if infection is present.
9. Insulin is necessary, if significant hyperglycemia occurs.
10. Aggressive respiratory care is provided for pulmonary infiltrates effusion and atelectasis.
11. Biliary drainage (drains and stents) results in decreased pain and increased weight gain.
12. Surgical interventions may be performed for diagnosis, drainage, resection or debridement.

Postacute Phase

- Antacids are given when the acute episode begins to resolve
- Oral feedings, low in fat and protein are initiated gradually
- Caffeine and alcohol are eliminated
- Medications (e.g. thiazide diuretics, glucocorticoids or oral contraceptives) are discontinued.

Nursing Management

Relieving Pain and Discomfort

1. Administer analgesics as prescribed. Current recommendation for pain management is parenteral opioids, including morphine, hydromorphone or fentanyl via patient controlled analgesia or bolus.
2. Frequently assess pain and the effectiveness of the pharmacological interventions.
3. Withhold oral fluids to decrease formation and secretion of secretin.
4. Use nasogastric suctioning to remove gastric secretions and relieve abdominal distention; provide frequent oral hygiene and care to decrease discomfort from the nasogastric tube and relive dryness of the mouth.
5. Maintain patient on bedrest to decrease metabolic rate and to reduce secretion of pancreatic enzymes; report increased pain (may be pancreatic hemorrhage or inadequate analgesic dosage).
6. Provide frequent and repeated, but simple explanations about treatment; patient may have clouded sensorium from pain, fluid imbalances and hypoxemia.
7. Improve breathing.
8. Maintain patient in semi-Fowler's position to decrease pressure on a diaphragm.
9. Change position frequently to prevent atelectasis and pooling of respiratory secretions.
10. Assess respiratory status frequently (pulse oximetry; ABG values) and teach patients techniques of coughing and deep breathing and the use of incentive spiromer.

Improving Nutritional Status

1. Assess nutritional status and note factors that alter the patient's nutritional requirements (e.g. temperature elevation, surgery drainage).
2. Monitor laboratory test results and daily weights.
3. Provide enteral nutrition or PN as prescribed.
4. Monitor glucose level every 4–6 hours.
5. Introduce oral feedings gradually as symptoms subside.
6. Avoid heavy meals and alcoholic beverages.

Maintain Skin Integrity

1. Assess the wound, drainage sites and skin carefully for signs of infection, inflammation and breakdown.
2. Carry out wound care as prescribed and take precautions to protect intact skin from contact with drainage; consult with a wound, ostomy and continence nurse as needed to identify appropriate skin care devices and protocols.
3. Turn patient every 2 hours; use of specialty beds may be indicated to prevent skin breakdown.

Monitoring and Managing Complications

Fluid and electrolyte disturbances

1. Assess fluid and electrolyte status by noting skin turgor and moistness of mucous membranes.

2. Weigh daily, measure all fluid intake and output.
3. Assess for other factors that may affect fluid and electrolyte status, including increased body temperature and wound drainage.
4. Observe for ascites and measure abdominal girth.
5. Administer IV fluids and blood or blood products to maintain volume and prevent or treat shock.
6. Report decreased blood pressure, reduced urine output and low serum calcium and magnesium.

Pancreatic necrosis

1. Transfer patient to intensive care unit for close monitoring.
2. Administer prescribed fluids, medications and blood products.
3. Assist with supportive management, such as mechanical ventilation.

Shock and multiple organ failure

1. Monitor patient for closely early signs of neurological, cardiovascular, renal and respiratory dysfunction.
2. Prepare for rapid changes in patient status, treatment and therapies, and responds quickly.
3. Inform family of status and progress of patient; allow time with patient.

Promoting Family- and Community-based Care

Teaching patients about self-care

1. Provide patient and family with facts and explanations of the acute phase of illness; provide necessary repetition and reinforcement. Offer verbal and written instructions materials.
2. Reinforce the need for a low-fat diet, avoidance of heavy meals and avoidance of alcohol.
3. Provide additional explanations on dietary modifications, if biliary tract disease is the cause.

Continuing care

1. Refer form home care (often indicated).
2. Assess the home situation and reinforce tract.
3. Provide information about resources and support particularly, if alcohol is the cause of acute pancreatitis.

CHRONIC PANCREATITIS

Chronic pancreatitis is an inflammatory characterized by progressive anatomic and functional destruction of the pancreas. Cells are replaced by fibrous tissue with repeated attacks of pancreatitis. The end result is obstruction of the pancreatic and common bile ducts and duodenum. In addition, there is atrophy of the epithelium of the ducts, inflammation and destruction of the secreting cells of malnutrition worldwide is the major causes. The incidence of pancreatitis among alcoholic is 50 times the rate in the non-drinking population.

Pathophysiology

The long-term alcohol consumption causes hypersecretion of the protein in pancreatic secretions, resulting in protein plugs and calculi within the pancreatic ducts. Alcohol has a direct toxic effect on the cells of the pancreas. Damage is more severe in patients with the diets low in protein and very high or very low in fat. Smoking is another factor in the development of chronic pancreatitis. Because heavy drinking usually smoke, it is difficult to separate the effects of the alcohol abuse and smoking.

Clinical Manifestations

1. Recurring attacks of severe upper abdominal and back pain accompanied by vomiting; opioids may not provide relief.
2. Risk of addiction to opiates is high because of the severe pain.
3. There may continuous severe pain or dull, nagging and constant pain.
4. Weight loss is a major problem.
5. Altered digestion (malabsorption) of foods (proteins and fats) results in frequent, frothy and foul smelling stools with a high fat content (steatorrhea).
6. As disease progresses, calcification of the gland may occur and calcium stones may form within the ducts.

Diagnostic Methods

1. Endoscopic retrograde cholangiopancreatography is the most useful study.
2. Various imaging procedures, including MRI, CT scans and ultrasound.
3. A glucose tolerance test evaluates pancreatic islet cell function.
4. Steatorrhea is best confirmed by laboratory analysis of fecal fat content.

Medical Management/Therapeutic Measures

1. Treatment is directed toward preventing and managing acute attacks, relieving pain and discomfort, and managing exocrine and endocrine insufficience of pancreatitis.
2. Endoscopy to remove pancreatic duct stones, correct strictures and drain cysts may be effective in selected patients to manage pain and relieve obstruction.
3. Pain and discomfort are relieved with analgesics. Yoga may be an effective non-pharmacological method of pain reduction and for relief of other coexisting symptoms.
4. Patient should avoid alcohol and foods that produce abdominal pain and discomfort. No other treatment will relieve pain if patient continues to consume alcohol.
5. Diabetes mellitus resulting from dysfunction of pancreatic islet cells is treated with diet, insulin or oral hypoglycemic agents. Patient and family are taught hazard of severe hypoglycemia related to alcohol use.
6. Pancreatic enzyme replacement therapy is instituted for malabsorption and steatorrhea.
7. Surgery is done to relieve abdominal pain and discomfort, restore drainage of pancreatic secretions and reduce frequency of attacks (pancreaticojejunostomy).
8. Morbidity and mortality after surgical procedures are highly because of patient's poor physical condition before surgery and concomitant occurrence of cirrhosis.

Nursing Management

Refer 'Acute Pancreatitis'.

CANCER OF THE PANCREAS

Cancer may develop in the head, body or tail of the pancreas. Symptoms vary depending on the location of the lesion and whether functioning insulin-secreting pancreatic islet cells are involved. It is very rare before the age of 45 years and most patient present in or beyond the sixth decade of life. Risk factors include cigarette smoking, exposure to industrialist chemicals or toxins in the environment and a high diet in the meat or both. Pancreatic cancer is also associated with diabetes mellitus, chronic pancreatitis and hereditary pancreatitis. Tumors that originate in the head of the pancreas are the most common and obstruct the common bile duct; functioning islet cell tumors are responsible for the syndrome of hyperinsulinism, particularly in islet cell tumors. The pancreatic carcinoma has a 5% survival rate at 5 years, regardless of the stage of disease at diagnosis.

Clinical Manifestations

1. Pain, jaundice or both are present in more than 80% of patients and along with weight loss, are considered classic signs of pancreatic carcinoma, but often do not appear until the disease is far advanced.
2. Rapid, profound and progressive weight loss.
3. Vague upper or midabdominal pain or discomfort unrelated to any GI function; radiates as a boring pain in the midback and is more severe at night and when lying in the supine position; pain is often progressive and severe. Ascites is common.
4. Symptoms of insulin deficiency (diabetes; glycosuria, hyperglycemia and abnormal glucose tolerance) may be an early sign of carcinoma.
5. Meals often aggravate epigastric pain.
6. Malabsorption of nutrients and fat-soluble vitamins, anorexia, and malaise, and clay-colored stools and dark urine are common with tumor in the head of the pancreas.
7. Gastrointestinal X-rays may show deformities in adjacent viscera related to pancreatic mass.

Diagnostic Measures

1. Spiral (helical) CT is more than 85%–90% accurate in the diagnosis and staging of pancreatic cancer and is currently the most useful preoperative imaging technique.
2. MRI, endoscopic, retrograde cholangiopancreatography (ERCP) endoscopic ultrasound (EUS), GI X-rays, percutaneous fine-needle biopsy, percutaneous transhepatic cholangiography (PTC), laparoscopy or intraoperative ultrasonography.
3. Glucose tolerance test to diagnose a pancreatic islet tumor.
4. Tumor markers are useful indicators of disease progression.

Medical Management/Therapeutic Measures

1. Surgical management is extensive to remove resectable localized tumors (e.g. pancreatectomy, whipple resection).
2. Radiation and chemotherapy may be used; intraoperative radiation therapy (IORT) or intestinal implantation of radioactive sources may be used for pain relief.

3. Diet high in protein with pancreatic enzymes, adequate hydration, vitamin K, and treatment of anemia with blood components and total PN may be instituted before surgery when indicated.
4. Treatment is often limited to palliative measures owing to widespread metastases especially to liver, lungs and bones.
5. A biliary stent may be used to relieve jaundice.

Nursing Management

Refer 'Preoperative and Postoperative Nursing Management' in Chapter 6 for additional information:

1. Provide pain management and attention to nutrition. Be alert for hypoglycemia in the patient with pancreatic islet tumor.
2. Assist patient to explore all aspects and effects of radiation therapy, chemotherapy or surgery on an individual basis.
3. Provide skin care and measures to relieve pain and discomfort associated with jaundice, anorexia and profound weight loss.
4. Monitor patient postoperatively: Vital signs, ABGs and pressures, pulse oximetry, laboratory values and urine output.
5. Provide emotional support to patient and family before, during and after treatment.
6. Discuss patient controlled analgesia (PCA) for severe, escalating pain.
7. If chemotherapy is elected, focus on teaching on prevention of side effects and complications of agents used.
8. If surgery was performed, teach patient about managing the drainage system and monitor for complications.
9. Teach patient and family strategies to prevent skin breakdown and relieve pain, pruritis and anorexia, including pancreatic enzymes, if indicated because of malabsorption and hyperglycemia. Monitor serum glucose levels, if patient has a pancreatic islet tumor.
10. Discuss palliative care with patient with patient and family to relieve discomfort, assist with care, and comply with end-of-life decisions.
11. Instruct family about changes in patient's status that should be reported to the physician.
12. Refer patient for home care for help dealing with problems, discomforts and psychological effects. Discharge to a long-term care setting with communication to staff about prior teaching.

CANCER OF THE LIVER

Few cancers originate in the liver. Primary liver tumors usually are associated with chronic liver disease, hepatitis B and C, and cirrhosis. Hepatocellular carcinoma (HCC), the most common type of primary liver tumor, usually cannot be resected because of rapid growth and metastasis elsewhere. Other types include cholangiocellular carcinoma and combined hepatocellular and cholangiocellular carcinoma. It found early, resection may be possible however, early detection is unlikely.

Cirrhosis, hepatitis B and C, and exposure to certain chemical toxins have been implicated in the etiology of hepatocellular carcinoma (HCC). Cigarette smoking, especially when combined with alcohol use, has also been identified as a risk factor. Other substances that have been implicated include aflatoxins and other similar toxin molds. Metastases from other primary sites, particularly the digestive system, breast and lung are found in the liver 2.5 times more frequently than tumors due to primary liver cancers.

Clinical Manifestations

- Early manifestations include pain (dull ache in upper right quadrant, epigastrium or back) weight loss, of strength anorexia and anemia
- Liver enlargement and irregular surface may be noted on palpation
- Jaundice is present only if larger bile ducts are occluded
- Ascites develops if such nodules obstruct the portal veins or if tumor tissue is seeded in the peritoneal cavity.

Diagnostic Findings

Diagnosis is made on the basis of clinical signs and symptoms, history and physical examination, and results of laboratory and X-ray studies, position emission tomography (PET) scans, liver scans, CT scans, ultrasound, MRI, arteriography, laparoscopy or biopsy, leukocytosis (increased WBC counts), erythrocytosis (increased red blood cell counts), hypercalcemia, hypoglycemia and hypocholesterolemia may also be seen on laboratory assessment. Elevated levels of serum α-fetoprotein (AFP) may be found.

Medical Management /Therapists Measures

Radiation Therapy

1. Intravenous or intra-arterial injection of antibodies tagged with radioactive isotopes that specifically attack tumor-associated antigens.
2. Percutaneous placement of a high-intensity source for interstitial radiation therapy.

Chemotherapy

1. Systemic chemotherapy; embolization of tumor vessels with chemotherapy.
2. Implantable pump to deliver high-concentration chemotherapy to the liver through hepatic artery.

Percutaneous Biliary Drainage

1. Percutaneous biliary drainage is used to bypass biliary ducts abstracted by the liver, pancreatic or bile ducts in patients with inoperable tumors or those who are poor surgical risks.
2. Complications include sepsis, leakage of bile, hemorrhage and reobstruction of the biliary system.
3. Observe patient for fever and chills, bile drainage around the catheter, changes in vital signs and evidence of biliary obstruction, including increased pain or pressure, pruritus and presence of jaundice.

Other Non-surgical Treatment Modalities

1. Hyperthermia: Heated by laser or radiofrequency energy directed to tumors to cause necrosis of the tumors, while sparing normal tissue.

2. Radiofrequency thermal ablation (tumor cell death from coagulation necrosis).
3. Immunotherapy: Lymphocytes with antitumor reactivity as administered.
4. Embolization (ischemia and necrosis of the tumor occur).
5. For multiple small lesions, ultrasound guided injection of alcohol promotes dehydration of tumor cells and tumor necrosis.

Surgical Management

Hepatic resection can be performed when the primary hepatic tumor is localized or when the primary site can be completely excised and the metastasis is limited. Capitalizing on the regenerative capacity of the liver cells, surgeons have successfully removed 90% of the liver. The presence of cirrhosis inhibits the ability of the liver to regenerate. In preparation for surgery the patient's nutritional, fluid and general physical, stamina are assessed, and efforts are undertaken to ensure the biophysical condition possible:

1. Removal of a lobe of the liver is the most common surgical procedure for excising a liver tumor.
2. In patients who are not candidates for resection or transplantation, ablation of HCC may be accomplished be chemicals such as ethanol or by physical means such as radiofrequency ablation or microwave coagulation.
3. Removing the liver and replacing it with a healthy donor organ is another way to treat liver cancer.

Nursing Management\Diagnosis

Refer 'Nursing Management' under 'Cancer' for additional information:

1. Assess for problems related to cardiopulmonary involvement, vascular complications, and respiratory and liver dysfunction.
2. Give careful attention to metabolic abnormalities (glucose, protein and lipids).
3. Provide close monitoring and care for the first 2 or 3 days.
4. Instruct patient and family about care of the biliary catheter and the potential complications and side effects of hepatic artery chemotherapy.
5. Instruct patient about the importance of follow-up visits to permit frequent checks on the response of patient and tumor to chemotherapy, condition of the implanted pump site and any toxic effects.
6. Encourage patient to resume activities as soon as possible, but caution patient to avoid activities that may damage the pump.
7. Provide reassurance and instructions to patient and family to reduce fear that the percutaneous biliary drainage catheter will fall out.
8. Provide verbal and written instructions as well as demonstration of biliary catheter care to patient and family; instruct in techniques to keep catheter site clean and dry to assess the catheter and its insertion site, and to irrigate the catheter to prevent debris and promote patency.
9. Refer patient for home care.
10. Collaborate with the healthcare team patient, and family to identify and implement pain management strategies.

11. Approaches to management of other problems: weakness, pruritus, inadequate dietary intake, jaundice and symptoms associated with metastasis.
12. Assist patient and family in making decisions about hospice care and initiate referrals. Encourage patient to discuss end-of-life care.

HEPATIC FAILURE FULMINANT

Fulminant hepatic failure is the clinical syndrome of sudden and severely impaired liver function in a previously healthy person. It is characterized by the development of first symptoms or jaundice within 8 weeks of the onset of disease. Three categories are frequently cited, i.e. hyperacute, acute and subacute. The hepatic lesion is potentially reversible, and survival rates are approximately 20%–50% depending greatly on the cause of liver failure. Those who do not survive die of massive hepatocellular injury and necrosis. Viral hepatitis a common cause; other causes include toxic drugs and chemicals metabolic disturbances and structural changes.

Clinical Manifestations

- Jaundice and profound anorexia
- Often accompanied by coagulation defects, renal failure and electrolyte disturbances, cardiovascular abnormalities, infection, hypoglycemia, encephalopathy and cerebral edema.

Management

- Liver transplantation (treatment of choice)
- Blood or plasma exchanges
- Liver support systems, such as hepatocytes within synthetic fiber columns, extracorporeal liver assist devices and bioartificial liver, until transplantation is possible.

10

Chapter Cardiovascular Nursing

HYPERTENSION (HYPERTENSIVE CRISIS)

Hypertension is defined as a systolic blood pressure (BP) greater than 140 mm Hg and a diastolic pressure greater than 90 mm Hg, based on two or more measurements. Hypertension can be classified as follow:

1. Normal: Systolic less than 120 mm Hg and the diastolic less than 80 mm Hg.
2. Prehypertension: Systolic 120–139 mm Hg; diastolic 80–89 mm Hg.
3. Stage 1: Systolic 140–159 mm Hg; diastolic 90–99 mm Hg.
4. Stage 2: Systolic > 160 mm Hg; diastolic > 100 mm Hg.

Hypertension is a major risk factor for the atherosclerotic cardiovascular disease, heart failure, stroke and kidney failure. Hypertension carries the risk for premature morbidity or mortality, which increases as systolic and diastolic pressure rise. Prolonged BP elevation damages blood vessels in target organs (heart, kidney, brain and eyes).

Types

Essential (Primary) Hypertension

In adult population with hypertension, between 90% and 95% have essential (primary) hypertension, which has no identifiable medical cause; it appears to be a multifactorial, polygenic condition. For high BP to occur, an increase in peripheral resistance and/or cardiac output must occur secondary to increased sympathetic stimulation, increased renal sodium reabsorption, increased renin-angiotensin-aldosterone system (RAAS) activity, decreased vasodilation of the arterioles, or resistance to insulin action.

Hypertensive emergencies and urgencies may occur in patients whose hypertension has been poorly controlled, whose hypertension has been undiagnosed or in those who have abruptly discontinued their medications.

Hypertension crisis or hypertensive emergency, exists when an elevated BP level must be lowered immediately (not necessarily to less than 140/90 mm Hg) to halt or prevent target organ damage. Hypertensive urgency exists when BP is very elevated, but there is no evidence of impending or progressive target organ damage. Oral agents [(β-adrenergic blocking agents (e.g. labetalol), angiotensin-converting enzyme (ACE) inhibitors (e.g. captopril), or α_2-agonists (e.g. clonidine)] can be administered with the goal of normalizing BP within 24–48 hours. Close hemodynamic monitoring of the patient's BP and cardiovascular status is required. Vital signs should be checked as often as 5 minutes.

Secondary Hypertension

Secondary hypertension is characterized by elevations in BP with a specific cause, such as narrowing of the renal arteries, renal parenchymal disease, hyperaldosteronism (mineralocorticoid hypertension); certain medications, pregnancy and coarctation of the aorta. Hypertension can also be acute, a sign of an underlying condition that causes a change in peripheral resistance or cardiac output.

Clinical Manifestations

1. Physical examination may reveal no abnormality other than high BP.
2. Changes in the retina with hemorrhage, exudates, narrowed arterioles and cotton-wool spots (small infarction).
3. Symptoms usually indicate vascular damage related to organ systems served by involved vessels.
4. Coronary artery disease (AD) with angina or myocardial infarction is the most common consequence.
5. Left ventricular hypertrophy may occur; heart failure ensues.
6. Pathological changes may occur in the kidney [nocturia and increased blood urea nitrogen (BUN) and creatinine levels].
7. Cerebrovascular involvement may occur [(stroke or transient ischemic attack (TIA), i.e. alternations in vision or speech, dizziness, weakness, a sudden fall, or transient or permanent hemiplegia)].

Diagnostic Measures

1. History and physical examination, including retinal examination, laboratory studies for organ damage, including urinalysis, blood chemistry (sodium, potassium, creatinine, fasting blood glucose, total and high-density lipoprotein); electrocardiogram (ECG) and echocardiography to assess left ventricular hypertrophy.
2. Additional studies, such as creatinine clearance, renin level, urine tests and 24-hour urine protein, may be performed.

Medical Management/Therapeutic Measures

1. The goal of any treatment program is to prevent death and complications by achieving and maintaining an arterial BP at or below 140/90 mm Hg (130/80 mm Hg for people with diabetes mellitus or chronic kidney disease), whenever possible.
2. Non-pharmacological approaches include weight reduction, restriction of alcohol and sodium, regular exercise and relaxation. A dietary approaches to stop hypertension (DASH) diet high in fruits, vegetables and low-fat dairy products has been shown to lower elevated pressures.
3. Select a drug class that has the greatest effectiveness, fewest side effects and best chance of acceptance by patient. Two classes of drugs available as first-line therapy are diuretics and beta blockers.
4. Promote compliance by avoiding complicated drug schedules.

Nursing Management

Nursing Assessment

1. Assess BP at frequent intervals; know baseline level. Note changes in pressure that would require a change in medication.
2. Assess for signs and symptoms that indicate target organ damage (e.g. anginal pain; shortness of breath, alterations in speech, vision or balance, nosebleeds, headaches, dizziness, or nocturia).

3. Note the apical and peripheral pulse rate, rhythm and character.
4. Assess extent to which hypertension has affected patient personally, socially or financially.

Nursing Diagnoses/Problems

Based on all the assessment data, major nursing diagnoses may include the following:

1. Deficient knowledge regarding the relationship between the treatment regimen and control of the disease process.
2. Noncompliance with therapeutic regimen related to side effects of prescribed therapy.

Collaborative problems/Potential complications: Left ventricular hypertrophy, myocardial infarction (MI), heart failure, transient ischemic attack (TIA), cerebrovascular accident (CVA), renal insufficiency and failure, retinal hemorrhage.

Planning and Goals/Objectives

The major goals for the patient include understanding of the disease process and its treatment, participation in a self-care program, and absence of complications.

The objectives include the following:

- Maintains adequate tissue perfusion
- Complies with self-care program
- Experiences no complications.

Nursing Interventions

Enhance Knowledge About Condition

1. Emphasize the concept of controlling hypertension (with lifestyle changes and medications) rather than curing it.
2. Arrange a consultation with a dietitian help to develop a plan for improving nutrient intake or weight loss.
3. Advise patient to limit alcohol intake and avoid use of tobacco.
4. Recommend support groups for weight control, smoking, cessation and stress reduction, if necessary.
5. Assist the patient to develop and adhere to an appropriate exercise regimen.

Promoting Family-based Care and Follow-up

Teach patient about self-care

1. Help the patient to achieve BP control through education about managing BP setting goal BP, and providing assistance with social support; encourage family members to support the patient's efforts to control hypertension.
2. Provide written information about the expected effects and side effects of medications; ensure patient understands importance of reporting side effects (and to whom) when they occur.
3. Inform patient that rebound hypertension can occur, if antihypertensive medications are suddenly stopped; advise patient to have an adequate supply of medication.
4. Inform the patient that some medications, such as beta blockers, may cause sexual dysfunction and that other medication are available if problem occur.

5. Encourage and teach patient to measure their BP at home; inform patient that BP varies continuously and the range within which their pressure varies should be monitored.

Continuing care

1. Reinforce importance of regular follow-up care.
2. Obtain patient history and perform physical examination at each clinic visit.
3. Assess for medication-related problems (orthostatic hypotension).
4. Provide continued education and encouragement to enable patients to formulate an acceptable plan that helps them have with their hypertension and adhere to the treatment plan.
5. Assist with behavior change by supporting patients in making small changes with each visit that move them toward their goals.

Gerontological Considerations

1. Compliance with the therapeutic program maybe more difficult for elderly people. The medication regimen can be difficult to remember and the expense can be a problem. Monotherapy (treatment with a single agent), if appropriate, may simplify the medications regimen and make it less expensive.
2. Ensure that the elderly patient understands the regimen and can see, read instructions, open the medication container, and get the prescription refilled.
3. Include family members of caregiver in the teaching program so that they understand the patient's needs, can encourage adherence to the treatment plan and know when, and whom to call if problems arise or information is needed.

Monitoring and Managing Potential Complications

- Assess all body systems, when patient returns for follow-up care to detect any evidence of vascular damage
- Question patient about blurred vision, spots or diminished visual acuity
- Report any significant findings promptly to determine whether additional studies or changes in medications are required.

Evaluation

Evaluation will be on the basis of expected patient outcomes/objectivities as mentioned in planning:

- Maintains adequate tissue perfusion
- Complies with self-care program
- Experiences no complications.

CORONARY ATHEROSCLEROSIS

Coronary atherosclerosis is the most common cause of cardiovascular disease in the United States and is characterized by an abnormal accumulation of lipid or fatty substances and fibrous tissue in the vessel wall. These substances block or narrow the vessel, reducing blood flow to the myocardium. Atherosclerosis involves a repetitious inflammatory response to injure the artery wall and subsequent alteration in the structural and biochemical properties of the arterial walls.

Risk Factors

- High blood cholesterol (hyperlipidemia)
- Cigarette smoking, tobacco use
- Elevated BP
- Hyperglycemia (diabetes mellitus)
- Metabolic syndrome
- Obesity
- Physical inactivity
- Positive family history (a first degree relative with cardiovascular disease at age 55 year or younger for males and at age 65 year or younger for females)
- Age (more than 45 year for men, more than 55 year for women)
- Gender (men develop cardiovascular disease at an earlier age do women)
- Race (higher incidence in African, Americans than in Caucasians).

Clinical Manifestations

Symptoms and complications develop according to the location and degree of narrowing of the arterial lumen, thrombus formation, and obstruction of blood flow to the myocardium. Symptoms include the following:

- Ischemia
- Chest pain; angina pectoris
- Atypical symptoms of myocardial ischemia (shortness of breath, nausea and weakness)
- Myocardial infarction
- Dysrhythmias, sudden death.

Diagnostic Measures

Identification of risk factors for coronary heart disease (CHD) primarily involves taking through history, including family history, physical examination (note BP and weight), and laboratory work (e.g. cholesterol levels) [low-density lipoproteins (LDL) to high-density lipoprotein (HDL), glucose].

Preventions

The major management goal is preventing of CHD, but modifiable risk factors-cholesterol abnormalities, tobacco use, hypertension and diabetes mellitus have been cited as major risk factors for CAD and its complications. As a result, they receive much attention in health promotion programs.

Medical Management

Refer 'Medical Management' under 'Angina Pectoris' and 'Myocardial Infarction' for additional information.

Nursing Management

Refer 'Nursing Management' under 'Angina Pectoris' and 'Acute Coronary Syndrome and Myocardial Infarction' for additional information.

ANGINA PECTORIS

Angina pectoris is a clinical syndrome characterized by paroxysms of pain or a feeling of pressure in the anterior chest. The cause is insufficient coronary blood flow, resulting in an adequate supply of oxygen to need the myocardial demand. Angina is usually a result of atherosclerotic heart disease and is associated with a significant obstruction of a major coronary artery. Factors affecting anginal pain are physical exertion, exposure to cold, eating a heavy meal, stress or any emotional provoking situation that increases BP, heart rate, and myocardial workload. Unstable angina is not associated with the above and may occur at rest.

Clinical Manifestations

1. Pain varies from a feeling of indigestion to a choking or heavy sensation in the upper chest ranging from discomfort to agonizing pain. The patient with diabetes mellitus may not experience severe pain with angina.
2. Angina is accompanied by severe apprehension and a feeling of impending death.
3. The pain is usually retrosternal, deep in the chest behind the upper or middle third of the sternum.
4. Discomfort is poorly localized and may radiate to the neck, jaw, shoulders and inner aspect of the upper arms (usually the left arm).
5. A feeling of weakness or numbness in the arms, wrists and hands, as well as shortness of breath, pallor, diaphoresis, dizziness or lightheadedness, nausea and vomiting, may accompany the pain. Anxiety may occur with angina.
6. An important characteristic of anginal pain is that it subsides when the precipitating cause is removed or with nitroglycerin.

Gerontological Considerations

The elderly person with angina may not exhibit the typical pain profile because of the diminished responses of neurotransmitters that occur with aging. Often, the presenting symptoms in the elderly are dyspnea. Sometimes, there are no symptoms ('silent' CAD), making recognition and diagnosis a clinical challenge. Elderly patients should be encouraged to recognize their chest pain-like symptom (e.g. weakness) as an indication that they should rest or take prescribed medications.

Diagnostic Measures

- Evaluate of clinical manifestations of pain and patient history
- Electrocardiogram changes (12-lead ECG) stress testing and blood tests
- Echocardiogram, nuclear scan or invasive procedures such as cardiac catheterization and coronary angiography.

Medical Management

The other objectives of the medical management of angina are the oxygen demand of the myocardium and to decrease or increase the oxygen supply. Medically, these objectives are met through pharmacological therapy and control of risk factors.

Alternatively, reperfusion procedures maybe used to restore the blood supply to the myocardium. These include percutaneous coronary intervention (PCI) procedures [e.g. percutaneous transluminal coronary angioplasty (PTCA), intracoronary stents and atherectomy] and coronary artery bypass graft (CABG).

Pharmacological Therapy

- Nitrates the mainstay of therapy (nitroglycerin)
- Beta-adrenergic blockers (metoprolol and atenolol)
- Calcium channel blockers/calcium ion antagonists (amlodipine and diltiazem)
- Antidotes and anticoagulant medications [Aspirin, clopidogrel, heparin, glycoprotein (GP) IIb/IIIa agents (O_2 therapy).

Nursing Management

Nursing Assessment

Catheter information about the patient's symptoms and activities, especially those that precede and precipitate attacks of angina pectoris. In addition, assess the patient's risk factors for CAD, the patient's response to angina. The patient's and family's understanding of the diagnosis, and adherence to the current treatment plan.

Nursing Diagnoses/Problems

- Ineffective cardiac tissues perfusion secondary to CAD as evidenced by chest pain or other prodromal symptoms
- Death anxiety
- Deficient knowledge about underlying disease and methods for avoiding complications
- Noncompliance, ineffective management of therapeutic regimen related to failure and accepts necessary lifestyle changes.

Collaborative problems/Potential complications: This include acute coronary syndrome (ACS) and/or MI, dysrhythmias, cardiac arrest, heart failure and cardiogenic shock.

Planning and Goals/Objectives

Goals include immediate and appropriate treatment when angina occurs, prevention of angina, reduction of anxiety, awareness of the disease process and understanding of the prescribed cares, adherence to the self-care program, and absence of complications. The objectives will be:

- Reports that pain is relieved promptly
- Reports decrease anxiety
- Understands way to avoid complications
- Complies with self-care program.

Nursing Interventions

Preoperative Teaching

1. Take immediate action, if patient reports pain or if the person's prodromal symptoms suggest anginal ischemia.
2. Direct the patient to stop all activities and sit or rest in bed in a semi-Fowler's position to reduce the oxygen requirements of the ischemic myocardium.

3. Measure vital signs and observe for signs of respiratory distress.
4. Administer nitroglycerin sublingually and assess the patient's response (repeat up to three doses).
5. Administer oxygen therapy, if the patient's respiratory rate is increased or if the oxygen saturation level is decreased.
6. If the pain is significant and continues after these interventions, the patient is further evaluated for acute MI and may be transferred to a higher-acuity nursing unit.

Reducing Anxiety and Depression

1. Explore implications that the diagnosis has for patient.
2. Provide essential information about the illness and methods of preventing progression.
3. Explain importance of following prescribed directives for the ambulatory patient at home.
4. Explore various stress reduction methods with patient (e.g. music therapy).
5. Preventing pain.
6. Review the assessment findings, identify the level of activity that causes the patient's pain or prodromal symptoms and plan the patient activities accordingly.
7. Factors that trigger angina episodes include:
   - Sudden or excessive exertion
   - Exposure to cold
   - Tobacco use
   - Heavy muscles
   - Excessive weight
   - Some over-the-counter (OTC) drugs, such as diet pills and nasal decongestants or drugs that increase heart rate and BP.

If the patient has pain frequently or with minimal activity alternates the patient's activities with rest periods. Balancing activity and rest is an important aspect of the educational plan for the patient and family.

Teaching Patient Self-care

1. Teaching program for the patient with angina is designed so that the patient and family understand the illness, identify the symptoms of myocardial ischemia, state the action to take when symptoms develop; discuss methods to prevent chest pain, and the advancement of CAD.
2. The goals of education are to reduce the frequency and severity of anginal attacks, to delay the progress of the underlying disease, if possible, to prevent complications.
3. Collaborate on a self-care program with patient, family or friends.
4. Plan activities to minimize angina episodes.
5. Teach patient that any pain unrelieved within 15 minutes by the usual methods, including nitroglycerin, should be treated at the closest emergency center. Patient should call 911 for assistance.

Evaluation

Evaluation will be on the basis of expected patient outcomes/ objectivities as mentioned in planning:

- Reports that pain is relieved promptly
- Reports decreased anxiety

- Understands ways to avoid complications and demonstrates freedom from complications
- Complies with self-care program.

ACUTE CORONARY SYNDROME AND MYOCARDIAL INFARCTION

Acute coronary syndrome (ACS) is an emergent situation characterized by an acute onset of myocardial ischemia that results in myocardial death, i.e. MI if definitive interventions do not occur promptly. Although, the terms coronary occlusion, heart attack and MI are used synonymously the preferred term is MI.

In unstable angina, there is reduced blood flow in a coronary artery, often due to rupture of an atherosclerotic plaque, but the artery is not completely occluded. This is an acute situation that is sometimes referred to as preinfarction angina because the patient will likely have an MI if prompt interventions do not occur.

In an MI, an area of the myocardium is permanently destroyed, typically because plaque rupture and subsequent thrombus formation result in complete occlusion of the artery. Vasospasm (sudden constriction or narrowing) of a coronary artery, decreased oxygen supply (e.g. from acute blood loss, anemia or low BP) and increased demand for oxygen of cocaine) are other causes of MI. In each case, a profound imbalance exists between myocardial oxygen supply and demand. An MI may be defined by the type, the location of the injury to the ventricular wall or by the point in time of the process of infarction (acute, evolving and old).

Clinical Manifestations

In many cases, the signs and symptoms of MI cannot be distinguished from those of unstable angina, hence, the evolution of the term ACS:

1. Chest pain that occurs suddenly and continues despite rest and medication is the primary presenting symptom.
2. Some patients have prodromal symptoms or a previous diagnosis of CAD, but about half report no previous symptoms.
3. Patient may present with a combination of symptoms, including chest pain, shortness of breath, indigestion, nausea and anxiety.
4. Patient may have cool, pale and moist skin; heart rate and respiratory rate maybe faster than normal. These signs and symptoms, which are caused by stimulation of the sympathetic nervous system, may be present only for a short time or may persist.
5. Patient history (description of presenting symptom; history of previous illness and family health history, particularly of heart disease). Previous history should also include information about patient's risk factors for heart disease.
6. Electrocardiography within 10 minutes of pain onset or arrival at the emergency department; echocardiography to evaluate ventricular function.
7. Cardiac enzymes and biomarkers (creatine kinase isoenzymes, myoglobin and troponin).

Medical Management/Therapeutic Measures

The goals of medical management are to minimize myocardial damage, preserve myocardial function and prevent complications such as lethal dysrhythmias and cardiogenic shock:

1. Reperfusion via emergency use of the PCI or thrombolytic medications.
2. Reduce myocardial oxygen demand and increase oxygen supply with medications, oxygen administration, and bedrest.
3. Coronary artery bypass or minimally invasive direct coronary artery bypass (MIDCAB).

Pharmacological Therapy

- Nitrates (nitroglycerin) to increase oxygen supply
- Anticoagulants (Aspirin, heparin)
- Analgesics (morphine sulfate)
- Angiotensin-converting enzyme inhibitors
- Beta blocker initially and a prescription to continue its use after hospital discharge
- Thrombolytics [alteplase (tPA, Activase) and reteplase (rPA, TNKase)]: Must be administered as early as possible after the onset of symptoms, generally within 3–6 hours.

Nursing Management

Nursing Assessment

Obtain baseline data on current status of patient for comparison with ongoing status. Include history of chest pain or discomfort, difficulty breathing (dyspnea), palpitations, unusual fatigue, faintness (syncope) or sweating (diaphoresis). Perform a complete physical assessment, which is crucial for detecting complications and any change in status. The examination should include the following:

1. Assess level of consciousness.
2. Evaluate chest pain (most important clinical finding).
3. Assess heart rate and rhythm; dysrhythmias may indicate not enough oxygen to the myocardium.
4. Assess heart sounds (S_3) can be an early sign of impending left ventricular failure.
5. Measure BP to determine response to pain and treatment; note pulse pressure, which maybe narrowed after an MI, suggesting ineffective ventricular contraction.
6. Assess bowel motility; mesenteric artery thrombosis is a potentially fatal complication.
7. Observe urinary output and check for edema; an early sign of cardiogenic shock in hypotension with oliguria.
8. Examine intravenous (IV) lines and sites frequently.

Nursing Diagnoses/Problems

1. Ineffective cardiac tissue perfusion related to reduced coronary blood flow.
2. Risk for imbalanced fluid volume.
3. Risk for ineffective peripheral tissue perfusion related to decreased cardiac output from left ventricular dysfunction.
4. Death anxiety.
5. Deficient knowledge about post-ACS self-care.

Potential complications: Acute pulmonary edema, heart failure, cardiogenic shock, dysrhythmias cardiac arrest, pericardial effusion and cardiac tamponade.

Planning and Goals/Objectives

The major goals of the patient include relief of pain or ischemic signs, (e.g. ST-segment changes) and symptoms, prevention of myocardial damage, absence of respiratory dysfunction, maintenance or attainment of adequate tissue perfusion, reduced anxiety, adherence to the self-care programs, and absence of early recognition of complications. The objective of that patient will:

- Experiences relief of angina
- Has stable cardiac and respiratory status
- Maintains adequate tissue perfusion
- Exhibits decreased anxiety
- Complies with self-care program
- Experiences absence of complications.

Nursing Interventions (Implementation)

Relieving Signs and Symptoms of Ischemia

1. Administer oxygen in tandem with medication therapy to assist relief of symptoms (inhalation of oxygen reduce pain associated with low levels of circulating oxygen).
2. Assess vital signs frequently as long as patient is experiencing pain.
3. Assist patient to rest back elevated or in cardiac chair to decrease chest discomfort and dyspnea.

Improving Respiratory Function

1. Assess respiratory function to detect early signs of complications.
2. Monitor fluid volume status to prevent overloading the heart and lungs.
3. Encourage patient to breathe deeply and change position often to prevent pooling fluid in lungs bases.

Promoting Adequate Tissue Perfusion

1. Keep patient on bed or chair, rest to reduce myocardial oxygen consumption.
2. Check skin temperature and peripheral pulses frequently to determine adequate tissue perfusion.

Reducing Anxiety

1. Develop a trusting and caring relationship with patient, provide information to the patient and family in an honest and supportive manner.
2. Ensure a quiet environment, prevent interruptions that disturb sleep, use a caring and appropriate touch relaxation technique use humor, and provide spiritual support consistent with the patient's beliefs. Music therapy and pet therapy may also be useful.
3. Provide frequent and private opportunities to share concerns and fears.
4. Provide an atmosphere of acceptance to help patient know that his/her feelings are realistic and normal.

Managing Complications

Monitor closely for cardinal signs and symptoms that signal onset of complications.

Promote Family-based Care and Follow-up

1. Identify the patient's priorities, provide adequate education about heart-healthy living and facilitate the patient's involvement in a cardiac rehabilitation program.
2. Work with the patient to develop a plan to meet specific needs to enhance compliance.
3. Provide home care referral if necessary.
4. Assist the patient with scheduling and keeping follow-up appointments and with adhering to the prescribed cardiac rehabilitation regimen.
5. Provide reminders about follow-up monitoring, including periodic library testing and ECG, as well as general health screening.
6. Monitor the patient's adherence to dietary restrictions and to prescribed medications.
7. If the patient is receiving home oxygen, ensure that the patient is using the oxygen as prescribed and appropriate home safety measures are maintained.
8. If the patient has evidence of heart failure secondary to an MI, appropriate home care guidelines for heart failure are followed.

Potential complications: Based on assessment data, potential complications that may develop include the following.

CARDIOGENIC SHOCK

Cardiogenic shock occurs when the heart's ability to contract or to pump blood is impaired, the supply of oxygen as inadequate for the heart and tissues. The cause of cardiogenic shock is known as either coronary or noncoronary. Coronary cardiogenic shock is more common that non-coronary cardiogenic shock and is seen most often in patients with acute myocardial infarction. Non-coronary causes of cardiogenic shock are related to conditions that stress the myocardium (e.g. severe hypoxemia, acidosis, hypoglycemia, hypocalcemia and tension pneumothorax) and conditions that result ineffective myocardial function (e.g. cardiomyopathies, valvular damage, cardiac tamponade, dysrhythmias).

Clinical Manifestations

- Classic signs include low BP rapid and weak pulse
- Dysrhythmias are common
- Angina pain may be experienced
- Hemodynamic instability
- Complaints of fatigue.

Medical Management/Therapeutic Measures

1. Goals of medical treatment include limiting further myocardial damage, preserving the health myocardium and improving cardiac function. It is necessary first to treat the oxygenation needs of the heart muscle, increasing oxygen supply to the heart muscle while reducing oxygen demands.
2. First-line treatment includes administering supplemental oxygen, controlling chest pain, administering fluids, administering vasoactive medications (e.g. dobutamine, nitroglycerin and dopamine) and antiarrhythmic medications.

3. Hemodynamic monitoring and laboratory marker monitoring are performed.
4. Mechanical cardiac support may be necessary.
5. Coronary cardiogenic shock may be treated with thrombolytic therapy, a PCI, coronary artery bypass graft surgery and/or intra-aortic balloon pump therapy.
6. Non-coronary cardiogenic shock may be treated with cardiac valve replacement, correction of dysrhythmia, correction of acidosis and electrolyte disturbances or treatment of the tension pneumothorax.

Nursing Management

Prevention

1. Early on, identify patients at risk for cardiogenic shock.
2. Promote adequate oxygenation to the heart muscle and decrease cardiac workload (e.g. conserve energy, relieve pain, administer oxygen).

Hemodynamic Monitoring

1. Monitor hemodynamic and cardiac status; maintain arterial lines and ECG equipment.
2. Anticipate need for medications, IV fluids and other equipment.
3. Promptly document report changes in hemodynamic cardiac and pulmonary status.

Medications and Fluids

1. Provide for safe and accurate administration of IV fluids and medications.
2. Monitor for desired effects and side effects (e.g. decreased BP after administering morphine or nitroglycerine, bleeding at arterial and venous puncture sites).
3. Monitor urine output, BUN and serum creatinine levels to detect any decrease in renal function.

Intra-aortic Balloon Counter Pulsations

1. Provide ongoing timing adjustments of the balloon pump for maximum effectiveness.
2. Perform frequent checks of neurovascular status of lower extremities.

Safety and Comfort

Take an active role in ensuring patient's safety and comfort and in reducing anxiety.

HYPOVOLEMIC SHOCK

Hypovolemic shock, the most common type of shock, is characterized by decreased intravascular volume. Hypovolemic shock can be caused by external fluid losses, as in traumatic blood loss or by internal fluid shifts, as in severe dehydration, severe edema, or ascites. Decreased blood volume results in decreased venous return and subsequent decreased ventricular filling, decreased stroke volume and cardiac output and decreased tissue perfusion.

Clinical Manifestations

- Fall in venous pressure rise in peripheral resistance and tachycardia
- Cold, moist skin pallor, thirst and diaphoresis
- Altered sensorium, oliguria, metabolic acidosis, tachypnea
- Most dependable criterion; level of arterial BP.

Medical Management

Goals of treatment are to restore intravascular volume, redistribute fluid volume and correct underlying cause. If the patient is hemorrhaging, bleeding is stopped by applying pressure or by surgery. Diarrhea and vomiting are treated with medications.

Fluid and Blood Replacement

1. At least two IV lines are inserted to administer fluid, medications and/or blood.
2. Lactated Ringer's solution, colloids or 0.9% sodium chloride solution (normal saline) are administered to restore intravascular volume.
3. Blood products are used only if other alternatives are unavailable or blood loss is extensive and rapid.

Redistribution of fluids: Positioning the patient properly assists fluids redistribution as modified. Trendelenburg position is recommended in hypovolemic shock. Elevation of the legs promotes the return of venous blood.

Medication Therapy

If fluid administration fails to reverse hypovolemic shock, then vasoactive medications that prevent cardiac failure are given. Medications are also administered to reverse the cause of the dehydration.

Nursing Management

1. Closely monitor patients at risk for fluid deficits (younger than 1 year or older than 65 year).
2. Assist with fluid replacement before intravascular volume is depleted.
3. Ensure safe administration of prescribed fluids, medications and document the effects.
4. Monitor and promptly report the signs of complications and effects of treatment. Monitor patient closely for adverse effects.
5. Monitor for cardiovascular overload, signs of difficulty breathing, pulmonary edema, hemodynamic pressure, vital signs arterial blood gases, serum lactate level, hemoglobin, hematocrit levels, fluid intake and output.
6. Reduce fear and anxiety about the need for an oxygen mask by giving patient explanations and frequent reassurance.

SEPTIC SHOCK

Septic shock, the most common type of circulatory shock is caused by widespread infection. Gram-negative bacteria are the most common pathogens. Other infectious agents, such as gram-positive bacteria (increasingly), viruses and fungi can also cause septic shock.

Risk Factors

Risk factors for septic shock include the increased use of invasive procedures and indwelling medical devices. The increased number of antibiotic resistant microorganisms and the increasingly older population. Other patients at risk are those with malnutrition or immunosuppression and those with chronic illness (e.g. diabetes mellitus, hepatitis).

Pathophysiology

Microorganism invasion causes an immune response. This immune response activates biochemical cytokines and mediators associated with an inflammatory response and produce a variety of effects leading to shock. The resulting increased in capillary permeability, with fluid loss from the capillaries and vasodilation, results in inadequate perfusion of oxygen, and nutrients to the tissues and cells.

Clinical Manifestations

In Early Stage

- Blood pressure may remain within normal limits (or hypertensive, but responsive to fluids)
- Heart and respiratory rates elevated
- High cardiac output with vasodilation
- Hyperthermia (febrile) with warm, flushed skin, bounding pulses
- Urinary output normal or decreased
- Gastrointestinal status compromised (e.g. nausea, vomiting, diarrhea or decreased bowel sounds)
- Subtle changes in mental status.

As Sepsis Progresses

- Low cardiac output with vasoconstriction
- Blood pressure drops
- Skin cool and pale
- Lower than normal body temperature
- Heart and respiratory rates rapid
- Anuria and multiple organ dysfunctions progressing to failure.

Diagnostic Measures

Septic shock maybe manifested by atypical or confusing clinical signs. Suspect septic shock in any elderly person who develops an unexplained acute confused state, tachypnea or hypotension.

Medical Management/Therapeutic Measures

1. Blood, sputum, urine and wound drainage specimens are collected to identify, and eliminate the cause of infection.
2. Potential routes of infection are eliminated (IV lines rerouted if necessary). Abscesses are drained and necrotic areas debrided.
3. Fluid replacement is instituted.
4. Broad-spectrum antibiotics are started. Recombinant human activated protein C (rhAPC) [drotrecogin alfa (Xigris)] administered to patients with end-organ dysfunction and high risk of death.
5. Aggressive nutritional supplementations (high protein) are provided. Enteral feedings are preferred.

Nursing Management

1. Identify patients at risk for sepsis and septic shock.
2. Carry out all invasive procedures with correct aseptic technique after careful hand hygiene.
3. Monitor IV lines, arterial and venous puncture sites, surgical incisions, trauma wounds, urinary catheters, and pressure ulcers for signs of infection.
4. Reduce patient's temperature when ordered for temperature higher than 40°C (104°F) or if the patient is uncomfortable by administering acetaminophen or applying a hypothermia blanket; monitor closely for shivering.
5. Administer prescribed IV fluids and medications.
6. Monitor and report blood levels [antibiotic, BUN, creatinine level, white blood cells (WBCs) count, hemoglobin, hematocrit levels and platelet count coagulation studies].
7. Monitor hemodynamic status, fluid intake and output, and nutritional status.
8. Monitor daily weights and serum albumin and prealbumin levels to determine daily protein requirements.

HEART FAILURE (COR PULMONALE)

Heart failure, sometimes referred to as congestive heart failure, is the inability of the heart to pump sufficient blood to meet the needs of the tissues for oxygen and nutrients. Heart failure is a clinical syndrome characterized by signs and symptoms of fluid overload or inadequate tissue perfusion. The underlying mechanism of heart failure involves impaired contractile properties of the heart (systolic dysfunction) of filling of the heart (diastolic) that leads to a lower than normal cardiac output. The low cardiac output can lead to compensatory mechanism that cause increased workload in the heart and eventual resistance to filling of the heart.

Heart failure is a progressive, life-long condition that is managed with lifestyle changes and medications to prevent episodes of acute decompensated heart failure, which are characterized by an increase in symptom, decreased cardiac output (CO) and low perfusion. Heart failure results from a variety of cardiovascular conditions, including chronic hypertension, CAD and valvular disease. These conditions can result in systolic failure, diastolic failure or both. Several systemic conditions (e.g. progressive renal failure and uncontrolled hypertension) can contribute to the development and severity of cardiac failure.

Clinical Manifestations

The signs and symptoms of heart failure can be related to which ventricle is affected. Left-sided heart failure (left ventricular failure) causes different manifestations than right-sided heart failure (right ventricular failure). In chronic heart failure; patients may have signs and symptoms of both left and right ventricular failure.

Left-sided Heart Failure

Most often precedes right-sided cardiac failure:

1. Pulmonary congestion, dyspnea, cough, pulmonary crackles and low oxygen saturation levels; an extra heart sound (S_3) or 'ventricular gallop' may be detected on auscultation.

2. Dyspnea on exertion (DOE), orthopnea, paroxysmal nocturnal dyspnea (PND).
3. Cough initially dry and nonproductive, may become moist over the time.
4. Large quantities of frothy sputum, which is sometimes pink (blood tinged).
5. Bibasilar crackles advancing to crackles in all lung fields.
6. Inadequate tissue perfusion.
7. Oliguria and nocturia.
8. With progression of heart failure: Altered digestion, dizziness, light headedness, confusion, restlessness, anxiety, pale or ashen, cool and clammy skin.
9. Tachycardia, weak, thread pulse and fatigue.

Right-sided Heart Failure

- Congestion of the viscera and peripheral tissues
- Edema of the lower extremities (dependent edema), hepatomegaly (enlargement of the liver), ascites (accumulation of fluid in the peritoneal cavity), anorexia, nausea, weakness and weight gain due to retention of fluid.

Diagnostic Measures

1. Assessment of ventricular function.
2. Echocardiogram, chest X-ray, ECG.
3. Cardiac stress testing, cardiac catheterization.
4. Laboratory studies, serum electrolytes, BUN, creatinine, thyroid stimulating hormone (TSH), complete blood count (CBC), brain natriuretic peptide (BNP) and routine urinalysis.

Medical Management/Therapeutic Measures

The overall goals of management of heart failure are relieved patient symptoms, to improve functional status quality of life and to extend survival. Treatment options vary according to the severity of the patient's condition it may include oral and IV medications, major lifestyle changes, supplemental oxygen implantation of assistive devices, and surgical approaches including cardiac transplantation. Lifestyle recommendation includes restriction of dietary sodium, avoidance of excessive fluid intake, alcohol and smoking; weight reduction when indicated and regular exercise.

Pharmacological Treatment

1. Intravenous (IV) infusions, nesiritide, milrinone, dobutamine.
2. Medications for diastolic dysfunction.
3. Possibly anticoagulants, medications that manage hyperlipidemia (stains).
4. Alone or in combination; vasodilators therapy ACE inhibitors, angiotensin II receptors blockers (ARBs), selective beta blockers, calcium channel blockers, diuretic therapy, cardiac glycosides (digitalis) and others.

Surgical Management

Surgical management includes coronary bypass surgery, PTCA, the innovative therapies as indicated (e.g. mechanical assist devices, transplantation).

Nursing Management

Nursing Assessment

The nursing assessment for the patient with heart failure focuses on observing for effectiveness of therapy and for the patient's ability to understand and implement self-management strategies. Signs and symptoms of pulmonary and systemic fluid overload are recorded and reported immediately:

1. Note report of sleep disturbances due to shortness of breath and number of pillows used for sleep.
2. Ask patient about edema, abdominal symptoms, altered mental status, activities of daily living and the activities that cause fatigue.
3. Respiratory: Auscultate lungs to detect crackles and wheezes. Note the rate and depth of respirations.
4. Cardiac: Auscultate for S_3 heart sound (sign heart beginning to fail); document heart rate and rhythm.
5. Assess sensorium and level of consciousness (LOC).
6. Periphery: Assess dependent parts of body for perfusion and edema, the liver for hepatojugular reflux and assess jugular venous distention.
7. Measure intake and output to detect oliguria or anuria; monitoring patient weight daily.

Nursing Diagnoses/Problems

- Activity intolerance and fatigue related to decreased CO
- Excess fluid volume related to the heart failure syndrome
- Anxiety related to breathlessness from inadequate oxygenation
- Powerlessness related to chronic illness and hospitalization
- Ineffective therapeutic regimen management related to lack of knowledge.

Potential complications: It may develop include hypotension, poor perfusion, cardiogenic shock, dysrhythmias, thromboembolism, pericardial effusion and cardiac tamponade.

Planning and Goals/Objectives

Major goal for the patient may include promoting activity and reducing fatigue, relieving fluid overload symptoms, decreasing anxiety or increasing the patient's ability to manage anxiety. Encouraging the patient to verbalize his/her ability to make decisions, and influence outcomes, and teaching the patient about the self-care program. The objectives include the following:

- Demonstrate tolerance for increased activity
- Maintains fluid imbalance
- Experience less anxiety
- Make sound decisions regarding care and treatment.

Nursing Interventions

Promoting Activity Tolerance

1. Monitor patient's response to activities. Instruct patient to avoid prolonged bedrest; patient should rest if symptoms are severe otherwise should resume regular activity.
2. Encourage patient to perform an activity more slowly than usual, for a shorter duration or with assistance initially.

3. Identify barriers that could limit patient's ability to perform an activity and discuss methods of pacing an activity (e.g. chop or peel vegetables while sitting at kitchen table rather than standing at the kitchen counter).
4. Take vital signs, especially pulse, before, during and immediately after an activity to identify whether they are within the predetermined range; heart rate should return to baseline within 3 minutes. If patient tolerates the activity, develop short-term and long-term goals to increase gradually the intensity, duration or frequency of activity.
5. Refer to cardiac rehabilitation program as needs, especially for patients with a recent MI, recent open heart surgery or increased anxiety.

Reducing Fatigue

1. Collaborate with patient to develop a schedule that promotes pacing and prioritization of activities. Encourage patient to alternate activities with period of rest and avoid having two significant energy-consuming activities occur on the same day or in immediate succession.
2. Explain that small frequent meals tend to decrease the amount of energy needed for digestion while providing adequate nutrition.
3. Help patient to develop a positive outlook focused on strengths, abilities and interests.

Managing Fluid Volume

1. Administer diuretics early in the morning so that diuresis does not disturb nighttime rest.
2. Monitor fluid status closely; auscultate lungs, compare daily body weights and monitor intake, and output.
3. Teach patient to adhere to a low-sodium diet by reading food labels and avoiding commercially prepared convenience foods.
4. Assist patient to adhere to any fluid restriction by planning the fluid distribution throughout the day, while maintaining dietary preferences.
5. Monitor IV fluids closely; contact physician or pharmacist about the possibility of double-concentration on of any medications.
6. Position patient or teach patient how to assume a position, that facilitates breathing (increase number of pillows, elevate head of bed), or patient may prefer to sit.
7. Assess for skin breakdown and institute preventive measures (frequent changes of position, positioning to avoid pressure, leg exercises).

Controlling Anxiety

1. Decreased anxiety so that patient's cardiac work is also decreased.
2. Administer oxygen during the acute stage to diminish the work of breathing and to increase comfort.
3. When patient exhibits anxiety, promote physical comfort and psychological support; a family member's presence may provide reassurance; pet visitation or animal-assisted therapy can be also beneficial.
4. When patient is comfortable, teach ways to control anxiety and avoid anxiety provoking situations (relaxation techniques).

5. Assist in identifying factor that contributes to anxiety.
6. Screen for depression, which often accompanies or results from anxiety.
7. In case of confusion and anxiety reactions that affect the patient's safety, the use of restraints should be avoided.
8. Restraints are likely to be resisted and resistance inevitably increases the cardiac workload.

Minimizing Powerlessness

1. Assess for factors contributing to a sense of powerlessness and intervene accordingly.
2. Listen actively to patient often; encourage patient to express concerns and questions.
3. Provide patient with decision-making opportunities with increasing frequency and significance; provide encouragement and praise while identifying patient's progress; assist patient to differentiate between factors that can be controlled, and those that cannot.

Monitoring and Managing Potential Complications

1. Many potential problems associated with heart failure therapy related to the use of diuretics.
2. Monitor for hypokalemia caused by diuresis (potassium depletion) signs are ventricular dysrhythmias, hypotension, muscle weakness and generalized weakness.
3. Monitor for hyperkalemia, especially with the use of inhibitors, ARBs or spironolactone.
4. Hyponatremia (deficiency of sodium in the blood) can occur, which results in disorientation, apprehension wetness fatigue, malaise and muscle cramps.
5. Volume depletion from excessive fluid loss may lead to dehydration and hypotension (ACE inhibitors and beta blockers may contribute to the hypotension).
6. Other problems associated with diuretics include increased serum creatinine and hyperuricemia (excessive uric acid in the blood) that leads to gout.

Promoting Family- and Community-based Care

Teaching patient self-care

1. Provide patient education and involve patient in implementing the therapeutic regimen to promote understanding, and compliance.
2. Support patient and family, encourage them to ask questions so that information can be clarified, and understanding enhanced.
3. Adapt teaching plan according to cultural factors.
4. Teach patient and family how the progression of the disease is influenced by compliance with the treatment of plan.

Continuing Care

1. Refer patient for home care if indicated (elderly patients or patients who have long-standing heart disease and whose physical stamina is compromised). The home care nurse

assesses the physical environment of the home and the patient's support system, and suggests adaptations in the home to meet patient's activity limitations.
2. Assess the physical environment of the home and makes suggestions for adapting the home environment to meet the patient's activity limitations.
3. Reinforce and clarify information about dietary changes and fluid restrictions. The need to monitor symptoms, daily body weights and the importance of obtaining follow-up health care.
4. Encourage patient to increase self-care and responsibility for accomplishing the daily requirements of the therapeutic regimen.
5. Refer to an heart failure clinic if necessary.

Evaluation

- Demonstrates tolerance for increased activity
- Maintains fluid balance
- Experiences less anxiety
- Makes sound decisions regarding care and treatment.

PERICARDITIS (CARDIAC TAMPONADE)

Pericarditis refers to an inflammation the pericardium, the membranous sac enveloping the heart. It may be primary or may develop in the course of variety of medical and surgical disorders. Some causes are unknown; other include infection (usually viral, rarely bacterial or fungal), connective tissue disorders, hypersensitivity states, diseases of adjacent structures, neoplastic disease, radiation therapy, trauma, renal disorders and tuberculosis (TB).

Pericarditis may be subacute, acute or chronic and may be classified by the layers of the pericardium becoming attached to each other (adhesive) or by what accumulates in the pericardial sac; serum (serous), pus (purulent), calcium deposits (calcific), clotting proteins (fibrous) or blood (sanguineous). Frequent or prolonged episodes of pericarditis may lead to thickening and decreased elasticity that restricts the heart's ability to fill properly with blood (constrictive pericarditis). The pericardium may also become calcified, which restricts ventricular contraction. Pericarditis can lead to an accumulation of fluid in the pericardial sac (pericardial effusion) and increased pressure on the heart, leading to calcified tamponade.

Clinical Manifestations

Pericarditis

1. Characteristic symptom is pain. Pain, which is felt over the precordium or beneath the clavicle and in the neck and left scapular region is aggravated by breathing, turning in bed, and twisting the body; it is relieved by sitting (or leaning forward).
2. The most characteristic sign of pericarditis is a creaky of scratchy friction rub heard most clearly at the left lower sternal border.
3. Other signs may include mild fever, increased WBC count, anemia, an elevated erythrocyte sedimentation rate (ESR) or C-reactive protein level, non-productive cough or cough.
4. Dyspnea and other signs and symptoms of heart failure may occur.

Tamponade

1. Falling BP, rising venous pressure (distended neck veins) and distant (muffled) heart sounds with pulsus paradoxus.
2. Shortness of breath, chest tightness or dizziness.
3. Anxious, confused and restless state.
4. Dyspnea, tachypnea and precordial pain.
5. Elevated central venous pressure (CVP).

Diagnostic Measures

Diagnosis is based on history, signs and symptoms; echocardiogram, ECG, computed tomography (CT) and magnetic resonance imaging (MRI) are useful diagnostic tools as well. Occasionally, a video-assisted pericardioscope guided biopsy of the pericardium or epicardium is performed.

Medical Management/Therapeutic Measures

Objectives of management are to determine the causes, to administer therapy for the specific cause (when known), and to detect signs and symptoms of cardiac tamponade.

Bedrest is instituted when cardiac output is impaired until fever, chest pain and friction rub have disappeared.

For Pericarditis

Analgesics and non-steroidal anti-inflammatory drug (NSAIDs) such as aspirin or ibuprofen (Motrin) are used to relieve pain and hasten reabsorption of fluid in rheumatic pericarditis. Colchicine may also be used as an corticosteroids (e.g. prednisone) may be prescribed, if the pericarditis is severe or if the patient does not respond to NSAIDs.

For Cardiac Tamponade

1. Thoracotomy for penetrating cardiac injuries.
2. Pericardiocentesis for pericardial fluid removal.
3. Surgical removal of tough encasing pericardium (pericardiectomy), if indicated.

Nursing Management

Nursing management skills are key to anticipating and identifying the trade of symptoms of cardiac tamponade, falling arterial pressure, rising venous pressure and distant heart sounds. Search diligently for a pericardial friction.

Nursing Assessment

1. Assess pain by observation and evaluation while varying positions of patient determine precipitating intensifying factors (pain influenced by respiratory movements).
2. Assess pericardial friction rub (a pericardial friction rub continuous, distinguish it from a pleural friction rub).
3. Ask patient to hold breath to help in differentiation audible on auscultation, synchronous with heartbeat, best heard at the left sternal edge in the fourth intercostal space where the pericardium comes into contact with the left chest wall, scratchy

or leathery sound, louder at the end of expiration and maybe best heard with patient in sitting position.

4. Monitor temperature frequently, because pericarditis causes an abrupt onset of fever in a previously afebrile patient.

Nursing Diagnoses

Acute pain related to inflammation of the pericardium.

Collaborative problems/Potential complications: Pericardial effusion and cardiac tamponade.

Planning and Goals/Objectives

The major goals of the patient may include relief of pain and absence of complications. The objective will be the patient:

- Free of pain
- Experiences no complications.

Nursing Interventions

Relieving Pain

- Advise bedrest or chair rest in a sitting upright and leaning forward position
- Instruct patient to resume activities of daily living as chest pain and friction rub abate
- Administer medications; monitor and record responses
- Instruct patient to resume bedrest, if chest pain and friction rub recur.

Monitoring and Managing Potential Complications

1. Observe for pericardial effusion, which can lead to cardiac tamponade; arterial pressure falls; systolic pressure falls while diastolic pressure remain stable; pulse pressure narrows; heart sounds progress from being distant to imperceptible.
2. Observe for neck vein distention and other signs of rising CVP.
3. Notify physician immediately upon observing any of the above symptoms and prepare for diagnostic echocardiography and pericardiocentesis. Reassure patient and continue to assess and record signs, and symptoms until physician arrives.

Evaluation

Evaluation is based on the objectives as stated above.

INFECTIVE ENDOCARDITIS

Infective endocarditis is a microbial infection of the endothelial surface of the heart. A deformity or injury of the endocardium leads to accumulation on the endocardium of fibrin and platelets (clot formation). Infectious organisms, usually staphylococci, streptococci, enterococci, pneumococci or *Chlamydia* invade the clot and endocardial lesion. Other causative microorganisms include fungi (e.g. *Candida*, *Aspergillus*) and *Rickettsia*.

Risk Factors

1. Prosthetic heart valves or structural cardiac defects [e.g. valve disorders, hypertrophic cardiomyopathy (HCM)].

2. Age: More common in older people, who are more likely to have degenerative or calcific valve lesion, reduced immunologic response to infection and the metabolic alterations associated with aging.
3. Intravenous drug use: There is a high incidence of staphylococcal endocarditis among IV drug users.
4. Hospitalization: Hospital-acquired endocarditis occurs most often in patients with debilitating disease or dwelling catheters and in those receiving hemodialysis or prolonged IV fluid or antibiotic therapy.
5. Immunosuppression: Patient taking immunosuppressive medications or corticosteroids are more susceptible to fungal endocarditis.

Clinical Manifestations

1. Primary presenting symptoms are fever and a heart murmur; fever may be intermittent or absent, especially in elderly patients. Patients receiving antibiotics or corticosteroids or those who have heart failure or renal failure.
2. Vague complaints of malaise, anorexia, weight loss, cough, back and joint pain.
3. A heart murmur may be absent initially, but develops in almost all patients.
4. Small, painful nodules (Osler's nodes) may be present in the pads of fingers or toes.
5. Irregular, red or purple, painless, flat macules (Janeway lesions) may be present on the palms, fingers, hands, soles and toes.
6. Hemorrhage with pale centers (Roth's spots) caused by emboli may be observed in the fundi of the eyes. Splinter hemorrhages (i.e. reddish brown lines and streaks) may be seen under the fingernails and toenails.
7. Petechiae may appear in the conjunctiva and mucous membranes.
8. Cardiomegaly, heart failure, tachycardia or splenomegaly may occur.
9. Central nervous system manifestations include headache temporary or transient cerebral ischemia and strokes.
10. Embolization may be presenting symptom, it may occur at any time and evolve other organ system embolic phenomena may occur.

Diagnostic Measures

1. A diagnosis of acute infective endocarditis is made when the onset of infection and resulting valvular destruction are rapid occurring within days to weeks.
2. Blood cultures.
3. Doppler or transesophageal echocardiography.

Complications

Complications include heart failure, cerebral vascular complications, valve stenosis or regurgitation, myocardial damage and mycotic aneurysms.

Management/Therapeutic Measures

Objectives of treatment are to eradicate the invading organism through adequate doses of an appropriate antimicrobial agent (continuous IV infusion for 2–6 week at home). Treatment measures include the following:

1. Isolating causative organism through serial blood cultures. Blood cultures are taken to monitor the course of therapy.
2. Monitoring patient's temperature for effectiveness of the treatment.
3. After recovery from the infectious process, seriously damaged valves may require debridement or replacement. For example, surgical valve replacement is required if heart failure develops, if patient has more than one serious systems embolic episode, if infection cannot be controlled of its recurrent or if infection is caused by a fungus.

Nursing Management

1. Provide psychological support, while patient is confined to hospital or home with restrictive IV therapy.
2. Monitor patient's temperature; a fever may be present for weeks.
3. Assess heart sounds for new or worsening murmur.
4. Monitor for signs and symptoms of systemic embolization or for patients with right heart endocarditis, signs and symptoms of pulmonary infarction, and infiltrates.
5. Assess for signs and symptoms of organ damage such as stroke CVA, brain attack meningitis, heart failure, MI, glomerulonephritis and splenomegaly.
6. Instruct patient and family about activity restrictions, medications, and signs and symptoms of infection.
7. Reinforce that antibiotic prophylaxis is recommended for patients who had infective endocarditis and who are undergoing invasive procedures.
8. If patient received surgical treatment, provide postsurgical care and instruction.
9. Refer to home care nurse to supervise and monitor IV antibiotic therapy in the home. For additional nursing interventions, refer Chapter 6 'Preoperative and Postoperative Nursing Management'.

RHEUMATIC ENDOCARDITIS

Acute rheumatic fever, which occurs most often in school-age children, may develop after an episode of group a β-hemolytic streptococcal pharyngitis. Patients with rheumatic fever may develop rheumatic heart disease as evidenced by a new heart murmur, cardiomegaly, pericarditis and heart failure. Prompt treatment of 'strep' throat with antibiotics can prevent the development of rheumatic fever. The *Streptococcus* is spread by direct contract with oral or respiratory secretions. Although the bacteria care the causative agents, malnutrition, overcrowding, poor hygiene and lower socioeconomic status may predispose individuals to rheumatic fever. The incidence of rheumatic fever in the United States and other developed countries has generally decreased, but the exact incidence is difficult to determine because the infection may go unrecognized and people may not seek treatment. Clinical diagnostic criteria are not standardized and autopsies are not routinely performed.

MITRAL REGURGITATION (INSUFFICIENCY)

Mitral regurgitation involves blood flowing back from the left ventricle into the left atrium during systole. Often, the edges of the mitral valve leaflets do not close during systole. There is a problem with one or more of the leaflets, the chordae tendineae, the annulus, or the papillary muscles. With each beat, the left ventricle forces some blood back into the left atrium, causing the atrium to dilate and hypertrophy. This backward flow of blood from the ventricle causes the lungs to become decongested, which adds strain to the right ventricle, resulting in cardiac failure.

Clinical Manifestations

1. Chronic mitral regurgitation is often asymptomatic, but acute regurgitation after MI usually presents as severe heart failure.
2. Dyspnea, fatigue and weakness are the most common symptoms.
3. Palpitations, shortness of breath on exertion and cough from pulmonary congestion also occur.

A systolic murmur is heard as a high pitched blowing sound at the apex. The pulse may be regular and of good volume or it may be irregular as a result of extrasystolic beats or atrial fibrillation. Doppler echocardiography is used to diagnose and monitor the progression of mitral regurgitation. Transesophageal echocardiography (TEE) provides the best images of the mitral valve.

Management

Management is the same as for heart failure. Surgical intervention consists of mitral valve replacement or valvuloplasty.

MITRAL STENOSIS

Mitral stenosis is the progressive thickening and contracture of the mitral valve leaflets and chordae tendineae that causes narrowing of the orifice and progressive obstruction to blood flow from the atrium into the left ventricle. Normally, the mitral valve opening is wide as three fingers. In cases of marked stenosis, the opening narrows to the width of a pencil. The left atrium dilates and hypertrophies because it has great difficulty moving blood into the ventricle and because of the increased blood volume the atria must now hold. Because there is no valve to protect the pulmonary veins from the backward flow of blood from the atrium, the pulmonary circulation becomes congested. The resulting high pulmonary pressure can eventually lead to right ventricular failure.

Symptoms

1. The first symptom is often dyspnea on exertion (due to pulmonary venous hypertension).
2. Progressive fatigue (result of low cardiac output), dry cough or wheezing, hemoptysis, palpitations, orthopnea, PND and repeated respiratory infections may be noted.
3. Weak and often irregular pulse (because of atrial fibrillation) may also be noted.

Nursing Assessment

- Doppler echocardiography is used to diagnose mitral stenosis
- Echocardiography and cardiac catheterization with angiography may be used to help determine the severity of the mitral stenosis.

Medical/Nursing Management

Refer 'Medical Management' and 'Nursing Management' under 'Heart Failure' for additional information. Additional management measures include the following:

- Congestive heart failure is treated
- Anticoagulants to decrease the risk for developing atrial thrombus
- Treatment of anemia if required
- Surgical intervention consists of valvuloplasty, usually a commissurotomy to open or rupture the fused commissures of the mitral valve
- Percutaneous transluminal valvuloplasty or mitral valve replacement maybe performed.

MITRAL VALVE PROLAPSE

Mitral valve prolapse is a dysfunction of the mitral valve leaflets that prevents the mitral valve from closing completely during systole. Blood then regurgitates from the left ventricle back into the left atrium. It occurs more frequently in women.

Clinical Manifestations

1. The syndrome may produce no symptoms or may progress rapidly and result in sudden death.
2. Patients may experience symptoms of fatigue, shortness of breath (not correlated with activity), lightheadedness, dizziness, syncope, palpitations, chest pain and anxiety.
3. Fatigue may be present regardless of the person's activity level and amount of rest or sleep.
4. During the physical examination, a mitral (systolic) click is identified. Presence of a click is an early sign that a valve leaflet is ballooning into the left atrium.
5. A murmur of mitral regurgitation maybe heard, if progressive valve leaflet stretching and regurgitation have occurred.
6. A few patient's experience signs and symptoms of heart failure if mitral regurgitation exists.

Medical Management

Medical management is directed at controlling symptoms:

- Dietary restrictions: Avoidance of alcohol, caffeine, smoking cessation
- Antiarrhythmic medications may be prescribed
- In advanced stages, mitral valve repair or replacement may be necessary.

Nursing Management

1. Teach patient about the diagnosis and the possibility that the disorder is hereditary.

2. Teach the patient how to minimize risk for infectious endocarditis, practicing good oral hygiene, obtaining routine dental care, avoiding body piercing and body branding, and not using toothpicks or other sharp objects in the oral cavity.
3. Explain the need to inform the healthcare provider about any symptoms that may develop.
4. Explain that alcohol, caffeine, ephedrine and epinephrine, which may be over the counter preparations, may stimulate dysrhythmias. Teach patient to read product labels to avoid these agents.
5. Explore possible diet, physical activity, sleep and other lifestyle factors that may correlate with symptoms.

AORTIC INSUFFICIENCY (REGURGITATION)

Aortic regurgitation is the flow of blood back into the left ventricle from the aorta during diastole. It may be caused by inflammatory lesions that deform the leaflets of the aortic valve, orifice, result from infective or rheumatic endocarditis, congenital abnormalities, diseases such as syphilis, a dissecting aneurysm that causes dilation or tearing of the ascending aorta, blunt chest, trauma, or deterioration of an aortic valve replacement. In many cases, the cause is unknown and is classified as idiopathic.

Clinical Manifestations

1. Develops without symptoms in most patients.
2. Earliest manifestations: Increased force of heartbeat, i.e. visible or palpable pulsations over the temporal arteries (head) and at the neck (carotid).
3. Exceptional dyspnea and fatigue.
4. Signs and symptoms of progressive left ventricular failure (orthopnea, paroxysmal nocturnal dyspnea).
5. Widened pulse pressure.
6. Water-hammer (Corrigan's) pulse (pulse strikes the palpating finger with quick, sharp strokes and then suddenly collapses).

Diagnostic Measures

The diagnostic may be confirmed by Doppler echocardiography (preferably transesophageal), radionuclide imaging, ECG, MRI and cardiac catheterization.

Medical Management

1. Advise patient to avoid physical exertion, competitive sports and isometric exercise.
2. Treat dysrhythmias and heart failure.
3. Medications usually prescribed first for patients with symptoms of aortic regurgitation are vasodilators such as calcium channel blockers [e.g. nifedipine, (Adalat, Procardia)] and ACE inhibitors [e.g. captopril (Capoten), enalapril (Vasotec), lisinopril (Prinivil, Zestril), ramipril (Altace) or hydralazine (Apresoline)].
4. The treatment of choice is aortic valvuloplasty or valve replacement, preferably performed before left ventricular failure occurs. Surgery is recommended for any patient with left ventricular hypertrophy, regardless of the presence or absence of symptoms.

Nursing Management

- Teach patient about wound care, diet, activity, medications and self-care
- Instruct patient on importance of antibiotic prophylaxis to prevent endocarditis
- Reinforce all new information and self-care instructions for 4–8 weeks after the procedure.

Refer Chapter 6 'Preoperative and Postoperative Nursing Management' for additional information.

AORTIC STENOSIS

Aortic valve stenosis is the narrowing of the orifice between the left ventricle and the aorta. In adults, the stenosis is often a result of degenerative calcifications or it may be a result of rheumatic endocarditis or cusp calcification of unknown cause. There is progressive narrowing of the valve orifice over a period of several years to several decades. The heart muscle increases in size (hypertrophy) in response to all degrees of obstruction; clinical signs of heart failure occur when compensatory mechanisms of the heart failure.

Clinical Manifestations

- Exceptional dyspnea
- Orthopnea, PND and pulmonary edema
- Dizziness and syncope (fainting)
- Angina pectoris
- Blood pressure possibly low, but usually normal
- Low pulse pressure (30 mm Hg or less)
- Physical examination: Loud rough, systolic murmur heard over the aortic area; vibration over the base of the heart.

Diagnostic Measures

- The 12-lead ECG and echocardiogram
- Left-sided heart catheterization.

Medical Management

Medications are prescribed to treat dysrhythmia or left ventricular failure. Definitive treatment for aortic stenosis is surgical replacement of the aortic valve. Patients, who are symptomatic and are not surgical candidates may benefit from one or two balloon percutaneous valvuloplasty procedures.

Nursing Management

Refer 'Preoperative and Postoperative Nursing Management' for additional information.

ARTERIAL EMBOLISM AND ARTERIAL THROMBOSIS

An arterial embolus is a vascular occlusion. It arises most commonly from thrombi that develop in the chamber of the heart as a result of atrial fibrillation, MI, infective endocarditis or chronic heart failure.

Arterial thrombosis is a slowly developing clot in a degenerated vessel that can itself occlude an artery. Thrombi also become detached and are carried from the left side of the heart into the arterial system, where they cause obstruction. The immediate effect is cessations of distal blood flow. Secondary vasospasm can contribute to ischemia. Emboli tend to lodge at arterial bifurcations and areas of atherosclerotic narrowing (cerebral, mesenteric, renal and coronary arteries). Acute thrombosis frequently occurs in patients with pre-existing ischemic symptoms.

Clinical Manifestations

The symptoms of arterial emboli depend primarily on the size of the embolus, the organ involved and the state of the collateral vessels:

1. Symptoms can generally be described as the six 'P's: Pain, pallor, pulselessness, paresthesia, poikilothermic (coldness) and paralysis.
2. The part of the limb below the occlusion is markedly colder and paler than the part above as a result of ischemia.
3. Sudden or acute onset of symptoms and apparent source for the embolus is diagnostic.
4. Two-dimensional transthoracic echocardiography or TEE, chest X-ray and ECG may reveal underlying cardiac disease.
5. Non-invasive duplex and Doppler ultrasonography can determine the presence and extent of underlying atherosclerosis, and arteriography maybe performed.

Medical Management/Therapeutic Measures

1. In cases of acute embolic occlusion, heparin therapy is initiated immediately, followed by emergency embolectomy as the surgical procedure of choice only, if the involved extremity is viable. Percutaneous thrombectomy devices, which require inserting a catheter into the obstructed artery, may also be used.
2. When collateral circulation is affected, the anticoagulant heparin is administered intravenously. Intra-arterial thrombolytic therapy may be administered with agents such as streptokinase, reteplase, staphylokinases or urokinase and others. Contraindications to peripheral thrombolytic therapy include active internal bleeding, cerebrovascular hemorrhage, recent major surgery, uncontrolled hypertension and pregnancy.

Nursing Management

1. Encourage movement of the leg to stimulate circulation and prevent stasis.
2. Continue anticoagulants to prevent thrombosis of the affected artery and to diminish development of subsequent thrombi.
3. Assess surgical incision frequently for potential hemorrhage.
4. Assess pulses, Doppler signals, ankle-brachial index (ABI), and motor and sensory function every hour for the first 24 hours, because significant changes may indicate reocclusion.

AORTIC ANEURYSM

An aneurysm is a localized sac or dilation formed at a weak point in the wall of the artery. It may be classified by its shape or form. The most common forms of aneurysms are saccular and fusiform. A saccular aneurysm projects from only one side of the vessel. If an entire arterial segment becomes dilated, a fusiform aneurysm is develops. Very small aneurysms due to localized infection are called mycotic aneurysm. Historically, the cause of abdominal aortic aneurysm is the most common type of degenerative aneurysm, has been attributed to atherosclerotic changes in the aorta. Occasionally in an aorta diseased by arteriosclerosis, a tear develops in the intima or the media degenerates resulting in a dissection. Arterial dissections are three times more common in men than in women and occur most commonly in the age group of 50–70 years. Aneurysms are serious because they can rupture leading to hemorrhage and death.

Thoracic aortic aneurysm occurs most frequently in men between the ages of 40 and 70 years. The thoracic area is the most common site for the development of a dissecting aneurysm. About one third of patients die from rupture. Abdominal aortic aneurysms are more common among Caucasians and affect men four times more often than women. These are most prevalent in elderly patients. Most of this aneurysm occurs below the renal arteries (infrarenal aneurysm).

Most abdominal aortic aneurysm occurs in patient between 62 and 90 years of age. Rupture is likely with coexisting hypertension and with aneurysms more than 6 cm wide. In most cases, at this point the chances of rupture are greater than the chance of each during surgical repair. If the elderly patient is considered at moderate risk of complications related to surgery or anesthesia, aneurysm is not repaired until it is at least 5.5 cm (2 inch) wide.

Clinical Manifestations

Thoracic Aortic Aneurysm

- Dyspnea, cough (paroxysmal and brassy)
- Hoarseness, stridor or weakness, or complete loss of the aphonia
- Dysphagia
- Dilated superficial veins on chest, neck or arms
- Edematous areas on chest wall
- Cyanosis
- Unequal pupils
- Constant boring pain, which may occur only when the patient is in the supine position (prominent symptom)
- Symptoms vary and depend on how rapidly the aneurysm dilates and affects the surrounding intrathoracic structures. Some patients are asymptomatic.

Abdominal Aortic Aneurysm

1. Only about 40% of patient's pain describing as tearing or 'ripping' in anterior chest or back, extending to shoulder, epigastric area, or abdomen (may be mistaken for acute MI).
2. Patient complaints of heart beating in abdomen, when lying or feeling abdominal throbbing.
3. Cyanosis and mottling of the toes is associated with thrombus.

Dissecting Aneurysm

1. Sudden onset with severe and persistent pain described on tearing or ripping in anterior chest or back extending to shoulders, epigastric area or abdomen (may be mistaken for MI).
2. Pallor, sweating and tachycardia.
3. Pressure elevated or markedly different from one arm to the other.

Diagnostic Measures

Aortic Aneurysm

Chest X-ray, computed tomography angiography (CTA) and TEE.

Abdominal Aortic Aneurysm

Palpation of pulsatile mass in the middle and upper abdomen (a systolic bruit may be heard over the mass); duplex ultrasonography or CTA is used to determine the size, length and location of the aneurysm.

Dissecting Aneurysm

Arteriography, CTA, TEE, duplex ultrasonography and magnetic resonance angiography (MRA).

Medical Management

Medical or surgical treatment depends on the type of aneurysm. For a ruptured aneurysm, prognosis is poor and surgery is performed immediately.

Pharmacological Management

When surgery can be delayed, medical measures include the following:

1. Strict control of BP.
2. Systolic pressure is maintained at 100–120 mm Hg with antihypertensive agents, including diuretics, beta blockers, ACE inhibitors, angiotensin II receptor antagonists and calcium channel blockers.

Surgical Management

An expanding or enlarging abdominal aortic aneurysm is likely to rupture. Surgery is the treatment of choice for abdominal aortic aneurysms more than 5.5 cm (2 inch) wide or those that are enlarging; the standard treatment has been open surgical repair of the aneurysm by resecting the vessel and sewing a bypass graft in place. An alternative for treatment an infrarenal abdominal aortic aneurysm is endovascular grafting, which involves the transluminal placement and attachment of sutureless aortic graft prosthesis across an aneurysm.

Nursing Management

Preoperative Assessment

1. Assessment is guided by anticipating a rupture (signs include persistent or intermittently back or abdominal pain that may be localized in the middle or lower abdomen or lower back) and by recognizing that the patient may have cardiovascular, cerebral, pulmonary, and renal impairment from atherosclerosis.
2. Assess functional capacity of all organ systems.
3. Implement medical therapies to stabilize patient.

Postoperative Assessment

1. Frequently monitor pulmonary, cardiovascular, renal and neurological status.

2. Monitor for complications: Arterial occlusion, hemorrhage, infection, ischemic bowel, renal failure and impotence.
3. Constant intense back pain, falling BP and increasing hematocrit level are signs of a rupturing abdominal aortic aneurysm. Hematomas into the scrotum, perineum, flank or penis indicate retroperitoneal rupture. Rupture into the peritoneal is rapidly fatal.

INTRACRANIAL ANEURYSM

An intracranial (cerebral) aneurysm is a dilation of the walls of a cerebral artery that develops as a result of weakness in the aortic wall. Its cause is unknown, but it may be due to atherosclerosis, a congenital defect of the vessel walls, hypertensive vascular disease, head trauma or advancing age. Most commonly affected areas are the internal carotid, anterior or posterior cerebral, anterior or posterior communicating and middle cerebral arteries. Symptoms are produced when the aneurysm presses on nearby cranial nerves or brain fissure or rupture, causing subarachnoid hemorrhage. Prognosis depends on the age and neurologic condition of the patient, associated diseases and the extent and location of the aneurysm.

Clinical Manifestations

1. Neurologic deficits (similar to those of ischemic stroke).
2. Rupture of the aneurysm causes sudden, unusually severe headache; often loss of consciousness for a variable period.
3. Pain and rigidity of the back of the neck and spine; and visual disturbances (visual loss, diplopia, ptosis). Tinnitus, dizziness and hemiparesis may also occur.
4. If the aneurysm leaks blood and forms a clot, patient may show little neurological deficit or may have severe bleeding, resulting in cerebral damage followed rapidly by coma and death.

Diagnostic Measures

Computed tomography scan or MRI, cerebral angiography and lumbar puncture are diagnostic procedures used to confirm an aneurysm.

Medical Management/Therapeutic Measures

1. Allow the brain to recover from the initial insult (bleeding).
2. Prevent or minimize the risk of rebleeding.
3. Prevent or treat other complications; rebleeding, cerebral vasospasm, acute hydrocephalus and seizures.
4. Provide bedrest with sedation to prevent agitation and stress.
5. Manage vasospasm with calcium channel blockers, such as nimodipine (Nimotop). Endovascular techniques may also be used.
6. Administer supplemental oxygen and maintain the hemoglobin and hematocrit at acceptable levels to assist in maintaining tissue oxygenation.
7. Institute surgical treatment (arterial bypass) or medical treatment to prevent rebleeding.
8. Manage increased intracranial pressure (ICP) by draining the cerebrospinal fluid (CSF) via ventricular catheter drainage.

9. Administer mannitol to reduce ICP, and monitor for signs of dehydration and rebound elevation of ICP.
10. Administer antifibrinolytic agents to delay or prevent dissolution of the clot if surgery is delayed or contraindicated.
11. Manage systemic hypertension with antihypertensive therapy, arterial hemodynamic monitoring, and stool softener to prevent straining and elevation of BP.

Nursing Management

Assessment

1. Perform a complete neurological assessment; level of consciousness, papillary reaction (sluggishness), motor and sensory function, cranial nerve deficits (extraocular eye movements, facial droop and ptosis), speech difficulties, visual disturbances or headache, and nuchal rigidity or other neurologic deficits.
2. Document and report neurologic assessment findings and assess, and report any changes in patient's condition.
3. Detect subtle changes, especially altered levels of consciousness (earliest signs of deterioration include mild drowsiness and slight slurring of speech).

Nursing Diagnoses

- Ineffective tissue perfusion (cerebral) related to bleeding or vasospasm
- Disturbed sensory perception due to the restriction of aneurysms precautions
- Anxiety due to illness or restrictions of aneurysm precautions.

Collaborative problems/Potential complications: Vasospasm, seizures, hydrocephalus, aneurysm rebleeding and hyponatremia.

Planning and Goals

Patients' goals include improved cerebral tissue perfusion, relief of sensory and perceptual deprivation, and relief of anxiety and absence of complications.

Nursing Interventions

Improving Cerebral Tissue Perfusion

1. Monitor closely for neurological deterioration and maintain neurologic flow record.
2. Check BP, pulse, level of consciousness, pupilating responses and motor function hourly; monitor respiratory status and report changes immediately.
3. Implement aneurysm precautions (immediate and absolute bedrest in quiet, non-stressful setting; restrict visitors, except for family).
4. The head of bed 15°–30° or as ordered.
5. Avoid any activity that suddenly increases BP or obstructs venous return (e.g. Valsalva maneuver and straining), instruct the patient to exhale during voiding or defecation to decrease strain, eliminate caffeine, administer all personal care and minimize external stimuli.

6. Apply antiembolism stockings or sequential compression devices. Observe legs for sign and symptoms of deep vein thrombosis (DVT) tenderness, redness, swelling, warmth and edema.

Relieving Sensory Deprivation

- Keep sensory stimulation to a minimum
- Explain restrictions to help reduce patient's sense of isolation.

Relieving Anxiety

- Inform patient of plan and care
- Provide support and appropriate reassurance to patient and family.

ARTERIOSCLEROSIS AND ATHEROSCLEROSIS

Arteriosclerosis or hardening of the arteries is the most common disease of the arteries. It is a diffuse process whereby the muscle fibers and the endothelial lining of the walls of small arteries and arterioles become thickened.

Atherosclerosis primarily affects the intima of the large and medium, sized arteries, causing changes that include the accumulation of lipids (atheromas), calcium, blood components, carbohydrates and fibrous tissue on the intimal layer of the artery. Although the pathological processes of arteriosclerosis and atherosclerosis differ, rarely does on occur without the other, and the terms often are used interchangeably. The most common direct results of atherosclerosis in the arteries include narrowing (stenosis) of the lumen and obstruction by thrombosis, aneurysm, ulceration, and rupture; ischemia and necrosis occur if the supply of blood, nutrients and oxygen is severely, and permanently disrupted.

Atherosclerosis can develop anywhere in the body, but is most common in bifurcation or branch areas of blood vessels.

Atherosclerosis lesions are of two types; fatty streak (composed of lipids and elongated smooth muscle cells) and fibrous plaques (predominantly found in the abdominal aorta and coronary, popliteal, and internal carotid arteries).

Risk Factors

Many risk factors are associated with atherosclerosis; the greater the number of risk factors, the greater the likelihood of developing the disease, i.e:

- The use of tobacco products (strongest risk factor)
- High fat intake (suspected risk factor, along with high serum cholesterol and blood lipids level)
- Hypertension
- Obesity, stress and lack of exercise
- Elevated C-reactive protein.

Clinical Manifestations

Clinical features depend on the tissue or organ affected; heart (angina and MI due to coronary atherosclerosis), brain (transient ischemic attacks and stroke due to cerebrovascular disease), peripheral vessels (include hypertension and symptoms of aneurysm of the aorta, renovascular disease, atherosclerotic lesions of the extremities).

Medical Management/Therapeutic Measures

1. The management of atherosclerosis involves modification of risk factors, a controlled exercise program to improve circulation and its functioning capacity, medication therapy, and interventional or surgical graft procedures (inflow or outflow procedures).
2. Several radiologic techniques are important adjunctive therapies to surgical procedures. They include arteriography, percutaneous transluminal angioplasty, and stents and stent-grafts.

BUERGER'S DISEASE (THROMBOANGIITIS OBLITERANS)

Buerger's disease is a recurring inflammation of the intermediate, and small arteries and veins of the lower and upper extremities. It results in thrombus formation and segmental occlusion of the vessels and is differentiated from other vessels diseases by its microscopic appearance. Buerger's disease occurs most often in men between 20 and 35 years of age and it has been reported in all races and in many areas of the world. There is considerable evidence that heavy smoking or chewing of tobacco is a causative or an aggravating factor.

Clinical Manifestations

1. Pain is the outstanding symptom (generally bilateral and symmetric with focal lesions). Patients complain of cramps in the feet, particularly the arches, after exercise (instep claudication). Pain is relieved by rest.
2. Burning pain aggravated by emotional disturbances, nicotine or chilling, digital rest pain (fingers or toes); and a feeling of coldness or sensitivity to cold may early symptoms.
3. Color changes (rubor) of the feet progress to cyanosis (in only one extremity or certain digits) that appears when the extremity is in a dependent position.
4. Various types of paresthesia may develop; radial and ulnar artery pulses are absent or diminished if upper extremities are involved.
5. Eventually ulceration and gangrene occur.

Diagnostic Measures

Segmental limb BP, duplex ultrasonography and contrast angiography are used to identify occlusions.

Medical Management/Therapeutic Measures

Main objectives are to improve circulation to the extremities, prevent the progression of the disease, and protect the extremities from trauma and infection. (Refer 'Medical Management' under 'Peripheral Arterial Occlusive Disease' for additional information). Treatment measures include the following:

1. Completely stopping use of tobacco.
2. Regional sympathetic block or ganglionectomy produces vasodilation and increases blood flow.
3. Conservative debridement of necrotic tissue is used in treatment of ulceration and gangrene.
4. If gangrene of a toe develops, usually a below knee amputation, or occasionally in above knee amputation is necessary.

Indications for amputation are worsening gangrene (especially if moist), severe pain during rest or severe sepsis.

5. Vasodilators are rarely prescribed (cause dilation of healthy vessels only).

Nursing Management

Refer 'Nursing Management' under 'Peripheral Arterial Occlusive Disease' for additional information.

RAYNAUD'S PHENOMENON

Raynaud's phenomenon is a form of intermittent arteriolar vasoconstriction that results in coldness, pain and pallor of the finger tips or toes. Primary or idiopathic Raynaud's disease occurs in absence of underlying disease. Secondary Raynaud's (Raynaud's syndrome) occurs in associated with an underlying disease, usually a connective tissue disorder, such as systemic lupus erythematosus, arterial lesions. Raynaud's phenomenon is most common in women between 16 and 40 years of age, and it occurs more frequently in cold climates and during the winter.

The prognosis for patients with Raynaud's phenomenon varies; some slowly improve, some become progressively worse and other shows no change. Raynaud's symptoms may be mild so that treatment is not required. However, secondary Raynaud's is characterized by vasospasm and fixed blood vessel obstruction that may lead to ischemia, ulceration, and gangrene.

Clinical Manifestations

1. Pallor brought on by sudden vasoconstriction followed by cyanosis and hyperemia (exaggerated reflow) due to vasodilation with a resultant red color (rubor); the progression follows the characteristic color change to white, blue and red.
2. Numbness tingling and burning pain occurs as color changes.
3. Involvement tends to be bilateral and symmetric, and may involve toes and fingers.

Medical Management

Avoiding the particular stimuli (e.g. cold, tobacco) that provoke vasoconstriction is a primary factor in controlling Raynaud's phenomenon. Calcium channel blockers [nifedipine (Procardia), amlodipine (Norvasc)] may be effective in relieving symptoms. Sympathectomy (interrupting the sympathetic nerves by removing the sympathetic ganglia or dividing their branches) may help some patients.

Nursing Management

1. Instruct patient to avoid situations that may be stressful or unsafe.
2. Advise patient to minimize exposure to cold, remain indoors as much as possible and wear protective clothing when outdoors during cold weather.
3. Reassure patient that serious complications (gangrene and amputation) are not usual.

4. Emphasize the importance of avoiding nicotine (smoking cessation without use of nicotine patches); assist in finding support group.
5. Advise patient to handle sharp object carefully to avoid injuring the fingers.
6. Inform patient about postural hypotension that may result from medications.

PERIPHERAL ARTERIAL OCCLUSIVE DISEASES

Arterial insufficiency of the extremities is found more often in men and predominantly in the legs. The age of onset and the severity are influenced by the type and atherosclerosis risk factors present. Obstructive lesions are predominantly confined to segments of the arterial system extending from the aorta, below the renal arteries to the popliteal artery.

Clinical Manifestations

Intermittent Claudication

1. Claudication is the hallmark of peripheral arterial occlusive disease, which insidious and described as aching, cramping, fatigue or weakness. Patient may report increased pain with ambulation.
2. Rest pain is persistent, aching or boring and is usually present in distal extremities with severe disease.
3. Elevation or horizontal placement of the extremity aggravates pain, lowering the extremity to a dependent position reduces pain.

Other Manifestations

1. Coldness or numbness in the extremities accompanies intermittent claudication.
2. Extremities may be cool and exhibit pallor on elevation or a ruddy, cyanotic color when in a dependent position.
3. Skin and nail changes, ulcerations, gangrene, and muscle atrophy may be evident.
4. Bruits may be auscultated and peripheral pulses may be diminished or absent.
5. Inequality of pulses between extremities or absence of a normally palpable pulse is a sign of peripheral arterial disease (PAD).
6. Nails may be thickened and opaque, and the skin shiny, atrophic, and dry with sparse hair growth.

Diagnostic Measures

The diagnosis of peripheral arterial occlusive disease may be made using continuous wave. Doppler and ankle-brachial index (ABI) tests, treadmill testing for claudication, duplex ultrasonography or other imaging studies previously described.

Medical Management/Therapeutic Measures

Key treatment measures include pharmacotherapy and surgery, pentoxifylline (Trental) and cilostazol (Pletal) are approved for the treatment of symptomatic claudication. Antiplatelet agents such as Aspirin or clopidogrel (Plavix) are used to prevent the formation of thromboemboli. Statin therapy can be used in some patients to reduce the incidence of new intermittent claudication symptoms. Surgery is reserved for treatment of severe and disabling claudication or when the limb is at risk of amputation because of tissue necrosis, and may include endarterectomy, bypass grafts, and vein grafts. Exercise programs combined with reduction and smoking cessation often improve activity limitations.

Nursing Management

Maintaining Circulation Postoperatively

1. The primary objective in postoperative management of patients who have had vascular procedures is to maintain adequate circulation through the arterial repair.
2. Check pulses, Doppler assessment, color and temperature, capillary refill, and sensory and motor function of the affected extremity and compare with those of the other extremity, record values initially in every 15 minutes and then at progressively longer intervals.
3. Perform Doppler evaluation of the vessels distal to the bypass graft for all postoperative vascular patients because it is more sensitive than palpation for pulses.
4. Monitor ABI every 8 hours for the first 24 hours.
5. Notify surgeon immediately if a peripheral pulse disappears, this may indicate thrombotic occlusion of the graft.

Monitoring and Managing Potential Complications

1. Monitor urine output (more than 30 mL/h), CVP, mental status, and pulse rate and volume to permit early recovery and treatment of fluid imbalances.
2. Instruct patient to avoid leg crossing and prolonged extremity dependence.
3. Teach patient to perform leg elevation and to exercise limbs while in bed to reduce edema.
4. Monitor for compartment syndrome (sever limb edema pain and decreased sensation).

Promoting Family- and Community-based Care

1. Assess patient's ability to manage independently or availability of family and friends to assist.
2. Determine patient's motivation to make lifestyle changes needed with chronic disease.
3. Assess patient's knowledge and ability to assess for postoperative complications, such as infection, occlusion of graft and decreased blood flow.
4. Determine if patient wants to stop smoking and encourage all efforts to do so.

VEIN DISORDERS

Vein disorders include venous thrombosis, thrombophlebitis, phlebothrombosis and DVT.

Although the vein disorders described here do not necessarily present an identical pathology for clinical purposes, these terms are often used interchangeably. The exact cause of venous thrombosis remains unclear, although three factors (Virchow's triad) are believed to play a significant role in its development—stasis of blood (venous stasis), vessel wall injury and altered blood coagulation.

Thrombophlebitis is an inflammation of the walls of the veins, often accompanied by formation of a clot. When a clot develops initially in the veins as a result of stasis or hypercoagulability, but without inflammation, the process is referred to as phlebothrombosis. Venous thrombosis can occur in any vein, but is most frequent in the veins of the lower extremities than the upper extremities. Both superficial and deep veins of the legs may be affected. Damage to the lining of blood vessels creates a site for clot formation and increased blood coagulability occurs in patients who abruptly stop taking anticoagulant medications and also occurs with oral contraceptive use and several blood dyscrasias. The danger associated with venous thrombosis is that parts of a clot can become detached and produce an embolic occlusion of the pulmonary blood vessels.

Risk Factors

- Obesity
- Advanced age
- Oral contraceptive use
- History of varicose veins, hypercoagulation, neoplastic disease, cardiovascular disease, or recent major surgery or injury.

Clinical Manifestations

1. Signs and symptoms are nonspecific.
2. Edema and swelling of the extremity resulting from obstruction of the deep veins of the leg; bilateral swelling may be difficult to detect (lack of size difference).
3. Skin over the affected leg may become warmer; superficial veins may become more prominent (cordlike venous segment).
4. Tenderness occurs later and detected by gently palpating the leg.
5. Homan's sign (pain in the calf after sharp dorsiflexion of the foot) is not specific for DVT because it can be elicited in any painful condition of the calf.
6. In some cases, signs of pulmonary embolus are the first indication of DVT.
7. Thrombus of superficial veins produces pain or tenderness redness and warmth in the involved area.
8. In massive iliofemoral venous thrombosis (phlegmasia cerulea dolens), the entire extremity becomes massively swollen, tense, painful and cool to touch.

Diagnostic Measures

1. History revealing risk factor such as varicose veins or neoplastic disease.
2. Doppler ultrasonography, duplex ultrasonography, air plethysmography and contrast phlebography (venography).

Preventions

Prevention is dependent on identifying risk factors for thrombus and on educating the patient about appropriate interventions.

Medical Management/Therapeutic Measures

Objectives of management are to prevent the thrombus from growing and fragmenting, resolve the current thrombus and prevent recurrence.

Pharmacological Therapy

1. Unfractionated heparin is administered for 5 days by intermittent or continuous IV infusion. Dosage is regulated by monitoring the activated partial thromboplastin time (APTT), the international normalized ratio (INR) and the platelet count. Low-molecular-weight heparin expensive than unfractionated heparin, but safer.
2. Oral anticoagulants [e.g. warfarin (Coumadin)] are given with heparin therapy.
3. Fondaparinux given subcutaneously for prophylaxis during major orthopedic surgery (hip replacement).
4. Thrombolytic (fibrinolytic) therapy (e.g. alteplase) is given within the first 3 days after acute thrombosis.
5. Throughout therapy, PTT, prothrombin time (PT), hemoglobin and hematocrit levels, platelet count, and fibrinogen level are monitored frequently. Drug therapy is discontinued if bleeding occurs and cannot be stopped.

Endovascular Management

Endovascular management is necessary for DVT, when anticoagulant or thrombolytic therapy is contraindicated, the danger of pulmonary embolism is extreme or venous drainage is so severely compromised that permanent damage to the extremity is likely. A thrombectomy may be necessary. A vena cava filter may be placed at the time of the thrombectomy.

Nursing Management

Assessing and Monitoring Anticoagulant Therapy

1. To prevent inadvertent infusion of large volumes of unfractionated heparin, which could cause hemorrhage, administer unfractionated heparin by continuous IV infusion using an electronic infusion device.
2. Dosage calculations are based on the patient's weight and any possible bleeding tendencies are detected by a pretreatment clotting profile; if renal insufficiency exists, lower doses of heparin are required.
3. Obtain periodic coagulation tests and hematocrit levels; heparin is in the effective or therapeutic, range when the APTT is 1.5 times the control.
4. Monitor oral anticoagulants, such as warfarin, by the PT or the INR. Because the full anticoagulant effect of warfarin is delayed for 3–5 days, it is usually administered concurrently with heparin until desired anticoagulation has been achieved (i.e. when the PT is 1.5–2 time normal or the INR is 2.0–3.0).

Monitoring and Managing Potential Complications

1. Assess for early signs of spontaneous bleeding (principal complication of anticoagulant therapy); bruises, nosebleeds and bleeding gums; administer IV injections of protamine sulfate to reverse effects of heparin and low-molecular weight heparin (LMWH) (less effective), administer vitamin K and/or infusion of fresh-frozen plasma or prothrombin concentrate to reverse effects of warfarin.
2. Monitor for heparin-induced thrombocytopenia by regularly monitoring platelet counts. Early signs include decreasing platelet count, the need for increasing doses of heparin to maintain the therapeutic level and thromboembolic or hemorrhagic complications (appearance of skin necrosis, skin discoloration, purpura and blistering). If thrombocytopenia does occur, perform platelet aggregation studies, discontinue heparin, and rapidly alternate anticoagulant therapy.
3. Close monitor the medication schedule, because oral anticoagulants interact with many other medications and herbal, and nutritional supplements.

Providing Comfort

1. Elevated affected extremity and apply warn, moist packs to reduce discomfort.
2. Encourage walking once anticoagulation therapy has been initiated (better than standing or sitting for long periods).
3. Recommend bed exercises, such as dorsiflexion of the foot against a footboard.
4. Provide additional pain relief with mild analgesic agents as prescribed.
5. Initiate compression therapy as prescribed to help improve circulation and increase comfort; graduated compression, stocking, external compression devices and wraps (e.g. short elastic wraps, Unna boot, CircAid), intermittent pneumatic compression devices.
6. With compression therapy, assess patient for comfort, inspect skin under device for signs of irritation or tenderness, and ensure that prescribed pressures are not exceeded.
7. Elderly patient may be unable to apply elastic stockings properly. Teach the family member who is to assist the patient to apply the stockings so that they do not cause undue pressure on any part of the feet or legs.
8. Any type of stockings can inadvertently become a tourniquet if applied incorrectly (i.e. rolled tightly at the top). In such instances, the stockings produce rather than prevent stasis. For ambulatory patients, graduated compression stockings are removed at night and reapplied before the legs are lowered from bed to the floor in the morning.
9. Positioning the body and encouraging exercise.
10. Elevate feet and lower legs periodically above heart level when on bedrest.
11. Perform early ambulation to help prevent venous stasis.
12. Encourage deep breathing exercises because they produce increased negative pressure in the thorax, which assists in emptying the large veins.

13. Once ambulatory, instruct the patient to avoid sitting for more than an hour at a time; encourage patient to walk at least 10 minutes in every 1–2 hours.
14. Instruct the patient to perform active and passive leg exercises as frequently as necessary when he/she cannot ambulate, such as during long car, bus, train, and plane trips.

Teaching Patient About Self-care

1. Teaching the patient how to apply graduated compression stockings and explain the importance of elevating the legs and exercising adequately.
2. Instruct patient on the purpose and importance of medications (correct dosage at specific times) and need for schedule blood tests to regulate medications.

CARDIOMYOPATHY

Cardiomyopathy is a heart muscle disease associated with cardiac dysfunction. It is classified according to the structural and functional abnormalities of the heart muscle; dilated cardiomyopathy (DCM) (most common), hypertrophic cardiomyopathy (HCM) (rare autosomal dominant condition), restrictive or constrictive cardiomyopathy (RCM), arrhythmogenic right ventricular cardiomyopathy (ARVC), and unclassified cardiomyopathies (different from or have characteristics of more than one of the other type). A patient may have pathology representing more than one of these classifications, such as patient with HCM developing dilations and symptoms of DCM. Ischemic cardiomyopathy is a term frequently used to describe an enlarged heart caused by CAD, which is usually accompanied by heart failure.

Pathophysiology

The pathophysiology of all cardiomyopathies is a series of events that culminate in impaired cardiac output. Decreased stroke volume stimulates the sympathetic nervous system and the renin-angiotensin-aldosterone response, resulting in increased systemic vascular resistance, and increased sodium and fluid retention, which places an increased workload on the heart. These alterations can lead to heart failure.

Clinical Manifestations

1. Presents initially with signs and symptoms of heart failure (shortness of breath on exertion fatigue).
2. May also report PND, cough and orthopnea.
3. Other symptoms include fluid retention, peripheral edema, nausea, chest pain, palpitations, dizziness and syncope with exertion.
4. With HCM, cardiac arrest (i.e. sudden cardiac death) may be the initial manifestations in young people.
5. Systemic venous congestion, jugular vein distention, pitting edema of dependent body parts, hepatic engorgement, tachycardia and extra heart sounds on physical examination.

Diagnostic Measures

1. Patient history, rule out other causes of failure.
2. Echocardiogram, cardiac MRI, ECG, chest X-ray, cardiac catheterization and possibly an endomyocardial biopsy.

Medical Management

Medical management is directed toward identifying and managing possible underlying or precipitating causes; correcting the heart failure with medications, a low-sodium diet and an exercise/rest regimen; and controlling dysrhythmias with antiarrhythmic medications and possibly with an implanted electronic device, such as an implantable cardioverter defibrillator.

Surgical Intervention

Surgical intervention (e.g. myectomy, heart transplantation) is considered when heart failure has progressed and treated.

In some cases, ventricular assist devices [e.g. a left ventricular assist device (LVAD)] are necessary to support the falling heart until a suitable donor becomes available.

Nursing Management

Nursing Assessment

1. Take detailed history of presenting signs and symptoms, and possible etiological factors.
2. Careful psychosocial history; identify family support systems and involve family in patient management.
3. Physical assessment directed towards signs and symptoms of heart failure. Evaluate vital signs (pulse pressure), weight and any gain/loss palpation for a shift to the left of the point of maximum impulse, auscultation for a systolic murmur and S_3 and S_4 heart sounds, pulmonary auscultation for crackles, measurement of jugular vein distention, and edema.

Nursing Diagnoses

1. Decreased cardiac output related to structural disorders secondary to cardiomyopathy or dysrhythmia.
2. Ineffective cardiopulmonary, cerebral, peripheral and renal tissue perfusion related to decreased peripheral blood flow.
3. Impaired gas exchange related to pulmonary congestion secondary to myocardial failure.
4. Activity intolerance related to decreased cardiac output and excessive fluid volume or both.
5. Anxiety related to change in health status and into functioning.
6. Powerless related to disease process.
7. Noncompliance with medication and diet therapies.

Collaborative problems/Potential complications: Heart failure, ventricular and atrial dysrhythmias, cardiac conduction defects, pulmonary or cerebral embolism, and valvular dysfunction.

Planning and Goals

The major goals for patients including improvement or maintenance of cardiac output, increased activity tolerance, reduction of anxiety, adherence to the self-care program, increasing power with decision-making and absence of complications.

Nursing Interventions/Implementation

Improving Cardiac Output

1. Assist patient into a resting position (usually sitting with legs down) during a symptomatic episode.
2. Administer oxygen if indicated.
3. Administer prescribed medications on time.
4. Promote low-sodium meals and adequate fluid intake.
5. Keep patient warm, and change positions frequently to stimulate circulation and reduce skin breakdown.

Increasing Activity Tolerance

1. Plan nurse care so that activities occur in cycles, alternating rest with activity.
2. Ensure that the patient recognizes the symptoms indicating the need for rest and actions to take when the symptoms occur.

Reducing Anxiety

1. Spiritual, psychological and emotional support may be indicated for patients, families, and significant others.
2. Provide patient with appropriate information about signs and symptoms.
3. Provide an atmosphere in which the patient feels free to verbalize concerns and receive assurance that their concerns are legitimate.
4. Assist patient to accomplish a goal, no matter how small to enhance a sense of well-being.
5. Provide time for the patient to discuss concerns, if facing death or awaiting transplantation; provide realistic hope.
6. Help the patient, family and significant others with anticipatory grieving.

Decreasing Sense of Powerlessness

1. Assist patient in identifying things he/she has lost (e.g. foods enjoyed).
2. Assist patient in identifying emotional responses to the loss (e.g. anger and depression).
3. Assist patient in identifying the amount of control that he/she still has on himself/herself (e.g. selecting food choices).

Promoting Family- and Community-based Care

Teaching patients about self-care

1. Teaching patients about the medications regimen, symptoms, monitoring and symptom management.
2. Help patient to balance lifestyle and work while accomplishing therapeutic activities.
3. Help patient cope with their disease status; help them to adjust to their lifestyles and implement a self-care program at home.

Continuing care

1. Reinforce previous teaching and perform ongoing assessment of the patient's symptoms and progress.
2. Assist in review lifestyle, and suggest strategies to incorporate therapeutic activities to balance lifestyle and work.
3. Stress the signs and symptoms that should be reported to the physician; teach the patient's family about cardiopulmonary resuscitation (CPR), if necessary.
4. Assess the psychological needs of the patient and family of ongoing basis.
5. Establish trust with patient and provide support during end-of-life, and in decision-making.
6. Refer the patient for home care and support if necessary.

Evaluation/Expected Patient Outcomes

- Maintains or improves cardiac function
- Maintains or increases activity tolerance
- Experiences reduction of anxiety
- Decrease sense of powerlessness
- Adheres to self-care program.

CARDIAC ARREST

Cardiac arrest occurs when the heart ceases to produce an effective pulse and circulate blood. It may be caused by a cardiac electrical event (i.e. dysrhythmia) such as ventricular fibrillation, progressive profound bradycardia or when there is no heart rhythm at all (systole). Cardiac arrest may follow respiratory arrest; it may occur when electrical activity is present, but there is ineffective cardiac contraction or circulating volume, which is called pulseless electrical activity (PEA). PEA can be caused by hypovolemia (e.g. with excessive bleeding), hypoxia, hypothermia, hyperkalemia, massive pulmonary embolism, myocardial infarction, and medication overdose (e.g. beta blockers and calcium channel blockers).

Clinical Manifestations

In cardiac arrest, consciousness, pulse and BP are lost immediately. Ineffective respiratory gasping may occur. The pupils of the eye begin dilating within 45 seconds. Seizures may or may not occur.

The risk of irreversible brain damage and death increases with every minute from time that circulating ceases. The interval varies with the age and underlying condition of the patient. During this period, the diagnosis of cardiac arrest must be made and measures must be taken immediately to restore circulation.

Management

- Initiate immediate CPR
- Institute follow-up monitoring once patient is resuscitated.

11

Chapter Orthopedic Nursing

SOFT TISSUE INJURIES

Strains

A strain is a soft tissue injury that occurs when a muscle or tendon is excessively stretched. The causes of strains include falls, excessive exercise and lifting heavy items without using proper body mechanics. Back and ankle injuries are common.

Clinical Manifestations

Strains may be mild, moderate or severe, i.e:

1. Mild: Minimal inflammation, i.e. swelling and tenderness.
2. Moderate: Partial tearing of muscles or tendons. It results in pain and inability to move the affected body part.
3. Severe: In this, muscle or tendon requires separation of muscles from muscle fibers, separation of tendon from muscle or tendon from bone.

Therapeutic Measures/Management

1. Use RICE, i.e. rest, ice, compression and elevation of strain injuries.
2. Injured area should be rested to protect it.
3. Ice should be applied to decrease pain, swelling and inflammation.
4. Applying an elastic bandage for compression.
5. Elevating the affected area to provide support and minimize swelling.
6. Once inflammation subside, heat applications increase blood flow for healing.
7. Activity is limited depending upon injury until soft tissues heal.
8. Administer anti-inflammation medication on prescribed.
9. Muscle relaxants must be used, if ordered.
10. Exercise may begin as early as possible according to severity.
11. Severe strains may need surgical repair care accordingly.

Sprains

A sprain is an excessive stretching of one or more ligaments than usually resulting from twisting movements during sports activity, exercise or fall.

Clinical Manifestations

1. Mild sprain: Involves tearing of just few ligament fibers and cause tenderness.
2. Moderate sprain: Here more fibers are torn, but the stability of joints is not affected. It is uncomfortable especially with activity.
3. Severe sprains: There is instability of joints and usually requires surgical interventions for tissue repair or grafting.
4. Pain and inflammation prevent mobility.

Therapeutic Measures/Management

1. Use RICE on strains until pain and swelling gets diminished.
2. Can use anti-inflammatory medication to control pain.
3. Moderate sprains need immobilization with brace or casts.

Dislocation

Dislocation is a common injury in which the ends of the bones are forced apart from their normal position. They are usually caused by trauma, as in falls or contact sports or by a disease such as rheumatoid arthritis. Any joint that is large or small, may be dislocated.

Clinical Manifestations

Severe pain along with lost range of motion of the joints and joint deformity occurs.

Therapeutic Measures/Management

1. Immediate medical treatment is required to preserve function.
2. Splint the extremity in the position found.
3. Apply ice and seek help.
4. Do not move the extremity because blood vessels, muscles and nerves could be damaged.

MUSCULOSKELETAL TRAUMA (CONTUSIONS, STRAINS, SPRAINS AND JOINT DISLOCATION)

Injury to one part of the musculoskeletal system results in malfunction of adjacent muscles, joints and tendons. The type and severity of injury affects the mobility of the injured area. Treatment of injury to musculoskeletal system involves providing support to the injured part until healing is completed.

A contusion is a soft tissue injury produced by blunt force (e.g. a blow, kick or fall). Many small blood vessels rupture and bleed into soft tissues (ecchymosis or bruising). A hematoma develops when the bleeding is sufficient to cause an appreciable collection of blood. Most contusions resolve in 1–2 weeks. A strain is a 'muscle pull' from overuse, overstretching or excessive stress. A sprain is an injury to the ligaments surrounding a joint, caused by a twisting motion or hyperextension (forcible) of a joint. A torn ligament loses its stabilizing ability. Blood vessels rupture and edema occurs. It includes local symptoms such as pain, swelling and discoloration.

A dislocation of a joint is a condition in which the articular surfaces of the bones forming the joint are no longer in anatomic contact. In complete dislocation, the bones are literally 'out of joint'. A subluxation is a partial dislocation of the articulating surfaces. Traumatic dislocations are orthopedic emergencies because the associated joint structures, blood supply and nerves are displaced, and may be entrapped with extensive pressure on them, if a dislocation or subluxation is not treated promptly, avascular necrosis (tissue death due to anoxia and diminished blood supply) may occur.

Strain includes soreness or sudden pain with local tenderness on muscle use and isometric contraction.

Sprain includes tenderness of the joint, painful movement, increased disability and pain in the first 2–3 hours after injury because of associated swelling and bleeding.

Dislocation or subluxation causes acute pain, change in the positioning of the joint, shortening of the extremity, deformity and decreased mobility.

Assessment

X-ray examination is used to evaluate for any bone injury.

Medical Management

1. Treatment of injury of the musculoskeletal system involves providing support for the injured part until healing is completed.
2. Treatment of contusions, strains and sprains consists of rest, applying ice, applying a compression bandage and elevate the affected part.
3. Severe sprains may require 1–3 weeks of immobilization before protected exercises are initiated.
4. Strains and sprains take weeks or months to heal. Splinting may be used to prevent reinjury.
5. With a dislocation, the affected joint needs to be immobilized, while the patient is transported to the hospital.
6. The dislocation is promptly reduced (i.e. displaced parts brought into normal position) to preserve joint function. Analgesia, muscle relaxants and possibly anesthesia are used to facilitate closed reduction.
7. The joint is immobilized by bandages, splints, casts or traction and is maintained in a stable position.
8. After reduction, gentle, progressive, active and passive movement is begun three to five times a day to preserve range of motion and restore strength.
9. The joint is supported between exercise sessions.

Nursing Management

1. Frequently assess and evaluate the injury, and complete full neurovascular assessment.
2. Educate the patient and family regarding proper exercises and activities as well as to look for dangerous signs and symptoms such as increasing pain (even with analgesics), 'numbness or tingling,' and increased edema in the extremity.
3. Ice or some form of moist or dry cold is applied intermittently for 20–30 minutes during the first 24–48 hours after injury to produce vasoconstrictions, which decrease bleeding, edema and discomfort. Avoid excessive cold because it could cause skin and tissue damage.
4. An elastic compression bandage controls bleeding, reduces edema and provides support for the injured tissues.
5. Elevation controls the swelling. If the sprain is severe (muscle fibers and disrupted ligaments), surgical repairs or immobilization may be necessary, so that joint will not lose its stability.
6. After the acute inflammatory stage (e.g. 24–48 hour after injury), heat may be applied intermittently (for 15–30 minute, four times a day) to relieve muscle spasm and to promote vasodilation, absorption and repair.
7. Depending on the severity of injury, progressive passive and active exercises may begin in 2–5 days.

CARPAL TUNNEL SYNDROME

Carpal tunnel syndrome (CTS) results in the compression of the median nerve within the carpal tunnel when swelling in the tunnel occurs. The swelling can result from edema, trauma, rheumatoid arthritis or repetitive hand movements, as used in some occupation, e.g. typing.

Clinical Manifestations

- Results in slow onset in fingers, hand and arm pain, and numbness
- Painful tingling and paresthesia may also be present
- Eventually, fine motor deficit and then muscles weakness.

Diagnostic Measures

- Signs and symptoms
- Positive Phalen's test (numbness with wrist flexion)
- Electromyography (EMG).

Therapeutic Measures

1. Treatment focus on relieving inflammation and restrict wrist flexion.
2. Splint ordered for patient to wear.
3. Medications to reduce pain and inflammation non-steroidal anti-inflammatory drugs (NSAIDs).
4. In some patients, surgery may be required to decompress the median nerves compression.

Nursing Management

1. Educate patient to prevent CTS, i.e. frequent short breaks during workday, interspersing ongoing tasks with repetitive movements throughout the day and using ergonomically appropriate device to minimize pressure in wrist.
2. Provide pain reliever as ordered.
3. If surgery is done, postoperatively elevate the patient hand.
4. Instruct the patient to use the splint as ordered for 2 weeks.
5. Lifting is restricted for several weeks.
6. Patient is taught to report neurovascular compromise such as numbness, tingling, coolness, lack of pulse, pale skin or nail beds or limited movements.
7. Instruct family members to assist patient in activities of daily living (ADL).

ROTATOR CUFF INJURY

Short tendons that are connected to muscles around the shoulder, form the rotator cuff. The cuff covers the top front and back of the shoulder. Muscle contraction causes these tendons to tighten and move or rotate the shoulder. Various injuries can occur.

The top tendons of the cuff and bursa may become impinged in a narrow space under the acromion bone. This causes inflammation when the arm is repeatedly moved forward and pain results. This also called chronic impingement syndrome. Over time, the tendon may finally tear from the bone.

Clinical Manifestations

- Shoulder aching, increased pain while lifting the arm
- Pain that is greater at night and weakness
- Limited range of motion.

Diagnosis

- Magnetic resonance imaging (MRI).

Therapeutic Measures

- For minor injury, resting the shoulder, applying ice packs physiotherapy is done
- For severe injury, following measures are needed:
  - Arthroscopic and/or small incisions surgery to relieve impingement or repair this tear
  - Sling or special brace to worn after surgery
  - Physical therapy for rehabilitation is often seen.

BURSITIS

Bursa (fluid-filled sacs) acts as a cushion between tendons during movement to prevent frictions between the bone and tendon. Several joints have bursas in shoulders, elbows, hip, knees, ankles and heels. Inflammation of bursa is called bursitis. It occurs from arthritis because of repetitive movements or sleeping on one side, which compress the shoulder bursae.

Clinical Manifestations

Aching pain, stiffness or burning pain over the joint area that worsens with activity.

Therapeutic Measures

1. Prevention: It is better to prevent bursitis by compression.
2. Teach patient to stretch and strengthen muscles, move frequently, avoid repetitive movements for long periods, use cushioned seats and avoid leaning on the elbows.
3. Usually pain is decreased in about a week.
4. If becomes chronic, i.e. lasts more than 6 months, then treatment includes:
   - Resting the joint
   - Application of ice for 20 minutes, several times a day until joints inflammation is gone
   - Switching to the heat, elevating the joint, ultrasound and massage
   - Can use NSAIDs or physical therapy.

FRACTURES

A fracture is a complete or incomplete disruption in the continuity of bone structure and is defined according to its type and extent. Fractures occur when the bone is subjected to stress that is greater than it can absorb. Fractures can be caused by a direct blow, crushing force, sudden twisting motion or even extreme muscle contraction.

When the bone is broken, adapted structures are also affected, resulting in soft tissue edema, hemorrhage into the muscle and joints, joint dislocation, ruptured tendons, severed nerves and damaged blood vessels. Body organs may be injured by the force that caused the rupture or by the fracture fragments. Fractures are classified into following types:

1. Complete fracture: A break across the entire cross section of the bone, which is frequently displaced.
2. Incomplete fracture: Also called greenstick fracture; break occurs only through part of the cross section of the bone.
3. Comminuted fractures: A break with several bone fragments.
4. Closed fracture or simple fracture: They does not produce a break in the skin.
5. Open fracture (compound or complex fracture): A break in which the skin or mucous membrane wound extend to the fractured bone. Open fractures are graded as follows:
   a. Grade I: A clean wound less than 1 cm long.
   b. Grade II: A larger wound without extensive soft tissue damage.
   c. Grade III: Wound is highly contaminated and has extensive soft tissue damage (most severe type).
6. Fractures may also be described according to anatomic placement of fragments, particularly if they are displaced or nondisplaced.
7. An intra-articular fracture extends into the joint surface of a bone.

Complications

Early complications include shock, fat embolism, compartment syndrome and venous thromboembolism [deep vein thrombosis (DVT), pulmonary embolism (PE)]. Delayed complications include delayed union, malunion, nonunion, avascular necrosis (AVN) of bone, reaction to internal fixation devices, complex regional pain syndrome (CRPS), formerly known as reflex sympathetic dystrophy (RSD) and heterotopic ossification.

Clinical Manifestations

1. The clinical signs and symptoms of a fracture include acute pain, loss of function, deformity, shortening of the extremity, crepitus, and localized edema and ecchymosis. Not all these are present in every fracture.
2. If fat embolism syndrome occurs with blockage of the small blood vessels that supply the brain, lungs, kidneys and other organs (sudden onset, usually occurring within 12–48 hour, but may occur up to 10 day after injury), the following may be noted—hypoxia, tachypnea, tachycardia pyrexia; dyspnea, crackles, wheezes, precordial chest pain, cough, large amount of thick white sputum. Hypoxia and blood gas values with PaO_2 below 60 mm Hg, with an early respiratory alkalosis and later respiratory acidosis mental status changes varying from headache and mild agitation to delirium and coma can occur. The chest radiograph exhibits a typical 'snowstorm' infiltrate. Eventually, acute pulmonary edema, acute respiratory distress syndrome (ARDS) and heart failure may develop.
3. With systemic embolization, the patient appears pale. Petechiae appear in the buccal membranes and conjunctival sacs on the hard palate, and over the chest and anterior axillary folds. Fever

[temperature above 39.5°C (103°F)] develops. Free fat may be found in the urine when emboli reach the kidneys. Acute tubular necrosis and renal failure may develop.

4. Compartment syndrome occurs when perfusion pressure falls below tissue pressure within a closed anatomic compartment. Acute compartment syndrome may produce deep, throbbing, unrelenting pain not controlled by opioids (can be due to a tight cast or constrictive dressing, or an increase in muscle compartment contents because of edema or hemorrhage). Cyanotic (blue-tinged) nail beds, and pale/dusky and cold fingers or toes are present; nail bed capillary refill times are prolonged (greater than 3 second) pulse may be diminished (Doppler effect) or absent; and motor weakness, paralysis and paresthesia may occur.
5. Manifestations of disseminated intravascular coagulation (DIC) include unexpected bleeding after surgery and bleeding from the mucous membranes, venipuncture sites, and gastrointestinal and urinary tracts.
6. Symptoms of infection may include tenderness, pain, reduces swelling, local warmth, elevated temperature and purulent drainage.
7. Nonunion is manifested by persistent discomfort and abnormal movement at the fracture site. Some risk factors include infection at the fracture site, interposition of tissue between the bone ends, inadequate immobilization or manipulation that disrupts callus formation, excessive space between bone fragments, limited bones contact and impaired blood supply resulting in AVN.
8. Manifestations of other complications may be noted (DVT, thromboembolism, PE).
9. Avoid testing for crepitus because testing can cause further tissue damage, subtle personality changes, restlessness, irritability or confusion in a patient who has sustained fracture are the indications for immediate blood gas studies.
10. Hip fractures frequently contribute to physical disability and are institutionalized among the elderly. Muscle weakness may have initially contributed to the fall and fracture. Stress and immobility related to the trauma predispose the older adults to atelectasis, pneumonia, sepsis, venous thromboembolism, pressure ulcers and reduce ability to cope with other health problems. Many elderly people hospitalized with hip fractures exhibit delirium as a result of the stress of the trauma, unfamiliar surroundings, sleep deprivation and medications. Because dehydration and poor nutrition may be present, the patient needs to be encouraged to consume adequate fluids and a healthy diet.

Diagnostic Measures

The diagnosis of a fracture depends on the symptoms, the physical signs and radiographic examination. Usually the patient reports an injury to the area.

Medical Management

Emergency Management

1. Immediately after injury, immobilize the body part before the patient is moved.

2. Splint the fracture, including joints adjacent to the fracture, to prevent movement of fracture fragments.
3. Immobilization of the long bones of the lower extremities may be accomplished by bandaging the legs together with the unaffected extremity serving as a splint for the injured one.
4. In an upper extremity injury, the arm may be bandaged to the chest or an injured forearm may be placed in a sling.
5. Assess neurovascular status distal to the injury, both before and after splinting, to determine adequacy of peripheral tissue perfusion and nerve function.
6. Cover the wound of an open fracture with a sterile dressing to prevent contamination of deeper tissues.

Reduction of Fractures

1. The fracture is reduced ('setting' the bone) using a closed method [manipulating and manual traction (e.g. splint or cast)] or an open method [surgical placement of internal fixation devices (e.g. metallic pins, wires, screws, plates, nails or rods)] to restore the fracture fragments to anatomic alignment and rotation. The specific method depends on the nature of the fracture.
2. After the fracture has been reduced, immobilization holds the bone in correct position and alignment until union occurs. Immobilization is accomplished by external or internal fixation.
3. The normal function is maintained and restored by controlling swelling, by elevating the injured extremity and applying ice as prescribed (restlessness, anxiety, and pain relief strategies, including use of analgesics). Isometric and muscle setting exercises are encouraged to minimize atrophy and to promote circulation. With internal fixation, the surgeon determines the amount of movement and weight-bearing stress in the extremity can withstand and prescribes the level of activity.

Management of Complication

1. Treatment of shock consists of stabilizing the fracture to prevent further hemorrhage, restoring blood volume and circulation, relieving the patient's pain, providing proper immobilization, and protecting the patient from further injury and other complications.
2. Prevention and management of fat embolism include immediate immobilization of fractures, adequate support for fractured bones during turning and positioning, and maintenance of fluid and electrolyte balance. Prompt initiation of respiratory support with prevention of respiratory and metabolic acidosis, and correction of homeostatic disturbances is essential. Corticosteroids as well as vasopressor medications may be given.
3. Compartment syndrome is managed by controlling the swelling by elevating the extremity to heart level or by releasing restrictive devices (dressings or cast). A fasciotomy (surgical decompression with excision of the fascia). The wound remains open and covered with moist sterile saline dressings for 3–5 days. The limb is splinted and elevated. Prescribed passive range of motion exercises may be performed.
4. Nonunion (failure of the ends of fractured bone to union) is treated with internal fixation, bone grafting (osteogenesis,

osteoconduction, osteoinduction), electrical bone stimulation or a combination of these.
5. Management of reaction to internal fixation devices involves protection from refracture related to osteoporosis, altered bones structure and trauma.
6. Management of CRPS involves elevation of the extremity, pain relief by range of motion exercises, and helping patient with chronic pain, disuse atrophy and osteoporosis. Avoid taking blood pressure or performing venipuncture in the affected extremity.
7. Other complications are treated as indicated.

Nursing Management

Managing Closed Fractures

1. Instruct the patient regarding the proper methods to control edema and pain (e.g. elevate extremity to heart level and take analgesic as prescribed).
2. Teach exercises to maintain the health of unaffected muscles and to strengthen muscles needed for transferring, and for using assistive devices (e.g. crutches, walker).
3. Teach patients how to use assistive devices safely.
4. Arrange to help patients modify their home environment as needed and to secure personal assistance, if necessary.
5. Provide patient teaching, including self-care, medication information, monitoring for potential complications and the need for continuing healthcare supervision.

Managing Open Fractures

1. The objectives of management are to prevent infection of the wound, soft tissue and bone, and to promote healing of bone and soft tissue. In an open fracture, there is a risk of osteomyelitis, tetanus and gas gangrene.
2. Administer intravenous (IV) antibiotics immediately upon the patient's arrival in the hospital along with tetanus toxoid, if needed.
3. Perform wound irrigation and debridement.
4. Elevate the extremity to minimize edema.
5. Assess neurovascular status frequently.
6. Take the patient's temperature at regular intervals and monitor for signs of infection.

Managing Fractures of Specific Sites

Maximum functional recovery is the goal of management. Fracture of the clavicle (collarbone) is a common injury that results from a fall or a direct blow to the shoulder. Monitor the circulation and nerve function of the affected arm, and compare with the unaffected arm to determine variations, which may indicate disturbances in neurovascular status. Caution the patient not to elevate the arm above shoulder level until the fracture has healed (about 6 week). Encourage the patient to exercise the elbow, wrist and fingers as soon as possible, and when prescribed, to perform shoulder exercises. Tell the patient that vigorous activity must be limited for 3 months.

Humeral neck

With humeral neck fractures (seen most frequently in older women after a fall on an outstretched arm), perform neurovascular assessment of the involved extremity to evaluate the extent of injury, and possible involvement of the nerves and blood vessels of the arm. Teach the patient to support the arm and immobilize it by a sling and swathe that secure the supported arm to the trunk. Begin pendulum exercises as soon as tolerated by the patient. Instruct the patient to avoid vigorous activity for an additional 10–14 weeks.

Inform the patient that residual stiffness, aching and some limitation of range of motion may persist for 6 or more months. When a humeral neck fracture is displaced with required fixation, exercises are started only after a prescribed period of immobilization.

With humeral shaft fractures, the nerves and brachial blood vessels may be injured, so neurovascular assessment is essential to monitor the status of the nerve or blood vessels. Use well-padded splints to initially immobilize the upper arm and to support the arm in 90 degrees of flexion at the elbow; use a sling or collar and cuff to support the forearm, and use external fixators to treat open fractures of the humeral shaft. Functional bracing may also be used for these fractures. Teach patient to perform pendulum shoulder exercises and isometric exercises, as prescribed.

Elbow

Elbow fractures (distal humerus) may result in injury to the median, radial or ulnar nerves. Evaluate the patient for paresthesia and signs of compromised circulation in the forearm and hand. Monitor closely for Volkmann's ischemic contracture (an acute compartment syndrome) as well as for hemarthrosis (blood in the joint). Reinforce information regarding reduction and fixation of the fracture and planned active motion when swelling has subsided and healing has begun. Explain care, if the arm is immobilized in a cast or posterior splint with a sling. Encourage active finger exercises. Teach and encourage patient to do gentle range of motion exercise of the injured joint about 1 week after internal fixation.

Radial head fractures are usually produced by a fall on the outstretched hand with the elbow extended. Instruct patient in use of a splint for immobilization. If the fracture is displaced, reinforce the need for postoperative immobilization of the arm in posterior plaster splint and sling. Encourage the patient to carry out a program of active motion of the elbow and forearm when prescribed.

Wrist

Wrist fractures [distal radius (Colles' fracture)] usually result from a fall on an open, dorsiflexed hand. They are frequently seen in elderly women with osteoporotic bones and weak soft tissues that do not dissipate the energy of a fall. Reinforce care of the cast, or with more severe fractures with wire insertion, teach incision care. Instruct patient to keep the wrist and forearm elevated for 48 hours after reduction. Begin active motion of the fingers and shoulder promptly by teaching patient to do the following exercises to reduce swelling and prevent stiffness:

1. Hold the hand at the level of the heart.
2. Move the fingers from full extension to flexion; hold and release. Repeat at least 10 times every hour when awake.
3. Use the hand in functional activities.
4. Actively exercise the shoulder and elbow, including complete range of motion exercise of both joints.

5. Assess the sensory function of the median nerve by pricking the distal aspect of the index finger, and assess the motor function by testing patient's ability to touch the thumb to the little finger. If diminished circulation and nerve function is noted, treat promptly.

Hand and fingers

Hand trauma often requires extensive reconstructive surgery. The objective of treatment is always to regain maximum function of the hand. With a non-displaced fracture, the finger is splinted for 3–4 weeks to relieve pain and protect fingertip from further trauma, but displaced fractures and open fractures may require open reduction with internal fixation, using wires or pins.

Evaluate the neurovascular status of the injured hand. Teach the patient to control swelling by elevating the hand. Encourage functional use of the uninvolved portions of the hand.

Pelvis

1. Pelvic fractures may be caused by falls, motor vehicle crashes or crush injuries. At least two thirds of these patients have significant and multiple injuries.
2. Monitor for symptoms including ecchymosis; tenderness over the symphysis pubis, anterior iliac spines, iliac crest, sacrum or coccyx; local edema; numbness or tingling of the pubis, genitals and proximal thighs; and inability to bear weight without discomfort.
3. Complete a neurovascular assessment of the lower extremities to detect injury to pelvic blood vessels and nerves. Examine urine for blood to assess for urinary tract injury. In male patients, do not insert a catheter until the status of the urethra is known. Monitor for diffuse and intense abdominal pain, hyperactive or absence of bowel sounds and abdominal rigidity and resonance (free air) or dullness to percussion (blood), which suggest injury to the intestines or abdominal bleeding.
4. If patient has a stable pelvic fracture, maintain patient on bedrest for a few days and provide symptoms management until the pain and discomfort are controlled.
5. Provide fluids, dietary fiber, ankle and leg exercises, antiembolism stockings to aid venous return, logrolling, deep breathing and skin care to reduce the risk of complications and to increase comfort.
6. Monitor bowel sounds. If patient has a fracture of the coccyx and experiences pain on sitting and with defecation, assist with sitz baths, as prescribed to relieve pain, and administer stool softeners to prevent the need to strain on defecation.
7. As pain resolves, instruct patient to resume activity gradually, using assistive mobility devices for protected weight bearing. Patients with unstable pelvic fractures may be treated with external fixation or open reduction and internal fixation (ORIF).
8. Promote hemodynamic stability and comfort, and encourage early mobilization.

Femur and hip

1. Femoral shaft fractures are most often seen in young adults involved in a motor vehicle crash or a fall from a high place. Frequently, these patients are associated with multiple traumas and develop shock from a loss of 2–3 units of blood.
2. Assess neurovascular status of the extremity, especially circulatory perfusion of the lower leg and foot (popliteal, posterior tibial, and pedal pulses and toe capillary refill time as well as Doppler ultrasound monitoring).

3. Note signs of dislocation of the hip and knee, and knee effusion, which may suggest ligament damage, and possible instability of the knee joint.
4. Apply and maintain skeletal traction or splint to achieve muscle relaxation and alignment of the fracture fragments before ORIF procedures, and later a cast brace.
5. Assist patient in minimal partial weight bearing when indicated and progress full weight bearing as tolerated.
6. Reinforce that the cast brace is worn for 12–14 weeks.
7. Instruct in and encourage patient to perform exercises of lower leg, foot, and toes on a regular basis. Assist patient in performing active and passive knee exercises as soon as possible, depending on the management approach and the ability of the fracture and knee ligaments.

Tibia and fibula

1. Tibia and fibula fractures (most common fractures below the knee) tend to result from a direct blow, falls with the foot in a flexed position, or a violent twisting motion
2. Provide instruction on the care of long leg walking cast of patellar tendon-bearing cast.
3. Instruct patient on care of a short leg cast or brace (in 3–4 week), which allows for knee motion.
4. Instruct patient in care of skeletal traction, if applicable. Encourage patient to perform hip, foot and knee exercises within the limit of immobilizing device.
5. Instruct patient to begin weight bearing when prescribed (usually in about 4–8 week).
6. Instruct patient to elevate extremity to control edema.
7. Perform continuous neurovascular evaluation.

Rib

Rib fractures occur frequently in adults and usually result in no impairment of function, but produce painful respirations. Assist patient to cough and take deep breaths by splinting the chest with hands or pillow during cough. Reassure patient that pain associated with rib fracture diminishes significantly in 3 or 4 days and the fracture heals within 6 weeks. Monitor for complications, which may include atelectasis, pneumonia, a flail chest, pneumothorax and hemothorax (refer specific disorder for nursing management).

RHEUMATOID ARTHRITIS

Rheumatoid arthritis (RA) is an inflammatory disorder of unknown origin that primarily involves the synovial membranes of the joints. Phagocytes produce enzymes within the joint. The enzymes breakdown collagen causing edema, proliferation of the synovial membrane and ultimately pannus the formation. Pannus destroys the cartilage and erodes the bone. The consequence is loss of articular surfaces and joint motion. Muscle fibers undergo degenerative changes. Tendon and ligament elasticity, and contractile power are lost. RA affects 1% of the population worldwide, affecting women two to four times more than men.

Clinical Manifestations

1. Clinical features are determined by the stage and severity of the disease.

2. Joints pain, swelling, warmth, erythema and lack of function are classic symptoms.
3. Palpation of joints reveals spongy or boggy tissue.
4. Fluid can usually be aspirated from the inflamed joint.

Characteristic Pattern of Joint Involvement

1. Begins with small joints in hand, wrists and feet.
2. Progressively involves knees, shoulder, hip, elbows, ankles, cervical spine and temporomandibular joints.
3. Symptoms are usually acute in onset, bilateral and symptomatic.
4. Joints may be hot, swollen and painful; joints stiffness often occurs in the morning.
5. Deformities of the hands and feet can result from misalignment and immobilization.

Extra-articular Features

1. Fever, weight loss, fatigue, anemia, sensory changes and lymph node enlargement.
2. Raynaud's phenomenon (cold- and stress-induced vasospasm).
3. Rheumatoid nodules, nontender and movable; found in subcutaneous tissue over bony prominences.
4. Arthritis, neuropathy, scleritis, pericarditis, splenomegaly and Sjögren's syndrome (dry eyes and mucous membranes).

Assessment

1. Several factors contribute to the RA diagnosis; rheumatoid nodules, joint inflammation detected on palpation, laboratory findings, extra-articular changes.
2. Rheumatoid factor is present in about three fourths of patients.
3. The red blood cell (RBC) count and C4 complement component are decreased; erythrocyte sedimentation rate is elevated.
4. C-reactive protein and antinuclear antibody test results may be positive.
5. Arthrocentesis and X-rays may be performed.

Medical Management/Therapeutic Measures

1. Treatment begins with education, a balance of rest and exercise, and referral to community agencies for support.
2. Early RA: Medication management involves therapeutic doses of salicylates or NSAIDs; includes new cyclooxygenase-2 (COX-2) enzyme blockers, antimalarials, gold, penicillamine or sulfasalazine; methotrexate; biologic response modifiers and tumor necrosis factor-alpha (TNF-α) inhibitors are helpful; analgesic agents for period of extreme pain.
3. Moderate, erosive RA: Formal program of occupational and physical therapy; an immunosuppressant such as cyclosporine may be added.
4. Persistent, erosive RA: Reconstructive surgery and corticosteroids.
5. Advanced unremitting RA: Immunosuppressive agents such as methotrexate, cyclophosphamide, azathioprine and leflunomide (highly toxic, can cause bone marrow suppression,

anemia, gastrointestinal (GI) tract disturbances, and rashes). Also promising for refractory RA is a Food and Drug Administration (FDA)-approved apheresis device—a protein A immunoadsorption column (Prosorba) that binds circulating immune system complex (IgG).

6. The RA patients frequently experience anorexia, weight loss and anemia, requiring careful dietary history to identify usual eating habits and food preferences. Corticosteroids may stimulate appetite and cause weight gain.
7. Low-dose antidepressant medications (amitriptyline) are used to re-establish adequate sleep pattern and manage pain.

Nursing Management

The most common issues for the patient with RA include pain, sleep disturbance, fatigue, altered mood and limit mobility. The patient with newly diagnosed RA needs information about the disease to make daily self-management decision and to cope with having a chronic disease.

Relieving Pain and Discomfort

1. Provide a variety of comfort measures (e.g. application of heat or cold; massage, position changes, rest; foam mattress, supportive pillow, splints; relaxation techniques, diversional activities).
2. Administer anti-inflammatory, analgesic and slow-acting antirheumatic medications, as prescribed.
3. Individualized medication schedule to meet patient's need for pain management.
4. Encourage verbalization of feelings about pain and chronically of disease.
5. Teach pathophysiology of pain and rheumatic disease and assist patient to recognize that pain often leads to unproven treatment methods.
6. Assist in identification of pain that leads to use of unproven methods of treatment.
7. Paleness: Subjective changes in pain.

Reducing Fatigue

1. Provide instruction about fatigue; describe relationship of disease activity to fatigue; describe comfort measures while providing them; develop and encourage a sleep routine, warm bath and relaxation techniques that promote sleep; explain importance of rest for relieving systematic, articular and emotional stress.
2. Explain how to use energy conservation techniques (pacing, setting priorities).
3. Identify physical and emotional factors that can cause fatigue, facilitate development of appropriate activity/rest schedule.
4. Encourage adherence to the treatment program.
5. To encourage a conditioning program.
6. Encourage adequate nutrition, including source of iron from and supplements.
7. Increasing mobility.
8. Encourage verbalization regarding limitations in mobility and need for occupational or physical therapy consultation.

Emphasize range of motion of affected joints; promote use of assistive ambulatory devices; explain use of safe footwear; use individual appropriate positioning/posture.
9. Assist to identify environmental barriers.
10. Encourage independence in mobility and assist as needed—allow ample time for activity; provide rest period after activity; reinforce principles of joint protection and work simplification.
11. Initiate referral to community health agency.

Facilitating Self-care

1. Assist patient to identify self-care deficits and factors that interfere with ability to perform self-care activities.
2. Develop a plan based on the patient's perceptions and priorities on how to establish and achieve goals to meet self-care needs, incorporating joint protection, energy conservation and work simplification concepts; provide appropriate assistive devices, allow patient to control timing of self-care activities; explore with the patient different ways to perform difficult tasks or ways to enlist the help of someone else.
3. Consult with community healthcare agencies when individuals have attained a maximum level of self-care, yet still have some deficits, especially regarding safety.

Improving Body Image and Coping Skills

1. Help patient identify elements of control over disease symptoms and treatment.
2. Encourage patient's verbalization of feelings, perceptions and fear.
3. Identify areas of life affected by disease. Answer the questions and dispel possible myths.
4. Develop a plan for managing symptoms and enlisting support of family and friends to promote daily function.

Monitoring and Managing Potential Complications

1. Help patient recognize and deal with side effects from medications.
2. Monitor for medication side effects, including GI tract bleeding or irritation, bone marrow suppression, kidney or liver toxicity, increased incidence of infection, mouth sores, rashes and changes in vision. Other signs and symptoms include bruising, breathing problems, dizziness, jaundice, dark urine, black or bloody stools, diarrhea, nausea and vomiting, and headaches.
3. Monitor closely for systemic and local infections, which often can be masked by high doses of corticosteroids.

Promoting Family- and Community-based Care

Teaching patients about self-care

1. Focus patient teaching on the disease, possible changes related to it, the prescribed therapeutic regimen, side effects of medications, strategies to maintain independence, and function and safety in the home.
2. Encourage patient and family to verbalize their concerns and ask questions.

3. Assess pain, fatigue and depression before initiating a teaching program, because they can interfere with patient's ability to learn.
4. Instruct patient about basic disease management and necessary adaptions in lifestyle.

Continuing Care

1. Refer for home care as warranted (e.g. frail patient with significant limited function).
2. Assess the home environment and its adequacy for patient safety and management of the disorder.
3. Identify any barriers to compliance and make appropriate referrals.
4. For patient at risk for impaired skin integrity, monitor skin and also instruct, provide or supervise the patient and family in preventing skin care measures.
5. Assess patient's need for assistance in the home and supervise health aides.
6. Make referrals to physical and occupational therapists; as problems are identified and limitations increase.
7. Alert patient and family to support services such as meals on wheels.
8. Assess patient's physical and psychological status, adequacy of symptom management, and adherence to the management plan.
9. Emphasize the importance of follow-up appointments to the patient and family.

OSTEOARTHRITIS (DEGENERATIVE JOINT DISEASE)

Osteoarthritis (OA), also known as degenerative joint disease; it is the most common and most frequently disabling joint disorders. It is characterized by a progressive loss of joint cartilage. Besides age, risk factors for OA include congenital and developmental disorders of the hip, obesity, previous joint damage, repetitive use (occupational or recreational), anatomic deformity and genetic susceptibility. The OA has been classified into primary (idiopathic) and secondary (resulting from previous joint injury or inflammatory disease). Obesity, in addition to being a risk factor for OA, increase symptoms of the disease OA peaks between fifth and sixth decades of life.

Clinical Manifestations

1. Pain, stiffness and functional impairment are primary clinical manifestations.
2. Stiffness is most common in the morning after awakening. It usually lasts less than 30 minutes and decreases with movement.
3. Functional impairment is due to pain on movement and limited joint motion when structural changes develop.
4. The OA occurs most often in weight-bearing joints (hips, knees, cervical and lumbar spine); finger joints are also involved.
5. Bony nodes may be present (painless unless inflamed).
6. X-ray study shows narrowing of joint space and osteophytes (spurs) at the joint margins and on the subchondral bone. These two findings together are sensitive and specific.

7. There is a weak correlation between joint pain and synovitis.
8. Blood tests are not useful in the diagnosis of this disorder.

Medical Management/Therapeutic Measures

Management focuses on slowing and treating symptoms because there is no treatment available that stops the degenerative joint disease process.

Preventive Measures

- Weight reduction
- Prevention of injuries
- Perinatal screening for congenital hip disease
- Ergonomic modifications.

Conservative Measures

- Heat, weight reduction, joint rest and avoidance of joint overuse
- Orthotic devices to support inflamed joints (splints, braces)
- Isometric and postural exercises, and aerobic exercises
- Occupational and physical therapy.

Pharmacological Therapy

- Acetaminophen, NSAIDs
- COX-2 enzyme blockers (for patients with increased risk for GI bleeding)
- Opioids and intra-articular corticosteroids
- Topical analgesics such as capsaicin and methyl salicylate
- Other therapeutic approaches—glucosamine and chondroitin, and viscosupplementation (intra-articular injection of hyaluronic acid).

Surgical Management

Use when pain is severe and function is lost, which include the following:
- Osteotomy
- Joint arthroplasty (replacement).

Nursing Management

The nursing care of the patient with OA is generally the same as the basic care plan for the patient with rheumatic disease (refer Rheumatoid Arthritis). Managing pain and optimizing functional ability are the major goals of nursing interventions, and helping patient understand their disease process and symptom patterns is critical to plan of care. It includes the followings:
1. Assist patients with management of obesity (weight loss and an increase in aerobic activity) and other health problems or diseases, if applicable.
2. Refer patient for physical therapy or to an exercise program. Exercises such as walking should be begun in moderations and increased gradually.
3. Provide and encourage use of canes or other assistive devices for ambulation as indicated.

GOUT/GOUTY ARTHRITIS

Gout is a heterogeneous group of inflammatory conditions related to genetic defect of purine metabolism and resulting in hyperuricemia.

Pathophysiology

In gout, there is an oversecretion of uric acid or a renal defect resulting in decreased excretion of uric acid, or a combination of both. Primary hyperuricemia may be due to severe dieting or starvation, excessive intake of food high in purines (shell-fish, organ meats) or hereditary. In secondary hyperuricemia, the gout is a clinical feature secondary to any of a number of genetic or acquired processes, including conditions with an increase in cell turnover (leukemia, multiple myeloma, psoriasis, some anemia) and an increase in cell breakdown.

Clinical Manifestations

Gout is characterized by deposits of uric acid in various joints. Four stages of gout can be identified namely asymptomatic hyperuricemia, acute gouty arthritis, intercritical gout and chronic tophaceous gout.

Characteristic Pattern of Gouty Arthritis

1. Acute arthritis of gout is most common early sign.
2. The metatarsophalangeal (MTP) joint of the big toe is most commonly affected; the tarsal area, ankle or knee may also be affected.
3. The acute attack may be triggered by trauma, alcohol ingestion, dieting, medications, surgical stress or illness.
4. Abrupt onset occurs at night, causing severe pain, redness, swelling and warmth over the affected joint.
5. Early attacks tend to subside spontaneously over 3–10 days without treatment.
6. The next attack may not come for months or years; at times, the attacks tend to occur more frequently, involving more joints, and last longer.
7. Tophi are generally associated with frequent and severe inflammatory episodes.
8. Higher serum concentrations of uric acid are associated with tophus formation.
9. Tophi occur in the synovium, olecranon bursa, subchondral bone, infrapatellar and Achilles tendons, subcutaneous tissue and overlying joints.
10. Tophi have also been found in aortic walls, heart valves, nasal and ear cartilage, eyelids, cornea and sclera.
11. Uric acid deposits may cause renal stones and kidney damage.

Diagnostic Methods

A definitive diagnosis of gouty arthritis is established by polarized light microscopy of the synovial fluid of the involved joint. Uric acid crystals are seen within the polymorphonuclear leukocytes in the fluid.

Medical Management

1. Colchicine (oral or parenteral) an NSAID such as indomethacin or a corticosteroid is prescribed to relieve an acute attack of gout.

2. Hyperuricemia, tophi, joint destructions and renal problems are treated after the acute inflammatory process has subsided.
3. Uricosuric agents, such as probenecid, correct hyperuricemia and dissolve deposited urate.
4. Allopurinol is effective when renal insufficiency or renal calculi are a risk.
5. Corticosteroids may be used in patients who have no response to other therapy.
6. Prophylactic treatment considered if patient experiences several acute episodes or there is evidence of tophi formation.

Nursing Management

Encourage patient to restrict consumption of foods high in purines, especially organ meats and to limit alcohol intake. Encourage patient to maintain normal body weight. These measures may help to prevent a painful episode of gout.

In acute episode of gouty arthritis, pain management is essential. Review medications with patient and family. Stress the importance of continuing medications to maintain effectiveness.

SYSTEMIC LUPUS ERYTHEMATOSUS

Systemic lupus erythematosus (SLE) is a chronic, inflammatory autoimmune collagen disease resulting from disturbed immune regulation that causes an exaggerated production of autoantibodies.

Pathophysiology

The SLE disturbance is brought about by some combination of genetic, hormonal (as evidenced by the usual onset during the childbearing years) and environmental factors (sunlight, thermal burns). Certain medications, such as hydralazine (Apresoline), procainamide (Pronestyl), isoniazid or INH (Nydrazid), chlorpromazine (Thorazine), and some antiseizure medications have been implicated in chemical or drug-induced SLE. Specifically, B cells and T cells both contribute to the immune response in SLE. The B cells are instrumental in promoting the onset and flares of the disease.

Clinical Manifestations

Onset is insidious or acute. The SLE can go undiagnosed for many years. The clinical course is one of exacerbations and remissions:

1. Classic symptoms: Fever, fatigue, weight loss and possibly arthritis, pleurisy.
2. Musculoskeletal system: Arthralgias and arthritis (synovitis) are common presenting features. Joint swelling, tenderness and pain on movement are common, accompanied by morning stiffness.
3. Integumentary system: Several different types are seen [e.g. subcutaneous lupus erythematosus (SCLE), discoid lupus erythematosus (DLE)]. A butterfly rash across the bridge of the nose and cheeks occurs in more than half of patients and may be a precursor to systemic involvement. Lesions worsen during exacerbations (flares) and may be provoked by sunlight or artificial ultraviolet light. Oral ulcers may involve buccal mucosa or hard palate.

4. Cardiovascular system: Pericarditis is the most common clinical cardiac manifestations. Women, who have SLE, are also at risk for early atherosclerosis. Papular, erythematous and purpuric lesions may occur on fingertips, elbows, toes and extensor surfaces of forearms or lateral sides of hands and may progress to necrosis.
5. Varied and frequent neuropsychiatric presentations generally demonstrated by subtle changes in behavior or cognitive ability.

Diagnostic Measures

Diagnosis is based on a complete history, physical examination and blood tests. No single laboratory test confirms SLE. Blood testing reveals moderate to severe anemia, thrombocytopenia, leukocytosis or leukopenia and positive antinuclear antibodies. Other diagnostic immunologic tests support, but do not confirm the diagnosis.

Medical Management

Treatment includes management of acute and chronic disease. Goals of treatment include preventing progressive loss of organ function, reducing the likelihood of acute disease, minimizing disease-related disabilities and preventing complications from therapy. Monitoring is preformed to assess disease activity and therapeutic effectiveness.

Medications

1. Non-steroidal anti-inflammatory drugs are used with corticosteroids to minimize corticosteroid requirements.
2. Corticosteroids are used topically for cutaneous manifestations.
3. The IV administration of corticosteroids is an alternative to traditional high-dose oral use.
4. Cutaneous, musculoskeletal and mild systemic features of SLE are managed with antimalarial drugs.
5. Immunosuppressive agents are generally reserved for the most serious forms of SLE that have not respond to conservative therapies.

Nursing Management

The nursing care of the patient with SLE is generally the same as that for the patient with rheumatic disease (Refer 'Nursing Management' under 'Arthritis, Rheumatoid'). The primary diagnoses address fatigue, impaired skin integrity, disturbed body image and deficient knowledge:

1. Be sensitive to the psychological reactions of the patient due to the changes and the unpredictable course of SLE; encourage participation in support groups, which can provide disease information, daily management tips and social support.
2. Teach patient to avoid sun and ultraviolet light exposure or to protect themselves with sunscreen and clothing.
3. Because of increased risk of involvement of multiple organ systems, teach patients about the importance of routine periodic screenings as well as health promotion activities.
4. Refer to dietician, if necessary.
5. Instruct the patient about the importance of continuing prescribed medications and address the changes and potential side effects that are likely to occur with their use.

6. Remind the patient of the importance of monitoring because of the increased risk of systemic involvement, including renal and cardiovascular effects.

BONE TUMORS

Neoplasms of the musculoskeletal system are of various types including osteogenic, chondrogenic, fibrogenic, muscle (rhabdomyogenic), and marrow (reticulum) cell tumors as well as nerve, vascular and fatty cell tumors. They may be primary tumors or metastatic tumors from primary cancers elsewhere in the body (e.g. breast, lung, prostate or kidney). Metastasis bone tumors are more common than primary bone tumors.

Types

Benign Bone Tumors

Benign bone tumors are slow growing, well circumscribed and encapsulated. They produce few symptoms and do not cause death. Benign primary neoplasms of the musculoskeletal system include osteochondroma, enchondroma, bone cyst (e.g. aneurysmal bone cyst), osteoid osteoma, rhabdomyoma and fibroma. Benign tumors of the bone and soft tissues are more common than malignant primary bone tumors.

Osteochondroma, the most common benign bone tumor, may become malignant. Enchondroma is a common tumor of the hyaline cartilage of the hand, femur, tibia or humeral. Osteoid osteoma is a painful tumor that occurs in children and young adults. Osteoclastomas (giant cell tumors) are benign for long periods, but may invade local tissue and cause destruction. These tumors may undergo malignant transformation and metastasize. Bone cysts are expanding lesions within the bone (e.g. aneurysmal and unicameral).

Malignant Bone Tumors

Primary malignant musculoskeletal tumors relatively arise from connective and supportive tissue cells [sarcoma or bone marrow elements (myelomas)]. Malignant primary musculoskeletal tumors include osteosarcoma, chondrosarcoma, Ewing's sarcoma and fibrosarcoma. Soft tissue sarcomas include liposarcoma, fibrosarcoma and rhabdomyosarcoma. Metastasis to the lungs is common. Osteogenic sarcoma (osteosarcoma) is the most common and is often fatal owing to metastasis to the lungs. It is seen most frequently in children, adolescents and young adults (in bone that grow rapidly); in older people with Paget's disease of the bone and in person's with prior history of radiation exposure. Common sites are distal femur, the proximal tibia and proximal humerus.

Chondrosarcoma the second most common primary malignant bone tumor, is a large, bulky tumor that may grow and metastasize slowly or very large, depending upon the characteristic of the tumor cells involved. Tumor sites may include pelvis, femur, humerus, spine, scapula and tibia. Tumors may occur after treatment.

Metastatic Bone Disease

Metastatic bone disease (secondary bone tumors) is more common than any primary malignant bone tumor. The most common primary sites of tumors that metastasize to bone are kidney, prostate, lung, breast, ovary and thyroid. Metastasized tumors most frequently attack the skull, spine, pelvis, femur and humerus, and often involve more than one bone.

Clinical Manifestations

Bone tumors present with a wide range of associated problems, such as:

1. Asymptomatic or pain (mild, occasional to constant, severe).
2. Varying degrees of disability at times; obvious bone growth.
3. Weight loss, malaise and fever may be present.
4. Spinal metastasis results in cord compression and neurologic deficits (e.g. progressive pain, weakness, gait abnormality, paraplegia, urinary retention, loss of bowel or bladder control).
5. May be diagnosed incidentally after pathological fracture CT scan, bone scan, myelography, MRI, arteriography X-ray studies.
6. Biochemical assays of the blood and urine (alkaline phosphatase levels are frequently elevated with metastatic carcinoma of the prostrate; hypercalcemia is present with breast, lung and kidney cancer bone metastases).
7. Surgical biopsy for histologic identification, staging based on tumor size, grade, location and metastasis.

Medical Management

The goal of treatment is to destroy or remove the tumor. This may be accomplished by surgical excision (ranging from local excision to amputation and disarticulation), radiation or chemotherapy.

1. Limb-sparing (salvage) procedures are used to remove the tumor and adjacent tissue; surgical removal of the tumor may, however, require amputation of the affected extremity.
2. Chemotherapy is started before and continued after surgery in an effort to eradicate micrometastatic lesions.
3. Soft tissue sarcomas are treated with radiation, limb-sparing excision and adjuvant chemotherapy.
4. Metastatic bone cancer treatment is palliative; therapeutic goal is to relieve pain and discomfort as much as possible while promoting quality of life.
5. Internal fixation of pathological fractures, arthroplasty or methyl methacrylate (bone cement) minimizes associated disability and pain in metastatic disease.

Nursing Management

1. Ask the patient about the onset and course of symptoms; assess the patient's understanding of the disease process, how the patient and the family have been coping and how the patient has managed the pain.
2. Gently palpate the mass and note its size and associated soft tissue swelling, pain and tenderness.
3. Assess patient's neurovascular status and range of motion of the extremity to provide baseline data for future comparison, evaluate the patient's mobility and ability to perform ADL.
4. Nursing care similar to that of other patients who have had skeletal surgery; monitor vital signs, assess blood loss; observe and assess for the development of complications such as DVT, pulmonary emboli, infection, contracture and disuse

atrophy; elevated affected part to reduce edema; and assess the neurovascular status of the extremity.
5. Teach the patient and family about the disease process and diagnostic and management regimens; explain diagnostic tests, treatments (e.g. wound care) and expected results (e.g. decreased range of motion, numbness, change of body contours) to help patient deal with the therapeutic regimen.
6. Assess pain and provide pharmacological and non-pharmacological pain management techniques to relieve pain and increase comfort level; work with the patient to design the most effective pain management regimen.
7. Prepare the patient and provide support during painful procedures.
8. Prescribe IV or epidural analgesics to be used during the early postoperative period; later, oral or transdermal opioid or non-opioid analgesics are indicated to alleviate pain; external radiation or systemic radioisotopes may be prescribed.
9. Support and handle the affected extremities gently; provide external supports (e.g. splints) for additional protection.
10. Ensure any prescribed weight-bearing restrictions are followed with help of physical therapist; teach the patient how to use assistive devices safely and how to strengthen unaffected extremities.
11. Encourage the patient and family to verbalize their fears, concerns and feelings; refer to psychiatric advanced practice nurse, psychologist, counselor or spiritual advisor, if necessary.
12. Assess the patient in dealing with changes in body image due to surgery and possible amputation; provide realistic reassurance about the future and resumption of role-related activities.
13. Encourage the patient to be as independent as possible.

BACK PAIN

Most back pain is caused by one of the many musculoskeletal problems, including acute lumbosacral strain, unstable submental ligaments and weak muscles, osteoarthritis of the spine, spinal stenosis, intervertebral disk problems and unique leg length, obesity, postural problems, structural problems, overstretching of the spinal supports and occasional depression may also result in back pain. Back pain due to musculoskeletal disorders usually is aggravated by activity, whereas pain due to other conditions is not. Older patients may experience back pain associated with osteoporotic vertebral osteoarthritis of the spine, spinal stenosis and spondylolisthesis, among other conditions.

Clinical Manifestations

1. Acute or chronic back pain (lasting more than 3 month). Evaluating improvement and fatigue.
2. Pain radiates down the leg (radiculopathy, sciatica); problems of these symptoms suggest nerve root involvement.
3. Spinal mobility, reflexes, leg length, leg motor strength and sensory perception may be affected.
4. Paravertebral muscle spasm (greatly increases muscle tone of back postural muscles) occurs with loss of normal lumbar chronic possible spinal deformity.

Diagnostic Measures

- Assess history and physical examination (back examination, neurologic testing)
- Spinal X-ray
- Bone scars and blood studies
- Computed tomography
- Magnetic resonance imaging
- Electro- and nerve-conduction studies
- Myelogram
- Ultrasound.

Medical Management

Most back pain is self-limited and resolves within 4 weeks with analgesics, rest and relaxation. Management focuses on relief of pain and discomfort, activity modification and patient education. Bedrest is recommended for 1–2 days, for a maximum of 4 days and only if pain is severe. Other effective non-pharmacological interventions include the applications of superficial heat and spinal manipulation. Cognitive-behavioral therapy (e.g. biofeedback), exercise regimen, spinal manipulations, physical therapy, acupuncture, massage and yoga are all effective non-pharmacological interventions for treating chronic low back pain, but not acute low back pain. They should avoid twisting, bending, lifting and reaching, all of which stress the back. A gradual return to activities and a program of low-stress aerobic exercises are recommended.

Medications

1. Acute low back pain: Non-prescription analgesic [e.g. acetaminophen (Tylenol)], NSAIDs [e.g. ibuprofen (Motrin)] and prescription muscle relaxants [e.g. cyclobenzaprine (Flexeril)].
2. Chronic low back pain: Tricyclic antidepressants [e.g. amitriptyline (Elavil)].
3. Other: Opioids (e.g. morphine), tramadol (Ultram), benzodiazepines [e.g. diazepam (Valium)] and gabapentin (Neurontin), i.e. prescribed for pain from radiculopathy.

Nursing Management

1. Encourage the patient to describe the discomfort (location, severity, duration, characteristics, radiation, associated weakness in the legs).
2. Obtain history of pain origin, previous pain control and how the back problem is affecting lifestyle, assess environmental variables, work situations and family relationships.
3. Observe patient's posture, position changes and gait.
4. Assess spinal curves, pelvic crest, leg length discrepancy and shoulder symmetry.
5. Palpate paraspinal muscles and note spasm and tenderness.
6. Note discomfort and limitations in movement when patient bends forward and laterally.
7. Elevate nerve involvement by assessing the deep tendon reflexes, sensations and muscle strength; back and leg pain on

straight leg is lifted upward with the knee extended suggests nerve root involvement.

8. Assess for obesity and perform nutritional assessment.
9. Assess patient's response to analgesic agents; evaluate and note patient's response to various pain management modalities.

Nursing Interventions

1. With severe pain, limit activity for 1–2 days.
2. Advise patient to rest on a firm, non-sagging mattress.
3. Help patient to increase lumbar flexion by elevating the head and thorax 30 degrees, using pillows or a foam wedge, and slightly flexing the knees supported on a pillow. Alternatively the patient can assume a lateral position with knees and hips flexed (curled position) with a pillow between the knees and legs, and a pillow supporting head.
4. Instruct the patient to get out of bed by rolling to one side and placing the legs down, while pushing the torso up, keeping the back straight.
5. After the patient achieves comfort, help patient gradually resume activities and initiate an exercise program; begin with low-stress aerobic exercise and then after 2 weeks, begin continuing exercises; each exercise period should begin with relaxation.
6. Encourage patient to adhere to the prescribed exercise program.
7. Encourage patient to improve postural and use good body mechanics, and to avoid excessive lumbar strain, twisting or discomfort (e.g. avoid activities such as horseback riding and weightlifting.
8. Teach patient how to stand, sit, lie and lift properly.
9. Shift weight frequently when standing and rest one foot on a low stool; wear low heals.
10. Sit with knees and hips flexed, and knees leveled with hips higher. Keep feet on floor. Avoid sitting on stools or chairs that do not provide firm back support.
11. Sleep on side with knees and hips flexed or supine with knees flexed and supported; avoid sleeping prone.
12. Lift objectives using thigh muscles, not back. Place feet hip width apart for a wide base of support, bend the knees, tighten the abdominal muscles and lift the object close to the body with a smooth motion. Avoid twisting and jarring motions.
13. Assist patient to resume former role-related responsibilities, when appropriate.
14. Refer patient to psychotherapy or counseling, if needed.
15. If patient is obese, assist with weight reduction through diet modification; note achievement and provide encouragement and positive reinforcement to facilitate adherence.

MUSCULAR DYSTROPHIES

Muscular dystrophies are a group of chronic muscle disorders characterized by a progressive weakening and wasting of the skeletal or voluntary muscles. Most are inherited. The pathological features include degeneration and loss of muscle fibers, variation in muscle fiber size, phagocytosis and regeneration, and replacement of muscle tissue among these diseases center on the genetic pattern of inheritance, the muscle involves the age at onset and the rate of disease progression.

Clinical Manifestations

1. Muscle wasting and weakness.
2. Gastrointestinal tract problems: Gastric dilation, rectal prolapse and fecal impaction.
3. Cardiomyopathy is a common complication in all forms of muscular dystrophy.

Medical Management

Treatment focuses on supportive care and prevention of complications. Supportive management is intended to keep patients active and functioning as normally as possible and to minimize functional deterioration. A therapeutic exercise program is individualized to prevent muscle tightness, contractures and disuse atrophy. Night splints and stretching exercises are employed to delay joint contractures (especially ankles, knees and hips). Braces may be used to fit with an orthotic jacket to improve sitting stability, reduce trunk deformity and support cardiovascular status. Spinal fusion may be performed to maintain spinal stability. All upper respiratory infections and fractures from falls are treated vigorously to minimize immobilization and to prevent joint contractures. Advise genetic counseling because of the genetic nature of this disease. Also advise patient to consult with appropriate caregivers for dental and speech problems and GI tract problems.

Nursing Management

The goals are to maintain function at optimal levels and enhance the quality of life:

1. Attend to patient's physical requirements, and emotional and development needs.
2. Actively involve patient and family in decision making, including end-of-life decisions.
3. During hospitalization, for treatment of complications, assess knowledge and expertise of patient, and family responsible for giving care in the home. Assist patient and family to maintain coping strategies used at home, while in hospital.
4. Provide patient and family with information about the disorder; it anticipates course and care, and management strategies that will optimize patient's growth and development, and physical and psychological status.
5. Communicate recommendations to all members of the healthcare team, so that they work toward the common goals.
6. Encourage patient to use self-help devices to achieve greater independence; assist adolescents to make transition to adulthood. Encourage education and job tracking as appropriate.
7. When teaching family to monitor patient for respiratory problems, give information regarding appropriate respiratory support, such as negative pressure devices and positive pressure ventilators.
8. Encourage range of motion exercises to prevent disabling contractures.
9. Assist family in adjusting home environment to maximize functional independence; patient may require manual or electric wheelchair, gait aids, seating systems, bathroom equipment, lifts, ramps and additional ADL aids.

10. Assess for signs of depression, prolonged anger, bargaining or denial and help patient to cope and adapt to chronic disease. Arrange for referrals to a psychiatric nurse clinician or other mental health professional, if indicated to assist patient to cope and adapt to the disease.
11. Provide a hopeful, supportive and nurturing environment.

OSTEOMALACIA

Osteomalacia is a metabolic bone disease characterized by inadequate mineralization of bone. The primary defect is a deficiency in activated vitamin D (calcitriol), which promotes calcium absorption from the GI tract and facilitates mineralization of bone. Osteomalacia may result from failed calcium absorption (malabsorption) or excessive loss of calcium (celiac disease, biliary tract obstruction, chronic pancreatitis, bowel resection) and loss of vitamin D (liver and kidney disease). Additional risk factors include severe renal insufficiency, hyperparathyroidism, prolonged use of antiseizures medications, malnutrition, and insufficient vitamin D (e.g. from inadequate dietary intake or inadequate sunlight exposure).

Clinical Manifestations

- Bone pain and tenderness
- Muscle weakness from calcium deficiency
- Waddling or limping gait; legs bowed in more advanced disease
- Pathological fractures
- Softened vertebrae becomes compressed, shortening the patient's trunk and deforming thorax (kyphosis)
- Weakness, unsteadiness, presenting risk of falls and fracture.

Diagnostic Measures

1. X-ray studies, bone biopsy shows increased osteoid (demineralized bone matrix).
2. Laboratory studies show low serum calcium and phosphorus levels, moderately elevated alkaline phosphatase level, decreased urine calcium and creatinine excretion.
3. Promote adequate intake of calcium and vitamin D, and a nutritious diet in disadvantaged elderly patients. Encourage patient to spend time in the sun; it reduces the incidence of fractures with prevention, identification and management of osteomalacia. When osteomalacia is combined with osteoporosis, the incidence of fractures increases.

Management

1. Physical, psychological and pharmaceutical measures are used to reduce the patient's discomfort and pain.
2. Underlying cause is corrected when possible (e.g. diet modifications, vitamin D, calcium supplements and sunlight).
3. If osteomalacia is caused by malabsorption, increased doses of vitamin D, along with supplemental calcium, are usually prescribed.
4. Exposure to sunlight may be recommended.

5. If osteomalacia is dietary in origin, a diet with adequate protein and increased calcium and vitamin D is provided.
6. Long-term monitoring is undertaken to ensure stabilization or reversal.
7. Orthopedic deformities may be treated with braces or surgery (osteotomy).

OSTEOPOROSIS

Osteoporosis is characterized by reduced bone mass, deterioration of bone matrix and diminished bone architectural strength. The bone resorption is greater than the rate of bone formation. The bones become progressively porous, brittle and fragile, and they fracture easily. Multiple compression fractures of the vertebrae result in skeletal deformity (kyphosis). This kyphosis is associated with loss of height. Patients at risk include postmenopausal women and small framed, non-obese Caucasian women.

Clinical Manifestations

Risk factors include inadequate nutrition, inadequate vitamin D and calcium, and lifestyle choices (e.g. smoking of caffeine intake and alcohol consumption), genetics and lacked physical activity. Age-related bone loss begins after peak bone mass is achieved (in fourth decade). Withdrawal of estrogens at menopause or oophorectomy causes decrease of calcitonin and accelerated bone resorption, which continues during menopausal years. Immobility contributes to the development of osteoporosis. Secondary osteoporosis is the result of medications or other conditions and diseases that affect bone metabolism. Specific disease states (e.g. corticosteroids, antiseizure medications) that place patient at risk, need to be identified and therapies instituted to reverse the development of osteoporosis.

Diagnostic Measures

1. Osteoporosis is identified on routine X-ray films when there has been 25%–40% demineralization.
2. Dual-energy X-ray absorptiometry (DEXA; DXA) provides information about spine and hip bone mass and bone mineral density (BMD).
3. Laboratory studies: Such as (e.g. serum calcium, serum phosphate, serum alkaline phosphate, urine calcium excretion, urinary hydroxyproline excretion, hematocrit, erythrocyte sedimentation rate (ESR) and X-ray studies are used to exclude other diagnosis.

Elderly people fail frequently as a result of environmental hazards, neuromuscular disorders, diminished senses and cardiovascular responses, and responses to medications. The patient and family need to include in planning for care and preventive management regimens. For example, the home environment should be assessed for safety and potential hazards (e.g. scatter rugs, cluttered rooms and stair, toys on the floor, pets underfoot). A safe environment is then be created (e.g. well-lighted staircases with secure and rails, grab bars in the bathroom, properly fitting underwear).

Medical Management

1. Adequate balance diet rich in calcium and vitamin D.
2. Increase calcium intake during adolescence, young adulthood and the middle years, or prescribe a calcium supplement with meals or beverages high in vitamin C.
3. Regular weight-bearing exercises to promote bone formation (20–30 minute aerobic exercises 3 day/week).
4. Other medications: The bisphosphonates alendronate (Fosamax), risedronate (Actonel), ibandronate (Boniva) and zoledronic acid (Reclast); calcitonin (Miacalcin); selective estrogen receptor modulators (SERMs) such as raloxifene.
5. Osteoporotic compression fractures of the vertebrae are managed conservatively. Patients who have not responded to first-line approaches to the treatment of vertebral compression fractures can be considered for percutaneous vertebroplasty or kyphoplasty (injection of polymethyl methacrylate bone cement into the fractured vertebra, followed by inflation of a pressurized balloon to restore the shape of the affected vertebra).

Nursing Management

The patient with a spontaneous vertebral fracture related to osteoporosis.

Assessment

To identify risk for and recognition of problems associated with osteoporosis, interview patient regarding family history, previous fractures, dietary consumption of calcium, exercise patterns, onset of menopause, and used of corticosteroids as well as alcohol, smoking and caffeine intake. On physical examination, observe for fracture, kyphosis of thoracic spine or shortened stature; explore any symptoms the patient is experiencing (e.g. back pain, constipation).

Nursing Diagnoses/Problems

1. Deficient knowledge of osteoporotic process and treatment regimen.
2. Acute pain related to fracture and muscle spasm.
3. Risk for constipation related to immobility or development of ileus.
4. Risk for injury; fracture related to osteoporosis bone.

Planning and Care

Major goals may include knowledge about osteoporosis and the treatment regimen, relief of pain, improved bowel elimination and absence of additional fracture.

Nursing Intervention

Promoting Knowledge of Osteoporosis

1. Focus on teaching patient about the factors influencing the development of osteoporosis, interventions to slow or arrest the process and measures to relieve symptoms.
2. Emphasize the need for sufficient calcium, vitamin D and weight-bearing exercise to slow the progression of osteoporosis.
3. Teach the patient about medication therapy.

Relieving Pain

1. Teach relief of back pain through bedrest and use of firm, non-sagging mattress, knee flexion, intermittently local heat and back rubs.
2. Instruct patient to move the trunk as a unit and avoid twisting; encourage good posture and good body mechanics.
3. Encourage patient to apply lumbosacral corset for immobilization and temporary support when out of bed.
4. Encourage the patient to gradually resume activities as pain diminishes.

Improving Bowel Elimination

1. Encourage patient to eat a high-fiber diet, increase fluids and use prescribed stool softeners.
2. Monitor patient's intake, bowel sounds and bowel activities, ileus may develop if the vertebral collapse involves T10–L2 vertebrae.

Preventing injury

1. Promote physical activity to strengthen muscles, prevent disuse atrophy and retard progressive bone demineralization.
2. Encourage patient to perform isometric exercises to strengthen trunk muscles.
3. Encourage walking, good body mechanics and good posture.
4. Instruct patient to avoid sudden bending, jarring and strenuous lifting.
5. Encourage outdoor activity in the sunshine to enhance body's ability to produce vitamin D.

Evaluation and Expected Patient Outcomes

- Acquires knowledge about osteoporosis and treatment regimen
- Achieves pain relief
- Demonstrates normal bowel elimination
- Experiences no new fractures.

OSTEOMYELITIS

Osteomyelitis is an infection of the bone. It may occur by extension of soft tissue injuries, direct bone contaminations (e.g. bone surgery, gunshot wound, hematogenous (blood) spread from other foci of infection. *Staphylococcus aureus* causes more than 50% of bone infections. Other pathogenic organism frequently found, include gram-positive organisms that include streptococci and enterococci, followed by gram-negative bacteria that include *Pseudomonas* species. Patients at risk include poorly nourished, elderly and patients who are obese; those with impaired immune systems and chronic illness (e.g. diabetes); and those on long-term corticosteroid therapy or immunosuppressive agents. The condition may be prevented by prompt treatment and management of focal and soft tissue infections.

Clinical Manifestations

1. When the infection is blood borne, onset is sudden, occurring with clinical manifestations of sepsis (e.g. chills, high fever, rapid pulse and general malaise).

2. Extremity becomes painful, swollen, warm and tender.
3. Patient may describe a constant pulsating pain that intensifies with movement (due to the pressure of collecting pus).
4. When osteomyelitis is caused by adjacent infection or direct contamination, there are no symptoms of sepsis; the area is swollen, warm, painful and tender to touch.
5. Chronic osteomyelitis presents with a non-healing ulcer that overlies the infected bone with a connecting sinus that will intermittently and spontaneously drain pus.

Diagnostic Measures

1. Acute osteomyelitis: Early X-ray films show only soft tissue swelling.
2. Chronic osteomyelitis: X-ray shows large, irregular cavities, a raised periosteum, sequestra or dense bone formations.
3. Radioisotope bone scans and MRI.
4. Blood studies and blood cultures.

Medical Management

1. Initial goal is to control and arrest the infective process.
2. General supportive measures (e.g. hydration, diet high in vitamins and proteins, correction of anemia) should be instituted; affected area is immobilized.
3. Blood and wound cultures are performed to identify organisms and select the antibiotic.
4. Intravenous antibiotic therapy is given around the clock; continues for 3–6 weeks.
5. Antibiotic medications are administered orally (on empty stomach) when infection appears to be controlled; the medication regimen is continued for up to 3 months.
6. Surgical debridement of bone is performed with irrigation; adjunctive antibiotic therapy is maintained.

Nursing Management

Assessment

1. Assess for risk factors (e.g. older age, diabetes, long-term steroid therapy) and for previous injury, infection or orthopedic surgery.
2. Observe for guarded movements of infected and generalized weakness due to systemic infection.
3. Observe for swelling and warmth of affected area, purulent drainage and elevated temperature.
4. Note that patients with chronic osteomyelitis may have minimal temperature elevations, occurring in the afternoon or evening.

Nursing Diagnoses

1. Acute pain related to inflammation and swelling.
2. Impaired physical mobility associated with pain, immobilization devices and weight-bearing limitations.
3. Risk for extension of infection; bone abscess formation.
4. Deficient knowledge about treatment regimen.

Planning and Goals

Major goals may include relief of pain, improved physical mobility within therapeutic limitations, control and eradication of infection, and knowledge of the treatment regimen.

Nursing Intervention

Relieving Pain

1. Immobilize affected part with splint to decrease pain and muscle spasm.
2. Monitor neurovascular status of affected extremity.
3. Handle affected part with great care to avoid pain.
4. Elevated affected part to reduce swelling and discomfort.
5. Administer prescribed analgesic agents and use other techniques to reduce pain.

Improving Physical Mobility

1. Teach the rationale for activity restrictions (bone is weakened by the infective process).
2. Gently move the joints above and below the affected part through their range of motions.
3. Encourage ADLs within physical limitations.

Controlling Infectious Process

1. Monitor response to antibiotic therapy. Observe intravenous sites for evidence of phlebitis or infiltration.
2. Monitor for signs of superinfection with long-term intensive antibiotic therapy (e.g. oral or vaginal candidiasis; loose or foul-smelling stools).
3. If surgery was necessary, ensure adequate circulation (wound suction, elevation of area, avoidance of pressure on grafted area); maintain immobility as needed; comply with weight-bearing restrictions. Change dressings using aseptic technique to promote healing and prevent cross-contamination.
4. Monitor general health and nutrition of patient.
5. Provide a balanced diet high in protein to ensure positive nitrogen balance and promote healing; encourage adequate hydration.

Promoting Home- and Community-based Care

Teaching patient about self-care

1. Advise patient and family to adhere strictly to the therapeutic regimen of antibiotics and preventions of falls or other injury that could result in fracture.
2. Teach patient and family how to maintain and manage the IV access site and IV administration equipment.
3. Provide in-depth medication education (e.g. drug name, dosage, frequency, administration rate, safe storage and handling, and adverse reactions), including need for laboratory monitoring.
4. Instruct patient to observe for and report elevated temperature, drainage, odor, signs of increased inflammation, adverse reactions and signs of superinfection.

Continuing care

1. Complete home assessment to determine patient's and family's ability to continue therapeutic regimen.
2. Refer for a home care nurse, if indicated.
3. Monitor patient for response to treatment, signs and symptoms of superinfection, and adverse drug reactions.
4. Stress importance of follow-up healthcare appointments and recommend age—appropriate health screening.

Expected Patient Outcomes

- Experiences pain relief
- Increases physical mobility
- Shows absence of infection
- Adheres to therapeutic plan.

12

Chapter Neurological Nursing

INCREASED INTRACRANIAL PRESSURE

Increased intracranial pressure (ICP) is the result of the amount of brain tissue, blood and cerebrospinal fluid (CSF) within the skull at any one time. The volume and pressure of these three components are usually in a state of equilibrium. Because, there is limited space for expansions within the skull, an increase in any of these components causes a change in the volume of the others by displacing or shifting CSF, increasing the absorption or diminishing the production of CSF, or decreasing cerebral blood volume. The normal ICP is 0–10 mm Hg with 15 mm Hg, the upper limit of normal. Although elevated ICP is most commonly associated with head injury, an elevated pressure may be seen secondary to brain tumors, subarachnoid hemorrhage and toxic and viral encephalopathies. Increased ICP from any cause decreases cerebral fusion, stimulates further swelling and may shift brain tissue resulting in herniation, a dire and frequently fatal event.

Clinical Manifestations

When ICP increases to the point where the brains ability to adjust has reached its limit, neural function is impaired. Increased ICP is manifested by changes in levels of consciousness and abnormal respiratory and vasomotor responses. The following are the signs and symptoms:

1. Lethargy is the earliest sign of increasing ICP. Slowing of speech and delay in response to verbal suggestions are early indicators.
2. Sudden change in condition such as restlessness (without apparent cause), confusion or increasing drowsiness has neurological significance.
3. As pressure increases, patient becomes stuporous and may react only to loud auditory or painful stimuli. This indicates serious impairment of brain circulation and immediate surgical interventions may be required. With further deterioration, coma and abnormal motor responses in the form of decortication, decerebration or flaccidity may occur.
4. When coma is profound, pupils are dilated and fixed, respirations are impaired and death is usually inevitable.
5. Decreases cerebral perfusion pressure (CPP) can result in a Cushings response and Cushing's triad (bradycardia, bradypnea and hypertension); widening pulse pressure is an ominous sign.

Diagnostic Methods

1. Computed tomography (CT) and magnetic resonance imaging (MRI) are most common diagnostic tests.
2. The ICP monitoring provides useful information (ventriculostomy, subarachnoid bolt/screw, epidural monitor and fiberoptic monitor).

Medical Management

Increased ICP is true emergency and must be treated promptly. Immediate management involves invasive monitoring of ICP, decreasing cerebral edema, lowering the volume of CSF or decreasing cerebral blood volume, while maintaining cerebral perfusion.

Pharmacological Therapy

1. Osmotic diuretics and possibly corticosteroids are administered, fluid is restricted, CSF is drained, fever is controlled [using antipyretics, hypothermia blanket, with chlorpromazine (Thorazine) to control shivering] and cellular metabolic demands are reduced (with barbiturates paralyzing agents).
2. If patient does not respond to conventional treatment, cellular metabolic demands may be reduced by administering high doses of barbiturates or administering pharmacological paralyzing agents such as pancuronium (Pavulon).
3. Patient requires care in a critical care unit.

Nursing Management

Assessment

1. Obtain patient history with subjective data including events leading to present illness.
2. Complete a neurological examination as patient's condition allows. Evaluate mental status, level of consciousness (LOC), cranial nerve function, cerebral function (balance and coordination), reflexes and motor and sensitivity function.
3. Ongoing assessment is more focused including pupil checks, assessment of selected cranial nerves, frequent measurements of vital signs and ICP, and use of the Glasgow coma scale.

Nursing Diagnoses/Problems

- Ineffective airway clearance related to diminished protective reflexes (cough, gag)
- Ineffective breathing patterns related to neurological dysfunction (brainstem compression, structural displacement)
- Ineffective cerebral tissue perfusion related to the effects of increased ICP
- Deficient fluid volume related to fluid restrictions
- Risk for infection related to ICP monitoring system (fiberoptic or intraventricular catheter).

Potential complications: Brainstem herniation, diabetes insipidus and syndrome of inappropriate antidiuretic hormone (SIADH) secretion.

Planning (Goals and Objectives)

The major goals of the patient may include maintenance of a patent airway, normalization of respiration and adequate cerebral tissue perfusion through reduction in ICP, restoration of fluid balance and absence of infection and complications.

Nursing Interventions (Implementation)

Maintaining Patent Airway

- Maintain patency of the airway; oxygenate patient before and after suctioning
- Discourage coughing and straining
- Auscultate lung fields for adventitious sounds every 8 hours
- Elevate the head of bed to clear secretions and improve venous drainage of the brain.

Achieving an Adequate Breathing Pattern

- Monitor constantly for respiratory irregularities
- Collaborate with respiratory therapist in monitoring arterial carbon dioxide pressure ($PaCO_2$) that is usually maintained below 30 mm Hg when hyperventilation is used
- Maintain continuous neurological observation record with repeated assessments.

Optimizing Cerebral Tissue Perfusion

1. Keep patient's head in a neutral (midline) position, maintained with the use of a cervical collar, if necessary to promote venous drainage. Elevation of the head is maintained at 30°–45° unless contraindicated.
2. Avoid extreme rotation and flexion of the neck because of compression or distortion of the jugular veins increases ICP.
3. Avoid extreme hip flexion: This position causes an increase in intra-abdominal and intrathoracic pressures, which produce a rise in ICP.
4. Rotating beds, turning sheets and holding the patient's head during turning may minimize the stimuli that increase ICP.
5. Instruct patient to avoid the Valsalva maneuver; instruct patient to exhale, while moving or turning in bed.
6. Provide stool softeners and high-fiber diet, if patient can eat; note any abdominal distention; avoid enemas and cathartics.
7. Avoid suctioning longer than 15 seconds; preoxygenated and hyperventilate on ventilator with 100% oxygen before suctioning.
8. Pace interventions to prevent transient increase in ICP. During nursing care, ICP should not rise above 25 mm Hg and should return to baseline within 5 minutes.
9. Maintain a calm atmosphere and reduce environmental stimuli; avoid emotional stress.

Maintaining Negative Fluid Balance

- Administer corticosteroids and dehydrating agents as ordered
- Assess skin turgor, mucous membranes, urine output and serum and urine osmolality for signs of dehydration
- Administer intravenous (IV) fluids by pump at a slow to moderate rate; monitor patients receiving mannitol for congestive failure
- Monitor vital signs to assess fluid volume status
- Insert dwelling catheter to assess renal and fluid status
- Monitor urine output every hour in the acute phase
- Give oral hygiene for mouth dryness.

Preventing Infection

1. Strictly adhere to the facilities written protocols for managing ICP monitoring systems.
2. Use aseptic technique at all times when managing the ventricular drainage system and changing drainage bag.
3. Check carefully for any loose connections that cause leaking, contamination of the ventricular system and contamination of CSF drainage for signs of infection (cloudiness or blood). Report the changes.
4. Monitor for signs and symptoms of meningitis such as fever, chills, nuchal (neck) rigidity and increasing or persistent headache.

Managing Potential Complications

1. Assess for and immediately report any of the following early signs or symptoms of increasing ICP: Disorientation, restlessness, increased respiratory effort, purposeless movements and mental confusion; pupillary changes and impaired extraocular movements; weakness in one extremity or on one side of the body; headache that is constant, increasing in intensity and aggravated by movement or straining.
2. Assess for and immediately report any of the following later signs and symptoms: LOC that continues to deteriorate until patient is comatose; decreased or erratic pulse rate and respiratory rate, increased blood pressure (BP) and temperature, widened pulse pressure, rapidly fluctuating pulse; altered respiratory patterns (Cheyne-Stokes breathing and ataxic breathing); projectile vomiting, hemiplegia, decorticate or decerebrate posturing; loss of brainstem reflexes.
3. The ICP elevation: Monitor ICP closely for continuous elevation or significant increase over baseline; assess vital signs and manifestations of increasing ICP.
4. Impending brain herniation: Monitor for increase in BP, decrease in pulse and change in pupillary response.
5. Diabetes insipidus requires fluid and electrolyte replacement and administration of vasopressin; monitor serum electrolytes for replacement.
6. The SIADH requires fluid restriction and serum electrolyte monitoring.

Evaluations

Evaluation is based on the objectives and expected patient outcomes:

- Maintain patent airway
- Attains optimal breathing pattern
- Demonstrates optimal cerebral tissue perfusion
- Attains desired fluid balance
- Has no sign of infection
- Remains free of complications.

HEAD INJURY (BRAIN INJURY)

Injuries to the head involve trauma to the scalp, skull and brain. A head injury may lead to conditions ranging from mild concussion to coma and death; the most serious form is known as a traumatic brain injury (TBI). The most common causes of TBI are falls (28%), motor vehicle crashes (20%), being struck by objects (19%) and assaults

(11%). Groups at highest risk for TBI are persons 15–19 years of age with a 2:1 male to female ratio. Adults 75 years of age or older have the highest TBI-related hospitalization and death rates.

Clinical Manifestations

Symptoms other than local depend on the severity and the anatomical location of the underlying brain injury:

1. Persistent, localized pain usually suggests fracture.
2. Fracture of the cranial vault may or may not produce swelling in that region.
3. Fractures of the base of the skull frequently produce hemorrhage from the nose, pharynx or ears and blood may appear under the conjunctiva.
4. Ecchymosis may be seen over the mastoid (Battle sign).
5. Drainage of CSF from the ears and the nose suggest basal skull fracture.
6. Drainage of CSF may cause serious infection (e.g. meningitis) through a tear in the dura mater.
7. Bloody spinal fluid suggests brain laceration or contusion.
8. Brain injury may have various signs including altered LOC, papillary abnormalities, altered or absent gag reflex, or corneal reflex, neurological deficits, change in vital signs (e.g. respiration pattern, hypertension, bradycardia), hyperthermia or hypothermia and sensory, vision or hearing impairment.
9. Signs of postconcussion syndrome may include headache, dizziness, anxiety, irritability and lethargy.
10. In acute or subacute subdural hematoma, changes in LOC, pupillary signs, hemiparesis, coma, hypertension, bradycardia and slowing respiratory rate are signs of expanding mass.
11. Chronic subdural hematoma may result in severe headache, alternating focal neurological signs, personality changes, mental deterioration and focal seizures.

Diagnostic Methods

- Physical examination and evaluation of neurological status
- Radiographic studies, X-ray, CT, MRI
- Cerebral angiography.

Scalp and Skull Injuries

1. Scalp trauma may result in an abrasion (brush wound), contusion, laceration or hematoma. The scalp bleeds profusely when injured. Scalp wounds are a portal of entry for intracranial infections.
2. Fracture of the skull is a break in the continuity of the skull caused by forceful trauma. Fractures may occur with or without damage to the brain. They are classified as simple, comminuted, depressed or basilar and may be open (dura is torn) or close (dura is not torn).

Medical Management

1. Non-depressed skull fractures generally do not require surgical treatment, but require close observation of patient.

2. Depressed skull fracture usually requires surgery with elevation of the skull and debridement, usually within 24 hours of injury.

Concussion (Brain Injury)

A cerebral concussion after head injury is a temporary loss of neurological function with no apparent structural damage. A concussion (also referred to as a mild TBI) may or may not produce a brief loss of consciousness. The mechanisms of injury are a usually blunt trauma form an acceleration-deceleration force, a direct blow or a blast injury. If brain tissue in the frontal lobe is affected, the patient may exhibit bizarre irrational behavior, whereas involvement of the temporal lobe can produce temporary amnesia or disorientation.

Nursing Management

1. Give information, explanations and encouragement to reduce postconcussion syndrome.
2. Instruct family to look for the following signs and notify physician or clinic; difficulty in awakening or speaking, confusion, severe headache, vomiting and weakness of one side of the body.

Contusion

A cerebral contusion is moderate to severe head injury in which the brain is bruised and damaged in a specific area because of severe acceleration-deceleration force or blunt trauma. The impact of the brain against the skull leads to a contusion. Contusions are characterized by LOC associated with stupor and confusion. Other characteristics can include tissue alteration and neurological deficit without hematoma formation, alternation in consciousness without localized signs, hemorrhage into the tissue that varies in size and in surrounded by edema. The effects of injury (hemorrhage and edema) peak after 18–36 hours. Patient outcome depends on the area and severity of the injury. Temporal lobe contusions carry a greater risk of swelling, rapid deterioration and brain herniation. Deep contusions are more often associated with hemorrhage and destruction of the reticular-activating fiber alternating arousal.

Diffuse Axonal Injury

Diffuse axonal injury results from widespread shearing and rotational forces that produce damage throughout the brain to axons in the cerebral hemisphere, corpus callosum and brainstem. The injured area may be diffuse with no identifiable focal lesion. The patient has no lucid intervals and experiences immediate coma, decorticate and decerebrate posturing and global cerebral edema. Diagnosis is made by clinical signs and by CT or MRI. Recovery depends on the severity of the axonal injury.

Intracranial Hemorrhage

Hematomas are collections of blood in the brain that may be epidural (above the dura), subdural (below the dura) or intracerebral (within the brain). Major symptoms are frequently delayed until the hematoma is large enough to cause distortion of the brain and increased ICP.

Epidural Hematoma (Extradural Hematoma or Hemorrhage)

Blood collects in the epidural space between the skull and dura mater. The hematoma can result from a skull fracture that causes a rupture or laceration of the middle meningeal artery. The artery that runs between the dura and skull inferior to a thin portion of temporal bone. Symptoms are caused by the pressure of the expanding hematoma. Usually, a momentary loss of consciousness at time of injury followed by an interval of apparent recovery, while compensation is no longer possible, sudden signs of herniation may appear including deterioration of consciousness and signs of focal neurological deficits (dilation and fixation of a pupil or paralysis of an extremity); the patient deteriorates rapidly.

Medical Management

Epidural hematoma is an extreme emergency because marked neurological deficit or respiratory arrest may occur within minutes. But holes are made to remove the clots and the bleeding point is controlled (craniotomy, drain insertion).

Subdural Hematoma

Blood collects between the dura and the underlying brain and is more frequently venous in origin. The most common cause is trauma, but it may also be associated with various bleeding tendencies (coagulopathies) or rupture of an aneurysm. Subdural hematoma may be acute (major head injury), subacute (sequelae of less contusions) or chronic (minor head injuries in the elderly may be a cause; signs and symptoms fluctuate and may be mistaken for neurosis, psychosis or stroke).

Intracerebral Hemorrhage and Hematoma

Bleeding occurs into the substance of the brain. Hematoma is commonly seen when forces are exerted to the head over a small area (missile injuries or bullet wounds; stab injury). It may also result from systemic hypertension causing degeneration and rupture of a vessel and saccular aneurysm; vascular anomalies; intracranial tumors; bleeding disorders such as leukemia, hemophilia, aplastic anemia and thrombocytopenia and complications of anticoagulant therapy. Its onset may be insidious with neurological deficits followed by headache.

Medical Management for Head Injury

Presume that a person with a head injury has a cervical spine injury until proven otherwise. From the scene of the injury, the patient is transported on a board with head and neck maintained is alignment with the axis of the body. Apply a cervical collar and maintain it until cervical spine X-rays have been obtained and the absence of cervical spine X-rays have been obtained and injury documented. All therapy is directed toward preserving brain homeostasis and secondary brain injury.

Nursing Management

Assessment

Obtain health history including time of injury, cause of injury, direction and force of the blow, LOC and condition following injury.

Detailed neurological information (LOC, ability to respond to verbal commands, if patient is conscious), response to light, corneal and gag reflexes, motor function and system assessment provide baseline data. The Glasgow coma scale serves as a guide for assessing LOCs base on three criteria:

1. Eye opening.
2. Verbal responses.
3. Motor responses to a verbal command or painful stimulus.

Monitoring vital signs

1. Monitor patient at frequent intervals to assess intracranial status.
2. Assess for increasing ICP including slowing of pulse, increasing systolic pressure and widening pulse pressure. As brain compression increases, vital signs are reversed, pulse and respiration become rapid and BP may decrease.
3. Monitor for rapid rise in body temperature; keep temperature below 38°C (100.4°F) to avoid increased metabolic demands of the brain.
4. Keep in mind that tachycardia and hypotension may indicate bleeding elsewhere in the body.

Assessing motor function

1. Observing spontaneous movements; ask patient to raise the lower extremities; compare strength and equality of the upper and lower extremities at periodic intervals.
2. Note presence or absence of spontaneous movement of the each extremity.
3. Determine patient's ability to speak; note quality of speech.
4. Assess responses to painful stimuli in absence of spontaneous movement; abnormal response carries a poorer prognosis.

Other neurological signs and observations

1. Evaluate spontaneous eye opening.
2. Evaluate size of pupils and reaction to light (unilaterally dilated and poorly responding pupils may indicate developing hematoma). If both pupils are fixed and dilated, it usually indicates overwhelming injury and poor prognosis.
3. The patient with a head injury may develop deficits such as anosmia (lack of sense of smell), eye movement abnormalities, aphasia, memory deficits and post-traumatic seizures or epilepsy.
4. Patients may be left with residual psychosocial deficits and may lack insight into their emotional responses.

Nursing Diagnoses/Problems

1. Ineffective airway clearance and impaired gas exchange related to brain injury.
2. Ineffective CPP and possible seizures.
3. Deficient fluid volume related to decreased LOC and hormonal dysfunction.
4. Imbalanced nutrition less than body requirements, related to increased metabolic demands, fluid restriction and inadequate intake.
5. Risk for injury (self-directed and directed at others) related to seizures, disorientation and restlessness or brain damage.
6. Risk for imbalanced body temperature related to damaged temperature regulating mechanisms in the brain.

7. Risk for impaired skin integrity related to bedrest, hemiparesis, hemiplegia and immobility or restlessness.
8. Disturbed thought processes (deficits in intellectual function, communications, memory and information processings) related to brain injury.
9. Disturbed sleep pattern related to brain injury and frequent neurological checks.
10. Interrupted family processes related to unresponsiveness of patient, unpredictability outcome, prolonged recovery period and the patient's residual physical disability and emotional deficit.
11. Deficit knowledge about brain injury, recovery and the rehabilitation process.

Potential complications: Decreased cerebral perfusion; cerebral edema and herniation; impaired oxygenation and ventilation; impaired fluid, electrolyte and nutritional balance and risk for post-traumatic seizures.

Planning (Goals and Objectives)

Goals may include maintenance of a patent airway, adequate CPP, fluid and electrolyte balance, adequate nutritional status, prevention of secondary injury, maintenance of normal body temperature, maintenance of skin integrity, improvement of cognitive function, prevention of sleep deprivation, effective family coping, increased knowledge about the rehabilitation process and absence of complications.

Nursing Interventions (Implementations)

Maintaining the Airway

1. Position the unconscious patient to facilitate drainage of secretions; elevate the head of bed 30° to decrease intracranial venous pressure.
2. Establish effective suctioning procedures.
3. Guard against aspiration and respiratory insufficiency.
4. Monitor arterial blood gases (ABGs) to assess adequacy of ventilation.
5. Monitor patient on mechanical ventilation for pulmonary complications [acute respiratory distress syndrome (ARDS) and pneumonia].

Maintaining Fluid and Electrolyte Balance

1. Fluid and electrolyte balance is particularly important in patients receiving osmotic diuretics those with SIADH secretion and those with post-traumatic diabetes insipidus.
2. Monitor serum and urine electrolyte levels (including blood glucose and urine acetone), osmolality and intake and output to evaluate endocrine function.
3. Record daily weights (which may indicate fluid loss from diabetes insipidus).

Promoting Adequate Nutrition

1. Parenteral nutrition (PN) via a central line or enteral feedings administered via a nasogastric or nasojejunal feeding tube may be used.

2. Monitor laboratory values closely in patients receiving PN.
3. Elevate the head of the bed and aspirate the enteral tube for evidence of residual feeding before administering additional feedings to prevent distention, regurgitation and aspiration, a continuous drip infusion or pump may be used to regulate the feeding.
4. Continue enteral or parenteral feedings until the swallowing reflex returns and the patient can meet caloric requirement orally.

Preventing Injury

1. Observe for restlessness, which may be due to hypoxia, fever and pain or a full bladder. Restlessness may also be a sign that the unconscious patient in regaining consciousness.
2. Avoid the restraints when possible because of straining can increase ICP.
3. Avoid bladder distention.
4. Protect patient from injury (padded side rails, hands wrapped in mitts).
5. Avoid using opioids for restlessness because they depress respiration, constrict pupils and alter LOC.
6. Keep environmental stimuli to a minimum.
7. Provide adequate lighting to prevent visual hallucinations.
8. Minimize disruption of patient's sleep/wake cycles.
9. Lubricate the patient's skin with oil or emollient lotion to prevent irritation due to rubbing against the sheet.
10. Use an external sheath catheter for incontinence because an indwelling catheter may produce infection.

Maintaining Body Temperature

1. Monitor temperature every 2–4 hours.
2. If temperature rises, try to identify the cause and administer acetaminophen and cooling blankets as prescribed to achieve normothermia.
3. Monitor for infection related to fever.

Maintaining Skin Integrity

1. Assess all body surfaces and document skin integrity in every 8 hours.
2. Turn patient and reposition in every 2 hours.
3. Provide skin care in every 4 hours.
4. Assist patient to get out of bed three times a day (when appropriate).

Improving Cognitive Functioning

1. Develop patient's ability to devise problem-solving strategies through cognitive rehabilitation overtime; use a multidisciplinary approach.
2. Be aware that there are fluctuations in orientation and memory and these patients are easily distracted.
3. Do not push to a level greater than patient's impaired cortical functioning allows because fatigue, anger and stress (headache, dizziness) may occur.

4. Level of cognitive function scale is frequently used to assess cognitive function and evaluate ongoing recovery from head injury.

Preventing Sleep Pattern Disturbance

1. Group nursing activities, so that the patient is disturbed less frequently.
2. Decrease environmental noise and dim room lights.
3. Provide strategies (e.g. back rubs) to increase comfort.

Supportive Family Coping

1. Provide family with accurate and honest information.
2. Encourage family to continue to set well-defined, mutual and short-term goals.
3. Encourage family counseling to deal with feelings of loss and helplessness, and provide guidance in the management of inappropriate behavior.
4. Refer family to support groups that provide a forum of networking, sharing problems and gaining assistance in maintaining realistic expectations and hope. The brain injury association provides information and other resources.
5. Assist patient and family in making decisions to end-of-life support and permit donation of organs.

Monitor and Managing Potential Complications

1. Take measures to control CPP (e.g. elevate the head of the bed and increase IV fluids).
2. Take measure for a patent airway, altered breathing pattern, hypoxemia and pneumonia. Assist with intubation and mechanical ventilation.
3. Provide enteral feedings, IV fluids and electrolytes or insulin as prescribed.
4. Initiate PN as ordered, if patient is unable to eat.
5. Assess carefully for development of post-traumatic seizures.

Promoting Family- and Community-based Care

Teaching patients about self-care

1. Reinforce information given to family about patient's condition and prognosis early in the course of head injury.
2. As patient's status changes overtime, focus teaching on interpretation and explanation of changes in patient's responses.
3. Instruct patient and family about limitations that can be expected and complications that may occur, if patient is to be discharged.
4. Explain to the patient and family, verbally and in writing, how to monitor the complications by merit or contacting the neurosurgeon.
5. Teach about self-care management strategies, if patient's status indicates.
6. Instruct about side effects of medications and importance.

Continuing care

1. Encourage patient to continue rehabilitation program after discharge. Improvement may take 3 or more years after injury

during which time the family and their coping skills need frequent assessment.
2. Encourage patient to return to normal activities gradually.
3. Remind the patient and family of the need for continuing health promotion and screening practices after the initial phase of care.

Evaluations

Evaluation is based on objectives, i.e. expected patient outcomes:
- Attains or maintains effective airway clearance, ventilation and brain oxygenation
- Achieves satisfactory fluid and electrolyte balance
- Attains adequate nutritional status
- Avoids injury
- Maintains normal body temperature
- Demonstrates intact skin integrity
- Shows improvement in cognitive function and improved memory
- Demonstrates normal sleep/wake cycle
- Demonstrates absence of complications
- Experiences no post-traumatic seizures
- Family demonstrates adaptive coping processes
- Patient and family participate in rehabilitation process as indicated.

MENINGITIS

Meningitis is an inflammation of the lining around the base and spinal cord caused by bacteria or viruses. Meningitis is classified as septic or aseptic. The aseptic form may be viral or secondary to lymphoma, leukemia or human immunodeficiency virus (HIV). The septic form is caused by bacteria such as *Streptococcus pneumoniae* and *Neisseria meningitidis.*

Pathophysiology

The causative organism enters the bloodstream, crosses the blood-brain barrier (BBB) and triggers an inflammatory reaction in the meninges. Independent of the causative agent, inflammation of the subarachnoid and pia mater occurs then ICP results. Meningeal infections generally originate in one of two ways, either through the bloodstream from other infections (cellulitis) or by direct extension (after traumatic injury to the facial bones). Bacterial of meningococcal meningitis also occur as an opportunistic infections in patients with acquired immunodeficiency syndrome (AIDS) and as complication of Lyme disease.

Bacterial meningitis is the most significant form. The common bacterial pathogens are *N. meningitidis* (meningococcal meningitis) and *S. pneumoniae,* accounting for 80% of cases of meningitis in adults. *Haemophilus influenzae* was once a common cause of meningitis in children, but because of vaccination infection with this organism is now rare in developed countries.

Clinical Manifestations

1. Headache and fever are frequently the initial symptoms; fever tends to remain high throughout the course of the illness; the headache is usually either steady or throbbing and very severe as a result of meningeal irritation.

2. Meningeal irritations results in a number of other well-recognized signs common to all types of meningitis:
   - Nuchal rigidity (stiff neck) is an early sign
   - Positive Kernig's sign: When lying with thigh flexed on abdomen, patient cannot completely extend leg
   - Positive Brudzinski's sign: Flexing patient's neck produced flexion of the knees and hips; passive flexion of lower extremity of one side produces similar movement for opposite extremity.
3. Photophobia (extreme sensitivity to light) is common.
4. Rash (*N. meningitidis*): Ranges from petechial rash with purpuric lesions to large areas of ecchymosis.
5. Disorientation and memory impairment; behavioral manifestations are also common. As the illness progresses, lethargy, unresponsiveness and coma may develop.
6. Seizures can occur and are the results of areas of irritability in the brain; ICP increases secondary to diffuse brain swelling or hydrocephalus; initial signs of increased ICP include decreased level of consciousness and focal motor deficits.
7. An acute fulminant infection occur in about 10% of patients with meningococcal meningitis producing signs of overwhelming septicemia; an abrupt onset of high fever, extensive purpuric lesions (over the face and extremities), shock and signs of disseminated intravascular coagulation (DIC) and death may occur within a few hours after onset of the infection.

Diagnostic Findings

1. Computed tomography or MRI to detect a shift in brain contents, which may lead to herniation prior to a lumbar puncture.
2. Key diagnostic tests are bacterial culture and Gram straining of CSF and blood.

Preventive Measures

The meningococcal conjugate vaccine be given to adolescents entering high school and to college freshmen living in dormitories. Vaccination should also be considered as an adjunct to antibiotic chemoprophylaxis for anyone living with a person who develops meningococcal infection. Vaccination against *H. influenzae* and *S. pneumoniae* should be encouraged for children and at risk adults.

People in close contact with patients with meningococcal meningitis should be treated with antimicrobial chemoprophylaxis using rifampin (Rifadin), ciprofloxacin hydrochloride or ceftriaxone sodium (Rocephin). Therapy should be started within 24 hours after exposure because a delay in initiation of therapy limits effectiveness of the prophylaxis.

Medical Management/Therapeutic Measures

1. Vancomycin hydrochloride in combination with one of cephalosporins (e.g. ceftriaxone sodium, cefotaxime sodium is administered by IV injection.
2. Dexamethasone (Decadron) has been shown to be beneficial as adjunct therapy in the treatment of acute bacterial meningitis and in pneumococcal meningitis.

3. Dehydration and shock are treated with fluid volume expanders.
4. Seizures, which may occur early in the course of the diseases are controlled with phenytoin (Dilantin).
5. Increased ICP is treated as necessary.

Nursing Management

Prognosis depends largely on the supportive care provided. Related nursing interventions include the following:

1. Assess neurological status and vital signs constantly. Determine oxygenation from ABG values and pulse oximetry.
2. Insert cuffed endotracheal tube (or tracheostomy) and position patient on mechanical ventilation as prescribed.
3. Assess BP (usually monitored using an arterial line) for incipient shock, which precedes cardiac or respiratory failure.
4. Rapid IV fluid replacement may be prescribed, but take care not to overhydrate patient because of risk of cerebral edema.
5. Reduce high fever to decrease load on heart and brain from oxygen demands.
6. Protect the patient from injury secondary to seizure activity or altered LOC.
7. Monitor daily body weight; serum electrolytes; urine volume, specific gravity and osmolality, especially if syndrome of SIADH is suspected.
8. Prevent complications associated with immobility such as pressure ulcers and pneumonia.
9. Institute infection control precautions until 24 hours after initiation of antibiotic therapy (oral and nasal discharge is considered infectious).
10. Inform family about patient's condition and permit family to be patient at appropriate intervals.

BRAIN ABSCESS

A brain abscess is a collection of infectious material within the tissue of the brain. Bacterial are the most common causative organism. An abscess can result from intracranial surgery, penetrating head injury or tongue piercing. Organism causing brain abscess may reach the brain by hematological spread from the lungs, gums, tongue or heart, or from a wound or intra-abdominal infections. It can be a complication in patients whose immune system has been suppressed through therapy or disease.

Clinical Manifestations

1. Generally, symptoms result from alterations in intracranial dynamics (edema, brain shift), infection or the location of the abscess.
2. Headache, usually worse in morning, is the most prevailing symptoms.
3. Fever, vomiting and focal neurological deficits (weakness and decreasing vision) occur as well.
4. As the abscess expands, symptoms of increased ICP such as decreasing LOC and seizures are observed.

Diagnostic Methods

1. Neuroimaging studies such as MRI or CT to identify the size and location of the abscess.
2. Aspiration of the abscess guided by CT or MRI to culture and identify the infectious organism.
3. Blood cultures, chest X-ray, electroencephalography (EEG).

Preventions

To prevent brain abscess, otitis media, mastoiditis, rhinosinusitis, dental infection and systemic infections should be treated promptly.

Medical Management

The goal is to eliminate the abscess. Treatment modalities include antimicrobial therapy, surgical incision or aspiration (CT-guided stereotactic needle). Medications used include corticosteroids to reduce the inflammatory cerebral edema and antiseizure medications for prophylaxis against seizures (phenytoin, phenobarbital). Abscess resolution is monitored by CT.

Nursing Management

Nursing interventions support the medical treatment, as do patient teaching activities that address neurosurgical procedures. Patients and families need to be advised of neurological deficits that may remain after treatment (hemiparesis, seizures, visual deficits and cranial nerve palsies). The nurse assesses the family's ability to express their distress at the patient's condition, copes with patient's illness and deficits and obtain support. Refer 'Nursing Management' under Associated Neurological Conditions (e.g. epilepsies, meningitis or ICP).

BRAIN TUMORS

A brain tumor is a localized intracranial lesion that occupies space within the skull. Primary brain tumors originate from cells and structures within the brain. Secondary or metastatic brain tumors develop from structures outside the brain [lung, breast, lower gastrointestinal tract, pancreas, kidney and skin (melanomas)] and occur in 10%–20% of all cancer patients. The highest incidence of brain tumors in adults occurs between the fifth and seventh decades. Brain tumors rarely metastasize outside the central nervous system (CNS), but death cause by impairing vital functions (respiration) or by increasing the ICP. Brain tumors may be classified into several groups such as those arising from the coverings of the brain (e.g. dural meningioma), those developing in or on the cranial nerves (e.g. acoustic neuroma), those originating within brain tissue (e.g. glioma) and metastatic lesions originating elsewhere in the body. Tumors of the pituitary and pineal glands and of cerebral blood vessels are also types of brain tumors. Tumors may be benign or malignant. A benign tumor may occur in a vital area and have effects as serious as a malignant tumor.

Types of Tumors

1. Gliomas, the most common brain neoplasms cannot be totally removed without causing damage because they spread by infiltrating into the surrounding neural tissue.
2. Meningiomas are common benign encapsulated tumors of arachnoid cells on the meninges. They are slow growing and occur most often in middle-aged women.
3. An acoustic neuroma is a tumor of the VIII cranial nerve (hearing and balance). It may grow slowly and attain considerable size before it is correctly diagnosed.
4. Pituitary adenomas may cause symptoms as a result of pressure on adjacent structures or hormonal changes such as hyperfunction or hypofunction of the pituitary.
5. Angiomas are masses compose largely of abnormal blood vessels and are found in or on the surface of the brain; they may never cause symptoms or they may give rise to symptoms of brain tumor. The walls of the blood vessels in angiomas are thin, increasing at risk for hemorrhagic stroke.

Clinical Manifestations

1. Increased ICP.
2. Headache, although not always present, is most common in the early morning and is made worse by coughing, straining, sudden movement. Headaches are usually described as deep, expanding or dull, but unrelenting. Frontal tumors produce a bilateral frontal headache; pituitary gland tumors produce bitemporal pain; in cerebellar tumors, the headache may be located in the suboccipital region at the back of the head.
3. Vomiting, seldom related to food intake, is usually due to irritation of the vagal centers in the medulla.
4. Papilledema (edema of the optic nerve) is associated with visual disturbances.
5. Personality changes and a variety of focal deficits including motor, sensory and cranial nerve dysfunction are common.

Signs and Symptoms

The progression of the signs and symptoms is important because it indicates tumor growth and expansion. The most common focal or localized symptoms are hemiparesis, seizures and mental status changes. Localized symptoms of different tumors are the following:

1. Tumor of the motor cortex: Seizure-like movements localized to one side of the body (Jacksonian seizures).
2. Occipital lobe tumors: Visual manifestations such as contralateral homonymous hemianopsia (visual loss in half the visual field on the opposite side of tumor) and visual hallucinations.
3. Tumors of the cerebellum: Dizziness, an ataxic staggering gait with tendency to fall toward side of lesion; marked muscle incoordination and nystagmus.
4. Tumors of the frontal lobe: Personality disorders, changes in emotional state and behavior and an apathetic mental attitude.
5. Tumors of the cerebellopontine angle: Usually, originate in sheath of acoustic nerve, tinnitus and vertigo then progressive

nerve deafness (VIII cranial nerve dysfunction); staggering gait, numbness and tingling of the face and tongue, progressing to weakness and paralysis of the face; abnormalities in motor function may be present.

Assessment and Diagnostic Methods

1. History of the illness and manner in which symptoms evolved.
2. Neurological examination indicating areas involved.
3. Positron emission tomography (PET), CT, MRI, computer-assisted stereotactic (three dimensional) biopsy, cerebral angiography, EEG and cytologic studies of the CSF.

Medical Management

A variety of medical treatments including chemotherapy and external-beam radiotherapy (EBRT) are used alone or in combination with surgical resection.

Surgical Management

The objective of surgical management is to remove or destroy the entire tumor without increasing the neurological deficit (paralysis, blindness) or to relieve symptoms by partial removal decompression. A variety of treatment modalities may be used; the specific approach depends on the type of tumor, its location and its accessibility. In many patients, combinations of these modalities are used.

Other Therapies

- Radiation therapy (the cornerstone of treatment of many brain tumors)
- Brachytherapy (the surgical implantation of radiation sources to deliver high doses at a short distance)
- The IV autologous bone marrow transplantation for marrow toxicity associated with high doses of drugs and radiation
- Gene-transfer therapy (currently being tested).

Nursing Management

1. Evaluate gag reflex and ability to swallow preoperatively.
2. Teach patient to direct food and fluids toward the unaffected side. Assist patient to an upright position to eat, offer a semisoft diet and have suction readily available, if gag response is diminished.
3. Rearses function postoperatively.
4. Perform neurological checks, monitor vital signs and maintain a neurological flowchart, and space nursing interventions to prevent rapid increase in ICP.
5. Reorient patient whenever necessary to person, time and place.
6. Reorienting devices (personal possessions, photographs, time and clock). Supervise and assist with self-care. Monitor and intervene to prevent injury.
7. Monitor patients with seizures.
8. Check motor function at intervals; assess sensory disturbance and evaluate speech.

CEREBROVASCULAR ACCIDENT (ISCHEMIC STROKE)

A cerebrovascular accident (CVA) is an ischemic stroke (brain attack) is a sudden loss of brain function resulting from disruption of the blood supply to a part of the brain. Stroke is primary cerebrovascular disorder in the United States. Strokes are usually hemorrhagic (15%) or ischemic/nonhemorrhagic.

Ischemic strokes are categorized according to their cause; large artery thrombotic strokes (20%), small penetrating artery cryogenic strokes (30%) and other (5%). Cryptogenic stokes have no known cause and other strokes result from causes such if illicit drug use, coagulopathies, migraine, and spontaneous dissection of the carotid or vertebral arteries. They result in interruption in the blood supply to brain, causing temporary or permanent loss of movement, thought, memory and speech, or sensation.

Risk Factors

Nonmodifiable

- Advanced age (older than 55 year)
- Gender (male)
- Race (African American).

Modifiable

- Hypertension
- Atrial fibrillation
- Hyperlipidemia
- Obesity
- Smoking
- Diabetes
- Asymptomatic carotid stenosis and valvular heart disease (e.g. endocarditis, prosthetic heart valves)
- Periodontal disease.

Clinical Manifestation

General signs and symptoms include numbness or weakness of face, arm, or leg (especially on one side of body); confusion or change in mental status; trouble speaking or understanding speech; visual disturbances; loss of balance, dizziness difficulty walking and or sudden severe headache.

Motor Loss

- Hemiplegia, hemiparesis
- Flaccid paralysis and loss of or decrease in the deep tendon reflexes (initial clinical features) followed by (after 48 hour) reappearance of deep reflexes and abnormally tone (spasticity).

Communication Loss

- Dysarthria (difficulty speaking)
- Dysphasia (impaired speech) or aphasia (loss of speech)
- Apraxia (inability to perform a previously learned activity).

Peripheral Disturbances and Sensory Loss

1. Visual perceptual dysfunction [homonymous (loss of half of visual field)].
2. Disturbances in visual-spatial relations (perceiving the origination of two or more objects in spatial areas), frequently in patient with right hemispheric damage.
3. Sensory losses: Slight impairment of touch or movement with loss of proprioception; difficulty in interrupting visual tactile and auditory stimuli.
4. Frontal lobe damage: Learning capacity, memory and other higher cortical intellectual functions may be impaired such as dysfunction may be reflected in a limited attention span, difficulties in comprehension, forgetfulness and lack of motivation.
5. Depression and other psychological problems such as emotional lability, hostility, frustration, resentment and lack of cooperation.

Diagnostic Methods

- History and complete physical and neurological examinations
- Non-contrast CT
- 12-lead electrocardiogram (ECG) and carotid ultrasound
- The CT angiography or MRI and angiography
- Transcranial Doppler flow studies
- Transthoracic or transesophageal echocardiography
- Xenon-enhanced CT
- Single photon emission CT (SPECT) scan.

Preventions

1. Help patient to alter risk factor for stroke; encourage patient to quit smoking, maintain a healthy weight, follow a healthy diet (including modest alcohol consumption) and exercise daily.
2. Prepare and support patient through carotid endarterectomy.
3. Administer anticoagulant agents as prescribed (e.g. low-dose heparin therapy).

Medical Management/Therapeutic Measures

1. Tissue plasminogen activator (TPA), unless indicated; monitor for bleeding.
2. Anticoagulation therapy.
3. Management of increased ICP; diuretics, maintain $PaCO_2$ to 30–35 mm Hg, position to avoid hypoxia (elevate the head of bed to promote venous drainage and to lowered increased ICP).
4. Possible hemicraniectomy for increased ICP from brain edema in very large stroke.
5. Intubation with an endotracheal tube to establish a patent activity, if necessary.
6. Hemodynamic monitoring (the goals for BP remain controversial for a patient who has not received thrombolytic therapy; antihypertensive treatment may be withheld unless the systolic BP exceeds 220 mm Hg or the diastolic BP exceeds 120 mm Hg).
7. Neurological assessment to determine if the stroke is evolving and if other acute complications are developing.

Management of Complications

- Decreased cerebral blood flow; pulmonary care, maintenance of a patent airway and administration of supplemental oxygen as needed
- Monitor for urinary tract infections (UTIs), cardiac dysrhythmia and complications of immobility.

Nursing Management

Assessment

During acute phase (1–3 day)

1. Weigh patient (used to determine medication dosages) and maintain a neurological flow sheet to reflect the following nursing assessment parameters.
2. Change in level of consciousness or responsiveness, ability to speak and orientation.
3. Presence or absence of voluntary or involuntary movements of the extremities such as muscle tone, body position and head position.
4. Stiffness or flaccidity of the neck.
5. Eye opening, comparative size of pupils and papillary reactions to lights and ocular position.
6. Color of face and extremities temperature and moisturized skin.
7. Quality and rates of pulse and respiration, i.e. ABGs body temperature and arterial pressure.
8. Volume of fluids ingested or administered and volume of urine excreted per 24 hours.
9. Signs of bleeding.
10. The BP maintained within normal limits.

Postacute phase

Assess the following function:

1. Mental status (memory, attention span, perception, orientation, affects and speech/language).
2. Sensation and perception (usually patient has decreased awareness of pain and temperature).
3. Motor control (upper and lower extremity movement), swallowing ability, nutritional and hydration status, skin integrity, activity tolerance and bowel and bladder function.
4. Continue focusing nursing assessment on impairment of function in patient's daily activities.

Nursing Diagnoses/Problems

1. Impaired physical mobility related to hemiparesis, loss of balance and coordination, spasticity and brain injury.
2. Acute pain related to hemiplegia and disuse.
3. Deficient self-care (bathing, hygiene, toileting, dressing, grooming and feeding related to stroke sequelae.
4. Disturbed sensory perception (kinesthetic, tactile or visual) related to altered sensory reception, transmission and/or integration.
5. Impaired swallowing.
6. Impaired urinary elimination related to flaccid bladder, detrusor instability confusion or difficulty in communicating.

7. Disturbed thought processes related brain damage.
8. Risk for impaired skin integrity related to hemiparesis or hemiplegia, decreased mobility.
9. Interrupted family processes related to catastrophic illness and caregiving burdens.
10. Sexual dysfunction related to neurological deficits or fear of failure.

Potential complications: Decreased cerebral blood flow due to increased ICP; inadequate oxygen delivery to the brain; pneumonia.

Planning and Goals

The major goals for the patient (and family) may include improved mobility, avoidance of shoulder pain, achievement of self-care, relief of sensory and perceptual deprivation, prevention of aspiration, continence of bowel and bladder, improved thought processes, achieving a form of communication maintain skin integrity, restored family functioning, improved sexual function and absence of complications. Goals are affected by knowledge of what the patient was like before the stroke.

Nursing Interventions/Implementations

Improving Mobility and Preventing Deformities

1. Position to prevent contractures, use measures to relieve pressure, assist in maintaining good body alignment and prevent compressive neuropathies.
2. Apply a splint at night to prevent flexion of affected extremity.
3. Prevent adduction of the affected shoulder with a pillow placed in the axilla.
4. Elevate affected arm to prevent edema and fibrosis.
5. Position fingers so that they are barely flexed; place hand in slight supination. If upper extremity spasticity is noted, do not use a hand roll, dorsal wrist splint may be used.
6. Change position every 2 hours; place patient in a prone position for 15–30 minutes several times a day.

Establishing and Exercise Program

1. Provide full range of motion four to five times a day to maintain joint mobility, regain motor control, prevent contractures in the paralyzed extremity, prevent further deterioration of the neuromuscular system and enhance circulation. If tightness occurs in any area, perform range of motion exercises more frequently.
2. Exercise is helpful in preventing venous stasis, which may predispose the patient to thrombosis and pulmonary embolus.
3. Observe for signs of pulmonary embolus or excessive cardiac workload during exercise period (e.g. shortness of breath, chest pain, cyanosis and increasing pulse rate). Supervise and support patient during exercises; plan frequent short periods of exercise, no longer periods; encourage patient to exercise unaffected side at intervals throughout the day.

Preparing form Ambulation

1. Start an active rehabilitation program when consciousness returns (all evidence of bleeding is gone, when indicated).
2. Teach patient to maintain balance in a sitting position then to balance while standing (use a tilt table, if needed).
3. Begin walking as soon as standing balance is achieved (use parallel bars and wheelchair available in anticipation of possible dizziness).
4. Keep training periods for ambulation short and frequent.
5. Initiate a full rehabilitation program even for elderly patients.

Preventing shoulder pain

1. Never lift patient by the flaccid shoulder or pull on the affected arm or shoulder.
2. Use proper patient movement and positioning (e.g. flaccid arm on a table or pillows when patient is seated, use of sling when ambulating).
3. Range of motion exercises are beneficial, but avoid overstrenous arm movements.
4. Elevate arm and hand to prevent dependent edema of the hand; administer analgesic agents as indicated.

Promote about Self-care

1. Encourage personal hygiene activities as soon as the patient can sit up; select suitable self-care activities that can be carried out with one hand.
2. Help patient to set realistic goals; add a new task daily, a sign first step, encourage patient to carry out all self-care activities on the unaffected side.
3. Make sure patient does not neglect affected side; provide assistive devices as indicated.
4. Improve morale by making sure patient is fully dressed during ambulatory activities.
5. Assist with dressing activities (e.g. clothing with Velcro closures; put garment on the affected side first); keep environment uncluttered and organized.
6. Provide emotional support and encouragement to prevent fatigue and discouragement.

Managing Sensory Perceptual Problems

1. Approach patient with decreased field vision on the side where visual perception is intact; place all visual stimuli on this side.
2. Teach patient to turn and look in the direction of the defective visual field to compensate for the loss; make eye contact with patient, and draw attention to affected side.
3. Increase natural or artificial lightning in the room; provide eyeglasses to improve vision.
4. Remind patient with hemianopsia of coughing, food dribbling out or pulling inside of the mouth, food retained for long periods in the mouth, or nasal regurgitation when swallowing liquids.
5. Consult with speech therapist to evaluate gag reflex assist in teaching alternate swallowing techniques, advice patient to take smaller boluses of food and inform patient of foods that are easier to swallow; provide thicker liquids or pureed diet as indicated.

6. Let patient sit upright, preferably on chair, when eating and drinking; advance diet as tolerated.
7. Prepare for gastrointestinal (GI) feedings through a tube if indicated, elevate the head of bed during feeding, slowly and ensure that cuff of tracheostomy tube is inflated (if applicable), monitor and report excessive retained or residual feeding.

Assisting with Nutrition (Feeding) and Attaining Bowel/Bladder Control

- Perform intermittent sterile catheterization during period of loss of sphincter control
- Analyze voiding pattern and offer urinal or bedpan on patient's voiding schedule
- Assist the male patient to an upright posture for voiding
- Provide high-fiber diet and adequate fluid intake (2–3 L/day), unless contraindicated
- Establish a regular time (after breakfast) for toileting.

Improve Thought Processes

1. Reinforce structured training program using cognitive perceptual retraining, visual imagery, reality orientation and cueing procedures to compensate for losses.
2. Support patient; observe performance and progress, give positive feedback, convey an attitude of confidence and hopefulness; provide other interventions as used for improving cognitive function after a head injury.

Improving Communication

1. Reinforce the individually tailored program.
2. Jointly establish goals with patient taking an active part.
3. Make the atmosphere conductive to communication, remaining sensitive to patient's reactions and needs and responding to them in appropriate manner; treat patient as an adult.
4. Provide strong emotional support and understanding to allay anxiety; avoid completing patient's sentences.
5. Be consistent in schedule, routines and repetitions. A written schedule, checklists and audiotapes may help with memory and concentration; a communication board may be used.
6. Maintain patient's attention when talking with patient, speak slowly and give one instruction at a time; allow patient time to process.
7. Talk to aphasic patients when providing care activities to provide social contact.

Maintaining Skin Integrity

1. Frequently assess skin for signs of breakdown with emphasis on bony areas and dependent body parts.
2. Employ pressure relieving devices; continue regular turning and positioning (every 2 hour minimally); minimize shear and friction when positioning.
3. Keep skin clean and dry, gently massage healthy dry skin and maintain adequate nutrition.

Improving Family Coping

1. Provide counseling and support to family.
2. Involve others in patient's care; teach stress management techniques and maintenance of personal health for family coping.
3. Give family information about the expected outcome of the stroke and counsel them to avoid doing things for patient that he/she can do.
4. Develop attainable goals for patient at home by involving the total healthcare team, patient and family.
5. Encourage everyone to approach patient with a supportive and optimistic attitude, focusing on abilities that remain; explain to family that emotional lability usually improves with time.

Helping the Patient to Cope up with Sexual Dysfunction

1. Perform in depth assessment to determine sexual history before and after the stroke.
2. Interventions for patient and partner focus on providing relevant information, education, reassurance, adjustment of medications, counseling regarding coping skills, suggestions for alternative sexual positions and means of sexual expression and satisfaction.

Promoting Family-based Care and Follow-up

1. Teach patient to resume as much self-care as possible; provide assistive devices as indicated.
2. Have occupational therapist make a home assessment and recommendation to help patient become more independent.
3. Coordinate care provided by numerous healthcare professionals, help family plan aspects of care.
4. Advise family that patient may tire easily, become irritable and upset by small events and show less interest in daily events.
5. Make referral for home speech therapy. Encourage family involvement. Provide family with practical instructions to help patient between speech therapy sessions.
6. Discuss patient's depression with physician for possible antidepressant therapy.
7. Encourage patient to attend community-based stroke clubs to give a feeling of belonging and fellowship with others.
8. Encourage patient to continue with hobbies, recreational and leisure interests and contact with friends to prevent social isolation.
9. Encourage family to support patient and give positive reinforcement.
10. Remind spouse and family to attend the personal health and well-being.

EPILEPSIES

The epilepsies is a symptom complex of several disorders of brain function characterized by recurring seizures. There may be associated with loss of consciousness, excess movement or loss of muscle tone, or movement and disturbances of behavior mood, sensation and perception. The basic problem is an electrical disturbance (dysrhythmia) in the nerve cells in section of brain, causing them to emit abnormal, recurring and uncontrolled electric discharges. The characteristic epileptic seizure is a manifestation of this excessive neuronal discharge. In most cases, the cause is unknown (idiopathic). Susceptibility to some types may be inherited. Epilepsies often follow many medical disorders, traumas and drug or alcohol intoxication. They are also associated with brain tumors, abscess and congenital malformations. Epilepsy affects an estimated 3% of people during their lifetime and most forms of epilepsy occur in childhood. Epilepsy is not synonymous with mental retardation or illness; it is not associated with intellectual level.

Clinical Manifestations

Seizures range from simple staring episodes to prolonged convulsive movements with loss of consciousness. Seizures are classified as partial, generalized and unclassified according to the area of brain involved. Aura, a premonitory or warning sensation may occur before a seizure (e.g. seeing a flashing light, hearing a sound).

Simple Partial Seizures

Only finger or hand may shake; the mouth may jerk uncontrollably; the patient may talk unintelligently may be dizzy or may experience unusual or unpleasant sights, sounds, odor, or taste all without loss of consciousness.

Complete Partial Seizures

The patient remains motionless or moves automatically, but inappropriately for time and place; may experience excessive emotions of fear, anger, elation or irritability and does not remember episode when it is over.

Generalized Seizures (Grand Mal Seizures)

1. Generalized seizures involve both hemispheres of the brain. There is intense rigidity of the entire body, followed by alterations of muscle relaxation and contraction (generalized tonic-clonic contraction).
2. Simultaneous contractions of diaphragm and chest muscles produce characteristic epileptic cry.
3. Tongue is chewed; patient is incontinent of urine and stool.
4. Convulsive movements last 1 or 2 minutes.
5. The patient then relaxes and lies in a deep coma, breathing noisily.

Postictal State

After the seizure, patients are often confused and hard to arouse, and may sleep for more hours. Many patients' complain of headache, sore muscles, fatigue and depression.

Diagnostic Methods

1. Development of history and physical and neurological examinations are done to determine the type, frequency and severity of seizures. Biochemical, hematological and serological studies are included.

2. The MRI is performed to detect structural lesions such as focal abnormalities cerebrovascular abnormalities and cerebral degenerative changes.
3. Electroencephalography aid to classifying the type of SPECT may be used to identify the epileptogenic zone.

Medical Management

The management of epilepsy and status epileptics is planned according to immediate and long-range needs and it is tailored to meet the patient's needs because some cases arise from brain damage and others are due to altered brain chemistry. The goals of treatment are to stop the seizures as quickly as possible, to ensure adequate cerebral oxygenation and to maintain a seizure free state, i.e:

1. An airway and adequate oxygenation (intubate, if necessary) are established as in an IV line for administering medications and obtaining blood samples for analysis.
2. Medications are used to achieve seizure control. Treatment is a single drug therapy.
3. The IV diazepam, lorazepam or fosphenytoin is administered slowly in attempt to halt the seizures. General with a short-acting barbiturate may be used, if treatment is unsuccessful.
4. To maintain a seizure-free state, other medications (phenobarbital) are prescribed after the initial seizure placed.
5. Surgery is indicated when epilepsy results from intracranial tumors, abscesses and cysts or vascular anomalies.
6. Surgical removal of epileptogenic focus is done for amount that originate in a well-circumscribed area of the brain that can be excised without producing significant neurological defects.

Nursing Management

Assessment

1. Obtain a complete seizure history. Ask about factors of events that precipitate the seizures; document alcohol intake.
2. Determine whether the patient has an aura before an epileptic seizure, which may indicate the origin of the seizure (originated in the occipital lobe).
3. Observe and assess neurological condition during and after a seizure. Assess vital and neurological signs continuously.
4. Patient may die from cardiac involvement or respiratory depression.
5. Assess effects of epilepsy on lifestyle.

Nursing Diagnoses/Problems

- Risk for injury related to seizure activity
- Fear related to possibility of having seizures
- Deficit knowledge about epilepsy and its control
- Ineffective coping related to stresses imposed by epilepsy.

Status epilepticus

Status epilepticus (acute, prolonged seizure activity) is a serious of generalized seizures that occur without full recovery of consciousness between attacks. The condition is a medical emergency that is characterized by continuous clinical or electrical seizures lasting at least 30 minutes. Repeated episodes of cerebral anoxia and edema may lead to irreversible and fatal brain damage. Common factors that precipitate status epilepticus include withdrawal of antiseizure medication, fever and concurrent infection.

Potential complications: Status epilepticus and toxicity related to medications.

Planning and Goals

Major goals include prevention of injury, control of seizures, achievement of a satisfactory psychosocial adjustment, acquisition of knowledge and understanding about the condition and absence of complications.

Nursing Interventions

General Care and Injury Prevention

1. Perform periodic physical examinations and laboratory tests for patients taking medications known to have toxic hematopoietic and genitourinary or hepatic effects.
2. Provide ongoing assessment and monitoring of respiratory and cardiac function.
3. Monitor the seizure type and general condition of patient.
4. Turn patient to side-lying position to assist in draining pharyngeal secretions.
5. Have suction equipment available, if patient aspirates.
6. Monitor IV line closely for dislodgment during seizures.
7. Protect patient from injury during seizures with padded side rails and keep under constant observation.
8. Do not restrain patient's movement during seizures. Do not insert anything in patient's mouth.

Reducing Fear of Seizures

1. Reduce fear that a seizure may occur unexpectedly be encouraging compliance with prescribed treatment. Emphasize that prescribed antiepileptic medications used to be taken on a continuing basis and is not habit forming.
2. Assess lifestyle and environment to determine factor that precipitate seizures such as emotional disturbances, environmental stressors and onset of menstruation or fever.
3. Encourage patient to avoid such stimuli.
4. Encourage patient to follow a regular and moderate routine in lifestyle, diet (avoiding excessive stimulant) exercise and rest (regular sleep patterns).
5. Advise patient to avoid photic stimulation (e.g. bright flickering lights, television viewing); dark glasses or contacting one eye help.
6. Encourage patient to attend classes on stress management.

Improving Coping Mechanisms

1. Understand that epilepsy imposes feelings of stigmatization, alienation, depression and uncertainty.
2. Provide counseling to patient and family to help them understand the condition and limitations imposed.
3. Encourage patient to participate in social and recreational activities.
4. Teach patient and family about symptoms and their management.

Providing Family-based Care

Teaching patient about self-care

1. Prevent or control gingival hyperplasia, a side effect of phenytoin (Dilantin) therapy by teaching patient to perform through oral hygiene and gum massage, and seek regular dental care.
2. Instruct patient to notify physician, if unable to take medications due to illness.
3. Instruct patient and family about medication side effects and toxicity.
4. Provide specific guidelines to assess and report signs and symptoms of medication overdose.
5. Teach patient to keep a drug and seizure chart, noting when medications are take and any seizure activity.
6. Instruct patient to take showers rather than tub baths to avoid drowning and to never swim alone.
7. Encourage realistic attitude toward the disease; provide facts concerning epilepsy.
8. Instruct patient to carry an emergency medical identifications card or wear an identification bracelet.
9. Advise patient to seek preconception and genetic counseling, if desired (inherited transmission of epilepsy has not been proved).

Continuing care

1. Financial considerations: Epilepsy Foundation of America offers a mail-order program for medications at minimum cost and access to life insurance as well as information on vocational rehabilitation and coping with epilepsy.
2. Vocational rehabilitation: The State Vocational Rehabilitation Agency, Epilepsy Foundation of America and federal and state agencies may be of assistance in cases of job discrimination.

Evaluations

Evaluation of care is based on objectives or expected outcomes:

- Sustains no injuries from seizure activity
- Indicates a decrease in fear
- Displays effective individual coping
- Exhibits knowledge and understanding of epilepsy
- Experiences no complications of seizures (injury) or complications of status epilepticus.

HEADACHE

Headache (cephalalgia) is one of the most common of all human physical complaints. Headache is actually a symptoms rather than a disease entity and may indicate organic disease (neurological), a stress responses, vasodilation (migraine), skeletal muscle tension (tension headache) or a combination of these factors. A primary headache is one for which no organic cause can be identified. These types of headache include migraine, tension-type and cluster headaches.

A secondary headache is a symptom associated with organic causes such as brain tumor or aneurysm, subarachnoid hemorrhage, stroke, severe hypertension, meningitis and head injury.

Examples of secondary headache include the following:

- Miscellaneous headaches associated with structural lesions
- Headache associated with head trauma
- Headache associated with vascular disorders (e.g. subarachnoid hemorrhage)

- Headache associated with non-vascular intracranial disorders (e.g. brain tumor)
- Headache associated with use of chemical substances or their withdrawal
- Headache associated with non-cephalic infection
- Headache associated with metabolic disorders (e.g. hypoglycemia)
- Headache or facial pain associated with disorder of the head or neck or their structures (e.g. acute glaucoma)
- Cranial neuralgia (persistent pain of cranial nerve origin).

Migraine Headache

Migraine is a complex symptoms characterized by periodic and recurrent attacks of severe headache. The cause of migraine has not been clearly demonstrated, but it is primarily a vascular disturbance that occurs more commonly in women and has strong familial tendencies. Onset typically occurs in puberty and the incidence is 18% in women and 6% in men.

Clinical Manifestations

Headache often begins in early morning (headache on awakening). The classic migraine attack can be divided into four phases are prodromal phase, aura, headache and recovery.

Prodromal Phase

- Present in 60% of patients with migraine headache
- Symptoms may occur consistently hours to days before onset of migraine
- Depression, irritability, feeling cold, food carving and anorexia, changes in activity level, increased urination and diarrhea or constipation may be noted with each migraine.

Aura Phase

- Occurs in a minority of patients and lasts less than 1 hour
- Focal neurological symptoms, predominantly visual disturbances (light flashes) occur and may be hemianoptic (occurring in half of the visual field)
- Numbness and tingling of lips, face or hands, mild confusion; slight weakness of an extremity and drowsiness and dizziness may be present.

Headache Phase

Headache phase occurring in 60% of patients involves a unilateral, throbbing headache that intensifies over several hours. Pain is severe and incapacitating often associated with photophobia, nausea and vomiting. Duration varies from about 4 to 72 hours.

Recovery Phase (Termination and Postdrome)

- Pain gradually subsides
- There is a period of muscles contraction in the neck and scalp with associated muscle ache and localized tenderness, exhaustion and mood changes

- Any physical exertion exacerbates the headache pain
- Patient may sleep for an extended period.

Assessment and Diagnostic Methods

- Physical assessment of head and neck
- Neurological examination
- Detailed health and headache assessment and history; medications history
- Cerebral angiography, CT or MRI, if abnormalities on neurological examination
- Electromyography (EMG) and laboratory tests [complete blood cell (CBC) count], electrolytes, glucose, creatinine erythrocyte sedimentation rate (ESR), electrolytes, glucose, creatinine and thyroid hormone levels.

Medical Management/Therapeutic Measures

Therapy is divided into abortive (symptomatic) and preventive approaches. Abortive approach is used for frequent attacks and is aimed at relieving or limiting a headache of onset or while in progress. Preventive approach is used for those who have frequent attacks at regular or predictable intervals and may have medical conditions that preclude abortive therapies.

Management of Acute Attack

Treatment varies greatly; close monitoring is indicated:

1. Triptans: Sumatriptan (Imitrex), naratriptan (Amerge), rizatriptan (Maxalt), zolmitriptan (Zomig) and almotriptan (Axert).
2. Ergotamine preparations may be effective if taken early. Ergotamine preparations may be taken by mouth [per (PO)], subcutaneous (SC) or intramuscular (IM) injection, sublingually, rectally, or they may be inhaled, Cafergot a combination of ergotamine and caffeine.

   Note: None of the triptans medications should be taken concurrently with medications containing ergotamine because of the potential for a prolonged vasoactive reaction.
3. Possibly, 100% oxygen by facemask for 15 minutes.
4. Symptomatic therapy includes analgesics, sedatives, antianxiety agents and antiemetic.

Preventive Medications

1. Daily use of medications thought to block the headache attack.
2. Beta blockers such as propranolol (Inderal) is widely used. Amitriptyline hydrochloride (Elavil), divalproex (Valproate), flunarizine (Sibelium) and serotonin antagonists (pizotyline) are also used.
3. Calcium antagonists used frequently (require several weeks until effective).
4. Several antiseizures medications are being evaluated for migraine prevention [e.g. topiramate (Topamax)].
5. Other prophylactic medication therapy may include ergotamine tartrate (occasionally), lithium, naproxen (Naprosyn) and methysergide.

Nursing Management

Relieving Pain

1. Attempt to abort headache early.
2. Provide comfort measures (e.g. a quiet, dark environment); elevate the head of bed 30°. Administer medications if non-pharmacological measures are ineffective.
3. Provide symptomatic treatment such as antiemetic indicated.

Promoting Family-based Care and Follow-up

Teaching patients about self-care

1. Teach that headaches, especially migraines are likely to occur when patient is ill, overtired or feeling stressed.
2. Educate patient about the type of headache, its mechanism (if known) and appropriate changes in lifestyle to avoid triggers.
3. Inform patient that regular sleep, meals, exercises, relaxation and avoidance of dietary triggers may be helpful in avoiding headaches.
4. Teach and reassure the patient with tension headaches that the headache is not the result of brain tumor (common unspoken fear).
5. Stress reduction techniques such as biofeedback, exercise programs and meditation may prove helpful.
6. Remind about the importance of following the prescribed treatment regimen, keeping follow-up appointments and participating in health promotion activities and recommend health screenings.

Continuing care

The National Headache Foundation provides a list of clinics in the United States and the names of physicians who are members of the American Association for the study of headaches.

Other Headache Types

Cluster Headache

Cluster headaches, another severe form of vascular headache are seen most frequently in men. The attacks come in cluster of one to eight daily with excruciating pain localized in the eye and orbit and radiating to the facial and temporal regions. The pain is accompanied by watering of the eye and nasal congestion lasting from 15 minutes to 3 hours and may have a crescendo-decrescendo pattern. They have been described as penetrating. They may be precipitated by alcohol, nitrates, vasodilators and histamines.

Cranial Arteritis

Inflammation of the cranial arteries is characterized by severe headache localized in the region of the temporal. The inflammation may be generalized or focal. This is of headache in the older population, particularly those than 70 years. Clinical manifestations include inflaming (e.g. heat, redness, swelling and tenderness or pain over involved artery). A tender, swollen or nodular temporal may be visible. Visual problems are caused by ischemia and involved structures. The headache is treated with corticosteroid drugs (do not stop abruptly) and analgesic agents.

Tension Headaches (Muscle Contraction Headache)

Emotional or physical stress may cause contraction of muscles in the neck and scalp resulting in tension headache. This is characterized by a steady, constant feeling of pressure that usually begins in the forehead, the temples or the neck. Tension headaches tend to be more chronic, severe and are probably the most common type of headache belief may be obtained by local heat, massage, analgesic, antidepressants and muscle relaxants. Reassure patient that the headache does not indicate a brain tumor and teach stress induction techniques (biofeedback, exercise, medication).

MULTIPLE SCLEROSIS

Multiple sclerosis (MS) is a chronic, degenerative, progressive disease of the CNS characterized by small patches of demyelination in the brain and spinal cord. Demyelination (destruction of myelin) results in impaired transmission of nerve impulses. MS may occur at any age, but typically manifests in young adults between the ages of 20 and 40 years; it affects women more frequently than men.

Pathophysiology

The cause of MS is not known, but a defective immune response probably plays a major role. In MS, sensitized T cells inhabit the CNS and facilitate the infiltration of other agents that damage immune system. The immune system attack leads to inflammation that destroys myelin and oligodendroglial cells that produce myelin in the CNS, plaques of sclerotic tissue appear on demyelinated axons, further interrupting the transmission of impulses. MS has various courses:

1. Benign course in which symptoms are so mild that patients do not seek health care or treatment.
2. Relapsing-remitting course (80%–85%) with complete recovery between relapses; 50% of these patients progress to a secondary progressive course in which disease progression occurs with or without relapses.
3. Primary progressive course (10%) in which disabling symptoms steadily increase with rare plateaus and temporary improvement may result in quadriparesis, cognitive dysfunction, visual loss and brainstem syndromes.
4. Progressive relapsing course (least common, about 5%), which is relapses with continuous disabling progression between exacerbations.

Clinical Manifestations

1. Signs and symptoms are varied and multiple and reflect the location of the lesion (plaque) or combination of lesions.
2. Primary symptoms: Fatigue, depression, weakness, numbness, difficulty in coordination, loss of balance and pain.
3. Assess how MS has affected the patient's lifestyle, how the patient is coping and what the patient would like to improve.

Nursing Management

Nursing Diagnoses/Problems

1. Improved bed and physical mobility related to weakness, muscle paresis spasticity.

2. Risk for injury related to sensory and visual impairment.
3. Impaired urinary and bowel elimination related to nervous system dysfunction.
4. Impaired verbal communication and risk for aspiration related to cranial nerve involvement.
5. Disturbed thought processes (loss of memory, dementia and euphoria) related to cranial nerve involvement.
6. Ineffective individual coping related to uncertainty of diagnosis.
7. Impaired home maintenance management related to physical, psychological and social limits imposed by MS.
8. Potential for sexual dysfunctions related to lesions or psychological reaction.

Planning (Goals and Objectives)

The major goals of the patient may include promotion of physical mobility, avoidance of injury, achievement of bladder and bowel continence, promotion of speech and swallowing mechanisms, improvement of cognitive function, development of coping strengths, improved home maintenance management and adaption to sexual dysfunction.

Nursing Interventions/Implementations

Promoting Physical Mobility

1. Encourage relaxation and coordination exercises to promote muscle efficiency.
2. Encourage progressive resistance exercise to strengthen weak muscles.
3. Encourage walking exercise to improve gait.
4. Apply warm packs to spastic muscles; avoid hot baths due to sensory loss.
5. Encourage daily exercises for muscle stretching to minimize joint contractures.
6. Encourage swimming, stationary bicycling and progressive weight bearing to relieve spasticity in legs.
7. Avoid hurrying patient in any activity because hurrying increases spasticity.
8. Encourage patient to work up to a point just short of fatigue.
9. Advise patient to take frequent short rest periods, preferably lying down and to prevent extreme fatigue.
10. Prevent complications of immobility by assessment and maintenance of skin integrity through coughing, and deep breathing exercises.

Preventing Injury

1. Teach patient to walk with feet wide apart to increase walking stability, if motor dysfunction causes incoordination.
2. Teach patient to watch the feet while walking if there is a loss of position sense.
3. Provide a wheelchair or motorized scooter if gait remains insufficient after gait training (walker, cane, braces, crutches, parallel bars and physical therapy).
4. Assess skin for pressure ulcers if patient is confined to wheelchair.

Enhancing Bladder and Bowel Control

1. Keep bedpan or urinal readily available because the need to void must be heeded immediately.
2. Set up a voiding schedule with gradual lengthening of time intervals.
3. Instruct patient to drink a measure amount of fluid every 2 hours and to attempt to void 30 minutes after drinking.
4. Encourage patient to take prescribed medications for bladder spasticity.
5. Teach intermittent self-catheterization, if necessary.
6. Provide adequate fluids, dietary fiber and a bowel-training program for bowel problems including constipation, fecal impaction and incontinence.

Managing Speech and Swallowing Difficulties

1. Arrange for evaluation by a speech therapist. Reinforce this instruction and encourage patient and family too.
2. Reduce the risk for aspiration by careful feeding, proper positioning for eating, having suction apparatus available.

Improving Sensory and Cognitive Function

1. Provide an eye patch or eyeglass occluder to block visual impulses of one eye when diplopia (double vision) occurs.
2. Advise patient about free talking book services.
3. Refer patient and family to a speech-language pathologist when mechanisms of speech are involved.
4. Provide compassion and emotional support to patient and family to adapt to new self-image and to cope with life disruption.
5. Keep a structured environment; use lists and other memory aids to help patient maintain daily routine.

Strengthening Coping Mechanisms

1. Alleviate stress and make referrals for counseling and support to minimize adverse effects of dealing with chronic illness.
2. Provide information on the illness to patient and family.
3. Help patient define problems and develop alternatives for management.

Improving Home Management

1. Suggest modifications that allow independence in self-care activities at home (raised toilet seat, bathing aids, telephone modifications, long-handle comb, tongs and modified clothing).
2. Maintain moderate environmental temperature; heat increases fatigue and muscle weakness and extreme cold may increase spasticity.

Promoting Sexual Function

Suggest a sexual counselor to assist patient and partner with sexual dysfunction (e.g. erectile and ejaculatory disorder in men; orgasmic dysfunction and adductor spasms of the thigh muscles in women; bladder and bowel incontinence; urinary tract infections).

Promoting Family-based Care and Follow-up

1. Teach patient and family about use of assistive devices, self-catheterization and administration of medications.
2. Assess patient and family to deal with new disabilities and changes as disease progresses.
3. Refer for home healthcare nursing assistance as indicated.
4. Assess changes in patient's health status and coping strategies, provide physical care to the patient if required, coordinate outpatient services and resources, and encourage health promotion, appropriate health screenings and adaption.
5. Encourage the patient to contact the primary care provide, if changes in the disease or its course are noted.
6. Encourage patient to contact the local MS society for services, publication and contact with other who have MS.

Evaluations

Evaluation is based on objectives or expected patient outcomes:

- Reports improved physical mobility
- Remains free of injury
- Attains or maintains improved bladder and bowel control
- Participates in strategies to improve speech and swallowing
- Compensates for altered thought processes
- Demonstrates improved coping strategies
- Adheres to plan for home maintenance management
- Adapts to changes in sexual function.

PARKINSON DISEASE

Parkinson disease is a slowly progressive degenerative neurological disorder affecting the brain centers that are responsible for control and regulation of movement. The degenerative or idiopathic form of Parkinson disease is the most common; there is also a secondary form with a known or suspected cause. The cause of the disease is mostly unknown, but research suggests several causative factors (e.g. genetics, atherosclerosis, viral infections and head trauma). The disease usually first appears in the fifth decade of life and is the fourth most common neurodegenerative disease.

Pathophysiology

Parkinson disease is associated with decreased levels of dopamine resulting from destruction of pigmented neuronal cells in the substantia nigra in the basal ganglia region of the brain. The loss of dopamine stores in this area of the brain results in more excitatory neurotransmitters than inhibitory neurotransmitters leading to an imbalance that affect its voluntary movements. Cellular degeneration causes impairment of the extrapyramidal tracts that control semiautomatic functions and coordinated movements; motor cells of the motor cortex and the pyramidal tracts are not affected.

Clinical Manifestations

The cardinal signs of Parkinson disease are tremor, rigidity, bradykinesia (abnormally slow movements) and postural instability:

1. Resting tremors: A slow, unilateral turning of the forearm and hand, and a pill-rolling motion of the thumb against the fingers; tremor at rest and increasing with concentration and anxiety.

2. Resistance to passive limb movement characterizes muscle rigidity; passive movement may cause the limb to move in jerky increments (lead pipe or cogwheel movements); stiffness of the arms, legs, face and posture are common; involuntary stiffness of passive extremity increases when another extremity is engaged in voluntary movement.
3. Impaired movement; bradykinesia included difficulty in initiating, maintaining and performing motor activities.
4. Loss of postural reflexes, shuffling gait, loss of balance (difficulty pivoting); postural and gait problems place the patient at increased risk for falls.

Other Characteristics

1. Autonomic symptoms that include excessive and uncontrolled sweating, paroxysmal flushing, orthostatic hypotension, gastric and urinary retention, constipation and sexual dysfunction.
2. Psychiatric changes may include depression, dementia, delirium and hallucinations; psychiatric manifestations include personality changes, psychosis, and acute confusion.
3. Auditory and visual hallucinations may occur.
4. Hypokinesia (abnormally diminished movement) is common.
5. As dexterity declines, micrographia (small handwriting) develops.
6. Mask-like facial expressions.
7. Dysphonia (soft, slurred, low pitched and less audible speech).

Diagnostic Methods

1. Patient's history and presence of two of the four cardinal manifestations such as tremor, rigidity, bradykinesia and postural changes.
2. The PET and SPECT scanning have been helpful in understanding the disease and advancing treatment.
3. Medical history, presenting symptoms, neurological examination and response to pharmacological management, and carefully evaluated when making the diagnosis.

Medical Management

Goal of treatment is to control symptoms and maintain functional independence, no approach prevents disease progressions:

1. Levodopa (Larodopa) is the most effective agent and the mainstay of treatment.
2. Anticholinergic agents to control tremor and rigidity.
3. Amantadine hydrochloride (Symmetrel) an antiviral agent to reduce rigidity, tremor and bradykinesia.
4. Dopamine agents [e.g. pergolide (Permax)], bromocriptine mesylate (Parlodel), ropinirole and pramipexole are used to postpone the initiation of carbidopa and levodopa therapy.
5. Monoamine oxidase inhibitors (MAOIs) to inhibit dopamine breakdown.
6. Catechol-O-methyltransferase (COMT) inhibitors to reduce motor fluctuation.
7. Antidepressant drugs.
8. Antihistamine drugs to allay tremors.

Surgical Management

1. Surgery to destroy a part of the thalamus (stereotactic thalamotomy and pallidotomy) to interrupt nerve pathways and alleviate tremor or rigidity.
2. Transplantation of neural cells from fetal tissue of human or animal source to re-establish normal dopamine release.
3. Deep brain stimulation with pacemaker-like brain implants to block nerve pathways in the brain that cause tremors.

Nursing Management

The nurse notes how the disease affects the patient's activities of daily living and functional abilities, and also observes for degree of disability and functional changes that occur throughout the day such as responses to medication. Observe the patient for quality of speech, loss of facial expression, swallowing deficits (drooling, poor head control, coughing), tremors, slowness of movement, weakness, forward posture, rigidity, evidence of slowness and confusion. The following questions may facilitate. Observations:

- Do you have leg or arm stiffness?
- Have you experienced any irregular jerking of your arms or legs?
- Have you ever been 'frozen' or rooted to the spot and unable to move?
- Does your mouth water excessively?
- Have you (or others) noticed yourself grimacing or making faces, or chewing movements?
- What specific activities do you have difficulty doing?

Nursing Diagnoses/Problems

- Impaired physical mobility related to muscle rigidity and motor weakness
- Self-care deficits (eating, drinking, dressing, hygiene and toileting) related to tremor and motor disturbance
- Constipation related to tremor and motor disturbance
- Constipation related to medication and reduced activity
- Imbalanced nutrition: Less than body requirements related to tremor, slowness in eating, difficulty in chewing and swallowing
- Impaired verbal communication related to decreased speech volume, slowness of speech and inability to move facial muscles
- Ineffective coping related to depression and dysfunction due to disease progression.

Other nursing diagnoses may include sleep pattern disturbances, deficient knowledge, risk for injury, risk for activity intolerance, disturbed thought processes and compromised family coping.

Planning and Goals

Patient goals may include improving functional mobility, maintaining independence in activities of daily livings (ADLs) achieving adequate bowel elimination, attaining and maintaining acceptable nutritional status, achievement effective communication and developing positive response mechanisms. The objectives will be that patient:

- Strives toward improved mobility
- Progresses toward self-care

- Maintains bowel function
- Attains improved nutritional status
- Achieves a method of communication
- Copes with effects of Parkinson disease.

Nursing Interventions/Implementations

Improving Mobility

1. Help patient plan progressive program of daily exercise to increase muscle strength, improve coordination and dietary, reduce muscular rigidity and prevent contraction. Encourage exercises for joint mobility (e.g. stationary walking).
2. Instruct in stretching and range of motion exercises to increase joint flexibility.
3. Encourage postural exercise to counter the tendency of the head and neck to draw forward and down. Teach patients to walk erect, watch the horizon, use a wide basal gait, swing arms with walking, heel-to-toe walking and practice marching to music. Also encourage breathing exercises while walking and frequent rest periods to prevent fatigue or frustrations.
4. Advise patient that warm baths and massage help relax muscles.

Enhancing Self-care Activities

- Encourage teach and support patient during ADL
- Modify environment to compensate for functional disabilities; adaptive devices may be useful
- Enlist assistance of an occupational therapist as indicated.

Improving Bowel Elimination

- Establish a regular bowel routine
- Increase fluid intake and eat foods with moderate fiber content
- Provide raised toilet seat for easier toilet use.

Improving Swallowing and Nutrition

1. Promote swallowing and prevent aspiration by having patient sit in upright position during meals.
2. Provide semisolid diet with thick liquids that are easier to swallow.
3. Teach patient to place the food on the tongue, close lips and teeth, lift the tongue up and then back and swallow; encourage patient to chew first on one side of the mouth and then the other.
4. Remind patient to hold head upright and to make a conscious effort to swallow to control buildup of saliva.
5. Monitor patient's weight on weekly basis.
6. Provide supplementary feeding and as disease progresses, tube feeding.
7. Consult a dietitian regarding patient's nutritional needs.

Encouraging Use of Assistive Devices

1. An occupational therapist can assist in identifying appropriate adaptive devices.
2. Useful devices may include an electric warming tray that keeps food hot and allows the patient to rest during the prolonged time

that it may take to eat; special utensils; a plate that is stabilized a non-spill cup and eating utensils.

Improving Communications

1. Remind the patient to face the listener, speak slowly and deliberately and exaggerate pronunciation of words; a small electronic amplifier is helpful if the patient has difficulty being heard.
2. Instruct the patient to speak in short sentences and take a few breaths before speaking.
3. Enlist a speech therapist to assist the patient.

Supporting Coping Abilities

1. Encourage faithful adherence to exercise and walking program; point out activities that are being maintained through active participation.
2. Provide continuous encouragement and reassurance.
3. Assist and encourage patient to set achievable goals.
4. Encouraging the patient to carry out the routine tasks to retain independence.

Promoting Family-based Care and Follow-up

1. The education plan should include a clear explanation of the disease and the goal of assisting the patient to remain functionally independent as long as possible. Make every effort to explain the nature of the disease and its management, to offset disabling associated and fears. The patient and family are also needed to know about the effects and side effects of medications and the importance of reporting side effects to the physician.
2. Acknowledge the stress, the family is facing, by living with family member who has disabilities.
3. Include others in the planning and counsel caregiver to learn stress reduction techniques; remind caregiver to include others in the caregiving process, obtain personal relief from responsibilities and have a yearly health assessment.
4. Allow family members to express feelings of frustrations, anger and guilt.
5. Remind the patient and family members of the importance of addressing health promotion needs such as screening for hypertension and stroke risk assessment.

Evaluations

Evaluation is based on the objectives or expected patient outcomes:

- Strives toward improved mobility
- Progresses toward self-care
- Maintains bowel function
- Attains improved nutritional status
- Achieves a method of communication
- Copes with effects of Parkinson disease.

MYASTHENIA GRAVIS

Myasthenia gravis (MG) is an automatic disorder affecting the myoneural junction. Antibodies directed at the acetylcholine receptor sites impair transmission of impulses across the myoneural junction. Therefore, fewer receptors are available for stimulation, resulting in voluntary muscle weakness that escalates with continued activity. Women are affected more frequently than men and they tend to develop with disease at an earlier age (20–40 year of age versus 60–70 year for men).

Clinical Manifestations

Myasthenia gravis is a purely motor disorder with no effect and sensation or coordination:

1. Initial manifestations involve ocular muscles (e.g. diplopia and ptosis).
2. Weakness of muscles of the face (resulting in a bland facial expression) and throat (bulbar symptoms), and generalized weakness.
3. Laryngeal involvement: Dysphonia (voice impairment) and increases the risk of choking and aspiration.
4. Generalized weakness that affects all extremities and the intercostal muscles resulting in decreasing vital capacity and respiratory failure.

Diagnostic Findings

1. Injection of edrophonium (Tensilon) is used to confirm the diagnosis (have atropine available for side effects). Improvement in muscle strength represents a positive test and usually confirms the diagnosis.
2. The MRI may demonstrate an enlarged thymus gland.
3. Tests include serum analysis for acetylcholine receptor and EMG to measure electrical potential of muscle cells.

Myasthenic crisis is an exacerbation of the disease process characterized by severe generalized muscle weakness and respiratory, and bulbar weakness may result in respiratory failure. Crisis may result from disease exacerbation or a specific precipitating event. The most common precipitator is respiratory infection others include medications change, surgery, pregnancy and medications that exacerbate myasthenia. A cholinergic crisis caused by overmedication with cholinesterase inhibitors is rare; atropine sulfate should be on hand to treat bradycardia or respiratory distress. Neuromuscular respiratory failure is the critical complication in myasthenic and cholinergic crisis.

Medical Management

Management of MG is directed at improving function and reducing and removing circulating antibodies. Therapeutic modalities include administration of anticholinesterase medications and immunosuppressive therapy, plasmapheresis, and thymectomy. There is no cure for MG; treatments do not stop the production of the acetylcholine receptor antibodies.

Pharmacological Therapy

Pyridostigmine bromide (Mestinon) is the first line of therapy. It provides symptomatic relief by inhibiting the breakdown of acetylcholine and increasing the relative concentration of available acetylcholine at the neuromuscular junction.

If pyridostigmine bromide does not improve muscles strength and control fatigue, the next agents used are the immunomodulating drugs. Immunosuppressive therapy aims to reduce the production of antireceptor antibody or remove it directly by plasma exchange. Corticosteroids are given to suppress the immune response, decreasing the amount of blocking antibody.

Other Treatment

Plasma exchange (plasmapheresis) produces a temporary reduction in the titer of circulating antibodies. Thymectomy (surgical removal of the thymus) produces substantial remission, either in patients with tumor or hyperplasia of thymus gland.

Nursing Management

1. Educate patient about self-care including mediation management, energy conservation, strategies to help with ocular manifestations and prevention and management of complications.
2. Ensure patient understands the actions of the medications and emphasize the importance of taking them on schedule, and the consequences of delaying medications; stress the signs and symptoms of myasthenic and cholinergic crisis.
3. Encourage patient to determine the best times for daily dosing by keeping a diary to determine fluctuation of symptoms and to learn when the medication is wearing off.
4. Teach the patient strategies to conserve energy (e.g. if the patient lives in a two story).
5. Help patient to identify optimal times for rest throughout the day.
6. Encourage the patient to apply for a handicapped license plate to minimize walking from parking spaces and to schedule activities to coincide with peak energy, and strength levels.
7. Instruct patient to schedule meal times to coincide with the peak effects of anticholinesterase medication; encourage rest before meals to reduce muscle fatigue; advise the patient to sit upright during meals with the neck slightly flexed to facilitate swallowing.
8. Encourage meals of soft foods in gravy or sauces; if choking occurs frequently suggest puree food with a pudding-like consistency. Supplemental feedings may be necessary in some patients to ensure adequate nutrition.
9. Ensure suction is available at home and that the patient and family are instructed in its use.
10. Instruct the patient to tape the eyes closed for short intervals and to regularly instill artificial tears; patients who wear eyeglasses can have 'crutches' attached (to help lift the eyelids); patching of one eye can help with double vision.
11. Remind the patient of importance of maintaining health promotion practices and of following healthcare screening recommendations.
12. Encourage patient to note and avoid factors that exacerbate symptoms and potentially cause crisis; emotional stress, infections (particularly respiratory infections), vigorous physical activity, some medications, and high environmental temperature.

13. Refer patient to the agencies, which can provide support groups, services and educational materials for patients and families.
14. Maintenance of stable blood levels of anticholinesterase medications is imperative to stabilize muscle strength. Therefore, the anticholinesterase medications must be administered on time. Any delay in administration of medications may exacerbate muscle weakness and make it impossible for the patient to take medications orally.

ALZHEIMER'S DISEASE

Alzheimer's disease (AD) is a progressive, irreversible, degenerative neurological disease that begins insidiously and is characterized by gradual losses of cognitive function and disturbances in behavior and affect. It is important to note that AD is not a normal part of aging.

Although the greatest risk factors for AD are increasing age, many environmental, dietary and inflammatory factors also may determine whether a person suffers from this cognitive disease. AD is a complex brain disorder caused by a combination of various factors that may include genetics, neurotransmitter changes, vascular abnormalities, stress hormones, circadian changes, head trauma and the presence of seizure disorders.

Alzheimer's disease can be classified into two types:
1. Familial or early-onset AD (which is rare and accounts for less than 10% of cases).
2. Sporadic or late-onset AD.

Clinical Manifestations

Symptoms are highly variable, some include the following:
1. In early disease, there is forgetfulness and subtle memory loss, although social skills and behavioral patterns remain intact. Forgetfulness is manifested in many daily actions with progression of the disease (e.g. the patient gets lost in a familiar environment or repeats the same stories).
2. When conversations become difficult, word-finding difficulties can occur.
3. Ability to formulate concepts and think abstractly disappears.
4. Patient may exhibit inappropriate impulsive behavior.
5. Personality changes are evident; patient may become depressed, suspicious, paranoid, hostile and combative.
6. Speaking skills deteriorate to non-sense syllables; agitation and physical activity increase.
7. Voracious appetite may develop from high activity level; dysphagia is noted with disease progression.
8. Eventually patient requires help with all aspects of daily living including toileting because incontinence occurs.
9. Terminal stage may last for months or years.

Diagnostic Findings

The diagnosis, which is one of exclusion, is confirmed at autopsy, but an accurate clinical diagnosis can be made in about 90% of cases:
1. Clinical symptoms are found through health history including physical findings and results from functional abilities assessments (e.g. mini-mental status examination).

2. Electroencephalography.
3. Computed tomography.
4. Magnetic resonance imaging.
5. Laboratory tests (CBC count, chemistry profile and vitamin B_{12} and thyroid hormone levels) and examination of the CSF.

Medical Management

Without a cure or a way to slow progression of AD, treatment relies on managing cognitive symptoms with cholinesterase inhibitors such as donepezil hydrochloride (Aricept), rivastigmine tartrate (Exelon), galantamine hydrobromide [Razadyne (formerly known as Reminyl)] and tacrine (Cognex). These drugs enhance acetylcholine uptake in the brain to maintain memory skills for a period of time. Donepezil and the newest medications memantine (Namenda) can be used for management of moderate to severe AD symptoms.

Nursing Management

Assessment

Obtain health history with mental status examination and physical examination, noting symptoms indicating dementia, report findings to physician. As indicated, assist with diagnostic evaluation, prompting calm environment to maximize patient safety and cooperation.

Nursing Diagnoses

- Impaired thought processes related to decline in cognitive function
- Risk for injury related to confused thought processes
- Imbalanced nutrition; less than body requirements related to cognitive decline
- Activity intolerance related to imbalance in activity/rest pattern
- Deficient self-care bathing/hygiene, feeding and toileting related to cognitive decline
- Impaired social interactions related to cognitive decline
- Deficient knowledge of family/caregiver related to care for patient as cognitive function declines
- Ineffective family processes related to decline in patients cognitive function.

Planning and Goals

Goals for the patient may include supporting cognitive function, physical safety, reduced anxiety and agitation, adequate nutrition, improved communication, activity tolerance, self-care, socialization and support and education of caregivers. The objectives will be that patient:

- Maintains cognitive, functional and social interaction abilities for as long as possible
- Patient remains free of injury
- Patient participates in self-care activities as much as possible
- Patient demonstrates minimal anxiety and agitation
- Patient is able to communicate (verbally or nonverbally)
- Patient's socialization and intimacy needs are met
- Patient receives adequate nutrition, activity and rest
- Patient and family caregivers are knowledgeable about condition and treatment and care regimens.

Nursing Interventions

Supporting Cognitive Function

- Provide a calm, predictable environment to minimize confusion and disorientation
- Help the patient to feel a sense of security with a quiet and pleasant manner; clear, sample explanations and use of memory aids and cues.

Promoting Physical Safety

1. Provide a safe environment (whether at home or in the hospital) to allow patient to move about as freely as possible and relieve family's worry about safety.
2. Prevent falls and other accidents by removing obvious hazards and providing adequate lighting; install handrails in the home.
3. Prohibit driving.
4. Allow smoking only with supervision.
5. Reduce wandering behavior with gentle persuasion and distraction. Supervise all activities outside the home to protect patient. As needed, secure doors leading from the house. Ensure that patient wears an identification bracelet or neck chain.
6. Avoid restraints because they may increase agitation.

Promoting Independence in Self-care Activities

- Simplify daily activities into short achievable steps so that patient feels a sense of accomplishment
- Maintain patient's personal dignity and autonomy
- Encourage patient to make choices when appropriate and to participate in self-care activities as much as possible.

Producing Anxiety and Agitation

- Provide emotional support to reinforce a positive self-image
- When skill losses occur, adjust goals to fit patient's declining ability and structure activities to help prevent agitation
- Keep the environment simple, familiar and noise-free limit changes
- Remain calm and unhurried, particularly for the patient who is experiencing a combative, agitated state known as catastrophic reaction (overreaction to excessive stimulation).

Improving Communication

- Reduce noises and distractions
- Use easy-to-understand sentences to convey messages.

Providing for Socialization and Intimacy Needs

- Encourage visits, letters and phone calls (visits should be brief and nonstressful with one or two visitors at a time)
- Encourage patient to participate in simple activities or hobbies
- Advise that the non-judgmental friendliness of a pet can provide satisfying activity and an outlet for energy
- Encourage spouse to talk about any sexual concerns and suggest sexual counseling, if necessary.

Promoting Adequate Nutrition

1. Keep mealtimes simple and calm; avoid confrontations.
2. Cut food into small pieces to prevent choking and convert liquids to gelatin to ease swallowing. Offer one dish at a time.
3. Prevent burns by serving typically hot food and beverages warm.

Balancing Activity and Rest

1. Offer music, warm milk or a back rub to help patient relax and fall asleep.
2. To enhance nighttime sleep, provide sufficient opportunities for daytime exercise. Discourage long periods of daytime sleeping.
3. Assess and address any unmet underlying physical or psychological needs that may prompt wandering or other inappropriate behavior.

Supporting Family-based Care

- Be sensitive to the highly emotional issues that the family is confronting
- Notify the local adult protective services agency if neglect or abuse is suspected
- Refer family to the Alzheimer's Association for assistance with family support groups, respite care and adult day care services.

Evaluations

Expected Patient Outcomes

- Patient maintains cognitive, functional and social interaction abilities for as long as possible
- Patient remains free of injury
- Patient participates in self-care activities as much as possible
- Patient demonstrates minimal anxiety and agitation
- Patient is able to communicate (verbally or nonverbally)
- Patient's socialization and intimacy needs are rest
- Patient and family caregivers are knowledgeable about condition and treatment and care regimens.

GUILLAIN-BARRÉ SYNDROME (POLYRADICULONEURITIS)

Guillain-Barré syndrome (GBS) results in the acute, rapid segmental demyelination of peripheral nerves and some cranial nerves, producing ascending weakness with dyskinesia (inability to execute voluntary movements), hyporeflexia and paresthesias (numbness). An antecedent event (most often a viral infection) precipitates clinical presentation.

Pathophysiology

Guillain-Barré syndrome results from an autoimmune (cell-mediated and humoral) attack on peripheral nerve myelin proteins (substances speeding condition of nerve impulses). The Schwann cell (which produces myelin in the peripheral nervous system) is spared in GBS, allowing for demyelination in the recovery phase of the disease.

Clinical Manifestations

1. Classic clinical features of GBS include are flexia and ascending weakness, although there may be variations in presentation. GBS does not affect cognitive function or level of consciousness.
2. Initial symptoms (include muscle weakness and diminished may progress of the lower extremities; hyporeflexia and weakness may progress to tetraplegia; demyelination of the nerves that innervate the diaphragm and intercostal muscles results in neuromuscular respiratory failure.
3. Sensory symptoms include paresthesias of the hands and feet and pain related to the demyelination of sensory fibers.
4. Optic nerve demyelination may result in blindness.
5. Bulbar muscle weakness related to demyelination of the glossopharyngeal and vagus nerves results in the inability to swallow or clear secretions.
6. Vagus nerve demyelination results in autonomic dysfunction manifested by instability of the cardiovascular system (tachycardia, bradycardia, hypertension or orthostatic hypotension).

Diagnostic Findings

1. Clinical presentation (symmetric weakness, diminished reflexes and upward progress in of motor weakness) and history of recent viral infection.
2. Changes in vital capacity and negative inspiratory force are assessed to identify impending neuromuscular respiratory failure.
3. Elevated protein levels are detected in CSF evaluation, without an increase in other cells.
4. Evoked potential studies demonstrate a progressive loss of nerve conduction velocity.

Medical Management

1. Guillain-Barré syndrome is considered a medical emergency; patient is managed in an intensive care unit.
2. Respiratory problems may require respiratory therapy or mechanical ventilation.
3. Elective intubation may be implemented before the onset of extreme respiratory muscle fatigue.
4. Anticoagulant agents and antiembolism stockings or sequential compression boots may be used to prevent thrombosis, and pulmonary emboli.
5. Plasmapheresis (plasma exchange) or intravenous immunoglobulin (IVIG) may be used directly to affect the peripheral antibody level.
6. Continuous ECG monitoring: Observe and treat cardiac dysrhythmias and other liable complications of autonomic dysfunction. Tachycardia and hypertension are treated with short-acting medications such as α-adrenergic blocking agents. Hypotension is managed by increasing the amount of IV fluid administered.

Nursing Management

Assessment (Ongoing and Critical)

Monitor the patient for life-threatening complications (respiratory failure, cardiac dysrhythmias, deep vein thrombosis (DVT) so that appropriate interventions can be initiated. Assess the patient's and family's ability to cope and their use of coping strategies.

Nursing Diagnoses/Problems

- Ineffective breathing pattern and impaired gas exchange related to rapidly progressive weakness and impending respiratory failure
- Impaired bed and physical mobility related to paralysis
- Imbalanced nutrition, less than body requirements related to inability to swallow
- Impaired verbal communication related to cranial nerve dysfunction
- Fear and anxiety related to loss of control and paralysis.

Potential complications: Respiratory failure and autonomic dysfunction.

Planning and Goals

Major goals include improved respiratory function, increased mobility, improved nutritional status, effective communication, decreased fear and anxiety and absence of complications.

Nursing Interventions/Implementations

Maintaining Respiratory Function

1. Encourage use of incentive spirometry and provide chest physiotherapy.
2. Monitor for changes in vital capacity and negative inspiratory force; if vital capacity falls, mechanical ventilation will be necessary (discuss the potential need for mechanical ventilation with the patient and family on admission, to provide time for psychological preparation and decision-making).
3. Suction to maintain a clear airway.
4. Assess BP and heart rate frequently to identify autonomic dysfunction.

Enhancing Physical Mobility

1. Provide passive range of motion exercises at least twice daily; support the paralyzed extremities in functional positions. Change patient's position at least every 2 hours.
2. Administer prescribed anticoagulant regimen to prevent DVT and pulmonary embolism, assist with physical therapy and position changes; use antiembolism stockings or sequential compression boots and provide adequate hydration.
3. Place padding over bony prominences such as elbow and heels to reduce the risk of pressure ulcers.

Providing Adequate Nutrition

1. Collaborate with physician and dietitian to meet patient's nutritional and hydration needs. Provide adequate nutrition to prevent muscle wasting.

2. Evaluate laboratory test results that may indicate malnutrition or dehydration (both of these conditions increase the risk of pressure ulcers).
3. If patient has paralytic ileus, provide IV fluids and parenteral nutrition as prescribed, and monitor for return bowel sounds.
4. Provide gastrostomy tube feedings if patient cannot swallow.
5. Assess the return of the gag reflex and bowel sounds before resuming oral nutrition.

Improving Communication

- Establish communication through lip reading, use of picture cards or eye blinking
- Collaborate with speech therapist, as indicated.

Reducing Fear and Anxiety

1. Refer patient and family to a support group.
2. Allow and encourage family members to participate in physical care of patient after providing instruction and support.
3. Provide patient with information about condition, emphasizing a positive appraisal of coping resources.
4. Encourage relaxation exercises and distraction techniques.
5. Create a positive attitude and atmosphere.
6. Encourage diversional activities to decrease loneliness and isolation. Encouraging visitors or volunteers to read to the patient, listening to music or books on tape and watching television are ways to alleviate the patient's sense of isolation.

Managing Potential Complications

1. Assess respiratory function at regular and frequent intervals; monitor respiratory rate, the quality of respirations and vital capacity.
2. Watch for breathlessness while talking, shallow and irregular breathing, use of accessory muscles, tachycardia, weak, cough and changes in respiratory pattern.
3. Monitor for and report cardiac dysrhythmias (through ECG monitoring), transient hypertension, orthostatic hypotension, DVT, pulmonary embolism, and urinary retention.

Promoting Family-based Care and Follow-up

1. Teach patient and family about the disorder and its generally favorable prognosis.
2. During the acute phase, instruct patient and family about strategies they can implement to minimize the effects of immobility and other complications.
3. Explain care and roles of patient and family in rehabilitation process.
4. Use an interdisciplinary effort for family or caregiver education (nurse, physician, occupational and physical therapy, speech therapist, and respiratory therapist).
5. Provide care in a comprehensive inpatient program or an outpatient program, if patient travel by care, or encourage a home program of physical and occupational therapy.
6. Support patient and family through long-recovery phase, and promote involvement for return of former abilities.

7. Remind or instruct patients and family members of the need for continuing health promotion and screening practices.

Evaluations

Evaluation is based on objectives of the care and expected outcomes:
- Maintain effective respirations and airway clearance
- Showing increasing mobility
- Receives adequate nutrition and hydration
- Demonstrates recovery of speech
- Shows lessening fear and anxiety
- Remains free of complications.

TRIGEMINAL NEURALGIA (TIC DOULOUREUX)

Trigeminal neuralgia, a condition affecting the V cranial nerve, is characterized by unilateral paroxysm of shooting and stabbing pain in the area innervated by any of the three branches, but most commonly the second and third branches of trigeminal nerve. The pain ends as abruptly as it starts and is described as a unilateral shooting and stabbing sensation. The unilateral nature of the pain is an important feature. Associated involuntary contraction of the facial muscles can cause sudden closing of the eye or twitching of the mouth, hence the former name tic douloureux (painful twitch). Trigeminal neuralgia occurs most often before 35 years of age. Pain-free intervals may last minutes, hours, days or longer. With advancing years, the painful episodes tend to become more frequent and agonizing. The patient lives in constant fear of attacks.

Pathophysiology

Although the cause is not certain, vascular compression and pressure are suggested causes. The disorder occurs more commonly in women and in people with MS compared with the general population.

Clinical Manifestations

Paroxysms are aroused by any stimulation of terminals of the affected nerve branches (e.g. washing the face, sharing, brushing teeth, eating and drinking). Patients may avoid these activities (behavior provides a cue to diagnosis).

Drafts of cold air and direct pressure against the nerve trunk may cause pain. Trigger points are areas where the slight touch immediately starts a paroxysm.

Diagnostic Methods

Diagnosis is based on characteristic behavior; avoiding stimulating trigger points areas (e.g. trying not to touch or wash the face, shave, chew, or do anything else that might cause an attack).

Medical Management

Antiseizure agents such as carbamazepine (Tegretol) reduce transmission of impulses at certain nerve terminals and relieve pain in most patients. Carbamazepine is given with meals. The patient is observed for side effects including nausea, dizziness, drowsiness and aplastic anemia. The patient is monitored for bone marrow depression during long-term therapy. Gabapentin and baclofen are also used to treat pain. If pain control is still not achieved, phenytoin (Dilantin) may be used as adjunctive therapy.

Surgical Management

In microvascular decompression of the trigeminal nerve, an intracranial approach (craniotomy) to decompress the trigeminal nerve is used. Percutaneous radiofrequency produces a thermal lesion on the trigeminal nerve. Although immediate pain relief is experienced, dysesthesia of the face and loss of the corneal reflex may occur. Use of stereotactic MRI for identification of the trigeminal nerve followed by Gamma Knife radiosurgery is being used at some medical centers. Percutaneous balloon microcompression disrupts large myelinated fibers in all three branches of the trigeminal nerve.

Nursing Management

1. Assist patient to recognize the factors that trigger excruciating facial pain (e.g. hot or cold food, or water, jarring motions). Teach patient how to lessen these discomforts by using cotton pads and room temperature water to wash face.
2. Instruct patient to rinse mouth after eating when toothbrushing causes pain and to perform personal hygiene during pain-free intervals.
3. Advise patient to take food and fluids at room temperature, so chew on unaffected side, and to ingest soft foods.
4. Recognize that anxiety, depression and insomnia often accompany chronic painful conditions, and use appropriate interventions and referrals.
5. Provide postoperative care by performing neurological checks as assess facial motor and sensory deficits. Instruct patient not to rub eye if the surgery results in sensory deficit to the affected side of the face because pain will not be felt in the event there is injury. Assess the eye for irritation or redness. Insert artificial tears, if prescribed, to prevent dryness to affected eye. Caution patient not to chew on the affected side until numbness diminishes. Observe patient carefully for any difficulty in eating and swallowing foods of different consistencies.

BELL'S PALSY

Bell's palsy (facial paralysis) is due to peripheral involvement of the VII cranial nerve on one side, which results in weakness or paralysis of the facial muscles. The cause is unknown, but possible causes may include ischemia, viral disease (herpes simplex, herpes zoster), autoimmune disease or a combination. Bell's palsy may represent a type of pressure paralysis in which ischemic necrosis of the facial nerve causes a distortion of the face, behind the ear and in the eye. The patient may experience speech difficulties and may be unable to eat on the affected side owing to weakness. Most patients recover completely and Bell's palsy rarely recurs.

Medical Management

The objectives of management are to maintain facial muscle tone and prevent or minimize denervation. Corticosteroid therapy (prednisone) may be initiated to reduce inflammation and edema, which reduces vascular compression and permits restoration of blood circulation to the nerve. Early administration of corticosteroids appears to diminish severity, relieve pain and minimize denervation. Facial pain is controlled with analgesic agents or heat applied to the involved side of the face. Additional modalities may include electrical stimulation applied to the face to prevent muscle atrophy or surgical exploration of the facial nerve. Surgery may be performed if a tumor is suspected for surgical decompression of the facial nerve and for surgical rehabilitation of a paralyzed face.

Nursing Management

Patients need reassurance that a stroke has not occurred and that spontaneous recovery occurs within 3–5 weeks in most patients. Teaching patient's with Bell's palsy to care themselves at home is an important nursing priority.

Teaching Eye Care

Because the eye usually does not close completely, the blink reflex is diminished, so the eye is vulnerable to injury from dust and foreign particles. Corneal irritation and ulceration may occur. Distortion of the lower lid alters the proper drainage of tears. Key teaching points include the following:

1. Cover the eye with a protective shield at night.
2. Apply eye ointment to keep eyelids closed during sleep.
3. Close the paralyzed eyelid manually before going to sleep.
4. Wear wraparound sunglasses or goggles to decrease normal evaporation from the eye.

Teaching About Maintaining Muscle Tone

1. Show patient how to perform facial massage with gentle upward motion several times daily when the patient can tolerate the massage.
2. Demonstrate facial exercises such as wrinkling the forehead, blowing out the cheeks and whistling in an effort to prevent muscle atrophy.
3. Instruct patient to avoid exposing the face to cold and drafts.

SPINAL CORD INJURY

Spinal cord injuries (SCIs) are major health problems. Most SCIs result from motor vehicle crashes. Other causes includes falls, violence (primarily from gunshot wounds) and recreational sporting activities. Half of the victims are between 16 and 30 years of age; most are males. Another risk factor is substance abuse (alcohol and drugs). There is a high frequency of associated injuries and medical complications. The vertebrae most frequently involved in SCIs are the fifth, sixth and seventh cervical vertebrae (C5–C7), the 12th thoracic vertebrae (T12) and the first lumbar vertebrae (L1). These vertebrae are the most susceptible because there is a greater range of mobility in the vertebral column in these areas. Damage to the spinal cord ranges from transient concussion (patient recovere fully) to contusion, laceration and compression of the cord substance (either alone or in combination), to complete transection of the cord (paralysis below the level of injury). Injury can be categorized as primary (usually permanent) or secondary (nerve fibers swell and disintegrate as a result of ischemia, hypoxia, edema and hemorrhagic lesions). Whereas a primary injury is permanent, a secondary injury may be reversible, if treated within 4–6 hours of the initial injury. The type of injury refers to extent of injury to the spinal cord itself.

Incomplete spinal cord lesions are classified according to the area of spinal cord damage; central, lateral, anterior or peripheral. A complete SCI can result in paraplegia (paralysis of the lower body) or tetraplegia (formerly quadriplegia—paralysis of all four extremities).

Clinical Manifestations

The consequence of SCI depends on the type and level of injury of the cord.

Neurological Level

The neurological level refers to the lowest level at which sensory and motor functions are normal. Signs and symptoms include the following:
- Total sensory and motor paralysis below the neurological level
- Loss of bladder and bowel control (usually with urinary retention and bladder distention)
- Loss of sweating and vasomotor tone
- Marked reduction of BP from loss of peripheral vascular resistance
- If conscious, patient reports acute pain in back or neck; patient may speak of fear that the neck or back is broken.

Respiratory Problems

- Related to compromised respiratory function; severity depends on the level of injury
- Acute respiratory failure is the leading cause of death in high cervical cord injury.

Diagnostic Measures

Detailed neurological examination, X-ray examinations (lateral cervical spine X-rays), CT, MRI and ECG (bradycardia and a systole are common in acute spinal injuries) are common assessment and diagnostic methods.

Complications

Spinal shock, serious complications of SCI is a sudden depression of reflex activity in the spinal cord (are flexia) below the level of injury. The muscles innervated by the part of the cord segment situated below the level of the lesion become completely paralyzed and flaccid, and the reflexes are absent. BP and heart rate fall as vital organs are affected. Part of the body below the level of the cord lesion are paralyzed and without sensation.

Medical Management

Acute Phase

Goals of management are to prevent further SCI and to observe for symptoms of progressive neurological deficits. The patient is resuscitated as necessary and oxygenation and cardiovascular stability are maintained. High-dose corticosteroids (methylprednisolone) may be administered to counteract spinal cord edema.

Oxygen is administered to maintain a high arterial PaO_2. Extreme care is taken to avoid flexing or extending the neck if endotracheal intubation in necessary. Diaphragm pacing (electrical stimulation of the phrenic nerve) may be considered for patient with high cervical spine injuries.

Spinal cord injury requires immobilization, reduction of dislocations and stabilization of the vertebral column. The cervical fracture is reduced and the cervical spine aligned with a form of skeletal traction (using skeletal tongs or calipers, or the halo vest technique). Weights are hung freely so as not to interfere with the traction.

Early surgery reduces the need for traction. The goals of surgical treatment are to preserve neurological function by removing pressure from the spinal cord and to provide stability.

Emergency Management

1. Immediate patient management at the accident scene is crucial. Improper handling can cause further damage and loss of neurological function.
2. Consider any victim of a motor vehicle crash, a diving or contact sports injury, a fall or any direct trauma to the head and neck as having an SCI until ruled out.
3. Initial care includes rapid assessment, immobilization, extrication, stabilization or control of life-threatening injuries and transportation to an appropriate medical facility.
4. Maintain patient to an extended positions (not sitting); no body part should be twisted or turned.
5. The standard of care is referral to a regional spinal injury center or trauma center for treatment in first 24 hours.

Management of Complications

Spinal and neurogenic shock

1. Intestinal decompression is used to treat bowel distention and paralytic ileus caused by depression of reflexes. This loss of sympathetic innervation causes a variety of other clinical manifestations including neurological shock signaled by decreased cardiac output, venous pooling in the extremities and peripheral vasodilation.
2. Patient who does not perspire on paralyzed portion of body requires close observation for early detection of an abrupt onset of fever.
3. Body defense are maintained and supported until the spinal shock abates, and the system has recovered from the traumatic insult (up to 4 month).
4. Special attention is paid to the respiratory system (may not be enough intrathoracic pressure to cough effectively). Special problems include decreased vital capacity, decreased oxygen levels and pulmonary edema.
5. Chest physiotherapy and suctioning are implemented to help clear pulmonary secretions. Patient is monitored for respiratory complications (respiratory failure, pneumonia).

Deep vein thrombosis and other complications

1. Patient is observed for DVT a complication of immobility (e.g. pulmonary embolism). Symptoms include pleuritic chest pain, anxiety, shortness of breath and abnormal blood gas values.
2. Low-dose anticoagulation therapy is initiated to prevent DVT and pulmonary embolism along with the use of antiembolism stockings or pneumatic compression devices. A permanent indwelling filter may be placed in the vena cava to prevent dislodged clots (emboli) from migrating to the lungs and causing pulmonary emboli.
3. Patient is monitored for autonomic hyperreflexia [characterized by pounding headache, profuse sweating, nasal congestion and piloerection (gooseflesh)] bradycardia and hypertension.
4. Constant surveillance is maintained for signs and symptoms of pressure ulcers and infection (urinary, respiratory local infection at pin sites).
5. The calves or thighs should never be massaged because of the danger of dislodging an undetected thromboemboli.

Nursing Management

Assessment

1. Observe the breathing pattern, assess strength of cough and auscultate lungs.
2. Monitor patient closely for any changes in motor or sensory function and for symptoms of progressive neurological damage.
3. Test motor ability by asking patient to spread fingers, squeeze examiner's head and move toes or turn the feet.
4. Evaluate sensation by pinching the skin or touching it lightly with a tongue blade, starting at shoulder and working down both sides; patient's eyes should be closed. Ask patient where sensation is felt.
5. Assess for spinal shock.
6. Palpate lower abdomen for signs of urinary retention and overdistention of the bladder.
7. Assess for gastric dilation and paralytic ileus due to atonic bowel.
8. Monitor temperature (hyperthermia may result due to autonomic disruption).

Nursing Diagnoses/Problems

1. Ineffective breathing patterns related to weakness or paralysis of abdominal and intercostal muscles, and inability to clear secretions.
2. Ineffective airway clearance related to weakness of intercostal muscles.
3. Impaired bed and physical mobility related to motor and sensory impairment.
4. Disturbed sensory perception related to the immobility and sensory loss.
5. Risk for impaired skin integrity related to the immobility or sensory loss.
6. Impaired urinary elimination related to inability to void spontaneously.
7. Constipation related to presence of atonic bowel as a result of autonomy disruption.

8. Acute pain and discomfort related to treatment and prolonged immobility.
9. The DVT.
10. Orthostatic hypotension.
11. Autonomic hyperreflexia.

Planning and Goals

Major patient goals may include improved breathing pattern and airway clearance, improved mobility, improved sensory and perceptual awareness, maintenance of skin integrity, relief of urinary retention, improved bowel function, promotion of comfort and absence of complications.

Nursing Interventions/Implementations

Promoting Adequate Breathing and Airway Clearance

1. Detect potential respiratory failure by observing patient, measuring vital capacity and monitoring oxygen saturation through pulse oximetry and ABG values.
2. Prevent retention of secretions and resultant atelectasis with early and vigorous attention to clearing bronchial and pharyngeal secretions.
3. Suction with caution because this procedure can stimulate the vagus nerve producing bradycardia and cardiac arrest.
4. Initiate chest physical therapy and assisted coughing to mobilize secretions, if the patient cannot cough effectively.
5. Supervise breathing exercise to increase strength and endurance of inspiratory muscles particularly the diaphragm.
6. Ensure proper humidification and hydration to maintain dyspnea.
7. Monitor respiratory status frequently.

Improving Mobility

1. Maintain proper body alignment at all times.
2. Reposition the patient frequently and assist patient out of bed as soon as the spinal column is stabilized.
3. Apply splints (various types) to prevent foot drop and trochanter rolls to prevent external rotation of the hip joints; reapply every 2 hours.
4. Patients with lesions above the midthoracic level may tolerate changes in position poorly; monitor BP when positions are changed.
5. Do not turn patient who is not on a rotating specialty bed unless physician indicates that it is safe to do so.
6. Perform passive range of motion exercises as soon as possible after injury to avoid complications, i.e. contracture and atrophy.
7. Provide a full range of motion at least four or five times daily to toes, metatarsal, ankles, knees and hips.
8. For patients who have a cervical fracture without neurological deficit reduction in traction followed by rigid immobilization for 6–8 weeks restores skeletal integrity. These patients are allowed to move gradually to an erect position. Apply neck brace or molded collar when the patient is mobilized after traction is removed.

Promoting Adaption to Disturbed Sensory Perception

1. Stimulate the area above the level of the injury through touch, aromas, flavorful food and beverages, conversation, and music.
2. Provide prism glasses to enable the patient to see from the supine position.
3. Encourage use of hearing aids, if applicable.
4. Provide emotional support; teach patient strategies to compensate for or cope with sensory deficits.

Maintaining Skin Integrity

1. Change patient's position for every 2 hours and inspect the skin, particularly under cervical collar.
2. Assess for redness or breaks in skin over pressure points; check perineum for soilage; observe catheter for adequate drainage; assess general body alignment and comfort.
3. Wash skin every few hours with a mild soap, rinse well and blot dry. Keep pressure sensitive areas well-lubricated and soft with bland cream or lotion.
4. Teach patient about pressure ulcers and encourage participation in preventive measures.

Maintaining Urinary Elimination

1. Perform intermittent catheterization to avoid overstretching the bladder and infection. If this is not feasible, insert an indwelling catheter.
2. Show family members how to catheterize and encourage them to participate in this facet of care.
3. Teach patient to record fluid intake, voiding pattern and amounts of residual urine after catheterization, characterization of urine, and any unusual feelings.

Improving Bowel Function

1. Monitor reactions to gastric intubation.
2. Provide a high-calorie, high-protein and high-fiber diet. Food amount may be gradually increased after bowel sounds resume.
3. Administer prescribed stool softener to counteract effects of immobility and analgesic agents, and institute a bowel program as early as possible.

Providing Comfort Measures

1. Reassure patient in halo traction that he/she will adapt to steel frame (i.e. feeling caged in and hearing noises).
2. Cleanse pin sites daily and observe for redness, drainage and pain; observe for loosening. If one of the pin becomes detached, stabilized the patient's head in a neutral position and have someone notify the neurosurgeon; keep a torque screwdriver readily available.
3. Inspect the skin under the halo vest for excessive perspiration, redness and skin blistering, especially on the bony prominences. Open vest at the sides to allow torso to be washed. Do not allow vest to become vest; do not use powder inside vest.

Monitoring and Managing Potential Complications

Thrombophlebitis
Refer to 'Medical Management' in text on 'Cardiovascular Disorders' in Chapter 10.

Orthostatic hypotension
Reduce frequency of hypotensive episodes by administering prescribed vasopressor medications. Provide antiembolism stockings and abdominal binder; allow time for slow position changes, and use tilt table as appropriate. Close monitoring of vital signs before and during position changes is essential.

Autonomic hyperreflexia

1. Perform a rapid assessment to identify and alleviate the cause of autonomic hyperreflexia and remove the trigger.
2. Place patient immediately in sitting position to lower BP.
3. Catheterize the patient to empty bladder immediately.
4. Examine skin for areas of pressure, irritation or broken skin.
5. As prescribed administer a ganglionic blocking agent such as hydralazine hydrochloride (Apresoline) if the above measures do not relieve hypertension and excruciating headache.
6. Label chart clearly and visibly; noting for risk for autonomic hyperreflexia.
7. Instruct patient in prevention and management measures. Inform patient with lesions above T6 that hyperreflexic episode can occur years after initial injury.

Promoting Family-based Care and Follow-up

1. Shift emphasis from ensuring that patient is stable and free of complications to specific assessment and planning for independence, and the skills necessary for activities of daily living.
2. Initially focus patient teaching on the injury and its effect on mobility, dressing and bowel, bladder, and sexual function. As the patient and family acknowledge, the consequences of the injury and the resulting disability, broaden the focus of teaching to address issue necessary for carrying out the tasks of daily living and taking charge of their lives.
3. Support and assist patient and family in assuming responsibility for increasing care and provide assistance in dealing with psychological impact of SCI and its consequences.
4. Coordinate management team and serve as liaison with rehabilitation centers and home care agencies.
5. Reassure female patients with SCI that pregnancy is not contraindicated and fertility is relatively unaffected, but that pregnant women with acute or chronic SCI pose unique management challenges.
6. Refer for home care nursing support as indicated or desired.
7. Refer patient to mental healthcare professional as indicated.

Evaluations

Evaluation is based on objectives of case or expected patient outcomes:

- Demonstrates improvement in gas exchange and clearance of secretions

- Moves within limits of dysfunction and demonstrates completion of exercises within functional limitations
- Demonstrates adaption to sensory and perceptual alterations
- Demonstrates optimal skin integrity
- Regains urinary bladder function
- Regains bowel function
- Reports absence of pain and discomfort
- Free of complications.

HUNTINGTON'S DISEASE

Huntington's disease is a chronic, progressive hereditary disease of the nervous system that results in progressive involuntary choreiform (dance like) movements and dementia. Researchers believe that glutamine abnormally collects in certain brain cell nuclei causing cell death. Huntington's disease affects men and women of all races. It is transmitted as an autosomal dominant genetic disorder. Therefore, each child of a parent with Huntington's disease has a 50% risk of inheriting the illness. Onset usually occurs between 35 and 45 years of age.

Clinical Manifestations

1. The most prominent clinical features are abnormal involuntary movements (chorea), intellectual decline and often and emotional disturbances.
2. Constant writhing, twisting and uncontrollable movements of the entire body occur as the disease progresses.
3. Facial movements produce tics and grimaces; speech becomes slurred, hesitant, often explosive and then eventually unintelligent.
4. Chewing and swallowing are difficult and aspiration and choking are dangers.
5. Gait becomes disorganized and ambulation is eventually impossible; patient is eventually confined to a wheelchair.
6. Bowel and bladder control is lost.
7. Progressive intellectual impairment occurs with eventual dementia.
8. Personality changes may result in nervous, irritable or impatient behaviors. During the early stages of illness, uncontrollable fits of anger; profound, often suicidal depressions apathy; anxiety, psychosis or euphoria.
9. Hallucinations, delusions and paranoid thinking may precede appearance of disjointed movements.
10. Patient dies in 10–20 years from heart failure (HF), pneumonia or infection, or as a result of a fall or choking.

Diagnostic Measures

1. Diagnosis is made based on the clinical presentation of characteristic symptoms, a positive family history and the known presence of a genetic marker, and exclusion of other causes.
2. A genetic marker for Huntington's disease has been located, it offers no hope of cure or even specific determination of onset.

Medical Management

No treatment stops or reverses the process; palliative care is given:

1. Thiothixene hydrochloride (Navane) and haloperidol decanoate (Haldol), while predominantly block dopamine receptors,

improve the chorea in many patients; antiparkinson medications such as levodopa (Larodopa) may provide temporary benefit to patients who present with rigidity.
2. Motor signs are continually assessed and evaluated. Akathisia (motor restlessness) in the overmedicated patient is dangerous and should be reported.
3. Psychotherapy aimed at allaying anxiety and reducing stress may be beneficial; antidepressants are given for depression or suicidal ideation; psychotic symptoms usually respond to antipsychotic medications.
4. Patient's needs and capabilities are the focus of treatment.

Nursing Management

1. Teach patient and family about medications including signs indicating need for change in dosage or medication.
2. Address strategies to manage symptoms (chorea, swallowing problems, ambulation problems or altered bowel, or bladder function).
3. Arrange for consultation with a speech therapist, if needed.
4. Provide supportive care as Huntington's exact enormous emotional, physical, social and functional tolls on every member of the patient's family.
5. Emphasize the need for regular follow-up.
6. Refer for home care nursing assistance, respite care, day care centers and eventually skilled long-term care to assist patient and family to cope.
7. Provide information about the Huntington's Disease Society of America, which gives information, referrals, education and support for research.

UNCONSCIOUS PATIENT

Unconscious is an altered LOC in which the patient is unresponsive to and unaware of environment stimuli, usually for a short duration. Coma is a clinical state—an unarousable, unresponsive condition in which the patient is unaware of self or the environment for prolonged periods (days to months or even years). Akinetic mutism is a state of unresponsiveness to the environment in which the patients make no voluntary movement. A persistent vegetative state is one in which the unresponsive patient resumes sleep-wake cycles after coma, but is devoid of cognitive or affective mental function. Locked in syndrome results from a lesion affecting the pons and results in paralysis and the inability to speak, but are used to indicate responsiveness. The causes of unconsciousness may be neurologic (head injury, stroke), toxicologic (drug overdose, alcohol intoxication) or metabolic (hepatic or renal failure, diabetic ketoacidosis).

Diagnostic Methods

1. Neurological examinations such as CT, MRI, PET, EEG, CT, SPECT to identify cause of loss of consciousness.
2. Laboratory test: Analysis of blood glucose, electrolytes, serum ammonia and liver function tests; blood urea nitrogen (BUN) levels; serum osmolality; calcium level; and partial thromboplastin, and prothrombin times.

3. Other studies may be used to evaluate serum ketones, alcohol and drug concentrations and ABGs.

Medical Management

The first priority is a patent and secure airway (intubation or tracheostomy) then circulatory status (carotid pulse, heart rate and impulse, BP) is assessed and adequate oxygenation maintained. An IV line is established to maintain fluid balance status and nutritional support is provided (feeding tube or gastrostomy). Neurological care is based on specific pathology. Other measures include drug therapy and measures to prevent complications.

Nursing Management

Assessment

1. Assess level of responsiveness (consciousness) using the Glasgow coma scale. Assess also the patient's ability to respond to verbally. Evaluate pupil size, equality and reaction to light; note movement of eyes.
2. Assess for spontaneous, purposeful or non-purposeful responses—decorticate posturing (arms, flexed, adducted and internally rotated, and legs in extension) or decerebrate posturing (extremities extended and reflexes exaggerated).
3. Rule out paralysis or stroke as cause of flaccidity.
4. Examine respiratory status, eye signs, reflexes and body function (circulation, respiration, elimination, fluid and electrolyte balance) in a systemic manner.

Nursing Diagnoses

- Ineffective airway clearance related to inability to clear respiratory secretions
- Risk for fluid volume deficit related to inability to ingest fluids
- Impaired oral mucous membrane related to mouth breathing, absence of pharyngeal reflex and inability to ingest fluids
- Risk for impaired skin integrity related to immobility or restlessness
- Impaired tissue integrity of the cornea is diminished or absent corneal reflex
- Ineffective thermoregulation (incontinence or retention) related to impairment in neurological sensing and control
- Bowel incontinence related to impairment in neurological sensing and control and also related to changes in nutritional delivery methods
- Disturbed sensory perception related to neurological impairment
- Interrupted family processes related to health crisis.

Potential complications: Respiratory distress failure, pneumonia, aspiration, pressure ulcer, deep vein thrombosis and contractures.

Planning (Goals and Objectives)

Goals of care during the unconscious period may include maintenance of a clear airway, protection from injury, attainment of fluid volume balance, achievement of intact mucous membranes, maintenance of normal skin integrity, absence of corneal irritation, attainment of effective thermoregulation, effective urinary elimination, bowel continence, accurate perception of environmental stimuli, maintenance of intact family or support system and absence of complications.

Nursing Interventions/Implementations

Maintaining the Airway

1. Establish an adequate airway and ensure ventilation.
2. Position patient in a lateral or semiprone position; do not allow patient to remain on back.
3. Remove secretions to reduce danger of aspiration; elevate head of bed to a 30° angle to prevent aspiration; provide frequent suctioning and oral hygiene.
4. Promote pulmonary hygiene with chest physiotherapy and postural drainage.
5. Auscultate chest every 8 hours to detect adventitious breath sounds or absence of breath sounds.
6. Maintain patency of endotracheal tube or tracheostomy; monitor ABGs; maintain ventilator settings.

Protect the Patient

1. Provide padded side rails for protection; keep two rails in the raised position during the day and three at night.
2. Prevent injury from invasive lines and equipment and identify other potential sources of injury such as restraints, tight dressings, environmental irritants damp bleeding or dressings and tubes and drains.
3. Protect the patient dignity and privacy; act as the patient's advocate.
4. If the patient begins to emerge from unconsciousness, every measure that is available and appropriate for calming and quieting the patient should be used. Any form of restraint is likely to be countered with resistance, leading to self-injury or to a dangerous increase in ICP. Therefore, physical restraints should be avoided if possible; a written prescription must be obtained if their use is essential for the patient's well-being.

Maintaining Nutritional Needs

1. Assess for hydration status: Examine tissue turgor and mucous membranes, assess intake and output trends and analyze laboratory data.
2. Meet fluid needs by giving required IV fluids and then nasogastric or gastrostomy feedings.
3. Give IV fluids and blood transfusions slowly if patient has an intracranial condition.
4. Never give oral fluids to a patient who cannot swallow; insert feeding tube for administration of enteral feedings.

Providing Mouth Care

1. Inspect mouth for dryness, inflammation and crusting; cleanse and rinse carefully to remove secretions and crusts, and keep membranes moist; apply petrolatum to lips.

2. Assess sides of mouth and lips for ulceration if patient has an endotracheal tube. Move tube to opposite side of mouth daily.
3. If the patient is intubated and mechanically ventilated, good oral care is also necessary; recent evidence shows that routine toothbrushing every 8 hours significantly decreases ventilator-associated pneumonia.

Maintaining Skin and Joint Integrity

1. Follow a regular schedule of turning and repositioning to prevent breakdown and necrosis of the skin, and to provide kinesthetic, proprioceptive, and vestibular stimulation.
2. Give passive exercise of extremities to prevent foot drop and eliminate pressure on toes.
3. Keep hip joints and legs in proper alignment with supporting trochanter rolls.
4. Position arms in abduction, fingers lightly flexed and hands in slight supination; assess heels of feet for pressure areas.
5. Specialty beds such as fluidized or low-air-loss beds may be used to decrease pressure on bony prominences.

Preserving Corneal Integrity

1. Cleanse eyes with cotton balls moistened with sterile normal saline to remove debris and discharge.
2. Instill artificial tears every 2 hours as prescribed.
3. Use cold compress as prescribed for periorbital edema after cranial surgery. Avoid contact with cornea.
4. Use eye patches cautiously because of potential for further corneal abrasions.

Maintaining Body Temperature

1. Adjust environment to promote normal body temperature.
2. Use prescribed measures to treat hyperthermia: Remove bedding, except light sheet; give acetaminophen as prescribed; give cools sponge baths, use hypothermia blanket and monitor frequently to assess response to therapy.
3. Take rectal or tympanic (unless contraindicated) body temperature.

Preventing Urinary Retention

1. Palpate or scan bladder at intervals to detect urinary retention.
2. Insert dwelling catheter if there are signs of urinary retention; observe for fever and cloudy urine; inspect urethral orifice for drainage.
3. Use external penile catheter (condom catheter) for male patients and absorbent pads for female patients if they can urinate spontaneously.
4. Initiate bladder training program as soon as conscious.
5. Monitor frequently for skin irritation and breakdown; implement appropriate skin care.

Promoting Bowel Function

1. Evaluate abdominal distention by listening for bowel sounds and measuring abdominal girth.

2. Monitor number and consistency of bowel movements; perform rectal examination for signs of fecal impaction; patient may require enema every other day to empty lower colon.
3. Administer stool softeners and glycerin suppositories as indicated.

Promoting Sensory Stimulation

1. Providing continuing sensory stimulation (e.g. auditory, visual, olfactory, gustatory, tactile, and kinesthetic activities) to help patient overcome profound sensory deprivation.
2. Make efforts to maintain usual day and night patterns of activity and sleep; orient patient to time and place every 8 hours.
3. Touch and talk to patient; encourage family and friends to do the same; avoid making any negative comments about patient's status in patient's presence. Avoid over-stimulating patient.
4. Explain to family that periods of agitation may be a sign of increasing patient awareness of the environment.
5. Introduce sounds from patient's usual environment if possible by means of audiotape and videotape.
6. Read favorite books and provide familiar radio and television programs to enrich environment.

Meeting the Family's Needs

1. Reinforce and clarify information about patient's condition to permit family members to mobilize their own adaptive capacities.
2. Encourage ventilation of feelings and concerns.
3. Support the family in decision-making process concerning posthospital management and placement or end-of-life care.

Managing Potential Complications

1. Monitor vital signs and respiratory function for signs of respiratory failure or distress.
2. Assess for adequate red blood cells to carry oxygen; total blood cell count and ABGs.
3. Initiate chest physiotherapy and suctioning to prevent respiratory complications such as pneumonia.
4. Perform oral care interventions for patient's receiving mechanical ventilation to decrease the incidence of pneumonia.
5. If pneumonia develops, obtain culture specimens to identify for selection of appropriate antibiotic.
6. Monitor for evidence of impaired skin integrity and implement strategies to prevent skin breakdown, and pressure ulcers.
7. Address factors that contribute to impaired skin integrity and undertake strategies to promote healing if pressure ulcers do develop.
8. Monitor for signs and symptoms of DVT (redness and swelling).

Evaluations

Evaluation is based on objectives of care and expected patient outcomes:

- Maintains clear airway and demonstrates appropriate breath sounds

- Experiences no injuries
- Attains or maintains adequate fluid balance
- Attains or maintains healthy oral mucous membranes
- Maintains normal skin integrity
- Has no corneal irritation
- Attains or maintains thermoregulation
- Has no urinary retention
- Has no diarrhea or fecal impaction
- Receives appropriate sensory stimulation
- Has family members who cope with crisis
- Avoids other complications.

AMYOTROPHIC LATERAL SCLEROSIS

Amyotrophic lateral sclerosis (ALS) is a disease of unknown cause in which there is a loss of motor neurons (nerve cells controlling muscles) in the anterior horns of the spinal cord and the motor nuclei of the lower brainstem. As these cells die, the muscle fibers that they supply undergo atrophic changes. The degeneration of the neurons may occur in both upper and lower motor neuron systems. Possible causes of ALS include autoimmune disease, free radical damage, oxidative stress and transmission of an autosomal dominant trait for familial ALS (5%–10%). In United States, it is often referred to as Lou Gehrig's disease. Death usually occurs from infection, respiratory failure or aspiration. The average time from onset to death is about 3–5 years.

Clinical Manifestations

Clinical manifestations of ALS depend on the location of the affected motor neurons. In most patients, the chief symptoms are fatigue, progressive muscle weakness, cramps, fasciculation (twitching) and incoordination.

Loss of Motor Neurons in Anterior Horns of Spinal Cord

- Progressive weakness and atrophy of the arms, trunk or leg muscles
- Spasticity: Deep tendon stretch reflexes are brisk and overactive
- Anal and bladder sphincters usually remain intact.

Weakness in Muscles Supplied by Cranial Nerves (25% of Patients in Early Stage)

- Difficulty talking, swallowing and ultimately breathing
- Soft palate and upper esophageal weakness causing liquids to be regurgitated through nose
- Impaired ability to laugh, cough or blow the nose.

Bulbar Muscle Impairment

- Progressive difficulty in speaking and swallowing, and aspiration
- Nasal voice and unintelligible speech
- Emotional liability
- Eventually, compromised respiratory function.

Diagnostic Methods

Diagnosis is based on signs and symptoms because no clinical or laboratory tests are specific for this disease. EMG and muscle biopsy studies, MRI and neuropsychological testing may be helpful.

Medical Management

No specific treatment for ALS is available. Symptomatic treatment includes the following:

1. Riluzole (Rilutek), a glutamate antagonist.
2. Baclofen, dantrolene sodium or diazepam for spasticity.
3. Mechanical ventilation (using negative-pressure ventilations) for alveolar hypoventilation; non-invasive positive-pressure ventilation is also an option.
4. Enteral feedings (percutaneous endoscopic gastrostomy PEG for patients with aspiration or swallowing difficulties.
5. Decisions about life support measures are based on patients and family understands of the disease, prognosis and implications of initiating such therapy.
6. Encourage patient to complete an advance directive or 'living will' to prevent autonomy.

Nursing Management

The nursing care of the patient with ALS is generally the same as the basic care plan for patients with degenerative neurological disorders (refer 'Myasthenia Gravis' in page no. 45). Encourage patient and family to contract suitable agency for information and support.

13

Chapter Hematological Nursing

MEGALOBLASTIC ANEMIA (VITAMIN B_{12} AND FOLIC ACID DEFICIENCY)

Anemia is caused by the deficiencies of vitamin B_{12} or folic acid, identical bone marrow and peripheral blood changes occur because both vitamins are essential for the normal deoxyribonucleic acid (DNA) synthesis.

Pathophysiology

Folic Acid Deficiency

Folic acid is stored as compounds referred to as folates. The folate stores in the body are much smaller than those of vitamin B_{12} and they are quickly depleted when the dietary intake of folate is deficient (within 4 month). Folate deficiency occurs in people who rarely eat uncooked vegetables. Alcohol increases folic acid requirements; folic acid requirements are also increased in patients with chronic hemolytic anemias and in women who are pregnant. Some patients with malabsorptive disease of the small bowel may not absorb folic acid normally.

Vitamin B_{12} Deficiency

A deficiency of vitamin B_{12} can occur in several ways; inadequate dietary intake is rare, but can develop in strict vegetarians who consume no meat or dairy products. Faulty absorption from the gastrointestinal (GI) tract is more common as with conditions such as Crohn's disease or after ileal resection, or gastrectomy and other cause is the absence of intrinsic factor. A deficiency may also occur, if disease involving the ileum or pancreas impairs absorption. The body normally has large stores of vitamin B_{12}, so years may pass before the deficiency results in anemia.

Clinical Manifestations

Symptoms of folic acid and vitamin B_{12} deficiencies are similar and the two anemias may coexist. Symptoms are progressive, although the course of illness may be marked by spontaneous partial remissions and exacerbations:

- Gradual development of sings of anemia (weakness, restlessness and fatigue)
- Possible development of a smooth, sore, red tongue and mild diarrhea (pernicious anemia)
- Mild jaundice, vitiligo and premature graying
- Confusion may occur; more often paresthesias in the extremities and difficulty keeping balance and loss of position sense
- Lack of neurological manifestations with folic acid deficiency alone
- Without treatment patients die, usually as a result of heart failure secondary to anemia.

Diagnostic Methods

- Schilling test (primary diagnostic tool)
- Complete blood count (CBC) [hemoglobin (Hgb) value as low as 4–5 g/dL, white blood cell (WBC) count 2,000–3,000 mm^3, platelet count fewer than 50,000 mm^3, very high mean corpuscular volume (MCV), usually exceeding 110 μm^3)]
- Serum levels of folate and vitamin B_{12} (folic acid deficiency and deficient vitamin B_{12}).

Medical Management

Folic Acid Deficiency

- Increase intake of folic acid in patient's diet and administer 1 mg folic acid daily
- Administer intramuscular (IM) folic acid for malabsorption syndromes
- Prescribe additional supplements as necessary because the amount in multivitamins may be inadequate to fully replace deficient body stores
- Prescribe folic acid for patients with alcoholism as long as alcohol intake continues.

Vitamin B_{12} Deficiency

1. Provide vitamin B_{12} replacement: Vegetarians can prevent or treat deficiency with oral supplements with vitamins or fortified soymilk; when the deficiency is due to more common defect in absorption or the absence of intrinsic factor replacement is by monthly IM injections of vitamin B_{12}.
2. A small amount of an oral dose of vitamin B_{12} can be absorbed by passive diffusion, even in the absence of intrinsic factor, but large doses (2 mg/day) are required, if vitamin B_{12} is replaced orally.
3. To prevent recurrence of pernicious anemia, vitamin B_{12} therapy must be continued for life.

Nursing Management

1. Assess patients at risk for megaloblastic anemia for clinical manifestations (e.g. inspect the skin, sclera and mucous membranes for jaundice, note vitiligo and premature graying).
2. Perform careful neurological assessment (e.g. note gait and stability, test position and vibration sense).
3. Assess need for assistive devices (e.g. cane, walkers) and need for support and guidance in managing activities of daily living and home environment.
4. Ensure safety when position sense, coordination and gait are affected.
5. Refer for physical or occupational therapy as needed.
6. When sensation is altered, instruct patient to avoid excessive heat and cold.
7. Advise patients to prepare bland, soft foods and to eat small amounts frequently.
8. Explain that other nutritional deficiencies such as alcohol-induced anemia, can induce neurological problems.
9. Instruct the patient in complete urine collections for the Schilling test. Also explain the importance of the test and of complying with the collection.

10. Teach the patient about chronicity of disorder and need for monthly vitamin B_{12} injections even when patient has no symptoms. Instruct patient how to self-administer injections, when appropriate.
11. Stress importance of ongoing medical follow-up and screening because gastric atrophy associated with pernicious anemia increases the risk of gastric carcinoma.

Refer 'Nursing Management' under heading 'Anemia' for additional information.

APLASTIC ANEMIA

Aplastic anemia is a rare disease caused by a decrease in or damage to marrow stem cells, damage to microenvironment within the marrow and replacement of the marrow with fat. The precise etiology is unknown, but it is hypothesized against the bone marrow resulting in bone marrow aplasia. Significant neutropenia and thrombocytopenia (i.e. a deficiency of platelets) also occur. Aplastic anemia can be congenital or acquired, but most cases are idiopathic. Infections and pregnancy can trigger it or it may be caused by certain medication, chemicals, or radiation damage. Agents that may produce marrow aplasia include benzene and benzene derivatives (e.g. paint remover). Certain toxic materials such as inorganic arsenic, glycol ethers, plutonium and radon have also been implicated as potential causes.

Clinical Manifestations

- Infection and the symptoms of anemia (e.g. fatigue, pallor, dyspnea)
- Retinal hemorrhages
- Purpura (bruising)
- Repeated throat infections with possible cervical lymphadenopathy
- Possible lymphadenopathies and splenomegaly sometimes occur.

Diagnostic Methods

Diagnosis is made by a bone marrow aspirate that shows an extremely hypoplastic or even aplastic (very few to no cells) marrow replaced with fat.

Medical Management

1. Those who are younger than 60 years, are otherwise healthy and have a compatible donor can be cured of the disease by a bone marrow transplant (BMT) or peripheral blood stem cell transplant (PBSCT).
2. In others, the disease can be managed with immunosuppressive therapy, commonly using a combination of antithymocyte globulin (ATG) and cyclosporine or androgens.
3. Supportive therapy plays a major role in the management of aplastic anemia. Any offending agent is discontinued. The patient is supported with transfusions of packed red blood cells (PRBCs).

Nursing Management

1. Assess patient carefully for signs of infection and bleeding, as patient with aplastic anemia are vulnerable to problems related to erythrocyte, leukocyte and platelet deficiencies.
2. Monitor for side effects of therapy, particularly for hypersensitivity reaction, while administering ATG.
3. If patients require long-term cyclosporine therapy, monitor them for long-term effects including renal or liver dysfunction, hypertension, pruritus, visual impairment, tremor and skin cancer.
4. Carefully assess each new prescription for drug-drug interactions, as the metabolism of ATG is altered by many other medications.
5. Ensure that patients understand the importance of not abruptly stopping immunosuppressive therapy.

Refer 'Nursing Management' under 'Anemia' for additional information.

ANEMIA

Anemia is a condition in which the hemoglobin concentration is lower than normal. It reflects the presence of fewer than the normal number of erythrocytes within circulation. As a result, the amount of oxygen delivered to body tissues is also diminished. Anemia is not a specific disease state, but a sign of an underlying disorder. It is by far the most common hematological condition. There are several kinds of anemia. A physiological approach classifies anemia according to whether the deficiency in erythrocytes is caused by a defect in their production (hypoproliferative anemia), by their destruction (hemolytic anemia), or by their loss (bleeding).

Clinical Manifestations

Aside from the severity of the anemia itself, several factors influence the development of anemia-associated symptoms; the rapidity with which the anemia has developed, the duration of the anemia (i.e. its chronicity), the metabolic requirements of patient, other concurrent disorders or disabilities (e.g. cardiac or pulmonary disease and complications or concomitant features) of the condition that produced the anemia. In general, the more rapidly an anemia develops, the more severe its symptoms. Pronounced symptoms of anemia include the following:

- Dyspnea, chest pain, muscle pain or cramping, tachycardia
- Weakness, fatigue, general malaise
- Pallor of the skin and mucous membranes (conjunctive, oral mucosa)
- Jaundice (megaloblastic or hemolytic anemia)
- Smooth, red tongue (iron-deficiency anemia)
- Beefy red, sore tongue (megaloblastic anemia)
- Angular cheilitis (ulceration of the corner of the mouth)
- Brittle, ridged, concave nails and pica (unusual craving for starch, dirt, ice) in patients with iron-deficiency anemia.

Diagnostic Methods

1. Complete hematological studies [e.g. hemoglobin, hematocrit, reticulocyte count and red blood cell (RBC) indices, particularly the MCV and RBC distribution width red cell distribution width (RDW)].

2. Iron studies [serum iron level, total iron-binding capacity (TIBC), percent saturation and ferritin)].
3. Serum vitamin B_{12} and folate levels; haptoglobin and erythropoietin levels.
4. Bone marrow aspiration.
5. Other studies as indicated to determine underlying illness.

Medical Management

Management of anemia is directed toward correcting or controlling the cause of anemia; if the anemia is severe, the erythrocytes that are lost or destroyed may be replaced with a transfusion of PRBCs.

Anemia is the most common hematological condition affecting elderly patients. The impact of anemia on function is significant. A review among the elderly has noted that fragility, decreased mobility and exercise performance, risk of falling, diminished cognitive function, increasing risk of developing dementia and major depression and lower muscle and bone density are associated with anemia.

Nursing Management

Assessment

1. Obtain a health history, perform a physical examination and obtain laboratory values.
2. Ask patient about extent and type of symptom experienced and impact of symptoms on lifestyle, meditory, alcohol intake and athletic endeavors (extremity).
3. Ask about family history of inherited anemias.
4. Perform nutritional assessment—ask about dietary habits resulting in nutritional deficiencies such as those vitamin B_{12} and folic acid.
5. Monitor relevant laboratory test results; note changes.
6. Assess cardiac status (symptoms of increased workload or heart failure): Tachycardia, palpitations, dyspnea, orthopnea, exertional dyspnea, cardiomegaly, hepatomegaly, peripheral edema.
7. Assess for GI function: Nausea, vomiting, diarrhea, melena or dark stools, occult blood, anorexia, women should be questioned about their menstrual periods (e.g. excessive menstrual flow, other vaginal bleeding and the use of iron supplements during pregnancy.
8. Assess for neurological deficits (important with pernicious anemia): Presence and extent of peripheral numbness and paresthesias, ataxia, poor coordination, confusion.

Nursing Diagnoses

1. Fatigue related to decreased hemoglobin and diminished oxygen-carrying capacity of the blood.
2. Altered nutrition less than body requirements related to inadequate intake of essential nutrients.
3. Altered tissue perfusion related to inadequate hemoglobin and hematocrit.
4. Noncompliance with prescribed therapy.

Potential complications: The following are potential complications:
- Heart failure
- Angina
- Paresthesias
- Confusion.

Planning (Goals and Objectives)

The major goals for the patient may include decreased fatigue, attainment or maintenance of adequate nutrition, maintenance of adequate tissue perfusion, compliance with prescribed therapy and absence of complications.

Nursing Interventions/Implementations

Managing Fatigue

- Assist patient to prioritize activities and establish a balance between activity and rest
- Encourage patient with chronic anemia to maintain physical activity and exercise to prevent deconditioning.

Maintaining Adequate Perfusion

- Monitor vital signs and pulse oximeter readings closely and adjust or withhold medications (antihypertensive) as indicated
- Administer supplemental oxygen, transfusions and intravenous (IV) fluids as ordered.

Promoting Compliance with Prescribed Therapy

1. Discuss with patients the purpose of their medication, how to take the medication and over what time period and how to manage any side effects; ensure patient knows that abruptly stopping some medications can have serious consequences.
2. Assist patient to incorporate the therapeutic plan into everyday activities, rather than merely giving the patient a list of instructions.
3. Provide assistance to obtain needed insurance coverage for expensive medications (e.g. growth factors) or to explore alternative ways to obtain these medications.

Monitoring and Managing Complications

- Assess patient with anemia for heart failure
- Perform a neurological assessment for patient with known or suspected megaloblastic anemia.

Evaluations

Evaluation of care is based on the objectives or expected patient outcomes:
- Reports less fatigue
- Attains and maintains adequate nutrition
- Maintains adequate perfusion
- No experiences or minimal complications.

IRON-DEFICIENCY ANEMIA

Iron-deficiency anemia typically results when the intake of dietary iron is inadequate for hemoglobin synthesis. It is the most common type of anemia in all age groups and it is most common anemia in the world. The most common cause of iron-deficiency anemia in men and postmenopausal women is bleeding from ulcers, gastritis, inflammatory bowel disease or GI tumors. The most common causes of iron-deficiency anemia is premenopausal women are menorrhagia (i.e. excessive menstrual bleeding) and pregnancy with inadequate iron supplementation. Patients with chronic alcoholism often have chronic blood loss from the GI tract, which causes iron loss and eventual anemia. Other causes include iron malabsorption, as seen after gastrectomy or with celiac disease.

Clinical Manifestations

- Symptoms of anemia
- Symptoms in more severe or prolonged cases: Smooth, sore tongue, brittle and ridged nails, angular cheilosis (mouth ulceration).

Diagnostic Methods

- Bone marrow aspiration
- Laboratory values including serum ferritin levels (indicates iron stores), blood cell count (hematocrit, RBC count, MCV), serum iron levels and TIBC.

Medical Management

1. Search for the cause, which may be a curable GI cancer or uterine fibroids.
2. Test stool specimens for occult blood.
3. People aged 50 years or older should have periodic colonoscopy endoscopy or X-ray examination of the GI tract to detect ulcerations, gastritis, polyps, or cancer.
4. Administer prescribed iron preparations (oral, intramuscular or IV).
5. Have patient continue iron preparations for 6–12 months.

Nursing Management

1. Administer IM or IV iron in some cases when oral iron is not absorbed, is poorly tolerated or is needed in large amounts.
2. Administer a small test dose before IM injection to avoid risk of anaphylaxis (greater with IM than with IV injections).
3. Advise patient to take iron supplements an hour before meals. If gastric distress occurs, suggest taking the supplement with meals and after symptoms subside, resuming between meal schedules for maximum absorption.
4. Inform patient that iron salts change stool to dark green or black.
5. Advise patient to take liquid forms of iron through a straw, to rinse the mouth with water and to practice good oral hygiene after taking this medication.
6. Teach preventive education because iron-deficiency anemia is common in menstruation and pregnant women.
7. Educate patient regarding foods high in iron (e.g. organ and other meats, bean, leafy green vegetables, raisins, molasses).

8. Instruct patient to avoid taking antacids or dairy products with iron (diminishes iron absorption).
9. Provide nutritional counseling for those whose normal diet therapy is inadequate.
10. Encourage patient to continue iron therapy for total therapy time (6–12 month), even when fatigue is no longer present.

Refer 'Nursing Management' under 'Anemia' for additional information.

SICKLE CELL ANEMIA

Sickle cell anemia is a severe hemolytic anemia resulting from the inheritance of the sickle hemoglobin (*HbS*) gene, which causes a defective hemoglobin molecule.

Pathophysiology

The defective hemoglobin molecule assumes a sickle shape when exposed to low-oxygen tension. These long, rigid RBCs become lodged in small vessels and can obstruct blood flow to body tissue. If ischemia or infarctions result, the patient may have pain, swelling and fever. The sickling process takes time; if the erythrocyte is again exposed to adequate amounts of oxygen (e.g. when it travels through the pulmonary circulation) before the membrane becomes too rigid, it can revert to a normal shape. For this reason, the 'sickling crises' are intermittent. The *HbS* gene is inherited with some people having the sickle cell trait (a carrier, inheriting one abnormal (gene) and some people having sickle cell disease (inheriting two abnormal genes). Sickle cell disease is found predominantly in people of African descent and less often in people who have descended from the Mediterranean countries, the Middle East or aboriginal tribes of India.

Clinical Manifestations

Symptoms of sickle cell anemia vary and are only somewhat based on the amount of HbS. Symptoms and complications results from chronic hemolysis or thrombosis are:

1. Anemia with hemoglobin values in the range of 7–10 g/dL.
2. Jaundice is characteristic, usually obvious in the sclera.
3. Bone marrow expands in childhood, sometimes causing enlargement of bones of the face and skull.
4. Tachycardia, cardiac murmurs and often cardiomegaly are associated with chronic anemia.
5. Dysrhythmias and heart failure may occur in adults.
6. Virtually any organ may be affected by thrombosis, but the primary sites involve those areas with slower circulation such as the spleen, lungs and central nervous system.
7. There is a severe pain in various parts of the body. All tissues and organs are vulnerable and susceptible to hypoxic damage or ischemic necrosis.
8. Sickle cell crisis: Sickle crisis, aplastic crisis or sequestration crisis.
9. Acute chest syndrome: Fever, cough, tachycardia and new infiltrates seen on the chest X-ray.
10. Pulmonary hypertension is a common sequelae of sickle cell disease and often the cause of death.

Diagnostic Findings

1. The patient with sickle cell trait usually has a normal hemoglobin level, hematocrit and blood smear.
2. In contrast, the patient with sickle cell anemia has a low-hematocrit level and sickled cells on the smear. The diagnosis is confirmed by hemoglobin electrophoresis.

Medical Management

Treatment of sickle cell anemia is the focus of continued research. However, aside from the equally important aggressive management of symptoms and complications, there are currently few primary treatment modalities for sickle cell diseases:

1. The PBSCT may cure sickle cell anemia, but is available to only as small subset of affected patients because of either the lack of compatible donor or because severe organ damage that may be already present in the patient is a contraindication for PBCT.
2. Pharmacological therapy: Hydroxyurea, a chemotherapy agent has been shown to be effective in increasing fetal hemoglobin (i.e. hemoglobin F) levels in patients with sickle cell anemia; arginine may be useful in managing pulmonary hypertension and acute chest syndrome.
3. Transfusion therapy: It has been shown to be highly effective in several situations (e.g. in an acute exacerbation of anemia, in the prevention of severe complications from anesthesia and surgery and in improving the response to infection, and in severe cases of acute chest syndrome).
4. Pulmonary function is monitored and pulmonary hypertension is treated early, if found. Infections and acute chest syndrome, which predispose to crisis are treated promptly. Incentive spirometry is performed to prevent pulmonary disease.
5. Fluid restriction may be beneficial. Corticosteroids may be useful.
6. Folic acid is administered daily for increased marrow requirement.
7. Supportive care involves pain management [Aspirin or non-steroidal anti-inflammatory drugs (NSAIDs), morphine and patient controlled analgesia], oral or IV hydration, physical and occupational therapy, physiotherapy, cognitive and behavioral intervention and support groups.

Nursing Management

Assessment

1. Questions patients in crisis about factors that could have precipitated the crisis and measures used to prevent crisis.
2. Assess all body systems with particular emphasis on pain (0–10 scale, quality and frequency), swelling, fever (all joint areas and abdomen).
3. Carefully assess respiratory system including breath sounds, oxygen saturation levels.
4. Assess for signs of cardiac failure [edema, increased point of maximal impulse and cardiomegaly (as seen on chest X-ray)].
5. Elicit symptoms of cerebral hypoxia by careful neurological examination.
6. Assess for signs of dehydration and history of fluid intake; examine mucous membranes, skin turgor, urine output, serum creatinine and blood urea nitrogen (BUN) values.

7. Assess for signs of any infectious process (examine chest and long bones, and femoral head because pneumonia and osteomyelitis are common).
8. Monitor hemoglobin, hematocrit and reticulocyte count and compare with baseline levels.
9. Assess current and past history of medical management, particularly chronic transfusion therapy, hydroxyurea use and prior treatment for infection.

Refer 'Nursing Management' under 'Anemia' for additional information.

Nursing Diagnoses

- Acute pain related to tissue hypoxia due to agglutination of sickled cells within blood vessels
- Risk for infection
- Risk for powerlessness related to illness induced helplessness
- Deficient knowledge regarding prevention of crisis.

Potential complications: Are as follows:

- Hypoxia, ischemia, infection, poor wound healing leading to skin breakdown and ulcers
- Dehydration
- Cerebrovascular accident (CVA), brain attack, stroke
- Anemia
- Acute and chronic renal failure
- Heart failure, pulmonary hypertension and acute chest syndrome,
- Impotence
- Poor compliance
- Substance abuse related to poorly managed chronic pain.

Planning (Goals and Objectives)

The major goals for the patient are relief of pain, decreased incidence of crisis, enhanced sense of self-esteem and power and absence of complications.

Nursing Interventions/Implementations

Managing Pain

1. Use patient's subjective description of pain and pain rating on a pain scale to guide the use of analgesic agents.
2. Support and elevate any joint that is acutely swollen until swelling diminishes.
3. Teach patient relaxation techniques, breathing exercises and distraction to ease pain.
4. When acute painful episode has diminished, implement aggressive measures to preserve function (e.g. physical therapy, whirlpool baths and transcutaneous nerve stimulation).

Preventing and Managing Infections

- Monitor patient for signs and symptoms of infection
- Initiate prescribed antibiotics promptly
- Assess patient for signs of dehydration
- Teach patient to take prescribed oral antibiotics at home, if indicated, emphasizing the need to complete the entire course of antibiotic therapy.

Promoting Coping Skills

- Enhance pain management to promote a therapeutic relationship based on mutual trust
- Focus on patient's strengths rather than deficits to enhance effective coping skills
- Provide opportunities for patient to make decisions about daily care to increase feelings of control.

Increasing Knowledge

1. Teach patient about situations that can precipitate a sickle cell crisis and take steps to prevent or diminish such crisis (e.g. keep warm, maintain adequate hydration and avoid stressful situations).
2. If hydroxyurea is prescribed for a woman bearing age, inform her that the drug can cure congenital harm to unborn children and advise about pregnancy prevention.

Monitoring and Managing Potential Complications

Management measures for many of the potential complications are delineated in the previous sections; additional measures should be taken to address the following issues.

Leg ulcers
- Protect the leg from trauma and contamination
- Use scrupulous aseptic technique to prevent nosocomial infections
- Refer to wound, ostomy and continence nurse, which may facilitate healing and assist with prevention.

Priapism leading to impotence
- Teach patient to empty the bladder at the onset of the attack, exercise and take a warm bath
- Inform patient to seek medical attention if an episode persists more than 3 hours.

Chronic pain and substance abuse
1. Emphasize the importance of complying with prescribed treatment plan.
2. Promote trust with patient through adequate management of acute pain during episodes of crisis.
3. Suggest to patient that receiving care from a single provider over time is much more beneficial than receiving care from physicians and staff in emergency department.
4. When a crisis arises, emergency department staff should contract patient's primary healthcare provider for optimal management.
5. Promote continuity of care and establish written contracts with patient.

Family-based Care and Follow-up

1. In value, the patient and his/her family in teaching about the disease, treatment, assessment and monitoring needed to detect complications. Also teach about vascular access device management and chelation therapy.
2. Advise healthcare providers, patients and families to communicate regularly.

3. Provide guidelines regarding when to seek urgent care.
4. Provide follow-up care for patient with vascular access devices, if necessary.

POLYCYTHEMIA

Polycythemia is an increased volume of RBCs. The hematocrit is elevated by more than 55% in men or more than 50% in women. Polycythemia is classified as either primary or secondary.

Secondary Polycythemia

Secondary polycythemia is caused by excessive production of erythropoietin. This may occur in response to a hypoxic stimulus as in chronic obstructive pulmonary disease (COPD) or cyanotic heart disease or in certain hemoglobinopathies in which the hemoglobin has an abnormally high affinity for oxygen, or it can occur from a neoplasm such as renal cell carcinoma. Management of secondary polycythemia involves treatment of the primary problem. If the cause cannot be corrected, phlebotomy may be necessary to reduce hypervolemia and hyperviscoscity.

Polycythemia Vera (Primary)

Polycythemia vera or primary polycythemia is a proliferative disorder of the myeloid stem cells. The bone marrow is hypercellular and the erythrocyte, leukocyte and platelet counts in the peripheral blood are elevated. Diagnosis is based on elevated erythrocyte mass, normal oxygen saturation level and often an enlarged spleen. The erythropoietin level may not be as low as would be expected with an elevated hematocrit.

Clinical Manifestations

Patients typically have a ruddy complexion and splenomegaly. The symptoms are due to the increased blood volume (headache, dizziness, tinnitus, fatigue, paresthesias and blurred vision) or to increase blood viscosity (angina, claudication, dyspnea and thrombophlebitis). Blood pressure and uric acid are often elevated and pruritus is another common and bothersome complication. Erythromelalgia (a burning sensation in the fingers and toes) may be reported.

Medical Management

The objective of management is to reduce the high RBC mass:

1. Phlebotomy is performed repeatedly to keep the hemoglobin within normal range; iron supplements are avoided.
2. Chemotherapeutic agents are used to suppress marrow function (may increase risk for leukemia).
3. Anagrelide (Agrylin) may be used to inhibit platelet aggregation and control the thrombocytosis related to polycythemia.
4. Interferon alpha-2b (Intron A) is the most effective treatment for managing the pruritus associated with polycythemia vera.
5. Antihistamines may be administered to control pruritus (not very effective).
6. Allopurinol is used to prevent gout attacks when the uric acid level is elevated.

Nursing Management

1. Assess risk factors for thrombotic complications and teach patient to recognize signs and symptoms of thrombosis.
2. Discourage sedentary behavior, crossing the legs and wearing tight or restrictive clothing (particularly stockings) to reduce the likelihood of DVT.
3. Advise patient to avoid Aspirin and medications containing Aspirin (if patient has a history of bleeding).
4. Advise patient to minimize alcohol intake, and avoid iron and vitamins containing iron.
5. Suggest a cool or tepid bath for pruritus, along with cocoa butter-based lotions and bath providing to relieve itching.

THROMBOCYTOPENIA

Thrombocytopenia (low-platelet count) is the most common cause of abnormal bleeding.

Pathophysiology

Thrombocytopenia can result from decreased production of platelets within the bone marrow or from increased destruction or consumption of platelets. Causes include failure a production as a result of hematological malignancies, myelodysplastic syndromes, metastatic involvement of bone marrow from solid tumors, certain anemias, toxins, medications, infection, alcohol and chemotherapy; increased destruction as a result of idiopathic thrombocytopenia purpura, lupus erythematosus, malignant lymphoma, chronic lymphocytic leukemia, medications, infections and sequestration and increased utilization such as results from disseminated intravascular coagulopathy (DIC).

Clinical Manifestations

1. With platelet count below 50,000/mm^3: Bleeding and petechiae.
2. With platelet count below 20,000/mm^3: Petechiae along with nasal and gingival bleeding after surgery or dental extraction.
3. With platelet count below 5,000/mm^3: Spontaneous and potentially fatal central nervous system hemorrhage or GI hemorrhage.

Diagnostic Methods

1. Bone marrow aspiration and biopsy if platelet deficiencies of secondary to decreased production.
2. Increased megakaryocytes (the cells from which platelet originate) and normal or even increased platelet production in bone marrow, when platelet destruction is the cause.

Medical Management

The management of secondary thrombocytopenia is usually treatment of the underlying disease. Platelet transfusions are used to raise platelet count and stop bleeding or preventive spontaneous hemorrhage, if platelet production is impaired. If excessive platelet destruction is the cause, the patient is treated as indicated for idiopathic thrombocytopenia purpura. For some patients, a splenectomy can be therapeutic, although it may not be an option for other patients (e.g. patients in whom the enlarged spleen is due to portal hypertension related to cirrhosis).

Nursing Management

Interventions focus on preventing injury (e.g. use soft toothbrush and electric razors, minimize needle stick procedures), stopping or slowing bleeding (e.g. pressure, cold) and administering medications and platelet as ordered, as well as patient teaching (refer 'Nursing Management' under 'Idiopathic Thrombocytopenic Purpura' for additional information).

HEMOPHILIA

Hemophilia is a relatively rare disease. There are two hereditary bleeding disorders that are clinically indistinguishable, but can be separated by laboratory tests, hemophilia A and hemophilia B. Hemophilia A is due to a genetic defect that results in deficient or defective factor VIII. Hemophilia B stems from a genetic defect that causes deficient or defective IX. Hemophilia A is about three times more common than hemophilia B. Both types are inherited as X-linked traits, so almost all affected people are males, females can be carriers, but are almost always asymptomatic. All ethnic groups are affected. The disease is usually recognized in early childhood, usually in toddlers. Mild hemophilia may not be diagnosed until trauma or surgery.

Clinical Manifestations

The frequency and severity of bleeding depend on the degree of factor deficiency and intensity of trauma:

1. Hemorrhage occurs into various body parts (large, spreading bruises and bleeding into muscles, joints and soft tissues) after even minimal trauma.
2. Most bleeding occurs in joints (most often in knees, elbows, ankles, shoulders, wrists and hips); pain in joints may occur before swelling and limitation of motion are apparent.
3. Chronic pain or ankylosing (fixation) of the joint may occur with recurrent hemorrhage; many patients are crippled by joint damage before adulthood.
4. Spontaneous hematuria and GI bleeding can occur. Hematomas within the muscles can cause peripheral nerve compression with decreased sensation, weakness and atrophy of the area.
5. The most dangerous site of hemorrhage is in the head (intracranial or extracranial); any head traumas require prompt evaluation and treatment.
6. Surgical procedures typically result in excessive bleeding at the surgical site; bleeding is most commonly associated with dental extraction.
7. Laboratory tests include clotting factor measurement and CBC count.

Medical Management

1. Factors VIII and IX concentrates are given when active bleeding occurs or as a preventive measure before traumatic procedures (e.g. lumbar puncture, dental extraction, surgery).

2. Plasmapheresis or concurrent immunosuppressive therapy may be required for patients who develop antibodies (inhibitors) to factor concentrates.
3. Aminocaproic acid may slow the dissolution of blood clots; desmopressin acetate (DDAVP) induces transient increase in factor VIII.
4. Desmopressin is useful in patient with mild forms of hemophilia A.

Nursing Management

1. Assist family and patient in coping with the condition because it is a chronic, places restriction on their lives and is an inherited disorder that can be passed to future generations.
2. From childhood, help patient to cope with the disease and to identify the positive aspects of their lives.
3. Encourage patients to be self-sufficient and to maintain independence by preventing unnecessary trauma.
4. Patients with mild factor deficiency that were not diagnosed until adulthood need extensive teaching about activity restrictions and self-care measures to diminish the chance of hemorrhage and complications of bleeding; emphasize safety at home and in the workplace.
5. Instruct the patients to avoid any agents that interfere with platelet aggregation such as Aspirin, NSAIDs, herbs, nutritional supplements and alcohol (also applies to over-the-counter medications).
6. Promote good dental hygiene as a preventive measures because dental extractions are hazardous.
7. Instruct patient that applying pressure to minor wound may be sufficient to control bleeding if the factor deficiency is not severe; avoid nasal picking.
8. Splints and other orthopedic devices may be useful in patients with joint or muscle hemorrhages.
9. Avoid all injections, minimize invasive procedures (e.g. endoscopy, lumbar puncture) or perform after administration of appropriate factor replacement.
10. Carefully assess bleeding during hemorrhagic episodes; patients at risk for significant compromise (e.g. bleeding into the respiratory tract or brain) warrant close observation and systematic assessment for emergent complications [e.g. respiratory distress, altered level of consciousness (LOC)].
11. If patient has had recent surgery, frequently and carefully assess the surgical site for bleeding; frequent monitoring of vital signs is needed until the nurse is certain that there is no excessive postoperative bleeding.
12. Patients who have been exposed to infections [e.g. human immunodeficiency virus (HIV) infections, hepatitis] through previous transfusions may need assistance in coping with the diagnosis and consequences.
13. Recommend genetic testing and counseling to female carriers so that they can make informed decisions regarding having children and managing pregnancy.
14. Advise patient to carry or wear medical identification.

DISSEMINATED INTRAVASCULAR COAGULATION

Disseminated intravascular coagulation (DIC) is a potentially life-threatening sign (not a disease itself) of a serious underlying disease mechanism. DIC may be triggered by a sepsis, trauma, cancer, shock, abruptio placentae, toxins or allergic reactions. The severity of DIC is variable, but is potentially life-threatening.

Pathophysiology

In DIC, the normal hemostatic mechanisms are altered so that tiny clots form within the microcirculation of the body. These clots consume platelets and clotting factors, eventually causing coagulation to fail and bleeding to result. This bleeding disorder is characterized by low platelet and fibrinogen levels; prolonged prothrombin time (PT), partial thromboplastin time (PTT) and thrombin time; and by elevated fibrin degradation products (D-dimers). The primary prognostic factor is the ability to treat the underlying condition that precipitated DIC.

Clinical Manifestations

Clinical manifestations of DIC are primarily reflected in compromised organ function or failure, usually a result of excessive clot formation (with resultant ischemia to all or part of the organ) or less, often, bleeding:

1. Patient may bleed from mucous membranes, venipuncture sites, and GI and urinary tracts.
2. Bleeding can range from minimal occult internal bleeding to profuse hemorrhage from all orifices.
3. Patients typically develop multiple organ dysfunction syndromes (MODS) and they may exhibit renal failure as well as pulmonary and multifocal central nervous system infarctions as a result of microthromboses, macrothromboses or hemorrhage.
4. Initially, the only manifestation is a progressive decrease in the platelet count, then progressively, the patient exhibits signs and symptoms of thrombosis in the organs involved. Eventually, bleeding occurs (at first subtle, advancing to frank hemorrhage). Signs and symptoms depend on the organs involved.

Diagnostic Findings

1. Clinically, the diagnosis of DIC is often established by a drop in platelet count, an increase in PT and activated partial thromboplastin time (aPTT), an elevation in fibrin degradation products and measurement of one or more clotting factors and inhibitors [e.g. antithromobin (AT)].
2. The International Society on Thrombosis and Haemostasis has developed a highly sensitive and specific scoring system using the platelet count, fibrin degradation products, PT and fibrinogen level to diagnose DIC. This system is also useful in predicting the severity of the disease and subsequent mortality.

Medical Management

The most important management issue is treating the underlying cause of DIC. A second goal is to correct the secondary effects of tissue ischemia by improving oxygenation, replacing fluids, correcting electrolyte imbalances and administering vasopressor medications. If serious hemorrhage occurs, the depleted coagulation factors and platelets may be replaced (cryoprecipitate to replace the fibrinogen, and factors V and VII; fresh-frozen plasma to replace other coagulation factors).

A heparin infusion, which is controversial management method, may be used to interrupt the thrombosis present. Other therapies include recombinant activated protein and AT infusions.

Nursing Management

1. Avoid procedures and activities that can increase intracranial pressure such as coughing and straining.
2. Closely monitor vital signs including neurological checks and assess for the amount of external bleeding.
3. Avoid medications that interfere with platelet function, if possible (e.g. β-lactam antibiotics, acetylsalicylic and NSAIDs).
4. Avoid rectal probes and rectal or intramuscular injection medications.
5. Use low pressure with any suctioning.
6. Administer oral hygiene carefully: Use sponge-tipped swabs salt or soda mouthrinses; avoid lemon-glycerin swabs, hydrogen peroxide and commercial mouthwashes.
7. Avoid dislodging any clots including those around IV sites, injection sites and so forth.
8. Assess skin with particular attention to bony prominence and skin folds.
9. Reposition carefully: Use pressure-reducing mattress and lambswool between digits and around ears, and soft absorbent material in skin folds as needed.
10. Perform skin care every 2 hours, administer oral hygiene carefully.
11. Use prolonged pressure (5 minute minimum) after essential injections.
12. Auscultate breath sounds every 2–4 hours.
13. Monitor extent of edema.
14. Monitor volume of IV medications and blood products, decrease volume of IV medications, if possible.
15. Administer diuretics agents as prescribed.

Assessment

Ineffective tissue perfusion related to microthrombi

- Assess neurological, pulmonary and skin systems
- Monitor response to heparin therapy; monitor fibrinogen levels
- Assess extent of bleeding
- Stop epsilon-aminocaproic acid, if symptoms of thrombosis occur.

Reducing fear and anxiety

- Identify previous coping mechanisms, if possible encourage patient to use them as appropriate
- Explain all procedures and rationale in terms that the patient and family can understand
- Assist family in supporting patient
- Use services from behavioral medicine and clergy, if desired.

IDIOPATHIC THROMBOCYTOPENIC PURPURA

Idiopathic thrombocytopenic purpura (ITP) also known as primary immune thrombocytopenic purpura is a disease affecting all ages, but is more common in children and young women. Although the precise cause remains unknown, viral infections sometimes precedes the disease in children. Other conditions (e.g. systemic lupus erythematosus, pregnancy) or medications (e.g. sulfa drugs) can also produce ITP.

Pathophysiology

In patients with ITP, antiplatelet autoantibodies that bind to the platelets are found in the blood. When the platelets are bound by the antibodies, the reticuloendothelial system (RES) or tissue macrophage system ingests the platelets, destroying them. The body attempts to compensate for this destruction by increasing platelet production within the marrow. There are two forms, acute (primarily in children) and chronic.

Clinical Manifestations

- Many patients have no symptoms
- Petechiae and easy bruising (dry purpura)
- Heavy menses and mucosal bleeding (wet purpura, high risk of intracranial bleeding)
- Platelet count generally below $20,000/mm^3$
- Acute form self-limiting, possibly with spontaneous remissions.

Diagnostic Findings

Usually, the diagnosis is based on the decreased platelet count and survival time and increased bleeding time and ruling out other causes of thrombocytopenia. Key diagnostic procedures include platelet count, CBC and bone marrow aspiration, which show an increase in megakaryocytes (platelet precursors). Many patients are infected with *Helicobacter pylori* (*H. pylori*). To date, effectiveness of *H. pylori* treatment in relation to management of ITP is unknown.

Medical Management

Primary goal of treatment is a safe platelet count. Splenectomy is sometimes performed (thrombocytopenia may return months or years later).

Immunosuppressive medications such as corticosteroids are the treatment of choice. The bone mineral density of patients receiving chronic corticosteroid therapy needs to be monitored. These patients may benefit from calcium and vitamin D supplementation or bisphosphonate therapy to prevent significant bone disease:

1. Intravenous gamma globulin (very expensive) and the chemotherapy agent vincristine are also effective.
2. Another approach involves using anti-D (WinRho) for patients who are Rh(D)-positive.
3. Thrombopoiesis-stimulating protein, AMG 531 has been successfully used to treat patient with chronic ITP.
4. Epsilon aminocaproic acid (EACA) (Amicar) may be useful for patients with significant mucosal bleeding who are refractory to other treatment modalities.
5. Platelet infusions are avoided except to stop catastrophic bleeding.

Nursing Management

1. Assess patient's lifestyle to determine the risk of bleeding from activity.
2. Obtain history of medication use including over-the-counter medications, herbs and nutritional supplements; recent viral illness or complications of headache, or visual disturbances (intracranial bleed). Be alert for sulfa-containing medications and medications that alter platelet function (e.g. Aspirin or other NSAIDs). Physical assessment should include a thorough search for signs of bleeding, neurological assessment and vital sign measurement.
3. Teach patient to recognize exacerbations of disease (petechiae, ecchymoses); how to contact healthcare personnel and the names of medications that induce ITP.
4. Provide information about medications (tapering schedule, if relevant), frequency of platelet count monitoring and medications to avoid.
5. To minimize bleeding, instruct patient to avoid all agents that interfere with platelet function. Avoid administering medications by injection or rectal route; rectal temperature measurements should not be performed.
6. Instruct patient to avoid constipation, the Valsalva maneuver and tooth flossing.
7. Encourage patient to use electric razor for shaving and soft-bristled toothbrushes instead of stiff-bristled brushes.
8. Advise patient to refrain from vigorous sexual intercourse when platelet count is less than 10,000/mm^3.
9. Monitor for complications including osteoporosis, proximal muscle wasting, cataract formation and dental caries.

LEUKEMIA

Leukemia is a malignancy of the blood-forming cells in the bone marrow.

Pathophysiology

The common feature of leukemias is an unregulated proliferation or accumulation of WBCs in the bone marrow. There is also proliferation in the liver and spleen and invasion of other organs such as meninges lymph nodes, gums and skin. The leukemias are commonly classified according to the stem cell line involved, either lymphoid or myeloid. Leukemia is also classified as acute (abrupt onset) or chronic (evolves over months to years). Its cause is unknown. There is some evidence that generic influence and viral pathogenesis may be involved. Bone marrow damage from radiation exposure or chemicals such as benzene and alkylating agents can also cause leukemia.

Clinical Manifestations

Cardial signs and symptoms include weakness and fatigue, bleeding tendencies, petechiae and ecchymoses, pain, headache, vomiting, fever and infection.

Diagnostic Findings

Blood and bone marrow studies confirm proliferation of WBCs (leukocytes) in the bone marrow.

Nursing Management

Assessment

1. Identify range of signs and symptoms reported by patient in nursing history and physical examination.
2. Assess results of blood studies, and report alterations of WBCs, absolute neutrophil count (ANC), hematocrit, platelet, creatinine and electrolyte levels, hepatic function test and culture results.

Nursing Diagnoses

1. Risk for infection and bleeding.
2. Risk for impaired skin integrity related to toxic effects of chemotherapy, alteration in nutrition and impaired mobility.
3. Impaired gas exchange.
4. Impaired mucous membranes from changes in epithelial lining of the GI tract from chemotherapy or antimicrobial medications.
5. Imbalanced nutrition: Less than body requirements related to hypermetabolic state, anorexia, mucositis, pain and nausea.
6. Acute pain and discomfort related to mucositis, leukocytic infiltration of systemic tissues, fever and infection.
7. Hyperthermia related to tumor lysis and infection.
8. Fatigue and activity intolerance related to anemia, infection and deconditioning.
9. Impaired physical mobility due to anemia, malaise, discomfort and protective isolation.
10. Risk for excess fluid volume related to renal dysfunction, hypoproteinemia, need for multiple IV medications and blood products.
11. Diarrhea due to altered GI flora, mucosal denudation, prolonged used of broad-spectrum antibiotics.
12. Risk for deficient fluid volume related to potential for diarrhea, bleeding, infection and increased metabolic rate.
13. Self-care deficits related to fatigue, malaise and protective isolation.
14. Anxiety due to knowledge deficit and uncertain future.
15. Disturbed body image related to change in appearance.
16. Grieving related to anticipatory loss and altered role functioning.
17. Risk for spiritual distress.
18. Deficient knowledge of disease process, treatment, complication management and self-care measures.

Potential complications: Infection, bleeding/disseminated intravascular coagulation (DIC), renal dysfunction, tumor lysis syndrome, nutritional depletion, mucositis, depression and anxiety.

Planning (Goals and Objectives)

The major goals of the patient may include absence of complications and pain, attainment and maintenance of adequate nutrition, activity tolerance, ability to provide self-care and to cope with the diagnosis and prognosis, positive body image and an understanding of the disease process and its treatment.

Nursing Interventions/Implementations

Preventing or Managing Bleeding

1. Assess for thrombocytopenia, granulocytopenia and anemia.
2. Report any increase in petechiae, melena, hematuria or nosebleeds.
3. Avoid trauma and injections; use small-gauge needles when analgesics are administered parenterally and apply pressure after injections to avoid bleeding.
4. Use acetaminophen instead of Aspirin and analgesia.
5. Give prescribed hormone therapy to prevent menses.
6. Manage hemorrhage with bedrest and transfuse RBCs, and platelets as ordered.

Preventing Infection

1. Infection is a major cause of death in leukemia patients.
2. Assess temperature elevation, flushed appearance, chills tachycardia and appearance of white patches in the mouth.
3. Observe for redness, swelling, heat or pain in eyes, ears, throat, skin joints, abdomen, and rectal and perineal areas.
4. Assess for cough and changes in character or color of sputum.
5. Give frequent oral hygiene.
6. Wear sterile gloves to start infusions.
7. Provide daily IV site care; observe for signs of infections.
8. Ensure normal elimination, avoid rectal thermometers, enemas and rectal trauma, avoid vaginal tampons.
9. Avoid catheterization is necessary.

The usual manifestations of infection are altered in patients with leukemia. Corticosteroid therapy may blunt the normal febrile and inflammatory responses to infection.

Managing Mucositis

1. Assess the oral mucosa thoroughly, identify and describe lesions and note color, and moisture (remove dentures first).
2. Assist patient with oral hygiene with soft-bristled toothbrush.
3. Avoid drying agents such as lemon-glycerin swabs and commercial mouthwashes (use saline or saline and baking soda).
4. Emphasize the importance of oral rinse medications to prevent yeast infections.
5. Instruct patient to cleanse the perirectal area after each bowel movement, monitor frequency of stools and stop stool softener with loose stool.

Improving Nutritional Intake

1. Give frequent oral hygiene (before and after meals) to promote appetite with oral anesthetics, caution patient to prevent self-injury and to chew carefully.
2. Maintain nutrition with palatable, small frequent feedings of soft non-irritating foods, provide nutritional supplements, as prescribed.
3. Record daily body weight, as well as intake and output to monitor fluid status.
4. Perform calorie counts and other more formal nutritional assessments.
5. Provide parenteral nutrition, if required.

Take Pain and Discomfort Measures

1. Administer acetaminophen rather than Aspirin for analgesia.
2. Sponge patient with cool water for fever, avoid cold water or ice packs, frequently change bedclothes and provide gentle back and shoulder massage.
3. Provide oral hygiene (for stomatitis) and assist the patient with use of patient-controlled analgesia (PCA) for pain.
4. Use creative strategies to permit uninterrupted sleep (a few hours). Assist the patient when awake to balance rest and activity to prevent deconditioning.
5. Listen actively to patients enduring pain.

Decreasing Fatigue and Deconditioning

1. Measure intake and output accurately; weigh the patient daily.
2. Assess for signs of fluid overdose or dehydration.
3. Monitor laboratory tests (electrolytes, BUN, creatinine and hematocrit) and replace blood, fluids, and electrolyte components as ordered and indicated.

Improving Self-care

- Encourage the patient to do as much as possible
- Listen empathetically to the patient
- Assist the patient to resume more self-care during recovery from treatment.

Managing Anxiety and Grief

1. Provide emotional support and discuss the impact of uncertain future.
2. Assess how much information patient wants to have regarding the illness, its treatment and potential complications; reassess at intervals.
3. Assist patient to identify the source of grief and encourage patient to allow time to adjust to the major life changes rendered by the illness.
4. Arrange to have communication with nurses across care settings to reassure patient that he/she has not been abandoned.

Encouraging Spiritual Well-being

- Assess the patient's spiritual and religious practices and offer relevant services
- Assist the patient to maintain realistic hope over the course of the illness (initially for a cure, in later stages for a quiet, dignified death).

Promoting Family-based Care and Follow-up

1. Ensure patients and their families to have a clear understanding of disease and complications (risk for infection and bleeding).
2. Teach family members about home care, while patient is still in the hospital, particularly vascular access device management, if applicable.
3. Maintain communication between the patient and nurses across care settings.

4. Provide specific instructions regarding when and how to seek care from the physician.

Terminal care

1. Respect the patient's choices about treatment including measures to prolong life and other end-of-life measures. Advance directives including living wills, provide patients with some measure of control during terminal illness.
2. Support families and coordinate home care services to alleviate anxiety about managing the patient's care in the home.
3. Provide respite for the caregivers and patient with hospice volunteers.
4. Provide the patient and caregivers assistance to cope with changes in their roles and responsibilities (i.e. anticipatory grieving).
5. Provide information on hospital-based hospice programs for patients to receive pallative care in the hospital when care at home is no longer possible.

Evaluation

Evaluation is based on objective care.

Excepted Patient Outcomes

- Shows no evidence of infection
- Experiences no bleeding
- Exhibits intact oral mucous membranes
- Attains optimal level of nutrition
- Reports satisfaction with pain and discomfort levels
- Experiences less fatigue and increases activity
- Maintains fluid and electrolyte balance
- Participates in self-care
- Copes with anxiety and grief
- Experiences absence of complications.

ACUTE LYMPHOCYTIC LEUKEMIA

Acute lymphocytic leukemia (ALL) results from an uncontrolled proliferation of immature cells (lymphoblasts) from the lymphoid stem cell. It is most common in young children; boys are affected more frequently than girls, with a peak incidence at 4 years of age. After age 15 years, ALL is uncommon. Therapy for this childhood leukemia has improved to the extent that about 80% of children survive at least 5 years:

1. Immature lymphocytes proliferate in marrow and impede development of normal myeloid cells.
2. Normal hematopoiesis is inhibited resulting in reduced numbers of leukocytes erythrocytes and platelets.
3. Leukocyte counts are low or high, but always include immature cells.
4. Manifestations of leukemic cell infiltration into other organs are more common with ALL than with other forms of leukemia and include pain from an enlarged liver of spleen and bone pain.

The central nervous systems are frequently a site for leukemic cells. Thus, patients may exhibit headache and vomiting because of meningeal involvement. Other extranodal sites include the testes and breasts.

Medical Management

1. Since ALL frequently invades the central nervous system, preventive cranial irradiation or intrathecal chemotherapy (e.g. methotrexate), or both are also a key part of the treatment plan.
2. Corticosteroids and vinca alkaloids are an integral part of the initial induction therapy. Typically, an anthracycline is included, sometimes with asparaginase (Elspar).
3. Once a patient is in remission, intensification therapy (consolidation) ensues. In the adult with ALL, allogeneic transplant may be used for intensification therapy. For those for whom transplant is not an option (or is reversed for relapse), a prolonged maintenance phase ensues, when lower doses of medications are given for up to 3 years.

Nursing Management

Refer 'Nursing Management' under heading 'Leukemia' for additional information.

CHRONIC LYMPHOCYTIC LEUKEMIA

Chronic lymphocytic leukemia (CLL) is a common cancer of older adulthood. The average age at diagnosis is 72 years. It is derived from a malignant clone of B lymphocytes. It was initially hypothesized that these cells can escape apoptosis (programmed cell death); however, this hypothesis is now being questioned. Most to the leukemia cells in CLL are fully mature, so it tends to be a mild disorder compared with the acute form. The disease is classified into three or four stages (two classification systems are in use). In the early stage, an elevated lymphocyte count is seen, it can exceed 100,000/mm^3. The disease is usually diagnosed during physical examination or treatment for another disease.

Clinical Manifestations

1. Many cases are asymptomatic.
2. Lymphocytosis is always present.
3. Erythrocyte and platelet counts may be normal or decreased.
4. Lymphadenopathy (enlargement of lymph nodes), which is to sometimes severe and painful, and splenomegaly may be noted.
5. The CLL patients can develop 'B symptoms'; fever, sweating (especially night) and unintentional weight loss. Infections are common.
6. Anergy (decreased or absent reaction to skin sensitivity tests) reveals the defect in cellular immunity.
7. In the later stages, anemia and thrombocytopenia may develop.

Medical Management

A major paradigm shift has occurred in CLL therapy. For years, there appeared to be no survival advantage in treating CLL in its early stages. However, with the advent of more sensitive means of assessing therapeutic response, it has been demonstrated that achieving a complete remission and eradicating even minimal residual disease results in improved survival:

1. The chemotherapy agent fludarabine (Fludara) and cyclophosphamide (Cytoxan) are often given in combination with the monoclonal antibody rituximab (Rituxan).

2. The monoclonal antibody alemtuzumab (Campath) is often used in combination with other chemotherapeutic agents when the disease is refractory to fludarabine, the patient has very poor prognostic markers or it is necessary to eradicate residual disease after initial treatment.
3. Prophylactic use of antiviral agents and antibiotics [e.g. trimethoprim/sulfamethoxazole (Bactrim, Septra)] for patients receiving alemtuzumab (at significant risk for infection).
4. The IV immunoglobulin may prevent recurrent bacterial infections in selected patients.

Nursing Management

Refer 'Nursing Management' under 'Leukemia' for additional information.

ACUTE MYELOID LEUKEMIA

Acute myeloid leukemia (AML) results from a defect in the hematopoietic stem cell that differentiates into all myeloid cells; monocytes, granulocytes (e.g. neutrophils, basophils, eosinophils), erythrocytes and platelets. AML can be further classified into seven different subgroups based on cytogenetic, histology and morphology (appearance) of the blasts. All age groups are affected; incidence rises with age and peaks at 67 years of age. It is the most common non-lymphocytic leukemia. Death usually occur secondary to infection or hemorrhage.

Clinical Manifestations

1. Most signs and symptoms evolve from insufficient production of normal blood cells: Fever and infection result from neutropenia, weakness and fatigue from anemia and bleeding tendencies form thrombocytopenia. Major hemorrhage occurs with a platelet count of less than $10,000/mm^3$. The most common sites of bleeding are GI, pulmonary and intracranial.
2. Proliferation of leukemic cells within organs leads to a variety of additional symptoms: Pain from an enlarged liver or spleen, hyperplasia of the gums and bone pain from expansion of marrow.
3. The AML has its onset without warning; symptoms develop over weeks or over months.
4. Peripheral blood shows decreased erythrocyte and platelet counts.
5. The leukocyte count is low, normal or high; the percentage of normal cells is usually vastly decreased.

Diagnostic Method

- Bone marrow specimen (excess of immature blast cells)
- The CBC count (decreased platelet count and erythrocyte count).

Medical Management

The objectives is to achieve complete remission, typically with chemotherapy (induction therapy), which in some instances results in remissions lasting a year or longer.

Chemotherapy

- Cytarabine (Cytosar, ara-C) and daunorubicin (Cerubidine)
- Mitoxantrone (Novantrone) or idarubicin (Idamycin)
- Sometimes etoposide (VP-16, VePesid) is added
- Consolidation therapy (postremission therapy with chemotherapy agents).

Supportive Care

- Administration of blood products
- Prompt treatment of infections
- Granulocyte-macrophage colony-stimulating factor [GM-CSF (sargramostim)] to decrease neutropenia
- Antimicrobial therapy and transfusions as needed
- Occasionally, hydroxyurea (Hydrea) may be used briefly to control the increase of blast cells.

Bone Marrow Transplantation

Bone marrow transplantation is used when a tissue match can be obtained. The transplantation procedure follows destruction and the leukemic marrow by chemotherapy.

Nursing Management

Refer 'Nursing Management' under heading 'Leukemia' for additional information.

CHRONIC MYELOID LEUKEMIA

Chronic myeloid leukemia is one of leukemia characterized by the Philadelphia chromosome and occurs most of ten in older adults.

Pathophysiology

Chronic myeloid leukemia (CML) arises from a mutation in the myeloid stem cells. A wide spectrum of cell types exists within the blood from blast forms through mature neutrophils. A cytogenetic abnormality termed the Philadelphia chromosome is found in 95% patients. CML is uncommon before 20 years of age, but the incidence increases with (mean age is 67 years). CML has three stages such as chronic, transformation and accelerated or blast crisis. Marrow expands into cavities of the long bones and cells are formed in the liver and spleen with resultant painful enlargement problems. Infection and bleeding are rare until the disease transformation to the acute phase.

Clinical Manifestations

- Many patients are asymptomatic and leukocytosis is detected by a CBC performed for some other reason
- Leukocyte count commonly exceeds 100,000/mm^3
- Patients with extremely high-leukocyte counts may be somewhat short of breath or slightly confused because of leukostasis
- Splenomegaly with tenderness and hepatomegaly are common
- Some patients have insidious symptoms such as malaise, anorexia and weight loss

- In the transforming phase, bone pain, fever, weight loss, anemia and thrombocytopenia are noted.

Medical Management

1. Oral formulation of a tyrosine kinase inhibitor, imatinib mesylate (Gleevec) is prescribed.
2. In those instances where imatinib (at conventional doses) does not elicit a molecular remission or when that remission is not maintained, other treatment options may be considered; the dosage of imatinib can be increased (with increased toxicity), another inhibitor of BCR-ABL can be used [e.g. dasatinib (Sprycel)] or allogeneic transplant can be used.
3. Bone marrow transplant and peripheral blood stem cell transplantation are additional strategies.
4. In the acute form of CML (blast crisis), treatment may resemble induction therapy for acute leukemia, using the same medications as for AML or ALL.
5. Oral chemotherapeutic agents typically hydroxyurea or busulfan (Myleran); leukapheresis [leukocyte count greater than 300,000/mm^3; an anthracycline chemotherapeutic agents e.g. daunomycin (Cerubidine)] for purely palliative approach (rare).

Nursing Management

Nursing management is similar to that for CLL (refer 'Nursing Management' under 'Leukemia' for additional information).

HODGKIN'S DISEASE LYMPHOMA

Hodgkin's disease is a rare cancer of unknown cause that is uncentric in origin and spreads along the lymphatic system. There is a familiar pattern associated with Hodgkin's as well as an association with the Epstein-Barr virus. It is somewhat more common in men and tends to peak in the early 20s and after 50s.

Pathophysiology

The Reed-Sternberg cell, a gigantic morphologically unique tumor cell that is thought to be of immature lymphoid origin, is the pathological hallmark and essential diagnostic criterion for Hodgkin's disease. Most patients with Hodgkin's disease have the types are currently designated 'nodular sclerosis' or 'mixed cellularity'. The nodular sclerosis type tends to occur more often in young women and at an earlier stage, but has a worse prognosis than the mixed cellularity subgroup, which occurs more commonly in men and causes more constitutional symptoms, but has a better prognosis.

Clinical Manifestations

1. Painless enlargement of the lymph nodes on one side of the neck. Individual nodes are firm and painless; common sites are the cervical, supraclavicular and mediastinal nodes.
2. Mediastinal lymph nodes may be visible on X-ray films and large enough to compress the trachea and cause dyspnea.
3. Pruritus is common and can be distressing; the cause is unknown. Herpes zoster infection is common.

4. Some patients experience brief, but severe pain after drinking alcohol, usually at the site of the tumor.
5. Symptoms may result from the tumor compressing other organs causing cough and pulmonary effusion (from pulmonary infiltrates), jaundice (from hepatic involvement or bile duct obstruction), abdominal pain (from splenomegaly or retroperitoneal adenopathy), or bone pain (from skeletal involvement).
6. Constitutional symptoms for prognostic purposes referred to as B symptoms, include fever (without chills), drenching sweats (particularly at night) and unintentional weight loss of more than 10% of body weight (found in 40% of patients and more common in advanced disease).
7. Mild anemia develops leukocyte count may be elevated or decreased, platelet count is typically normal, unless the tumor has invaded the bone marrow, suppressing hematopoiesis; impaired cellular immunity (evidenced by an absence of or decreased response to skin sensitivity tests such as candidal infection, mumps) may be noted.

Diagnostic Methods

1. Since many manifestations are similar to those occurring with infection, diagnostic studies are performed to rule out an infectious origin for the disease.
2. Diagnosis is made by means of an excisional lymph node biopsy and the finding of the Reed-Sternberg cell.
3. Assessment for any 'B symptoms,' physical examination to evaluate the lymph node chains as well as the size of the spleen and liver.
4. Chest X-ray and a computed tomography (CT) of the chest, abdomen and pelvis; positron emission tomography (PET) scans to identify residual disease.
5. Laboratory tests: CBC platelet count, erthrocyte sedimentation rate (ESR), and liver and renal function studies.
6. Bone marrow biopsy and sometimes bilateral biopsies.
7. Bone scans may be performed.

Medical Management

Treatment is determined by the stage of the disease instead of the histological type:

1. Chemotherapy followed by radiation therapy is used in early stage disease.
2. Combination chemotherapy with doxorubicin (Adriamycin), bleomycin (Blenoxane), vinblastine (Velban), and dacarbazine (DTIC), referred to as ABVD and is often considered the standard treatment for more advanced disease.
3. Chemotherapy is often successful in obtaining remission even when relapse occurs. Transplant is used for advanced or refractory disease.

Nursing Management

1. Address the potential development of a second malignancy with the patient when treatment decisions are made. It is also important to tell patients that Hodgkin's lymphoma is often curable.

2. Encourage patients to reduce other factors that increase the risk of developing second cancers such as use of tobacco and alcohol and exposure to environmental carcinogens and excessive sunlight.
3. Screen for late effects of treatment [e.g. immune dysfunction, herpes infections (zoster and varicella); pneumococcal sepsis].
4. Provide education about relevant self-care strategies and disease management.

Refer 'Nursing Management' under 'Cancer' for additional information about nursing interventions for patients undergoing chemotherapy and radiation treatments.

MULTIPLE MYELOMA

Multiple myeloma is a malignant disease of the most mature form of B lymphocyte, i.e. the plasma cell.

Pathophysiology

Plasma cells secrete immunoglobulins, proteins necessary for antibody production in fight infection. The malignant plasma cells produce an increased amount of specific immunoglobulin that is nonfunctional. Functional types of immunoglobulin are still produced by non-malignant plasma cells, but in lower than normal quantity. The median 5-year survival rate for newly diagnosed patients is 33%.

Clinical Manifestations

1. The classic presenting symptom of multiple myeloma is bone pain, usually in the back or ribs. Pain increases with movement and decreases with rest, patients report that they have less pain on awakening, but more during the day.
2. Severe bone destruction causing vertebral collapse and fractures, including spinal fractures, which can impinge on the spinal cord and result in spinal cord compression.
3. Hypercalcemia may develop and renal failure may also occur.
4. Anemia is a reduced number of leukocytes and platelets (late stage).
5. Neurological manifestations (e.g. spinal cord compression).
6. Hyperviscocity manifested by bleeding from the nose or mouth, headache, blurred vision, paresthesias or heart failure.

Diagnostic Methods

1. An elevated monoclonal protein spike in the serum (via serum protein electrophoresis) urine (via urine protein electrophoresis) or light chain (via serum free light chain analysis) is considered to be a major criterion in the diagnosis of multiple myeloma.
2. The diagnosis of myeloma is confirmed by bone marrow biopsy.

The incidence of multiple myeloma increases with age. The disease rarely occurs before age 40 years. Closely investigate any back pain, which is a common presenting complaint.

Medical Management

1. For those who are not candidates for transplant, chemotherapy.
2. Corticosteroids, particularly dexamethasone (Decadron) often combined with other agents [e.g. melphalan (Alkeran) thalidomide (Thalomid), lenalidomide (Revlimid) and bortezomib (Velcade)].
3. Radiation therapy in combination with systemic treatment such as chemotherapy.
4. Vertebroplasty often performed when lytic lesions result in vertebral compression fractures.
5. Some bisphosphonates such as pamidronate (Aredia) and zoledronic acid (Zometa) have been shown to strengthen bone in multiple myeloma by diminishing survival of osteoclasts.
6. Plasmapheresis when patients have signs and symptoms of hyperviscosity.
7. Narcotic analgesics, thalidomide and bortezomib for refractory disease and severe pain.
8. Administer medications as recommended for pain relief.
9. Carefully monitor for renal function and assess for gastritis.
10. Educated about activity restrictions (e.g. lifting no more than 10 lb, use of proper body mechanics), braces are occasionally needed to support the spinal column.
11. Teach patient to recognize and report signs and symptoms of hypercalcemia.
12. Observe for bacterial infections (pneumonia); instruct patient in appropriate infection prevention measures.
13. Maintain mobility and use strategies that enhance venous return (e.g. antiembolism stockings, avoid crossing the legs).

LYMPHEDEMA AND ELEPHANTIASIS

Lymphedema is classified as primary (congenital malformations) or secondary (acquired obstruction). Tissues in the extremities swell because of an increased quantity of lymph that result from an obstruction of the lymphatic vessels. It is specially marked when the extremity is in a dependent position. The most common type is congenital lymphedema (lymphedema praecox) caused by hypoplasia of the lymphatic system of the lower extremity. It is usually seen in women and appears first between the ages of 15 and 25 years. The obstruction may be in both the lymph nodes and the lymphatic vessels. At times, it is seen the arm after a radical mastectomy and in the leg in association with varicose veins or a chronic thrombophlebitis (from lymphagitis). Lymphatic obstruction caused by a parasite (filariasis) is seen frequently in the tropics. When chronic swelling is present, there may be frequent bouts of infection (high fever and chills) and increased residual edema after inflammation resolves. These lead to chronic fibrosis, thickening of the subcutaneous tissues and hypertrophy of the skin. The condition in which chronic swelling of the extremity recedes only slightly with elevation is referred to as elephantiasis.

Medical Management

1. Active and passive exercise to assist in moving lymphatic fluid into the bloodstream and also manual lymphatic drainage (a massage technique).

2. External compression devices; custom-fitted elastic stockings, when patient is ambulatory.
3. Strict bedrest with leg elevation to help mobilize fluids.
4. Manual lymphatic drainage in combination with compression bandages, exercises, skin care, pressure gradient sleeves and pneumatic pumps (depending on the severity and stage of the lymphedema).
5. Diuretic therapy, initially with furosemide (Lasix) to prevent fluid overload and other diuretic therapy palliatively for lymphedema.
6. Antibiotic therapy, if lymphangitis or cellulitis is present.

Surgical Management

Excision of the affected subcutaneous tissue and fascia with skin grafting to cover the defect or surgical relocation of superficial lymphatic vessels into the deep lymphatic system by means of buried flap to provide a conduit for lymphatic drainage.

Nursing Management

1. If the patient undergoes surgery, provide standard postsurgical care of skin grafts and flaps, elevate the affected extremity and observe for complications constantly (e.g. flap necrosis, hematoma or abscess under the flap, cellulitis).
2. Instruct patient or caregiver to inspect the dressing's daily unusual drainage or any inflammation around the wound margin should be reported to the surgeon.
3. Inform patient that there may be a loss of sensation in the skin graft area.
4. Instruct patient to avoid the application of heating pads of exposure to sun to prevent burns or trauma to the area.

14

Chapter Endocrinological Nursing

GROWTH HORMONE HYPERSECRETION

Excess secretion of growth hormone can be caused by pituitary hyperplasia, a benign pituitary tumor or excess of growth hormone-releasing hormone (GHRH) due to hypothalamic dysfunction. Sometimes, tumor in the other parts of the body secret ectopic growth hormone (GH) or GHRH.

ACROMEGALY

Acromegaly occurs on a result of over secretion of GH in an adult. Bones increase in size, leading the enlargement of facial features, hands and feet. Long bones grow width not in length. Subcutaneous tissue increases causing fleshy appearance. Internal organ and glands enlarge, and impaired glucose tolerance.

Clinical Manifestations

- First symptom noticed in a change in ring or shoe size
- The nose, jaw, brow, hands and feet enlarge
- Teeth may be displaced causing difficulty chewing
- Tongue become thick causing difficulty in speaking and swallowing (dysphagia)
- It may develop sleep apnea
- Vertebral changes leads to kyphosis
- Visual disturbances due to pressure of tumor on optic nerve
- Headaches due to pressure on brain
- Diabetes mellitus been GH increases blood sugar may increase workload on pancreases
- Osteoporosis or erectile dysfunction, amenorrhea.

Diagnostic Methods

- Serum GH levels
- Radiographs
- Blood glucose test.

Therapeutic Measures

- Treat the cause
- Hypophysectomy if required.

Nursing Management

1. Teach the patient and family about disease and treatment.
2. Nursing care of the patient undergoing hypophysectomy.

Medical Management

1. Surgical removal through a trans-sphenoidal approach is the treatment of choice.

2. Stereotactic radiation therapy is used to deliver the external beam radiation therapy to the tumor with minimal effect on normal tissue.
3. Conventional radiation therapy and the use of bromocriptine (dopamine agonist) and octreotide (somatostatin analogue) inhibit production or release of growth hormone.
4. Hypophysectomy is used to remove primary tumors surgically.

PITUITARY TUMORS

Pituitary tumors are of three principal types, representing an overgrowth of eosinophilic cells, basophilic cells (hyperadrenalism), or chromophobic cells (cells with no affinity for either eosinophilic or basophilic stains). They are usually benign.

Clinical Manifestations

Eosinophilic Tumors Developing Early in Life

1. Gigantism: Patient may be more than 7 feet tall and large in all proportions.
2. Patient is weak and lethargic, hardly able to stand.

Eosinophilic Tumors Developing in Adulthood

1. Acromegaly (excessive skeletal growth of the feet, hands, superciliary ridge, molar eminences, nose and chin).
2. Enlargement of every tissue and organ of the body.
3. Severe headaches and visual disturbances because the tumors exert pressure on the optic nerves.
4. Loss of color discrimination, diplopia (double vision) or blindness of a portion of the field of vision.
5. Decalcification of the skeleton, muscular weakness and endocrine disturbances, similar to those occurring in hyperthyroidism.

Basophilic Tumors

Cushing's syndrome, masculinization and amenorrhea in females, truncal obesity, hypertension, osteoporosis and polycythemia.

Chromophobic Tumors (90% of Pituitary Tumors)

Symptoms of hypopituitarism include the following:
1. Obesity and somnolence.
2. Fine, scanty hair, dry, soft skin, a pasty complexion and small bones.
3. Headaches, loss of libido and visual defects progressing to blindness.
4. Polyuria, polyphagia, lowering of the basal metabolic rate and subnormal body temperature.

Diagnostic Methods

- History and physical examination (visual field assessment)
- Computed tomography (CT) and magnetic resonance imaging (MRI)
- Serum levels of pituitary hormone.

Medical Management

Refer 'Nursing Management' described for 'Acromegaly'.

SYNDROME OF INAPPROPRIATE ANTIDIURETIC HORMONE SECRETION

The syndrome of inappropriate antidiuretic hormone (SIADH) secretion refers to excessive antidiuretic hormone (ADH) secretion from the pituitary gland even in the face of subnormal serum osmolality. Patients with this disorder cannot excrete dilute urine. They retain fluids and develop sodium deficiency (dilution hyponatremia). SIADH is often of non-endocrine origin. The syndrome may occur in patients with bronchogenic carcinoma (malignant lung cells synthesize and release ADH). Other causes include severe pneumonia, pneumothorax, other disorders of lungs and malignant tumors that affect other organs. Disorders of the central nervous system (head injury, brain surgery or tumor or infection) are thought to produce SIADH by direct stimulation of the pituitary gland. Some medications (vincristine, diuretics, phenothiazines, tricyclic antidepressants) and nicotine have been implicated in SIADH.

Medical Management

The SIADH is generally managed by eliminating the underlying cause if possible and restricting fluid intake. Diuretics are used with fluid restriction to treat severe hyponatremia.

Nursing Management

1. Monitor fluid intake and output, daily weight, urine and blood chemistries, and neurological status.
2. Provide supportive measures and explanations of procedures and treatments to assist patient to deal with this disorder.

ACUTE AND SUBACUTE THYROIDITIS

Thyroiditis (inflammation of the thyroid) can be acute, subacute or chronic. Each type is characterized by inflammation, fibrosis or lymphocytic infiltration of the thyroid gland. Acute thyroiditis is a rare disorder caused by infection of the thyroid gland. The causes are bacteria (*Staphylococcus aureus* most common), fungi, mycobacteria or parasites. Subacute cases may be granulomatous thyroiditis (de Quervain's thyroiditis) or painless thyroiditis (silent thyroiditis or subacute lymphocytic thyroiditis). This form often occurs in the postpartum period and is thought to be a reaction.

Clinical Manifestations

Acute Thyroiditis

- Anterior neck pain and swelling, fever, dysphagia and dysphonia
- Pharyngitis or pharyngeal pain
- Warmth, erythema and tenderness of the thyroid gland.

Subacute Thyroiditis

1. Myalgias, pharyngitis, low-grade fever and fatigue, which progress to a painful swelling in the anterior neck that lasts 1–2 months and then disappears spontaneously without residual effect.

2. Thyroid enlarges symmetrically and may be painful.
3. Overlying skin is often reddened and warm.
4. Swallowing may be difficult and uncomfortable.
5. Symptoms such as irritability, nervousness, insomnia and weight loss (manifestations of hyperthyroidism) are common.
6. Chills and fever may occur.
7. Painless thyroiditis are caused due to the symptoms of hyperthyroidism or hypothyroidism are possible.

Management

Acute Thyroiditis

1. Antimicrobial agents and fluid replacement.
2. Surgical incision and drainage if abscess is present.

Subacute Thyroiditis

1. Control of inflammation; non-steroidal anti-inflammatory drugs (NSAIDs) to relieve neck pain.
2. Beta-blocking agents to control symptoms of hyperthyroidism.
3. Oral corticosteroids to relieve pain and reduce swelling; do not usually affect the underlying cause.
4. Follow-up monitoring.
5. Painless thyroiditis: Treatment is directed at symptoms and yearly follow-up is recommended to determine the patient's need for treatment of subsequent hypothyroidism.

CHRONIC THYROIDITIS (HASHIMOTO'S THYROIDITIS)

Chronic thyroiditis occurs most frequently in women aged 30–50 years and is termed Hashimoto's disease or chronic lymphocytic thyroiditis. Diagnosis is based on the histological appearance of the inflamed gland. The chronic forms are usually not accompanied by pain, pressure symptoms or fever, and thyroid activity is usually normal or low. Cell-mediated immunity may play a significant role in the pathogenesis of chronic thyroiditis. A genetic predisposition also appears to be significant in its etiology. If untreated, the disease slowly progresses to hypothyroidism.

Management

Objectives of treatment are to reduce the size of the thyroid gland and to prevent hypothyroidism:

1. Thyroid hormone therapy is prescribed to reduce thyroid activity and production of thyroglobulin.
2. Thyroid hormones are given when the hypothyroid symptoms are present.
3. Surgery is performed when pressure symptoms persist.

THYROID STORM (THYROTOXIC CRISIS)

Thyroid storm (thyrotoxic crisis) is a form of severe hyperthyroidism, usually of abrupt onset and characterized by high fever (hyperpyrexia), extreme tachycardia and altered mental state, frequently appears as delirium. Thyroid storm is a life-threatening condition that is usually precipitated by stress, such as injury, infection, surgery, tooth extraction, insulin reaction, diabetic ketoacidosis, pregnancy, digitalis intoxication, abrupt withdrawal of antithyroid drugs, extreme emotional stress or vigorous palpation of the thyroid. These factors precipitate thyroid storm in the partially controlled or completely untreated patient with hyperthyroidism. Untreated thyroid storm is almost always fatal, but with proper treatment the mortality rate can be reduced substantially.

Clinical Manifestations

1. High fever (hyperpyrexia) above 38.5°C (101.3°F).
2. Extreme tachycardia (more than 130 beats/min).
3. Exaggerated symptoms of hyperthyroidism with disturbances of a major system, such as gastrointestinal (weight loss, diarrhea, abdominal pain) or cardiovascular (edema, chest pain, dyspnea, palpitations).
4. Altered neurological or mental state, which frequently appears as delirium psychosis, somnolence or coma.

Medical Management

Immediate objectives are to reduce body temperature and heart rate and prevent vascular collapse:

1. A hypothermia mattress or blanket, ice packs, cool environment, hydrocortisone, and acetaminophen (Tylenol).
2. Humidified oxygen is administered to improve tissue oxygenation and meet high metabolic demands, and respiratory status is monitored by arterial blood gas analysis or pulse oximetry.
3. Intravenous fluids containing dextrose are administered to replace glycogen stores.
4. Hydrocortisone is given to treat shock or adrenal insufficiency.
5. Propylthiouracil (PTU) or methimazole is given to impede formation of thyroid hormone.
6. Hydrocortisone to treat shock or adrenal insufficiency.
7. Iodine is administered to decrease output of thyroxine (T4) from thyroid gland.
8. Sympatholytic agents are given for cardiac problems. Propranolol, combined with digitalis has been effective in reducing cardiac symptoms.

Note: Salicylates are not used in the management of thyroid storm because they displace thyroid hormone from binding proteins and worsen the hypermetabolism.

Nursing Management

Observe patient carefully and provide aggressive, and supportive nursing care during and after acute stage of illness. Care provided for the patient with hyperthyroidism is the basis for nursing management of patients with thyroid storm.

CANCER OF THE THYROID

Cancer of the thyroid is less prevalent than other forms of cancer. The most common type, papillary adenocarcinoma accounts for more than half of thyroid malignancies; it starts in childhood or early adult life, remains localized and eventually metastasizes. When papillary adenocarcinoma occurs in an elderly patient, it is more aggressive. Risk factors include female gender and external irradiation of the head, neck or chest in infancy and childhood. Other types of thyroid cancer include follicular adenocarcinoma, medullary, anaplastic and thyroid lymphoma.

Clinical Manifestations

Lesions that are single, hard and fixed on palpation or associated with cervical lymphadenopathy suggest malignancy.

Diagnostic Methods

- Needle biopsy or aspiration biopsy of thyroid gland
- Thyroid function tests
- Ultrasound, MRI, CT, thyroid scans, radioactive iodine uptake studies and thyroid suppression tests.

Medical Management

1. Treatment of choice is surgical removal (total or near-total thyroidectomy).
2. Modified or extensive radical neck dissection is done if lymph nodes are involved.
3. Radioactive iodine is used to eradicate residual thyroid tissue.
4. Thyroid hormone is administered in suppressive doses after surgery to lower the levels of thyroid-stimulating hormone (TSH) to a euthyroid state.
5. Lifelong thyroxine is required, if remaining thyroid tissue is inadequate to produce sufficient hormone.
6. Radiation therapy is administered by several routes.
7. Chemotherapy is used only occasionally.

Nursing Management

Refer 'Nursing Management' described for 'Cancer' for additional information:

1. Inform the patient about the purpose of any preoperative tests and explain what preoperative preparations to except; teaching includes demonstrating to the patient how to support the neck with the hands after surgery to prevent stress on the incision.
2. Provide postoperative care (e.g. assess and reinforce surgical dressings, observe for bleeding, monitor pulse and blood pressure for signs of internal bleeding, assess respiratory status, assess intensity of pain and administer analgesics as prescribed).
3. Monitor and observe for potential complications such as hemorrhage, hematoma formation, edema of the glottis and injury to recurrent laryngeal nerve.
4. Teach patient and family about signs and symptoms of possible complications and those that should be reported; suggest strategies for managing postoperative pain at home and for increasing humidification.
5. Explains to the patient and family the need for rest, relaxation and nutrition, patient can resume former activities and responsibilities once recovered from surgery.
6. Refer for home care, if indicated.

HYPERTHYROIDISM (GRAVES' DISEASE)

Hyperthyroidism is the second most common endocrine disorder, and Graves' disease is the most common type. It results from an excessive output of thyroid hormones due to abnormal stimulation of the thyroid gland by circulating immunoglobulins. The disorder affects women eight times more frequently than men and peaks between the second and fourth decades of life. It may appear after an emotional shock, stress or infection, but the exact significance of these relationships is not understood. Other common causes include thyroiditis and excessive ingestion of thyroid hormone (e.g. from the treatment of hypothyroidism).

Clinical Manifestations

Hyperthyroidism presents a characteristic group of signs and symptoms (thyrotoxicosis):

1. Nervousness (emotionally hyperexcitable), irritability apprehensiveness; inability to sit quietly; palpitations; rapid pulse on rest and exertion.
2. Poor tolerance of heat; excessive perspiration; skin that is flushed, with a characteristic salmon color, and likely to be warm, soft and moist.
3. Dry skin and diffuse pruritus.
4. Fine tremor of the hands.
5. Exophthalmos (bulging eyes) in some patients.
6. Increased appetite and dietary intake, progressive loss of weight, abnormal muscle fatigability, weakness, amenorrhea and changes in bowel function (constipation or diarrhea).
7. Pulse range between 90–160 beats per minute; systolic (but not diastolic) blood pressure elevation (increased pulse pressure).
8. Atrial fibrillation; cardiac decompensation in the form of congestive HF, especially in the elderly.
9. Osteoporosis and fracture.
10. Cardiac effects may include sinus tachycardia or dysrhythmias, increased pulse pressure and palpitations; myocardial hypertrophy and HF may occur if the hyperthyroidism is severe and untreated.
11. May include remissions and exacerbations, terminating with spontaneous recovery in a few months or years.
12. May progress relentlessly, causing emaciation, intense nervousness, delirium, disorientation and eventually HF.
13. Thyroid gland is enlarged; it is soft and may pulsate; a thrill may be felt and bruit heard over thyroid arteries.
14. Laboratory tests show a decrease in serum TSH, increased free T4 and an increase in radioactive iodine uptake.

Elderly patients commonly present with vague and non-specific signs and symptoms. The only presenting manifestations may be anorexia and weight loss, absence of ocular signs or isolated atrial fibrillation (new or worsening HF or angina is more likely to occur in elderly than in younger patients). These signs and symptoms may mask the underlying thyroid disease. Spontaneous remission of hyperthyroidism is rare in the elderly. Measurement of TSH uptake is indicated in elderly patients with unexplained physical or mental deterioration. Use of radioactive iodine is generally recommended for treatment of thyrotoxicosis rather than surgery unless an enlarged thyroid gland in pressing on the airway. Thyrotoxicosis must be radiation may precipitate thyroid storm, which has a mortality rate of 10% in the elderly. The β-adrenergic blocking agents may be indicated. Use these agents with extreme caution and monitor closely for granulocytopenia. Modify dosages of other medications because of the altered rate of metabolism in hyperthyroidism.

Medical Management

Treatment is directed toward reducing thyroid hyperactivity to relieve symptoms and prevents complications. Different forms of treatment available are:

- Radioactive iodine therapy for destructive effects on the thyroid gland
- Antithyroid medications
- Surgery
- Adjunctive therapy.

Radioactive Iodine

1. Radioactive iodine (^{131}I) is given to destroy the overactive thyroid cells (most common treatment in elderly).
2. The ^{131}I is contraindicated in pregnancy and nursing mothers because radioiodine crosses the placenta and is secreted in breast milk.

Antithyroid Medications

1. The objective of pharmacotherapy is to inhibit hormone synthesis or release and reduce the amount of thyroid tissue.
2. The most commonly used medications are propylthiouracil (Propacil, PTU) and methimazole (Tapazole) until patient is euthyroid.
3. Maintenance dose is established, followed by gradual withdrawal of the medication over the next several months.
4. Antithyroid drugs are contraindicated in late pregnancy because of a risk for goiter and cretinism in the fetus.
5. Thyroid hormone may be administered to put the thyroid to rest.

Adjunctive Therapy

1. Potassium iodine, Lugol's solution and saturated solution of potassium iodide (SSKI) may be added.
2. Beta-adrenergic agents may be used to control the sympathetic nervous system effects that occur in hyperthyroidism; for example, propranolol is used for nervousness, tachycardia, tremor, anxiety and heat tolerance.

Surgical Interventions

1. Surgical intervention (reserved for special circumstances) removes about five sixths of the thyroid tissue.
2. Surgery to treat hyperthyroidism is preformed after thyroid function is returned to normal (4–6 week).
3. Before surgery, patient is given propylthiouracil until signs of hyperthyroidism have disappeared.
4. Iodine is prescribed to reduce thyroid size and vascularity and blood loss. Patient is monitored carefully for evidence.
5. Risk for relapse and complications necessities long-term follow-up of patient undergoing treatment of hyperthyroidism.

Nursing Management

Assessment

1. Obtain a health history, including family history of hyperthyroidism, and note of irritability or increased emotional reaction and the impact of these changes on patient's interaction with family, friends and co-workers.
2. Assess stressors and patient's ability to cope with stress.
3. Evaluate nutritional status and presence of symptoms; note excessive nervousness and changes in vision and appearance of eyes.
4. Assess and monitor cardiac status periodically (heart rate, blood pressure, heart sounds and peripheral pulses).
5. Assess emotional state and psychological status.

Nursing Diagnoses/Problems

1. Imbalanced nutrition: Less than body requirement related to exaggerated metabolic rate, excessive appetite and increased gastrointestinal activity.
2. Ineffective coping related to irritability, hyperexcitability, apprehension and emotional instability.
3. Low self-esteem related to changes in appearance, excessive appetite and weight loss.
4. Altered body temperature.

Potential complications: They are:
- Thyrotoxicosis or thyroid storm
- Hypothyroidism.

Planning (Goals and Objective)

Goals of the patient may be improved nutritional status, improved coping ability, improved self-esteem, maintenance of normal body temperature and absence of complications.

Nursing Interventions/Implementation

Improving Nutritional Status

1. Provide several small, well-balanced meals (up to six meals a day) to satisfy patient's increased appetite.
2. Replace food and fluids lost through diarrhea and diaphoresis and control diarrhea that results from increased peristalsis.
3. Reduce diarrhea by avoiding highly seasoned foods and stimulants such as coffee, tea, cola and alcohol; encourage high-calorie, high-protein foods.
4. Provide quite atmosphere during mealtime to aid digestion.
5. Record weight and dietary intake daily.

Enhancing Coping Measures

1. Reassure the patient that the emotional reactions being experienced are a result of the disorder and that with effective treatment those symptoms will be controlled.
2. Reassure family and friends that symptoms are expected to disappear with treatment.

3. Maintain a calm, unhurried approach and minimize stressful experiences.
4. Keep the environment quiet and uncluttered.
5. Provide information regarding thyroidectomy and preparatory pharmacotherapy to alleviate anxiety.
6. Assist patient to take medications as prescribed and encourage adherence to the therapeutic regimen.
7. Repeat information often and provide written instructions as indicated due to short attention span.

Improving Self-esteem

1. Convey to patient an understanding of concerns regarding problems with appearance, appetite and weight, and assist in developing coping strategies.
2. Provide eye protection if patient experiences eye changes secondary to hyperthyroidism; instruct regarding correct instillation of eye drops or ointment to soothe the eyes and protect the exposed cornea. Discourage smoking.
3. Make arrangements for the patient to eat alone, if desired and if embarrassed by the large meals consumed.

Maintaining Normal Body Temperature

1. Provide a cool, comfortable environment and fresh bedding and gown as needed.
2. Give cool baths and provide cool fluids; monitor body temperature.

Managing Potential Complications

1. Monitor closely for signs and symptoms indicative of thyroid storm.
2. Assess cardiac and respiratory function; vital signs, cardiac output, ECG monitoring, arterial blood gases (ABGs), pulse oximetry.
3. Administer oxygen to prevent hypoxia, to improve tissue oxygenation and to meet the high metabolic demands.
4. Give intravenous (IV) fluids to maintain blood glucose levels and replace lost fluids.
5. Administer antithyroid medications to reduce the thyroid hormone levels.
6. Administer propranolol and digitalis to treat cardiac symptoms.
7. Implement strategies to treat shock if needed.
8. Monitor for hyperthyroidism; encourage continued therapy.
9. Instruct patient and family about the importance of continuing therapy indefinitely after discharge and about the consequences of failing to take medications.

Promoting Family-based Care and Follow-up

1. Instruct how and when to take prescribed medications.
2. Teach patient how the medication regimen fits in with the broader therapeutic plan.
3. Provide an individualized written plan of care for use at home.
4. Teach patient and family about the desired effects and side effects of medications.
5. Instruct patient and family about which adverse effects should be reported to physician.

6. Teach patient about what to expect from thyroidectomy if this is to be performed.
7. Teach patient to avoid situations that have the potential of stimulating thyroid storm.
8. Refer to home care for assessment of the home and family environment.
9. Stress long-term follow-up care because of the possibility of hypothyroidism after thyroidectomy or treatment with antithyroid drugs or radioactive iodine.
10. Assess for changes indicating return to normal thyroid function; assess for physical signs of hyperthyroidism and hypothyroidism.
11. Remind the patient and family about the importance of health promotion activities and recommended health screening.

Evaluations

Evaluation is based on the objectives/expected patient outcomes:

1. Shows improved nutritional status.
2. Demonstrates effective coping methods in dealing with family, friends and co-workers.
3. Achieves increased self-esteem.
4. Maintains normal body temperature.
5. Displays absence of complications.

HYPOTHYROIDISM AND MYXEDEMA

Hypothyroidism results from suboptimal levels of thyroid hormone. Refers to dysfunction of the thyroid gland (more than 95% of cases); central, due to failure of the pituitary gland, hypothalamus or both; secondary or pituitary, which is due entirely to a pituitary disorder; and hypothalamic or tertiary, due to a disorder of the hypothalamus resulting in inadequate secretion of TSH from decreased stimulation by thyrotropin-releasing hormone (TRH). Hypothyroidism occurs most often in older women. Its causes include autoimmune thyroiditis (Hashimoto's thyroiditis, most common type in adults); therapy for hyperthyroidism (radioiodine, surgery or antithyroid drugs); radiation therapy for head and neck cancer; infiltrative diseases of the thyroid (amyloidosis and scleroderma); iodine deficiency; and iodine excess. When thyroid deficiency is present at birth, the condition is known as cretinism.

'Myxedema' is the term, which refers to the accumulation of mucopolysaccharide in the subcutaneous and other interstitial tissue and it is used only to describe the extreme symptoms of severe hypothyroidism.

Clinical Manifestations

1. Extreme fatigue.
2. Hair loss, brittle nails, dry skin, and numbness and tingling of fingers.
3. Husky voice and hoarseness.
4. Menstrual disturbances (e.g. menorrhagia or amenorrhea); loss of libido.
5. Severe hypothyroidism: Subnormal temperature and pulse rate; weight gain without corresponding increase in food intake; cachexia.

6. Thickened skin, thinning hair or alopecia; expressionless and mask-like facial features.
7. Sensation of cold in a warm environment.
8. Subdued emotional responses as the condition progresses; dulled mental processes and apathy.
9. Slowed speech; enlarged tongue, hands and feet; constipation; possibly deafness.
10. Advanced hypothyroidism; personality and cognitive changes, pleural effusion, pericardial effusion and respirate.
11. Hypothermia: Abnormal sensitivity to sedatives, opiates and anesthetic agents (these drugs are given with extreme caution).
12. Severe hypothyroidism: Elevated serum cholesterol level atherosclerosis, coronary artery disease and poor left ventricular function.
13. Myxedema coma (rare).

The higher prevalence of hypothyroidism in the elderly population may be related to alternations in immune function with age. Depression, apathy or decreased mobility or activity may be the major initial symptom. In all patients with hypothyroidism, the effect of analgesic agents, sedatives and anesthetic agents are prolonged; special caution is necessary in administering these agents to elderly patients because of concurrent changes in liver and renal function. Thyroid hormone replacement must be started with low doses and gradually increased to prevent serious cardiovascular and neurological side effects, such as angina. Regular testing of serum TSH is recommended for people older than 60 years. Myxedema and myxedema coma generally occur in patients older than 50 years.

Medical Management

The primary objective is to restore a normal metabolic state by replacing thyroid hormone. Additional treatment in severe hypothyroidism consists of maintaining vital functions, monitoring ABG values and administering fluids cautiously because of the danger of water intoxication, which includes:

1. Synthetic levothyroxine (Synthroid or Levothroid) is the preferred preparation.
2. External heat application is avoided because it increases oxygen requirements and may lead to vascular collapse.
3. Concentrated glucose may be given if hypoglycemia is evident.
4. If myxedema coma is present, thyroid hormone is given intravenously until consciousness is restored.

Interaction of Thyroid Hormones with Other Drugs

1. Thyroid hormones increase blood glucose levels, which may necessitate adjustment in doses of insulin or oral hypoglycemic agents.
2. Thyroid hormone many increase the pharmacological effect of digitalis, glycosides, anticoagulants and indomethacin, requiring careful observation and assessment for side effects of these drugs.
3. The effects of thyroid hormone may be increased by phenytoin and tricyclic antidepressants.

Patient with unrecognized hypothyroidism undergoing surgery are at increased risk for intraoperative hypotension, postoperative congestive HF and altered mental status. Myocardial ischemia or infarction may occur in response to therapy in patients with severe, long-standing hypothyroidism or myxedema coma. Be alert for signs of angina, especially during the early phase of treatment and discontinue administration of thyroid hormone immediately if symptoms occur.

Nursing Management

Promoting Family-based Care and Follow-up

Oral and written instructions should be provided regarding the following:

1. Desired actions and side effects of medications.
2. Correct medications administration.
3. Importance of continuing to take the medications as prescribed even after symptoms improve.
4. When to seek medical attention.
5. Importance of nutrition and diet to promote weight loss and normal bowel patterns.

The patient and family should be informed that many of the symptoms observed during the course of the disorder will disappear with effective treatment:

1. Monitor the patient's recovery and ability to cope with the recent changes, along with patient's physical and cognitive status, and the patient's and family's understanding of the instructions provided before hospital discharge.
2. Document and report to the patient's primary healthcare provider subtle signs and symptoms that may indicate either inadequate or excessive thyroid hormone.

HYPOPARATHYROIDISM

The most common cause of hypoparathyroidism is inadequate secretion of parathyroid hormone after interruption of the blood supply or surgical removal of parathyroid gland tissue during thyroidectomy, parathyroidectomy or radical neck dissection. Atrophy of the parathyroid glands of unknown etiology is a less common cause. Symptoms are due to deficiency of parathormone that results in an elevation of blood phosphate (hyperphosphatemia) and decrease in blood calcium (hypocalcemia) levels.

Clinical Manifestations

1. Tetany is the chief symptom.
2. Latent tetany; numbness, tingling and cramps in the extremities; stiffness in the hands and feet.
3. Overt tetany; bronchospasm, laryngeal spasm, carpopedal spasm, dysphagia, photophobia, cardiac dysrhythmias and seizures.
4. Other symptoms: anxiety, irritability, depression and delirium. ECG changes and hypotension may also occur.

Diagnostic Findings

1. Latent tetany is suggested by a positive Trousseau's sign or a positive Chvostek's sign [tetany noted with serum calcium 5–6 mg/dL (1.2–1/5 mmol/L) or lower].
2. Diagnosis is difficult because of vague symptoms; laboratory studies show increased serum phosphate; X-rays of bone show

increased density and calcification of the subcutaneous or paraspinal basal ganglia of the brain.

Medical Management

1. Serum calcium level is raised to 9–10 mg/dL (2.2–2.5 mmol/L).
2. When hypocalcemia and tetany occur after thyroidectomy, IV calcium glauconite is given immediately. Sedatives (pentobarbital) may be administered. Parenteral parathormone may be given, watching for an allergic reaction and changes in serum calcium levels.
3. Neuromuscular irritability is reduced by providing an environment that is free of noise, drafts, bright lights or sudden movements.
4. Tracheostomy or mechanical ventilation and bronchodilating medications may become necessary, if the patient develops respiratory distress.
5. Chronic hypoparathyroidism is treated with a diet high in calcium and low in phosphorus. Patient should avoid milk, products, egg yolk and spinach.
6. Oral calcium tablets and vitamin D preparations and aluminum hydroxide or aluminum carbonate may be given.

Nursing Management

1. Detecting early signs of hypocalcemia and anticipate signs of tetany, seizures and respiratory difficulties.
2. Keep calcium gluconate at the bedside; if patient has a cardiac disorder, is subject to dysrhythmias or is receiving digitalis the calcium gluconate is administered slowly and cautiously.
3. Provide continuous cardiac monitoring and careful assessment; calcium and digitalis increase systolic contraction and also potentiate each other; this can produce potentially fatal dysrhythmias.
4. Teach patient about medications and diet therapy, the reason for high calcium and low phosphate intake, and the symptoms of hypocalcemia and hypercalcemia.
5. Direct patient to contact physician if symptoms occur.

HYPOPITUITARISM

Hypopituitarism a hypofunction of the pituitary gland can result from disease of the pituitary gland itself or disease of the hypothalamus; the result is essentially the same. Hypopituitarism also may result from destruction of the anterior lobe of the pituitary gland and from radiation therapy to the head and neck area. The total destruction of the pituitary gland by trauma, tumor or vascular lesions removes all stimuli that are normally received by the thyroid, the gonads and the adrenal glands. The results in extreme weight loss, emaciation, atrophy of all endocrine glands and organs, hair loss, impotence, amenorrhea, hypometabolism and hypoglycemia. Coma and death occur if the missing hormones are not replaced.

CUSHING'S SYNDROME

Cushing's syndrome result from excessive, rather than deficient, adrenocortical activity. It is commonly caused by use of corticosteroid medications and is frequently the result of excessive corticosteroid production secondary to hyperplasia of the adrenal cortex. It may be caused by several mechanisms, including a tumor of the pituitary gland or less commonly an ectopic malignancy that produces adrenocorticotropic hormone (ACTH). Regardless of the cause, the normal feedback mechanisms that control the function of the adrenal cortex becomes ineffective, resulting in oversecretion of glucocorticoids, androgens and possibly mineralocorticoid. Cushing's syndrome occurs five times more often in women ages 20–40 years than in men.

Clinical Manifestations

1. Arrested growth, weight gain and obesity, musculoskeletal changes and glucose intolerance.
2. Classic features: Central type obesity, with a fatty 'buffalo hump', in the neck and supraclavicular areas, a heavy trunk and relatively thin extremities; skin is thin, fragile, easily traumatized with ecchymoses and striae.
3. Weakness and lassitude; sleep is disturbed because of altered diurnal secretion of cortisol.
4. Excessive protein catabolism with muscle wasting and osteoporosis; kyphosis, backache and compression fraction of the vertebrae are possible.
5. Retention of sodium and water, producing hypertension and heart failure.
6. 'Moon-faced' appearance, oiliness of skin and acne.
7. Increased susceptibility to infections slow healing of minor cuts and bruises.
8. Hyperglycemia or over diabetes.
9. Virilization in females (due to excess androgens) with appearance of masculine traits and recession of feminine traits (e.g. excessive hair on face, breasts, atrophy, menses cease, clitoris enlarges and voice deepens); libido is lost in males and females.
10. Changes occur in mood and mental activity; psychosis may develop and distress, and depression are common.
11. If Cushing's syndrome is the result of a pituitary tumor, visual disturbance is possible because of pressure on the optic chiasm.

Diagnostic Methods

1. Overnight dexamethasone suppression test to measure plasma cortisol level (stress, obesity, depression and medications may falsely elevate results).
2. Laboratory studies (e.g. serum sodium, blood glucose, serum potassium, plasma, urinary); 24-hour urinary free cortisol level.
3. Ultrasound, CT or MRI may localize adrenal tissue and detect adrenal tumors.

Medical Management

Treatment is usually directed at the pituitary gland because most cases are due to pituitary tumors rather than tumors of the adrenal cortex:

1. Surgical removal of the tumor by trans-sphenoidal hypophysectomy is the treatment of choice (80% success rate).
2. Radiation of the pituitary gland is successful, but takes several months for symptom control.
3. Adrenalectomy is performed in patients with primary adrenal hypertrophy.

4. Postoperatively, temporary replacement therapy with hydrocortisone may be necessary until the adrenal glands begin to respond normally (may be several months).
5. If bilateral adrenalectomy was performed, lifetime replacement of adrenal cortex hormones is necessary.
6. Adrenal enzyme inhibitors (e.g. metyrapone, aminoglutethimide, mitotane, ketoconazole) may be used with ectopic ACTH-secreting tumors that cannot be totally removed; monitor closely for inadequate adrenal function and side effects.
7. If Cushing's syndrome results from exogenous corticosteroids, taper the drug to the minimum level or use alternate-day therapy to treat the underlying disease.

Nursing Management

Assessment

1. Focus on the effects on the body of high concentrations of adrenal cortex hormones.
2. Assess patient's level of activity and ability to carry out routine and self-care activities.
3. Observe for skin for trauma, infection, breakdown, bruising and edema.
4. Note changes in appearance and patient's responses to these changes; family is good source of information about patient's emotional status and changes in appearance.
5. Assess patient's mental function, including mood, response to questions, depression and awareness of environment.

Nursing Diagnoses/Problems

1. Risk for injury related to weakness.
2. Risk for infection related to altered protein metabolism and inflammatory response.
3. Self-care deficits related to weakness, fatigue, muscle wasting and altered sleep patterns.
4. Impaired skin integrity related to edema, impaired bleeding.
5. Disturbed body image related to altered appearance impaired sexual functioning and decreased activity level.
6. Disturbed thought processes related to mood swings, irritability and depression.

Potential complications: They are:

- Addisonian crisis
- Adverse effects on adrenocortical activity.

Planning (Goals and Objectives)

Major goals include decreased risk of injury, decreased risk of infection, increased ability to carry out self-care activities improved skin integrity, improved body image, improved mental function and absence of complications.

Nursing Interventions/Implementation

Decreased Risk of Injury

1. Provide a protective environment to prevent falls, fractures, and other injuries to bones and soft tissues.

2. Assist the patient who is weak in ambulating to prevent falls or colliding into furniture.
3. Recommend foods high in protein, calcium, and vitamin D to minimize muscle wasting and osteoporosis; refer to dietitian for assistance.

Decreased Risk of Infection

1. Avoid unnecessary exposure to people with infections.
2. Assess frequently for subtle signs of infections (corticosteroids mask signs of inflammation and infection).

Preparing Patient for Surgery

Monitor blood glucose levels, and assess stools for blood because diabetes mellitus and peptic ulcer are common problems (refer also 'Preoperative Preparation' under 'Preoperative and Postoperative Nursing Management' in Chapter 6).

Encouraging Rest and Activity

Encourage moderate activity to prevent complications of immobility and promote self-esteem. Plan rest periods throughout the day and promote a relaxing, quiet environment for rest and sleep.

Promoting Skin Integrity

1. Use meticulous skin care to avoid traumatizing fragile skin.
2. Avoid adhesive tape, which can teat and irritate the skin.
3. Assess skin and bony prominences frequently.
4. Encourage and assist patient to change positions frequently.

Improving Body Image

1. Discuss the impact that changes have had on patient's self-concept and relationships with others. Major physical changes will disappear in time if the cause of Cushing's syndrome can be treated.
2. Weight gain and edema may be modified by a low-carbohydrate and low-sodium diet; a high protein intake can reduce some bothersome symptoms.

Improving Thought Processes

1. Explain to patient and family the cause of emotional instability, and help them cope with mood swings, irritability and depression.
2. Report any psychotic behavior.
3. Encourage patient and family members to verbalize feelings and concerns.

Managing Complications

1. Adrenal hypofunction and addisonian crisis: Monitor for hypotension; rapid, weak pulse; rapid respiratory rate; pallor; and extreme weakness. Note factors that may have led to crisis (e.g. stress, trauma, surgery).

2. Administer IV fluids and electrolytes and corticosteroids before, during and after surgery or treatment as indicated.
3. Monitor for circulatory collapse and shock present in addisonian crisis; treat promptly.
4. Assess fluid and electrolyte status by monitoring laboratory values and daily weight.
5. Monitor blood glucose level and report elevations to physician.

Teaching Patients Self-care

1. Present information about Cushing's syndrome verbally and in writing to patient and family.
2. If indicated, stress to patient and family that stopping corticosteroid use abruptly and without medical supervision can result in adrenal insufficiency and reappearance of symptoms.
3. Emphasize the need to keep an adequate supply of the corticosteroid to prevent running out to skipped dose this could result in addisonian crisis.
4. Stress need for dietary modifications to ensure adequate calcium intake without increasing risk for hypertension, hyperglycemia and weight gain.
5. Teach patient and family to monitor blood pressure, blood glucose levels and weight.
6. Stress the importance of wearing a medical alert bracelet and notifying other health professionals (e.g. dentist) that he/she has Cushing's syndrome.
7. Refer for home care as indicated to ensure safe environment with minimal stress and risk for falls, and other side effects.
8. Emphasize importance of regular medical follow-up and ensure patient is aware of side and toxic effects of medications.

Evaluations/Expected Patient Outcomes

- Has decreased risk of injury
- Has decreased risk of infection
- Increases participation in self-care activities
- Attains or maintains skin integrity
- Achieves improved body image
- Exhibits improved mental functioning
- Experiences no complications.

ADDISON'S DISEASE (ADRENOCORTICAL INSUFFICIENCY)

Addison's disease occurs when the adrenal cortex function is inadequate to meet the patient's need for cortical hormones. Autoimmune for idiopathic atrophy of the adrenal glands is responsible for the vast majority of cases. Other causes include surgical removal of both adrenal glands. Inadequate secretion of ACTH form the primary pituitary gland also results in adrenal insufficiency. Therapeutic use of corticosteroids is the most common cause of adrenocortical insufficiency. Symptoms may also result from sudden cessation of exogenous adrenocortical hormonal therapy, which interferes with normal feedback mechanisms.

Clinical Manifestations

Chief clinical manifestations include muscle weakness, anorexia, gastrointestinal (GI) symptoms, fatigue, emaciation, dark pigmentation of the skin and mucous membranes, hypotension, low blood glucose, low serum sodium and high serum potassium. The onset usually occurs with non-specific symptoms. Mental changes (depression, emotional liability, apathy, and confusion) are present in 60%–80% of patients. In severe cases, disturbance, of sodium and potassium metabolism may be marked by depletion of sodium and water, and severe chronic dehydration.

Addisonian Crisis

The medical emergency develops as the disease progresses. Signs and symptoms include the following:

1. Cyanosis and classic signs of circulatory shock; pallor, apprehension, rapid and weak pulse, rapid respirations and low blood pressure.
2. Headache, nausea, abdominal pain, diarrhea, confusion and restlessness.
3. Slight overexertion, exposure to cold, acute infections or a decrease in salt intake may lead to circulatory collapse, shock and death.
4. Stress of surgery or dehydration from preparation for diagnostic tests or surgery may precipitate addisonian or hypotensive crisis.

Diagnostic Findings

Greatly increased plasma ACTH (more than 22.0 pmol/L); serum cortisol level lower than normal (less than 165 nmol/L) or in low-normal range; decreased blood glucose (hypoglycemia) and sodium (hyponatremia) levels, increased serum potassium concentration (hyperkalemia) and increased WBC count (leukocytosis).

Medical Management

Immediate treatment is directed toward combating circulatory shock:

1. Restore blood circulating, administer fluids and corticosteroids, monitor vital signs, and place patient in a recumbent position with legs elevated.
2. Administer IV hydrocortisone, followed by 5% dextrose in normal saline.
3. Vasopressor amines may be required if hypotension persists.
4. Antibiotics may be administered if infection has precipitated adrenal crisis.
5. Oral intake may be initiated as soon as tolerated.
6. If adrenal gland does not regain function, lifelong replacement of corticosteroids and mineralocorticoids is required.
7. Dietary intake should be supplemented with salt during times of GI losses of fluids through vomiting and diarrhea.

Nursing Management

Assessment

Assessment focuses on fluid imbalanced and stress:

1. Monitor blood pressure and pulse rate as the patient moves from a lying, sitting and standing position to assess for inadequate fluid volume.
2. Assess skin color and turgor.

3. Assess history of weight changes, muscle weakness and fatigue.
4. Ask patient and family about onset of illness or increased stress that may have precipitated crisis.

Monitoring and Managing Addisonian Crisis

1. Monitor for signs and symptoms indicative of addisonian crisis, which can include shock; hypotension; rapid, weak pulse; rapid respiratory rate; pallor; and extreme weakness.
2. Advise patient to avoid physical and psychological stressors such as cold exposure overexertion, infection and emotional distress.
3. Immediately treat patient with addisonian crisis with IV administration of fluid, glucose and electrolytes, especially sodium; replacement of missing steroid hormones and vasopressors.
4. Anticipate and meet the patient's needs to promote return to a precrisis state.

Restoring Fluid Balance

1. Encourage the patient to consume foods and fluids that assist in restoring, and maintaining fluid and electrolyte balance.
2. Along with dietitian, help the patient to select foods high in sodium during GI tract disturbances and in very hot weather.
3. Instruct the patient and family to administer hormone replacement as prescribed and to modify the dosage during illness and other stressful situations.
4. Provide written and verbal instructions about the administration of mineralocorticoid (Florinef) or corticosteroid (prednisone) as prescribed.

Improving Activity Tolerance

1. Avoid unnecessary activities and stress that might precipitate a hypotensive episode.
2. Detect signs of infection or presence of stressors that may have triggered the crisis.
3. Explain rationale for minimizing stress during acute crisis.

Promoting Family-based Care and Follow-up

1. Give patient and family explicit verbal and written instructions about the rationale for replacement therapy and proper dosage.
2. Teach patient and family how to modify drug dosage and increase salt intake in times of illness, very hot weather and stressful situations.
3. Instruct patient to modify diet and fluid intake; to maintain fluid and electrolyte balance.
4. Provide patient and family with preloaded, single-injection syringes of corticosteroid for use in emergencies and instruct when and how to use.
5. Advise patient to inform healthcare providers (e.g. dentists) of steroid use.
6. Urge patient to wear a medical alert bracelet and to carry information at all times about the need for corticosteroids.
7. Teach patient and family signs of excessive or insufficient hormone replacement.

8. If patient cannot return to work and family responsibilities after hospital discharge refer to home healthcare nurse to assess the patient's recovery, monitor hormone replacement and evaluate stress in the home.
9. Assess patient's and family's knowledge about medication therapy and dietary modifications.
10. Assess the patient's plans for follow-up visits to clinic or physician's office.
11. Remind the patient and family about the importance of participating in health promotion activities and health screening.

PHEOCHROMOCYTOMA

A pheochromocytoma is a tumor (usually benign) that originates from the chromaffin cells of the adrenal medulla. In 90% of patients, the tumor arises in the medulla; in the remaining patients, it occurs in the extra-adrenal chromaffin located in or near the aorta, ovaries, spleen or other organs. It occurs at any age, but peak incidence is between 40 and 50 years of age; it affects men and women equally and has familial tendencies. Ten percent of the tumors are bilateral and 10% are malignant. Although uncommon, it is one cause of hypertension that is usually cured by surgery, but without detection and treatment it is usually fatal.

Clinical Manifestations

1. The typical triad of symptoms is headache, diaphoresis and palpitations in the patient with hypertension.
2. Hypertension (intermittent or persistent) and other cardiovascular disturbances are common.
3. Other symptoms may include tremor, headache, flushing and anxiety.
4. Hyperglycemia may result from conversion of liver and muscle glycogen to glucose due to epinephrine secretion, insulin may be required to maintain normal blood glucose levels.

Symptoms of Paroxysmal Form of Pheochromocytoma

1. Acute, unpredictable attacks, lasting seconds or several hours, during which patient is extremely anxious, tremulous and weak; symptoms usually begin abruptly and subside slowly.
2. Headache, vertigo, blurring of vision, tinnitus, air hunger and dyspnea.
3. Polyuria, nausea, vomiting, diarrhea, abdominal pain and feeling of impending doom.
4. Palpitations and tachycardia.
5. Life-threatening blood pressure elevation (> 250/150 mm Hg).
6. Postural hypotension (decrease in systolic blood pressure, lightheadedness, dizziness on standing).

Diagnostic Methods

1. Measurements of urine and plasma levels of catecholamines and metanephrine (MN), a catecholamine metabolite, are the most direct and conclusive tests for overactivity of the adrenal medulla.

2. A clonidine suppression test may be performed if the results of plasma and urine tests of catecholamines are inconclusive.
3. Imaging studies [e.g. ^{131}I-metaiodobenzylguanidine (MIBG) scintigraphy, CT and MRI, ultrasound] to localize the pheochromocytoma and to determine whether more than one tumor is present.

Medical Management

1. Bedrest with the head of the bed elevated is recommended.
2. The patient may be moved to the intensive care unit for close monitoring of ECG changes and careful administration of α-adrenergic blocking agents [e.g. phentolamine (Regitine)] or smooth muscle relaxants [e.g. sodium nitroprusside (Nipride)] to lower the blood pressure quickly.
3. Treatment is surgical removal of the tumor, usually with adrenalectomy (hypertension usually subsides with treatment); patient preparation includes control of blood pressure and blood volumes; usually this is carried out over 4–7 days.
4. Patient is hydrated before, during and after surgery; use of sodium nitroprusside (Nipride) and α-adrenergic blocking agents may be required during and after surgery.
5. Postoperative corticosteroid replacement is required after bilateral adrenalectomy.
6. Careful attention is directed toward monitoring and treating hypertension and hypoglycemia.
7. Several days after surgery, urine and plasma levels of catecholamines and their metabolites are measured to determine whether the surgery was successful.

Nursing Management

1. Monitor ECG changes, arterial pressures, fluid and electrolyte balance, and blood glucose levels.
2. Encourage patient to schedule follow-up appointments to ensure that pheochromocytoma does not recur undetected.
3. Instruct the patient about the purpose of corticosteroids, the medication schedule, and the risks of skipping doses or stopping their administration abruptly.
4. Teach the patient and family how to measure the patient's blood pressure and when to notify the physician about the changes in blood pressure.
5. Give verbal and written instructions on collecting 24-hour urine specimen.
6. Refer for home care nurse if indicated.
7. Give encouragement and support, because patient may be fearful of repeated attacks.

DIABETES INSIPIDUS

Diabetes insipidus is a disorder of the posterior lobe of the pituitary gland that is characterized by a deficiency of antidiuretic hormone (ADH) (vasopressin). Excessive thirst (polydipsia) and large volumes of dilute urine characterize the disorder. It may occur secondary to head trauma, brain tumor or surgical ablation or irradiation of the pituitary gland. It may also occur with infections of the central nervous system (meningitis, encephalitis, tuberculosis) or with tumors (e.g. metastatic disease, lymphoma of the breast or lung). Another cause of diabetes insipidus is failure of the renal tubules to respond to ADH; this nephrogenic form may be related to hypokalemia, hypercalcemia and a variety of medications [e.g. lithium, demeclocycline (Declomycin)].

The disease cannot be controlled by limiting fluid intake, because the high-volume loss of urine continues even without fluid replacement. Attempts to restrict fluids cause the patient to experience an insatiable craving for fluid and to develop hypernatremia and severe dehydration.

Clinical Manifestations

1. Polyuria: Enormous daily output of very dilute urine (specific gravity 1.001–1.005). Primary diabetes insipidus may have an abrupt onset or an insidious onset in adults.
2. Polydipsia: Patient experiences intense thirst, drinking 2–20 liter of fluid daily, with a special craving for cold water.
3. Polyuria continues even without fluid replacement.
4. If diabetes insipidus in inherited, the primary symptoms may begin at birth; in adults, onset may be insidious or abrupt.

Diagnostic Findings

1. Fluid deprivation test: Fluids are withheld for 8–12 hours until 3%–5% of the body weight is lost. Inability to increase specific gravity and osmolality of the urine during test is characterized of diabetes insipidus.
2. Other diagnostic procedures include concurrent measurements of plasma levels of ADH and plasma, and urine osmolality as well as a trail of desmopressin (synthetic vasopressin) therapy and IV infusion of hypertonic saline solution.

Medical Management

The objectives of therapy are:

1. To replace ADH (which is usually a long-term therapeutic program).
2. To ensure adequate fluid replacement.
3. To identify and correct the underlying intracranial pathology.

Nephrogenic causes require different management approaches.

The medication used includes the following:

1. Desmopressin (DDAVP), administered intranasally, one of two administrations daily to control symptoms.
2. Intramuscular administration of ADH (vasopressin tannate in oil) every 24–96 hours to reduce urinary volume (shake vigorously or warm; administer in the evening; rotate injection sites to prevent lipodystrophy).
3. Clofibrate (Atromid-S), a hypolipidemic agent, has been found to have an antidiuretic effect on patients who have some residual hypothalamic vasopressin; chlorpropamide (Diabinese) and thiazide diuretics are also used in mild forms of the disease because they potentiate the action of vasopressin.
4. Thiazide diuretics, mild salt depletion and prostaglandin inhibitors [ibuprofen (Advil, Motrin), indomethacin (Indocin) and Aspirin] are used to treat the nephrogenic form of diabetes insipidus.

Nursing Management

1. Instruct the patient and family members about follow-up care and emergency measures.
2. Provide specific verbal and written instructions, including the actions and adverse effects of all medications; demonstrate correct medication administration and observe return demonstrations.
3. Advise patient to wear a medical identification bracelet and to carry medication information about this disorder at all times.

DIABETES MELLITUS

Diabetes mellitus is a group of metabolic disorders characterized by elevated levels of blood glucose (hyperglycemia) resulting from defects in insulin secretion, insulin action or both. Three major acute complications of diabetes related to short-term imbalances in blood glucose levels are hypoglycemia, diabetic ketoacidosis (DKA) and hyperglycemia may contribute to chronic microvascular complications (kidney and eye disease) and neuropathic complications. Diabetes is also associated with an increased occurrence of macrovascular diseases, including coronary artery disease (myocardial infarction), cerebrovascular disease (stroke) and peripheral vascular disease.

Types of Diabetes

Type 1 (Formerly Insulin-dependent Diabetes Mellitus)

1. About 5%–10% of patients with diabetes have type 1 diabetes. It is characterized by destruction of the pancreatic β-cells due to genetic, immunological and possibly environmental (e.g. viral) factors. Insulin injections are needed to control the blood glucose levels.
2. Type 1 diabetes has a sudden onset, and usually before the age of 30 years.

Type 2 (Formerly Non-insulin-dependent Diabetes Mellitus)

1. About 90%–95% of patients with diabetes have type 2 diabetes. It results from a decreased sensitivity to insulin (insulin resistance) or from a decreased amount of insulin production.
2. Type 2 diabetes is first treated with diet and exercise, and then with oral hypoglycemic agents as needed.
3. Type 2 diabetes occurs most frequently in patient older than 30 years and in patients with obesity.

Gestational Diabetes Mellitus

1. Gestational diabetes is characterized by any degree of glucose intolerance with onset during pregnancy (second or third trimester).
2. Risks for gestational diabetes include marked obesity, a personal history of gestational diabetes, glycosuria or a strong family history of diabetes. High-risk ethnic groups include Hispanic Americans and Pacific Islanders. It increases their risk for hypertensive disorders of pregnancy.

Clinical Manifestations

1. Polyuria, polydipsia and polyphagia.
2. Fatigue and weakness, sudden vision changes, tingling of numbness in hands or feet, dry skin lesions or wounds that are slow to heal and recurrent infections.
3. Onset of type 1 diabetes may be associated with sudden weight loss or nausea, vomiting or stomach pains.
4. Type 2 diabetes results from a slow (over years), progressive glucose intolerance and results in long-term complications of diabetes goes undetected for many years (e.g. eye disease, peripheral neuropathy, peripheral vascular disease). Complications may have developed before the actual diagnosis is made.
5. Signs and symptoms of DKA include abdominal pain, nausea, vomiting, hyperventilation and a fruity breath odor. Untreated DKA may result in altered level of consciousness, coma and death.
6. High blood glucose levels fasting plasma glucose levels 126 mg/dL or more, or random plasma glucose or 2-hour postload glucose levels more than 200 mg/dL.
7. Evaluation for complications.

Preventions

For patients who are obese (especially those with type 2 diabetes) weight loss is the key to treatment and the major preventive factor for the development of diabetes.

Complications of Diabetes

Complications, which are associated with diabetes are classified as acute and chronic.

Acute Complications

Acute complications occur from short-term imbalances in blood glucose and include the following:

- Hypoglycemia
- Diabetic ketoacidosis
- Hyperosmolar hyperglycemic nonketotic syndrome.

Chronic Complications

Chronic complication generally occurs 10–15 years after the onset of diabetes mellitus. The complications include the following:

1. Macrovascular (large vessel) disease: Affects coronary, peripheral vascular and cerebral vascular circulations.
2. Microvascular (small vessel) disease; affects the eyes (retinopathy) and kidneys (nephropathy); control blood glucose levels to delay or avoid onset of both microvascular and macrovascular complications.
3. Neuropathic disease: Affects sensory motor and autonomic nerves and contributes to such problems as impotence and foot ulcers.

Because the incidence of elevated blood glucose levels increases with advancing age, elderly adults should be advised that physical activity that is consistent and realistic is beneficial to those with diabetes. Advantages of exercise include a decrease in hyperglycemia, a general sense of well-being and better use of ingested calories, resulting in weight reduction. Consider physical impairment from other chronic diseases when planning exercise regimen for elderly patients with diabetes.

Medical Management

The main management of treatment is to normalize insulin activity and blood glucose levels to reduce the development of vascular and neuropathic complications. The therapeutic goal within each type of diabetes is to achieve normal blood glucose levels (euglycemia) without hypoglycemia and without seriously disrupting the patient's usual activities. There are five components of management for diabetes: nutrition, exercise monitoring, pharmacological therapy and education:

1. Primary treatment of type 1 diabetes is insulin.
2. Primary treatment of type 2 diabetes is weight reduction.
3. Exercise is important in enhancing the effectiveness of insulin.
4. Use of oral hypoglycemic agents if diet and exercise are not successful in controlling blood glucose levels. Insulin injections may be used in acute situations.
5. Because treatment varies throughout the course because of changes in lifestyles, and physical and emotional status as well as advances in therapy, continuously assess and modify treatment plan as well as daily adjustments in therapy. Education is needed for both patient and family.

Nutritional Management

Details are to achieve and maintain blood glucose, and blood pressure levels in the normal range (or as close to normal as safely possible), and a lipid and lipoprotein profile that reduces the risk for vascular disease; to prevent, or at least slow, the rate of development of chronic complications, to address individual nutrition needs; and to maintain the pleasure of eating only limiting food choices when indicated by scientific evidence:

1. Meal plan should consider the patient's food preferences, lifestyle, usual eating times, and ethnic and cultural background.
2. For patients who require insulin to help control blood glucose levels, consistency is required in maintaining calories and carbohydrates consumed at different meals.
3. Initial education addresses the importance of consistent eating habits, the relationship of food and insulin, and the provision of an individualized meal plan. In-depth follow-up education then focuses on management skills, such as eating at restaurants; reading food labels; and adjusting the meal plan for exercise, illness and special occasions.

Calorie Requirements

1. Determine basic calorie requirements, taking into consideration age, gender, body weight, and height factor and factoring in degree of activity.
2. Long-term weight reducing basic calorie intake by 500–1,000 cal from calculated basic caloric requirements.
3. The American Diabetes and American Dietetic Association recommend that for all levels of calorie intake, 50%–60% of calories derived from carbohydrates, 10%–20% from fat, and the remaining 10%–20% from protein. Using food combinations to lower the glycemic response (glycemic index) can be useful.

Carbohydrate counting and the food guide pyramid can be useful tools.

Nursing Management

Nursing management of patients with diabetes can involve treatment of a wide variety of physiological disorders, depending on the patient's health status and whether the patient is newly diagnosed or seeking care for an unrelated health problem. Because all patients with diabetes must master the concepts and skills necessary for long-term management and avoidance of potential complications of diabetes, a solid educational foundation is necessary for competent self-care and is ongoing focus of nursing care.

Providing Patient Education

Diabetes mellitus is a chronic illness that requires a lifetime of special self-management behaviors. Nurses play a vital role in identifying patients with diabetes, assessing self-care skills, providing basic education, reinforcing the teaching provided by the specialists and referring patients for follow-up care after discharge.

Developing a Diabetic Teaching Plan

1. Determine how to organize and prioritize the vast amount of information that must be taught to patients with diabetes. Many hospitals and outpatient diabetes centers have devised written guidelines, care plans, and documentation forms that may be used to document and evaluate teaching.
2. The American Association of Diabetes Educators recommends organizing education using the following seven tips for managing diabetes; healthy eating, being active, monitoring, taking medication, problem solving, healthy coping and reducing risks.
3. Another general approach is to organize information and bills into two main types basic, initial (survival) skills and information, and in-depth (advanced) or continuing educations.
4. Basic information is literally what patients must know to survive (e.g. to avoid severe hypoglycemic or acute hypoglycemic complications after discharge) and includes pathophysiology, treatment modalities, recognition treatment, and prevention of acute complications, and other pragmatic information (e.g. where to buy and store insulin how to contact physician).
5. In-depth and continuing education involves teaching more detailed information related to survival skills as well as teaching preventive measures for avoiding long-term diabetic complications, such as foot care, eye care, general hygiene, and risk factor management (e.g. blood pressure control and blood glucose normalization). More advanced continuing education may include alternative methods for insulin delivery.

Assessing Readiness to Learn

1. Assess the patient's (and family's) readiness to learn; assess the patient's coping strategies, and reassure the patient and family that feelings of depression and shock are normal.

2. Ask the patient and family about their major concerns of fears in order to learn about any misinformation that may be contributing to anxiety; provide simple, direct information to dispel misconceptions.
3. Evaluate the patient's social situation for factors that may influence the diabetes treatment and education plan (e.g. low literacy level, limited financial resources or lack of health insurance, presence or absence of family support, typical daily schedule and neurological deficits).

Teaching Experienced Patients

1. Continue to assess the skills and self-care behaviors of patients who have had diabetes for many years, including direct observation of skills, not just the patient's self-report of self-care behaviors.
2. Ensure these patients are fully aware of preventive measures related to foot care eye care, and risk factor management.
3. Encourage patient to discuss feelings and fears related to complications; provide appropriate information regarding diabetic complications.

Determining Teaching Methods

1. Maintaining flexibility with regard to teaching approaches; a teaching method for one patient might not work for another.
2. If desired, use various tools to complement teaching (e.g. booklets, video tapes).
3. Written handouts should match the patient's learning needs including different languages, low-literacy information, large print and reading level.
4. Encourage patients to continue learning about diabetes care by participating in activities sponsored by local hospitals and diabetes organizations; inform patient that magazines and web sites with information on diabetes management are available.

Teaching Patients to Self-administer Insulin

Insulin injections are self-administered into the subcutaneous tissue with the use of special insulin syringes. Basic information includes explanations of the equipment, insulin and syringes, and how to mix insulin.

Storing insulin: Vials not in use, including spare vials, should be refrigerated; extremes of temperature should be avoided; insulin should not be allowed to freeze and should not be kept in direct sunlight or in a hot car; insulin vial in use should be kept at room temperature (for up to 1 month). Instruct patient to always have a spare vial of the type or types of insulin needed. Also instruct patient to thoroughly mix any cloudy insulin by gently inverting the vial or rolling it between the hands before drawing the solution into a syringe or a pen and to discard any bottles of intermediate-acting insulin showing evidence of flocculation (a frosted, whitish coating inside the bottle).

Selecting syringes: Syringes must be matched with the insulin concentration (U-100 is standard in the United States); currently, three sizes of U-100 insulin syringes are available (1 mL syringes that hold 100 units, 0.5 mL syringes that hold 50 units, and 0.3 mL syringes that hold 30 units). Small syringes allow patient who require small amount of insulin to measure and draw up the amount of insulin accurately. Patients who require large amount of insulin use large syringes. Smaller syringes (marked and unit increments) may be easier to use for patients with deficits. Very thin patients and children may require smaller needles.

Mixing insulin: The most important issues are—how patients be consistent in technique, so as not to draw up the wrong dose in error or the wrong type of insulin, and if that patients not inject one type of insulin into the bottle containing a different type of insulin. Patients who have difficulty mixing insulin may use a premixed insulin, have prefilled syringes prepared or take two injections.

Withdrawing insulin: Most (if not all) of the printed materials available on insulin dose preparation instruct patients to inject air into the bottle of insulin equivalent to the number of units of insulin to be withdrawn; this is to prevent the formation of a vacuum inside the bottle, which would make it difficult to withdraw the proper amount of insulin.

Selecting and rotating the injection site: The four main areas for injects are abdomen (fast absorption) upper arms (posterior surface), thighs (anterior surface) and hips (slowest absorption). Systemic rotation of injections sites within an anatomic area is recommended; encourage the patient to use all available injection sites within one area rather than randomly rotating sites from area to area. The patient should try not to use the same site more than once in 2–3 weeks.

Preparing the skin: Usage of alcohol to cleanse the skin is not recommended, but patients who have learned this technique often continue to use it. Caution these patients to allow the skin to dry after cleansing with alcohol to avoid carrying it into the tissues, which can result in a localized reddened area and a burning sensation.

Inserting the needle: The correct technique is based on the need for the insulin to be injected into the subcutaneous tissue; inject that is too deep or too shallow may affect the rate of absorption. A 90° insertion angle is best for most patients. Aspiration is generally not recommended with self-injection of insulin.

Disposing of syringes and needles: Insulin syringes and pens, needles and lancets should be disposed according to the local regulations. If community disposal programs are unavailable, used sharps should be place in a puncture-resistant container. Instruct patient to contact local trash authorities for instructions about proper disposal of filled containers.

Promoting Family-based Care and Follow-up

Promoting self-care

1. If problems exist with glucose control or with the development of preventable complications, assess the reasons for the patient's ineffective management of the treatment regimen; do not assume that problems with diabetes management are related to the patient's willful decisions to ignore self-management; problem may be correctable simply through providing complete information and ensuring that the patient understands the information.
2. Assess for certain physical (e.g. decreased visual acuity) or emotional factors (e.g. denial, depression) may be impairing the patient's ability to perform self-care skills.
3. Help patient whose family, personal or work problems may be of higher priority than self-care to establish priorities.

4. Assess the patient for infection or emotional stress, which may lead to elevated glucose levels despite adherence to the treatment regimen.
5. Promote self-care management skills by addressing any underlying factors that may affect diabetic control, simplifying and/or adjusting the treatment regimen, establishing a specific plan or contract with the patient, providing positive reinforcement, helping patient identify personal motivating factors and encouraging the patient to pursue life goals and interests.

Continuing care

1. Age, socioeconomic level, existing complications, type of diabetes and comorbid conditions all may dictate the frequency the follow-up visits.
2. In addition to individualized follow-up appointments, remind the patient to participate in recommended health promotion activities (e.g. immunization) and age-appropriate health, screenings (e.g. pelvic examinations, mammograms).
3. Encourage all patients with diabetes to participate in support groups.

DIABETIC KETOACIDOSIS

Diabetic ketoacidosis is caused by an absence or markedly inadequate amount of insulin. This results in disorders in the metabolism of carbohydrates, protein and fat. The three main clinical features of DKA are:

1. Hyperglycemia, due to decreased use of glucose by the cells and increased production of glucose by the liver.
2. Dehydration and electrolyte loss, resulting from polyuria, with a loss of up to 6.5 liter of water and up to 400–500 mEq each of sodium, potassium and chloride over 24 hours.
3. Acidosis, due to an excess breakdown of fat to fatty acids and production of ketone bodies, which also acids.

Three main causes of DKA are decreased or missed dose of insulin, illness or infection, and initial manifestations of undiagnosed or untreated diabetes.

Clinical Manifestations

1. Polyuria and polydipsia (increased thirst).
2. Blurred vision, weakness and headache.
3. Orthostatic hypotension in patients with volume depletion.
4. Frank hypotension and weak, rapid pulse.
5. Gastrointestinal symptoms, such as anorexia, nausea/vomiting and abdominal pain (may be severe).
6. Acetone breath (fruity odor).
7. Kussmaul's respirations; hyperventilation with very deep, but not labored respirations.
8. Mental status varies widely from patient to patient (alert to lethargic or comatose).

Diagnostic Findings

1. Blood glucose level: 300–800 mg/dL (may be lower or higher).

2. Low serum bicarbonate level: 0–15 mEq/L.
3. Low pH: 6.8–7.3.
4. Low $PaCO_2$: 10–30 mm Hg.
5. Sodium and potassium levels may be low, normal or high depending on amount of water loss (dehydration).
6. Elevated creatinine, blood urea nitrogen (BUN) and hematocrit values may be seen with dehydration. After rehydration, continued elevation in the serum creatinine and BUN levels suggests underlying renal insufficiency.

Medical Management

In addition to treating hyperglycemia, management of DKA is aimed at correcting dehydration, electrolyte loss and acidosis.

Rehydration

Patients may need as much as 6–10 L of IV fluid [0.9% normal saline (NS) is administered at a high rate of 0.5–1 L/h for 2–3 hour] to replace fluid loss caused by polyuria, hyperventilation, diarrhea and vomiting. Hypotonic (0.45%) NS solution may be used for hypertension or hypernatremia and for those at risk for heart failure. This is the fluid of choice (200–500 mL/h for several additional hour) after the first few hours, provided that blood glucose levels reaches 300 mg/dL (16.6 mmol/L) or less, the IV solution may be changed to dextrose 5% in water (D5W) to prevent a precipitous decline in the blood glucose level. Plasma expanders may be used to correct severe hypotension that does not respond to IV fluid treatment.

Restoring Electrolytes

Potassium is the main electrolyte of concern in treating DKA. Cautions, but timely replacement of potassium is vital for avoiding severe cardiac dysrhythmias that occur with hypokalemia.

Because a patient's serum potassium level may drop quickly as a result of rehydration and insulin treatment, potassium replacement must begin once potassium levels drop to normal.

Reversing Acidosis

Acidosis of DKA is reversed with insulin, which inhibits the breakdown of fat. Insulin (only regular insulin) is infused at a slow, continuous rate (e.g. 5 units per hour). IV fluid solutions with higher concentrations of glucose, such as NS solution (e.g. D5NS, D5, 45NS), are administered when blood glucose levels reach 250–300 mg/dL (13.8–16.6 mmol/L), to avoid too rapid a drop in the blood glucose level. IV insulin must be infused continuously until subcutaneous administration of insulin can be resumed. However, IV insulin must be continued until the serum bicarbonate level improves and patient can eat.

Nursing Management

Assessment

1. Monitor the electrocardiogram (ECG) for dysrhythmias indicating abnormal potassium levels.

2. Assess vital signs (especially blood pressure and pulse), arterial blood gases, breath sounds, and mental status every hour and record on a flow sheet.
3. Include neurological status check as part of the hourly assessment as cerebral edema can be severe and sometimes fatal outcomes.

Nursing Diagnoses/Problems

1. Risk for fluid volume deficit related to polyuria and dehydration.
2. Fluid and electrolyte imbalance related to fluid loss or shifts.
3. Deficient knowledge about diabetes self-care skills/information.
4. Anxiety related to loss of control, fear of inability to manage diabetes, misinformation related to diabetes, fear of diabetes complications.

Potential complications: They are:

- Fluid overload, pulmonary edema and heart failure
- Hypokalemia
- Hyperglycemia and ketoacidosis
- Hypoglycemia
- Cerebral edema.

Planning (Goals and Objectives)

The major goals for the patient may include maintenance of fluid and electrolyte balance, optimal control of blood glucose levels, ability to perform diabetes survival skills and self-care activities and absence of complications.

Nursing Interventions/Implementation

Maintaining Fluid and Electrolyte Balance

1. Measure intake and output.
2. Administer IV fluids and electrolyte as prescribed; encourage oral fluid intake and when permitted.
3. Monitor laboratory values of serum electrolytes (especially sodium and potassium).
4. Monitor vital signs hourly for signs of dehydration (tachycardia, orthostatic hypotension) along with assessment of breath sounds, level of consciousness, presence of edema and cardiac status (ECG rhythm strips).

Enhancing Knowledge About Diabetes Management

1. Carefully assess the patients understanding of and adherence to the diabetes management plan.
2. Explore factors that may have leads to the development of DKA with the patient and family.
3. If the patient's management differs from those identified in the diabetes management plan, discuss their relationship to the development of DKA, along with early manifestations of DKA.
4. If other factors (e.g. trauma, illness, surgery or stressed to implicated, describe appropriate strategies to respond to these and similar situations in the future so the patient can avoid developing life-threatening complications. Reteach survival skills to patients who may not be able to recall them.
5. If necessary, explore reasons a patient has omitted insulin or oral antidiabetic agents that have been prescribed and address

issues to prevent future recurrence and readmissions for treatment of these complications.

6. Teach (or remind) the patient about the need for maintaining blood glucose at a normal level, and teaching about diabetes management and survival skills.

Managing Potential Complications

Fluid overload: Monitor the patient closely during treatment by measuring vital signs, and intake and output at frequent intervals; initiate central venous pressure monitoring and hemodynamic monitoring to provide additional measures of fluid status; focus physical examination on assessment of cardiac rate and rhythm, breath sounds, venous distention, skin turgor, and urine output, monitor fluid intake, along with urine, monitor fluid intake and keeps careful records of IV and other fluid intake, along with urine output measurement hypokalemia—ensure cautions replacement of potassium, however, prior to administration, it is important to ensure that a patient's kidneys are functioning; because of the adverse effects of hypokalemia on cardiac function, monitor cardiac rate, cardiac rhythm, ECG and serum potassium levels.

Cerebral edema: Assist with gradual reduction of the blood glucose levels; use an hourly flow sheet enable close monitoring of the blood glucose level, serum electrolyte levels, urine output, mental status and neurological signs. Take precautions to minimize activities that could increase intracranial pressure.

Educating Patient About Self-care

1. Teach patient survival skills, including treatment modalities (diet, insulin administration, monitoring of blood glucose and for type 1 diabetes monitoring urine ketones); recognition, treatment and prevention of DKA.
2. Teaching should also address those factors leading to DKA.
3. Arrange follow-up education with a home care nurse and dietician or an outpatient diabetes education center.
4. Reinforce the importance of self-monitoring, and of monitoring and follow-up by primary healthcare providers; remind the patient about the importance of keeping follow-up appointments.

Evaluations

Evaluation is based on objectives/expected outcomes:
- Achieves fluid and electrolyte balance
- Demonstrates knowledge about DKA
- Has absence of complications.

HYPERGLYCEMIC HYPEROSMOLAR NONKETOTIC SYNDROME

Hyperglycemic hyperosmolar nonketotic syndrome (HHNS) is a serious condition in which hyperglycemia and hyperosmolarity predominate with alternations of the sensorium (sense of awareness). Ketosis is minimal or absent. The basic biochemical defect is lack of effective insulin (insulin resistance).

Pathophysiology

Persistent hyperglycemia causes osmotic diuresis, resulting in water and electrolyte losses. Although there is not enough insulin to prevent hyperglycemia, the small amount of insulin present is enough to prevent fat breakdown. This condition occurs most frequently in older people (50–70 year of age) who have no known history of diabetes or who have type 2 diabetes. The acute development of the condition can be traced to some precipitating event, such as an acute illness [e.g. pneumonia, cerebrovascular accident (CVA)], medications (e.g. thiazides) that exacerbate hyperglycemia or treatments such as dialysis.

Clinical Manifestations

- History of days to weeks of polyuria with adequate fluid intake
- Hypotension, tachycardia
- Profound dehydration (dry mucous membranes, poor skin turgor)
- Variable neurological signs (alterations of sensorium, seizures, hemiparesis).

Diagnostic Methods

1. Laboratory tests, including blood glucose, electrolytes, BUN, CBC count, serum osmolality and ABGs.
2. Clinical picture of severe dehydration.

Medical Management

The overall treatment of HHNS is similar to that of DKA—fluids, electrolytes and insulin:

1. Start fluid treatment with 0.9% or 0.45% normal saline, depending on sodium level and severity of volume depletion.
2. Central venous or hemodynamic pressure monitoring may be necessary to guide fluid replacement.
3. Add potassium to replacement fluids when urinary output is adequate; guided by continuous ECG monitoring and laboratory determinations of potassium.
4. Insulin is usually given at a continuous low rate to treat hyperglycemia.
5. Dextrose is added to replacement fluids when the glucose levels decreases to 250–300 mg/dL.
6. Other therapeutic modalities are determined by the underlying illness and results of continuing clinical and laboratory evaluation.
7. Treatment is continued until metabolic abnormalities are corrected and neurological symptoms clear (may take 3–5 day for neurological symptoms to resolve).

Nursing Management

Refer 'Nursing Management' under 'Diabetes Mellitus' and 'Diabetic Ketoacidosis' for additional information:

1. Assess vital signs, fluid status and laboratory values. Fluid status and urine output are closely monitored because of the high risk of renal failure secondary to severe dehydration.
2. Because HHNS tends to occur in older patients, the physiology changes to occur with aging should be considered.

3. Careful assessment of cardiovascular, pulmonary and renal function throughout the acute and recovery phases of HHNS is important.

HYPOGLYCEMIA (INSULIN REACTION)

Hypoglycemia (abnormally low blood glucose level) occurs when the blood glucose falls below 50–60 mg/dL. It can be caused by too much insulin or oral hypoglycemic agents, too little food or excessive physical activity. Hypoglycemia may occur at any time. It often occurs before meals, especially if meals are delayed or if snacks are omitted. Middle-of-the-night hypoglycemia may occur because of peaking evening neutral protamine Hagedorn (NPH) or Lente insulin, especially in patients who have not eaten a bedtime snack.

Elderly people frequently live alone and may not recognize the symptoms of hypoglycemia. With decreasing renal function it takes longer for oral hypoglycemic agents to be excreted by the kidneys. Teach patient to avoid skipping meals because of decreased appetite or financial limitations. Decreased visual acuity may lead to errors in insulin administration.

Clinical Manifestations

1. The symptoms of hypoglycemia may be grouped into two categories: Adrenergic symptoms and central nervous system symptoms.
2. Hypoglycemic symptoms may occur suddenly and unexpectedly and vary from person to person.
3. Patients who have blood glucose in the hyperglycemic range (200 mg/dL or greater) may feel hypoglycemic with adrenergic symptoms when blood glucose quickly drops to 120 mg/dL [6.6 mmol/dL (2.7 mmol/L)].
4. A decreased hormonal (adrenergic) response to hypoglycemia may occur in patient's who have had diabetes for many years. Patient must perform blood glucose checks frequently.
5. As the glucose falls, the normal surge of adrenaline does not occur and patient does not feel the usual adrenergic symptoms (sweating and shakiness).

Mild Hypoglycemia

The sympathetic nervous system is stimulated, producing sweating, tremor, tachycardia, palpitations, nervousness and hunger.

Moderate Hypoglycemia

Moderate hypoglycemia produces impaired function of the central nervous system, including inability to concentrate, headache, lightheadedness, confusion, memory lapses, numbness of the lips and tongue, slurred speech, impaired coordination, emotional changes, irrational or combative behavior, double vision and drowsiness or any combination of these symptoms.

Severe Hypoglycemia

In severe hypoglycemia, central nervous system function is further impaired. The patient needs the assistance of an another for treatment. Symptoms may include disoriented behavior, seizures, difficulty arousing from sleep or loss of consciousness.

Diagnostic Methods

Measurement of serum glucose levels.

Medical Management

1. The usual recommendation is 15 g of a fast-acting concentrated source of carbohydrate orally (e.g. three or four commercially prepared glucose tablets; 4–6 oz of fruit juice or 6–10 candies, 2–3 tsp sugar or honey).
2. Patient should avoid adding table sugar to juice, even 'unsweetened' juice, which may cause a sharp increase in glucose, resulting in hyperglycemia hours later.
3. Treatment is repeated if the symptoms persist more than 10–15 minutes after initial treatment; patient is retested in 15 minutes and retreated if blood glucose level is less than 70–75 mg/dL.
4. Patient should eat a snack contain protein and starch (milk, or cheese and crackers) after the symptoms resolve or should eat a meal or snack within 30–60 minutes.

Management of Hypoglycemia in the Unconscious Patient

1. Glucagon, 1 mg subcutaneously or intramuscularly for patients who cannot swallow or who refuse treatment patient may take up to 20 minutes to regain consciousness. Give a concentrated source of carbohydrate followed by snack when awake.
2. From 25 to 50 mL of 50% dextrose in water is administered intravenously to patients who are unconscious or unable to swallow (in a hospital setting).

Nursing Management

1. Teach patients to prevent hypoglycemia by following a consistent, regular pattern for eating, administering insulin, an exercising. Advise patient to consume between meal an bedtime snacks to counteract the maximum insulin effect.
2. Reinforce that routine blood glucose tests are performed that changing insulin requirements may be anticipated and the dosage adjusted.
3. Encourage patients taking insulin to wear an identification bracelet or tag indicating they have diabetes.
4. Instruct patient to notify after severe hypoglycemia and use of glucagon.
5. Teach family that hypoglycemia can cause irrational and unintentional behavior.
6. Teach patient the importance of performing self-monitoring of blood glucose on a frequent and regular basis.
7. Teach patients with type 2 diabetes who take oral sulfonylurea agents that symptoms of hypoglycemia may also develop.
8. Patients with diabetes should carry a form of simple sugar with them at all times.
9. Patient is discouraged from eating high calorie, high-fat dessert food to treat hypoglycemia, because high-fat snack may slow absorption of the glucose.

15

Chapter Urological Nursing

URINARY TRACT INFECTIONS

Urinary tract infections (UTIs) refer to invasion of the urinary tract by bacteria. Normally, the urinary tract is sterile above the urethra. UTI are the second most common bacterial disease. Lower UTI includes urethritis, prostrates and cystitis, upper UTI includes pyelonephritis and urethritis. Infections may result in chronic kidney disease, sepsis and/or damage to the kidney.

Urinary tract infections are caused most often by ascending infection, starting on the external urinary meatus and progressing toward bladder and kidneys. Most UTI caused by *Escherichia coli,* which is commonly found in feces. The predisposing factors include the following:

1. Stasis of urine in the bladder due to obstruction, e.g. clamped catheter or simply from not voiding.
2. Contamination in the perineal and urethral areas can be from fecal soiling or from sexual intercourse or from infection on the area vaginitis, epididymitis, or prostatitis.
3. Instrumentation or having instrument, or tubes inserted into the urinary meatus can cause infection, e.g. catheterization, indwelling catheter.
4. Faulty valves that do not maintain one-way flow can cause reflux of urine from the urethra to the bladder or to bladder to ureter, e.g. congenital or previous infection.
5. Previous UTI's.
6. Women are more susceptive due to short-length urethra and also proximity to anus and vagina or due to pregnancy (second and third trimester).
7. In older adults due to diminished immune response, e.g. diabetes mellitus, neurogenic bladder.

Clinical Manifestations

- Urinary urgency, frequency, dysuria
- Flank pain, fever, chills
- Costovertebral tenderness
- Cloudy urine with casts, bacteria and white blood cells (WBCs)
- Urine positive for nitrates.

Diagnostic Measures

- Urinalysis culture greater than 100,000 bacteria
- Elevated WBCs
- Elevated sedimentation rate (ESR)
- Increased neutrophils.

Complications

Complications of urinary tract infections are pyelonephritis, urosepsis, chronic kidney disease.

Therapeutic Measures

- Antibiotic therapy sensitive to organisms cultured from urine
- Force fluids.

Nursing Management

- Encouraging fluids at 2–3 L/day to flush bacteria
- Give antimicrobial therapy as ordered
- Teach patient to finish all prescribed medications to prevent further infection
- Give antispasmodic as ordered to relieve bladder irritability and pain
- Administer antipyretics as ordered to relieve fever, pain, discomfort
- Encourage voiding every 3 hours to empty bladder, reduce stasis, bacterial count
- Teach patient avoid cola, coffee, tea, alcohol as they are irritants
- Apply heat to suprapubic area to relieve discomfort
- Instruct patient to empty bladder as soon as urge is felt and after sexual intercourse to flush bacteria out of the body
- Avoid substances such as bubble bath and scented toilet paper
- Teach patient to practice good perineal hygiene and wipe front to back to reduce risk of reinfection
- Teach patient to wear cotton underwear to reduce perineal moisture
- Monitor urinary elimination including frequency, consistency, volume and color
- Teach signs and symptoms of complication and report.

CYSTITIS

Cystitis (lower UTI) is an inflammation of the urinary bladder. The most common route of infection is transurethral, often from fecal contamination, ureterovesical reflux or the use of a catheter or cystoscope. Bacteria may enter the urinary tract in three ways, by the transurethral route (ascending infection), through the bloodstream (hematogenous spread) or by means of a fistula from the intestine (direct extension). Cystitis occurs more often in women, particularly sexually active women. Cystitis in men is secondary to some other factor (e.g. defected prostrate, epididymitis or bladder stones).

Clinical Manifestations

- Urgency, frequency, burning and pain on urination
- Nocturia, incontinence and back, suprapubic or pelvic pain
- Hematuria
- With complicated UTIs (e.g. patients with indwelling catheters), symptoms can range from asymptomatic bacteriuria to a gram-negative sepsis with shock.

Diagnostic Methods

1. Urine cultures, colony counts, cellular studies
2. Leukocyte esterase (LE) test and nitrite testing
3. Test for sexually transmitted disease (STD)

4. Computed tomography (CT) and transrectal ultrasonography; cystourethroscopy may be indicated to visualize the ureters or to detect strictures, calculi or tumors.
5. Elderly patients often lack the typical symptoms of UTI and sepsis. Non-specific symptoms such as altered sensorium, lethargy, anorexia, new incontinence, hyperventilation and low-grade fever may be the only clues to cystitis in these patients.

Medical Management

Management of UTIs typically involves drug therapy and patient education. The nurse teaches the patient about prescribed medication, regimens and infection prevention measures. In acute stages on:

1. Ideal treatment is an antibacterial agent that eradicates bacteria from the urinary tract with minimal effects on head and vaginal flora.
2. Medications may include cephalexin (Keflex), Co-trimoxazole (TMP-SMX, Bactrim Septra), nitrofurantoin (macrodantin Furadantin), ciprofloxacin (Cipro), Levaquin and Phenazopyridine (Pyridium).
3. Occasionally, ampicillin or amoxicillin (but *E. coli* has developed resistance to these agents).
4. About 20% of women treated for uncomplicated UTI experience a recurrence.
5. Recurrence in men is usually due to persistence of the same organism; further evaluation and treatment are indicated. Reinfection of women with new bacteria is more common than persistence of the initial bacteria.
6. If diagnostic evaluation reveals no structural abnormalities, patient may be instructed to begin treatment on own testing urine with a dipstick whenever symptoms occur, and in contact healthcare provider only with persistence of symptoms, at the occurrence of fever or if the number of treatment episodes exceeds four in a 6-month period.
7. Long-term use of antimicrobial agents, decreases risk of infection.

Nursing Management

- Take careful history of urinary signs and symptoms
- Assess for pain and urinary frequency, urgency and hesitancy and changes in urine
- Determine usual pattern of voiding to detect factors that may predispose patient to infection
- Assess for infrequent emptying of the bladder, association of symptoms of UTIs with sexual intercourse, contraceptive practices and personal hygiene
- Check for urine for volume, color, concentration, cloudiness and odor.

Nursing Diagnoses

- Acute pain related to infection within the urinary tract
- Deficient knowledge related to factors disposing to infection and recurrence, detection and prevention of recurrence and pharmacological therapy.

Potential complications: Sepsis, renal failure, which may occur as the long-term result of either an extensive infective or inflammatory process.

Planning (Goals and Objectives)

Goals of the patient may include relief of pain and discomfort, increased knowledge of preventive measures and treatment modalities and absence of complications.

Nursing Interventions/Implementations

Relieving Pain

- Use antispasmodic drugs to relieve bladder irritability and pain
- Relieve pain and spasm with analgesic agents and heat to the perineum
- Encourage patient to drink liberal amounts of fluid (water is best)
- Instruct patient to avoid urinary tract irritants (e.g. coffee, tea, citrus, spices, colas, alcohol)
- Encourage frequent voiding (every 2–3 hour).

Managing Complications

1. Recognize and teach patient to recognize the signs and symptoms of UTIs early; initiate prompt treatment.
2. Manage UTIs with appropriate antimicrobial therapy, liberal fluids, frequent voiding and hygiene measures.
3. Instruct patient to notify physician if fatigue, nausea, vomiting or pruritus occurs.
4. Provide for periodic monitoring of renal function and evaluation for strictures, obstructions or stones.
5. Avoid indwelling catheters, if possible; remove at early opportunity. Use strict aseptic technique if an indwelling catheter is necessary.
6. Check vital signs and level of consciousness for impending sepsis.
7. Report positive blood cultures and elevated WBC count.

Promoting Family-based Care

1. Teach patient health-related behaviors that help to prevent recurrent UTIs including practicing careful personal hygiene, increasing fluid intake to promote voiding and dilution of urine, urinating regularly and more frequently and adhering to the therapeutic regimen.
2. Teaching should meet the patient's individual needs.

Evaluation

Evaluation is based on objectives and expected patient outcomes:

- Experiences relief of pain
- Explains UTIs and their treatment.

ACUTE PYELONEPHRITIS

Pyelonephritis (upper UTI) is a bacterial infection of the renal pelvis, tubules and interstitial tissue of one or both kidneys. Causes involve either the upward spread of bacteria from the bladder or spread from systemic sources reaching the kidney via the bloodstream. An incompetent ureterovesical valve or obstruction occurring in the urinary tract increases the susceptibility of the kidneys to infection. Bladder tumors, strictures, benign prostatic hyperplasia and urinary stones are some potential causes of obstruction that can lead to infection. Pyelonephritis may be acute or chronic.

Clinical Manifestations

- Chills, fever, leukocytosis, bacteriuria and pyuria
- Low-back pain, flank pain, nausea and vomiting, headache malaise and painful urination are common findings
- Pain and tenderness in the area of the costovertebral angle
- Symptoms of lower urinary tract such as urgency and frequency, are common.

Diagnostic Methods

- Ultrasound or CT
- An intravenous (IV) pyelogram may be indicated with pyelonephritis of functional and structural renal abnormalities are suspected
- Urine culture and sensitivity tests
- Radionuclide imaging with gallium, if other studies not conclusive.

Medical Management

1. For outpatients, a 25-weeks course of antibiotics is recommended. Commonly prescribed agents include some of the same medications prescribed for the treatment of UTIs.
2. Pregnant women may be hospitalized for 2–3 days of parenteral antibiotic therapy. Oral antibiotic agents may be prescribed once the patient is afebrile and showing clinical improvement.
3. After the initial antibiotic regimen, the patient may need antibiotic therapy for up to 6 weeks, if a relapse occurs. A follow-up urine culture is obtained 2 weeks after completion of antibiotic therapy to document clearing of the infection.
4. Hydration with oral or parenteral fluids is essential in all patients with UTIs, when there is adequate kidney function.

Nursing Management

The plan of care is the same as that for upper UTIs.

CHRONIC PYELONEPHRITIS

Repeated bouts of acute pyelonephritis may lead to chronic pyelonephritis.

Complications

Complications of chronic pyelonephritis include end-stage renal disease (from progressive loss of nephrons secondary to chronic inflammation and scarring), hypertension and formation of kidney stones (from chronic infection with urea-splitting organisms).

Clinical Manifestations

- Patient usually has no symptoms of infection unless an acute exacerbation occurs
- Signs and symptoms include fatigue, headache and poor appetite, polyuria, excessive thirst and weight loss may result
- Persistent and recurring infection may produce progressive scarring of kidney, resulting in renal failure.

Diagnostic Methods

- Intravenous urography
- Measurement of blood urea nitrogen (BUN), creatinine levels and creatinine clearance.

Medical Management

Long-term use of prophylactic antimicrobial therapy may help limit recurrence of infections and renal scarring. Impaired renal function alters the excretion of antimicrobial agents and necessities careful monitoring of renal function, especially if the medications are potentially toxic to the kidneys.

Nursing Management

The plan of care is the same as that for upper UTIs. They are:
- If patient is hospitalized, encourage fluids (3–4 L/day) unless contraindicated
- Monitor and record intake and output
- Assess body temperature every 4 hours and administers antipyretic and antibiotic agents as prescribed
- Teach preventive measures and early recognition of symptoms
- Stress the importance of taking antimicrobial medications exactly as prescribed, along with the need for keeping follow-up appointments.

URETHRITIS

Both sexually and non-sexually transmitted microorganism can cause urethritis in men and women:
1. In men inflammation of the urethra, prostate and epididymis can result in different painful and frequent urination and a urethral discharge, which may be clear, cloudy or yellow.
2. In female partner of men with urethritis also suffer from urethritis and they develop mucopurulent cervicitis (MPC) and variety of other symptoms of particular infections. Some causative agents for urethritis include *Neisseria gonorrhoeae, Chlamydia trachomatis, Ureaplasma urealyticum, Trichomonas vaginalis, Candida albicans* and herpes simplex.

Therapeutic Measure

Treat the cause and nursing care accordingly.

CHRONIC GLOMERULONEPHRITIS

Chronic glomerulonephritis may be due to repeated episodes of acute nephritic syndrome, hypertensive nephrosclerosis, hyperlipidemia, chronic tubulointerstitial injury, or hemodynamically mediated glomerular sclerosis.

Pathophysiology

The kidneys are reduced as little a one fifth of their normal size and consist of largely fibrous tissue. The cortex layer shrinks to 1–2 mm in thickness or less, scarring occurs and the branches of the renal artery are thickened. The resulting severe glomerular damage can progress to stage five chronic kidney disease (CKD) and require renal replacement therapies.

Clinical Manifestations

Symptoms are variable. Some patients with severe disease have no symptoms for many years:

- Hypertension or elevated BUN and serum creatinine levels are detected
- General symptoms such as loss of weight and strength, increasing irritability and an increased need to urinate at night (nocturia); headaches, dizziness and digestive disturbances are also common.

Renal Insufficiency and Chronic Renal Failure

1. Patient appears poorly nourished with a yellow-gray pigmentation of the skin, periorbital and peripheral edema and pale mucous membranes.
2. Blood pressure is normal or severely elevated.
3. Retinal findings include hemorrhage, exudates, narrowed tortuous arterioles and papilledema.
4. Anemia causes pale membranes.
5. Cardiomegaly, gallop rhythm, distended neck veins and other signs of heart failure may be present.
6. Crackles in lungs.
7. Possibly, peripheral neuropathy with diminished deep tendon reflexes.
8. Neurosensory change occurs late in the illness, resulting in confusion and limited attention span. Other late signs include pericarditis with pericardial friction rub and pulsus paradoxus.

Diagnostic Findings

On laboratory analysis, the following abnormalities may be found:

1. Urinalysis: Fixed specific gravity of 1.010, variable proteinuria and urinary casts.
2. Blood studies related to renal failure progression: Hyperkalemia, metabolic acidosis, anemia, hypoalbuminemia, decreased serum calcium and increased serum phosphorus and hypermagnesemia.
3. Impaired nerve conduction and mental status changes.
4. Chest X-ray: Cardiac enlargement and pulmonary edema.
5. Electrocardiography (ECG): Normal or may reflect left ventricular hypertrophy.
6. The CT and magnetic resonance imaging (MRI) show a decrease in the size of the renal cortex.

Medical Management

The treatment of ambulatory patients is guided by symptoms:

1. If hypertension is present, the blood pressure is lowered with sodium and water restriction, antihypertensive agents or both.
2. Weight is monitored daily and diuretic medications are prescribed to treat fluid overload.
3. Proteins of high-biological value are provided to support good nutritional status (dairy products, eggs, meats).
4. Urinary tract infections are treated promptly.
5. Dialysis is considered early in the course of disease to keep patient in optimal physical condition, prevent fluid and electrolyte imbalances and minimize the risk of complications of renal failure.

Nursing Management

1. Observe for common fluid and electrolyte disturbances in renal disease; report changes in fluid and electrolyte status and in cardiac and neurological status.
2. Give emotional support throughout the disease and treatment course by providing opportunities for patient and family to verbalize concerns. Answer questions and discuss options.
3. Educate patient and family about prescribed treatment plan and the risk of noncompliance. Explain about need for follow-up evaluations of blood pressure, urinalysis for protein and casts, blood for BUN and creatinine.
4. If long-term dialysis is needed, teach the patient and family about the procedure, how to care for the access site, dietary restrictions and other necessary lifestyles modifications.
5. Refer to community health or home care nurse for assessment of patient progress and continued education about problems to report to healthcare provider.
6. Remind patient and family about the importance of participation in health promotion activities including health screening.
7. Instruct patient to inform all healthcare providers about the diagnosis of glomerulonephritis.

NEPHROTIC SYNDROME

Nephrotic syndrome is a primary glomerular disease characterized by proteinuria, hypoalbuminemia, diffuse edema, high-serum cholesterol and hyperlipidemia. It is seen in any condition that seriously damages the glomerular capillary membrane, causing increased glomerular permeability with loss of protein in the urine. It occurs with many intrinsic renal diseases and systemic disease that causes glomerular damage. It is not specific glomerular disease, but a constellation of clinical findings that result from the glomerular damage.

Clinical Manifestations

1. Major manifestations are edema. It is usually soft, pitting and commonly occurs around the eyes (periorbital), independent area (sacrum, ankles and hands) and in the abdomen (ascites).
2. Patients may also exhibit malaise, headache, irritability.

Diagnostic Methods

1. Protein electrophoresis and immunoelectrophoresis to determine type of proteinuria exceeding 3.5 g/day.
2. Urine may contain increased WBCs and granular and epithelial casts.
3. Needle of biopsy of the kidney may be performed for histological examination to confirm diagnosis.

Medical Management

Treatment is focused on treating the underlying disease state causing proteinuria, slowing progression of CKD and relieving symptoms. Typical treatment includes diuretics for edema, angiotensin-converting enzyme (ACE) inhibitors to reduce proteinuria and lipid-lowering agents for hyperlipidemia.

Nursing Management

1. In early stages, management is similar to that of acute glomerulonephritis.
2. As the disease worsens, management is similar to that of end-stage renal disease (ESRD).
3. Provide adequate instruction about the importance of following all medication and dietary regimens so that the patient's condition can remain stable as long as possible.
4. Convey the patient about importance of communicating any health-related change to their healthcare providers as soon as possible so that appropriate medication and dietary changes can be made before further changes occur within the glomeruli.

ACUTE NEPHRITIC SYNDROME

Acute nephritic syndrome is the clinical manifestations of glomerular inflammation. Glomerulonephritis is an inflammation of the glomerular capillaries that can occur in acute and chronic forms.

Pathophysiology

Antigen-antibody complexes in the blood are trapped in the glomeruli, stimulating inflammation and producing injury to the kidney. Glomerulonephritis may also follow impetigo (infection of the skin) and acute viral infections [upper respiratory tract infection, mumps and varicella zoster virus, Epstein-Barr virus, hepatitis B and human immunodeficiency virus (HIV) infections].

Clinical Manifestations

1. Primary presenting features of an acute glomerular inflammation are hematuria, edema, azotemia, an abnormal concentration of nitrogenous wastes in the blood, and proteinuria or excess protein in the urine (urine may appear cola colored).
2. Some degree of edema and hypertension is present in most patients.
3. The BUN and serum creatinine levels may increase as urine output decreases; anemia may be present.
4. In the more severe form of the disease, headache, malaise and flank pain may occur.

5. Elderly patients may have circulatory overload; dyspnea, engorged neck veins, cardiomegaly and pulmonary edema.

Diagnostic Findings

1. Primary presenting features; microscopic or gross (macroscopic) hematuria.
2. Patients with an immunoglobulin (Ig) A nephropathy have an elevated serum IgA and low to normal complement levels.
3. Electron microscopy and immunofluorescent analysis help to identify the nature of the lesions; however, a kidney biopsy may be needed for definitive diagnosis.

Medical Management

Management consists primarily of treating symptoms, attempting to preserve kidney function and treating complications promptly. Treatment includes using corticosteroids, managing hypertension and controlling proteinuria. Pharmacological therapy depends on the cause of acute glomerulonephritis. If residual streptococcal infection is suspected, penicillin is the agent of choice. However, other antibiotic agents may be prescribed. Dietary protein is restricted when renal insufficiency and nitrogen retention (elevated BUN) develop. Sodium is restricted when the patient has hypertension, edema and heart failure.

Nursing Management

Although most patients with acute uncomplicated glomerulonephritis are cared for as outpatients, nursing care is important in every setting.

Providing Care in the Hospital

- Give patient carbohydrates liberally to provide energy and reduce the catabolism of protein
- Carefully measure and record intake and output; give fluids on the basis of the patient's fluid losses and daily body weight
- Provide patient education about the disease process and explanations of laboratory and other diagnostic tests
- Prepare the patient for safe and effective self-care at home.

Promoting Family-based Care and Follow-up

1. Educate patient toward symptom management and monitoring for complications.
2. Review fluid and diet restrictions with the patient to avoid worsening of edema and hypertension.
3. Instruct the patient verbally and in writing to notify the physician, if symptoms of renal failure occur (e.g. fatigue, nausea, vomiting, diminishing urine output) or at the first sign of any infection.
4. Stress to the patients the importance of follow-up evaluation of blood pressure, urinalysis for protein, and BUN and serum creatinine levels to determine, if the disease has progressed.
5. Refer for home care, if indicated to assess the patient's progress and detect early signs and symptoms of renal insufficiency.
6. Review with the patient the dosage, desired action and adverse effects of medications and the precautions to be taken.

CANCER OF KIDNEYS (RENAL TUMORS)

The most common type of renal carcinoma arises from the renal epithelium and accounts for more than 85% of all kidney tumors. These tumors may metastasize early to the lungs, bone, liver, brain and contralateral kidney. One quarter of patients have metastatic disease at the time of diagnosis. Risk factors include gender (male) tobacco use, occupational exposure to industrial chemicals, obesity and dialysis.

Clinical Manifestations

1. Many tumors are with symptoms and are discovered as a palpable abdominal mass on routine examination.
2. The classic triad occurring in only 10% of patients, is hematuria, pain and a mass in the flank.
3. The sign usually first calls attention to the tumor is painless hematuria, either intermittent or microscopic of continuous and gross.
4. Dull pain occurs in the back from pressure due to compression of the ureter, extension of the tumor or hemorrhage into the kidney tissue.
5. Colicky pain occurs, if a clot or mass of tumor cells passes down the ureter.
6. Symptoms from metastasis may be the first manifestations of renal tumor including unexplained weight loss, increasing weakness and anemia.

Diagnostic Methods

- The IV urography
- Cystoscopic examination
- Nephrotomography, renal angiography
- Ultrasonography
- Computed tomography (CT).

Medical Management

The goal of management is to eradicate the tumor before metastasis occurs:

1. Radical nephrectomy is the preferred treatment including removal of the kidney (and tumor), adrenal gland, surrounding fat and Gerota's fascia and lymph nodes.
2. Radiation therapy, hormonal therapy or chemotherapy may be used with surgery.
3. Immunotherapy may be helpful; allogeneic stem cell transplantation may be indicated, if no response to immunotherapy.
4. Nephron-sparing surgery (NSS) (partial nephrectomy) may be used for some patients.
5. Renal artery embolization may be used in metastasis to occlude the blood supply to the tumor and kill the tumor cells. Post infection syndrome of flank and abdominal pain, elevated temperature and gastrointestinal (GI) complications is treated with parenteral analgesics, antiemetics, restricted oral intake, and IV fluids.
6. Biological response modifiers (BRMs) such as interleukin-2 (IL-2).

Nursing Management

1. Monitor for infection resulting from use of immunosuppressant agents.
2. After surgery, give frequent analgesia for pain and muscle soreness.
3. Assist the patient with turning, coughing, use of incentive spirometry and deep breathing to prevent atelectasis and other pulmonary complications.
4. Support patient and family in coping with diagnosis and uncertainties about outcome and prognosis.
5. Teach patient to inspect and care for the incision and perform other general postoperative care.
6. Inform patient of limitations on activities, lifting and driving.
7. Teach patient about correct use of pain medications.
8. Provide instructions about follow-up care and need to notify physician about fever, breathing difficulty and wound drainage, blood in urine, pain or swelling of legs.
9. Encourage patient to eat a healthy diet and to drink adequate liquids to avoid constipation and to maintain an adequate urine volume.
10. Instruct patient and family in need for follow-up care to detect signs of metastases; evaluate all subsequent symptoms with possible metastases in mind.
11. Emphasize that a yearly physical examination and chest X-ray thought life are required for patients who have had surgery for renal carcinoma.
12. With follow-up chemotherapy, educate patient and family thoroughly including treatment plan or chemotherapy protocol, what to expect with visits and how to notify the physician. Explain the need for periodic evaluation of renal function (creatinine clearance, BUN and creatinine).
13. Refer to home care nurse as needed to monitor and support patient and coordinate services and resources needed.

Refer 'Nursing Process': 'The Patient with Cancer' under 'Cancer' for additional information.

URETHRAL STRICTURES

A urethra stricture is a narrowing of the lumen of the urethra caused by scar tissue. It may be due to rising incidence of STDs, gonococcal and chlamydial infections. It may be acquired from injuries or infections.

Clinical Manifestation

- Prone to develop UTI due to diminished urinary stream.

Therapeutic Measures

- Mechanical dilation of urethral urologist
- If strictures continues often dilation surgical repair urethroplasty.

Nursing Management

- Assist in dilation process
- Administer pain medication as ordered
- Care of indwelling catheter

- Give antimicrobial medication to prevent risk for infection as prescribed
- Advice patient to prevent UTI as in.

NEPHROSCLEROSIS

Nephrosclerosis refers to hardening of the kidney associated with hypertension and disease of the renal arterioles. In other words hypertension damage the kidneys by causing sclerotic changes in the small arteries and arterioles such an atherosclerosis with thickening and hardening of renal blood vessels. These changes results in a decreased blood supply to the kidneys. The remaining nephrons try to compensate with vasodilation to increase blood flow to glomeruli, which results increased glomerular pressure and filtration, which thicken blood vessels.

Clinical Manifestations

- High pressure causes the vessels to weaken and hemorrhage
- Large areas of kidney damaged leads to:
  - Proteinuria, hyaline casts in the urine
  - Symptoms of chronic kidney disease—decreased urine output, kidney injury symptoms, fatigue, nausea and vomiting, shortness of breath, platelet dysfunction.

Therapeutic Measures

- The patient is placed on antihypertensive medications (stronger ones)
- Low-sodium diet
- Dialysis may be used to maintain life.

Nursing Management

- Help patient to learn much about the control of hypertension
- Patient should taught to symptoms of chronic kidney disease and seek medical help
- Take care of patient who lost renal function, i.e. dialysis and other measures.

RENAL CALCULI

Renal calculi are hard, usually small stones that form somewhere in the renal structures. The stones are masses of crystals and protein that form where the urine becomes supersaturated with a salt capable of forming solid crystals. Symptoms occur when the stones become impacted in the urinary tract. Calcium phosphate, magnesium, ammonia uric acid and cysteine is common urinary salts.

Clinical Manifestations

- Costovertebral angle pain, groin pain, renal colic
- Flank pain radiating to genitalia
- Hematuria, anuria, restlessness, pallor, temperature increase
- Diminished or absent bowel sounds with ileus.

Complications

Shock, sepsis, hydronephrosis, hydroureter and kidney disease.

Diagnostic Measures

- Urinalysis, crystals and urine pH
- 24-hours renal creatinine clearance
- Creatinine, BUN
- Kidney, ureter and bladder (KUB) reveals most renal calculi
- Retrograde pyelography, ultrasound.

Therapeutic Measures

- Treat pain to prevent shock
- Chemolysis—stone dissolution using infusion of chemical solutions
- Surgery—lithotripsy, nephrolithotomy, pyelolithotomy, percutaneous nephrostomy tube.

Nursing Management

- Ask severity, location and duration of pain using pain scale
- Monitor patency of drains and catheter in pre- and post-operative patients
- Encourage fluid intake unless contraindicated
- Administer pain medications as ordered
- Apply heat to flank area to reduce pain and promote comfort
- Monitor vital signs and BP and observe perioperative bleeding
- Strain urine through gauze or strictures to identify stones
- Monitor urine amount, color, clarity and odor to ensure patency
- Ambulate, if possible
- Teach patient to maintain fluid balance, take medication promptly and report any signs of infection, pain, etc. (refer Management of Urolithiasis for additional information).

UROLITHIASIS

Urolithiasis refers to stones (calculi) in the urinary tract. Stones are formed in the urinary tract when the urinary concentration of substances such as calcium oxalate, calcium phosphate and uric acid increases. Stones vary in size from minute granular deposits to the size of an orange. Factors that favor formation of stones include infection, urinary stasis and periods of immobility all of which slow renal drainage and alter calcium metabolism. The problem occurs predominantly in the third to fifth decades and affects men more often than women.

Clinical Manifestations

Manifestations depend on the presence of obstruction, infection and edema. Symptoms range from mild to excruciating pain and discomfort.

Stones in Renal Pelvis

- Intense, deep ache in costovertebral region
- Hematuria and pyuria

- Pain that radiates anteriorly and downward bladder in female and toward testes in male
- Acute pain, nausea, vomiting, costovertebral area tenderness (renal colic)
- Abdominal discomfort, diarrhea.

Ureteral Colic (Stones Lodged in Ureter)

- Acute, excruciating, colicky, wave-like pain, radiating down the thigh to the genitalia
- Frequent desire to void, but little urine passed; usually contains blood because of the abrasive action of the stone (known as ureteral colic).

Stones Lodged in Bladder

- Symptoms of irritation associated with urinary tract infection and hematuria
- Urinary retention, if stone obstructs bladder neck
- Possible urosepsis if infection is present with stone.

Diagnostic Methods

- Diagnosis is confirmed by X-rays of the KUB or by ultrasonography, IV urography or retrograde pyelography
- Blood chemistries and a 24-hours urine test for measurement of calcium, uric acid, creatinine, sodium, pH and total volume
- Chemical analysis is performed to determine stone composition.

Medical Management

Basic goals to eradicate the stone, determine the stone type, prevent nephron destruction, control infection and relieve any obstruction that may be present.

Medication and Nutritional Therapy

1. Opioid analgesic agents (to prevent shock and syncope) and non-steroidal anti-inflammatory drugs (NSAIDs).
2. Increased fluid intake to assist in stone passage, unless patient is vomiting; patients with renal stones should drink 8–10 glasses of water daily or have IV fluids prescribed to keep the urine dilute.
3. For calcium stones: Reduced dietary protein and sodium intake, liberal fluid intake, medications to acidify urine such as ammonium chloride with thiazide diuretics, if parathormone production is increased.
4. For uric stones: Low purine and limited protein diet; allopurinol (Zyloprim).
5. For cystine stones: Low-protein diet, alkalization of urine and increased fluids.
6. For oxalate stones: Dilute urine; limited oxalate intake (spinach, strawberries, rhubarb, chocolate, tea, peanuts and wheat bran).

Stone Removal Procedures (Surgery)

1. Ureteroscopy: Stones fragmented with use of laser, electrohydraulic lithotripsy or ultrasound and then removed.

2. Extracorporeal shock wave lithotripsy (ESWL).
3. Percutaneous nephrostomy; endourological methods.
4. Electrohydraulic lithotripsy.
5. Chemolysis (stone dissolution): Alternative for those who are poor risks for other therapies, refuse other methods, or have easily dissolved stones (struvite).
6. Surgical removal is performed in only 1%–2% of patients.

Nursing Management

Assessment

1. Assess for pain and discomfort including severity, location and radiation of pain.
2. Assess for associated symptoms including nausea, vomiting, diarrhea and abdominal distention.
3. Observe for signs of urinary tract infection (chills, fever, frequency and hesitancy) and obstruction (frequent urination of small amounts, oliguria or anuria).
4. Observe urine for blood; strains for stones or gravel.
5. Focus history on factors that predispose patient to urinary tract stones or that may have precipitated current episode or renal or ureteral colic.
6. Assess the patient's knowledge about renal stones and measures to prevent recurrence.

Nursing Diagnoses/Problems

- Acute pain related to inflammation, obstruction and abrasion of the urinary tract
- Deficiency knowledge regarding prevention of recurrence of renal stones.

Potential complications: Infection and urosepsis (from urinary tract infection and pyelonephritis) and obstruction of the urinary tract by a stone or edema, with subsequent acute renal failure.

Planning (Goals and Objectives)

Major goals may include relief of pain and discomfort, prevention of recurrence of renal stones and absence of complications.

Nursing Interventions/Implementations

Relieving Pain

- Administer opioid analgesics (IV or intramuscular) with IV NSAID as prescribed
- Encourage and assist patient to assume a position of comfort
- Assist patient to ambulate to obtain some pain relief
- Monitor pain closely and report promptly increases in severity.

Managing Complications

- Encourage increased fluid intake and ambulation
- Begin IV fluids, if patient cannot take adequate oral fluids
- Monitor total urine output and patterns of voiding
- Encourage ambulation as a means of moving the stone through the urinary tract

- Strain urine through gauze
- Crush any blood clot passed in urine and inspect sides of urinal and bedpan for clinging stones
- Instruct patient to report any increase in pain
- Monitor vital signs for early indications of infection; infections should be treated with the appropriate antibiotic agent before efforts are made to dissolve the stone.

Promoting Family-based Care

1. Explain causes of kidney stones and ways to prevent recurrence.
2. Encourage patient to follow a regimen to avoid further stone formation including maintaining a high-fluid intake.
3. Encourage patient to drink enough to excrete 3,000–4,000 mL of urine every 24 hours.
4. Recommend that patient have urine cultures every 1–2 months the 1st year and periodically thereafter.
5. Recommend that recurrent urinary infection be treated vigorously.
6. Encourage increased mobility whenever possible; discourage excessive ingestion of vitamins (especially vitamin D) and minerals.
7. If patient has surgery, instruct about the signs and symptoms of complications that need to reported to the physician; emphasize the importance of follow-up to assess kidney function and to ensure the eradication or removal of all kidney stones to the patient and family.
8. If patient had ESWL, encourage patient to increase fluid intake to assist in the passage of stone fragments; inform the patient to expect hematuria and possibly a bruise on the treated side of the back; instruct patient to check his/her temperature daily and notify the physician if the temperature is greater than 38°C (about 101°F) or the pain is unrelieved by the prescribed medication.
9. Provide instructions for any necessary home care and follow-up.

Providing Home and Follow-up Care After Extracoreal Shock Wave Lithotripsy

1. Instruct patient to increase fluid intake to assist passage of stone fragments (may take 6 week to several month after procedure).
2. Instruct patient about signs and symptoms of complications such as fever, decreasing urinary output and pain.
3. Inform patient that hematuria is anticipated, but should subside in 24 hours.
4. Give appropriate dietary instructions based on composition of stones.
5. Encourage regimen to avoid further stone formation; advise the patient to adhere to prescribed diet.
6. Teach patient to take sufficient fluids in the evening to prevent urine from becoming too concentrated at night.
7. Closely monitor the patient to ensure that treatment has been effective and that no complications have developed.
8. Assess the patient's understanding of ESWL and possible complications; assess the patient's understanding of factors that increase the risk of recurrence of renal calculi and strategies to reduce those risks.

9. Assess the patient's ability to monitor urinary pH and interpret the results during follow-up visits.
10. Ensure that patient understands the signs and symptoms of stone formation, obstruction and infection and the importance of reporting these signs promptly.
11. If medications are prescribed for the prevention of stone formation, explain their actions, importance and side effects to the patient.

Evaluation

Evaluation is done according to objectives of care and expected patient outcomes:
- Reports relief of pain
- States increased knowledge of health-seeking behaviors to prevent recurrence
- Experiences no complications.

HYDRONEPHROSIS

Hydronephrosis is distention of the renal pelvis and calices. It is result from untreated obstruction of the urine flow in the urinary tract. The kidney enlarges as urine collects in the pelvis and kidney tissue. Obstruction of urine flow can be from a stricture in urethra or ureter, from kidney stones, from a tumor or from an enlarged prostate. Because of the unrelieved obstruction, urine backups and distends the ureters and then progresses to kidney.

Clinical Manifestations

- Onset of obstruction is gradual, patient initially asymptomatic
- Usually patient develops UTI, i.e. symptoms of frequency, urgency, dysuria
- As it progresses, flank and back pain and chronic kidney disease symptoms develops.

Therapeutic Measures

- Initial removal of obstruction by intervening indwelling catheter
- Long-term measures—relieve obstruction from strictures, stones, tumor or enlarged prostrate (surgery)
- Stents, nephrostomy may be required.

Nursing Management

According procedure performed.

RENAL TRAUMA

Renal trauma is the most common injury to the urinary system. The kidney are highly vascular and have a lot of mobility, so they are vulnerable to vascular and tissue damage.

The main causes of trauma to the kidney, ureter and bladder include motor vehicle accidents, sport injuries, falls, gunshot wounds and stabbing.

Diagnosis

- History of the injury and inspections of the abdomen and flank for asymmetry and bruising and swelling
- Urinalysis, intravenous pyelogram (IVP), ultrasound, CT, MRI.

Clinical Manifestations

- Flank pain and hematuria
- If bladder trauma, hematuria, abdominal pain, inability to void, shock.

Therapeutic Measures

- Treatment depends on the extent of injury, i.e. pelvic hemotoma
- Bedrest to surgical interventions
- Urinary or suprapeutic catheter should be in place till bladder heals.

Nursing Measures

- Measuring intake and output
- Monitoring vital signs
- Providing IV fluids and pan relief.

CANCER OF BLADDER

Cancer of the urinary bladder is more common in people older than 55 years, affects men more often than women (4:1) and is more common in Caucasians than in African-Americans. Bladder tumors usually arise at the base of the bladder, and involve the ureteral orifices and bladder neck. Tobacco use continues to a leading risk factor for all urinary tract cancers. People who smoke develop bladder cancer twice as often as those who do not smoke. Cancers arising from the prostrate, colon and rectum in males, and from the lower gynecological tract in females may metastasize to the bladder.

Clinical Manifestations

- Visible, painless hematuria is the most common symptom
- Infection of the urinary tract is common and produces frequency and urgency
- Any alteration in voiding or change in the urine is indicative
- Pelvic or back pain may occur with metastasis.

Diagnostic Methods

Biopsies of the tumor and adjacent mucosa are definitive, but the following procedures are also used:

- Cystoscopy (the mainstay of diagnosis)
- Excretory urography
- Computed tomography (CT)
- Ultrasonography
- Bimanual examination under aesthesia
- Cytological examination of fresh urine and saline bladder washings

- Newer diagnostic tools such as bladder tumor antigens, nuclear matrix proteins, adhesion molecules, cytoskeletal proteins and growth factors are being studied.

Medical Management

Treatment of bladder cancer depends on the grade of tumor, the stage of tumor growth, and the multicentricity of the tumor. Age and physical, mental and emotional status are considered in determining treatment.

Surgical Management

1. Transurethral resection (TUR) or fulguration for simple papillomas with intravesical bacille Calmette-Guérin (BCG) is the treatment of choice.
2. Monitoring of benign papillomas with cytology and cystoscopy periodically for the rest of patient's life.
3. Simple cystectomy or radical cystectomy for invasive or multifocal bladder cancer.
4. Trimodal therapy [transurethral resection (TUR), radiation and chemotherapy] to avoid cystectomy remains investigational in the United States.
5. Chemotherapy with a combination of methotrexate (Rheumatrex), 5-fluorouracil (5-FU), vinblastine (Velban), doxorubicin (Adriamycin) and cisplatin (Platinol) has been effective in producing partial remission of transitional cell carcinoma of the bladder in some patients.
6. Intravesical BCG (effective with superficial transitional cell carcinoma).

Radiation Therapy

1. Radiation of tumor preoperatively to reduce microextension and viability.
2. Radiation therapy in combination with surgery to control inoperable tumors.
3. Hydrostatic therapy: For advanced bladder cancer or patient with intractable hematuria (after radiation therapy).
4. Formalin, phenol or silver nitrate instillations to achieve relief of hematuria and strangury (slow and painful discharge of urine) in some patients.

Investigational Therapy

The use of photodynamic techniques in treating superficial bladder cancer is under investigation.

Nursing Management

Refer 'Nursing Management' for the patient undergoing cancer surgery, radiation, and chemotherapy under 'cancer' for additional information.

ACUTE RENAL FAILURE

Renal failure, when the kidneys are unable to remove metabolic waste and perform their regulatory functions. Acute renal failure (ARF) is a rapid loss of renal function due to damage to the kidneys. Three major categories of ARF are prerenal (hypoperfusion, as from volume depletion disorders, extreme vasodilation or impaired cardiac performance), intrarenal [parenchymal damage to the glomeruli or kidney tubules, as from burns, crush injuries, infections, transfusion reaction, or nephrotoxicity, which may lead to acute tubular necrosis (ATN)] and postrenal (urinary tract obstruction, as from calculi, tumor, strictures, prostatic hyperplasia or blood clots).

Clinical Stages

- Initiation period: Initial insult and oliguria
- Oliguria period (urine volume less than 400 mL/day): Uremic symptoms first appear and hyperkalemia may develop
- Dieresis period: Gradual increase in urine output, signaling beginning of glomerular filtration recovery, laboratory values stabilize and start to decrease
- Recovery period: Improving renal function (may take 3–12 month).

Clinical Manifestations

- Critical illness and lethargy with persistent nausea, vomiting and diarrhea
- Skin and mucous membranes are dry
- Central nervous system manifestations: Drowsiness, headache, muscle twitching, seizures
- Urine output scanty to normal: Urine may be bloody with low-specific gravity
- Stead rise in BUN may occur depending on degree of catabolism; serum creatinine values increases with disease progression
- Hyperkalemia may lead to dysrhythmias and cardiac arrest
- Progressive acidosis, increase in serum phosphate concentrations and low-serum calcium levels may be noted
- Anemia from blood loss due to uremic GI lesions, reduced RBC life span and reduced erythropoietin production.

Diagnostic Methods

- Urine output measurements
- Renal ultrasonography, CT and MRI
- Creatinine, electrolyte analyses, BUN.

About half of all patients who develop ARF during hospitalization are older than 60 years. The etiology of ARF in older adults includes prerenal causes such as dehydration, intrarenal causes such as nephrotoxic agents (e.g. medications, contrast agents) and complications of major surgery. Suppression of thirst, enforced bedrest, lack of access to drinking water, and confusion all contribute to the older patient's failure to consume adequate fluids, and may lead to dehydration further compromising already decreased renal function.

Acute renal failure in the elderly is also often seen in the community setting. Nurses in the ambulatory setting need to be aware of the risk. All medications need to monitored for potential side effects that could result in damage to the kidney either through reduced circulation or nephrotoxicity. Outpatient procedures that require fasting or a bowel preparation may cause dehydration and therefore require careful monitoring.

Medical Management

Treatment objectives are to restore normal chemical balance and prevent complications until renal tissues are repaired and renal function is restored. Possible causes of damage are identified and treated:

1. Fluid balance is managed on the basis of daily weight, serial measurements of central venous pressure, serum and urine concentrations, fluid losses, blood pressure and clinical status. Fluid excesses are treated with mannitol, furosemide or ethacrynic acid to initiate dieresis and prevent or minimize subsequent renal failure.
2. Blood flow is restored to the kidneys with use of IV fluids, albumin or blood product transfusions.
3. Dialysis (hemodialysis, hemofiltration or peritoneal dialysis) is started to prevent complications including hyperkalemia, metabolic acidosis, pericarditis and pulmonary edema.
4. Cation-exchange resins (orally or by retention enema).
5. Dextrose IV, 50% insulin and calcium replacement for the patient who is hemodynamically unstable (low blood pressure, changes in mental status, dysrhythmia).
6. Shock and infection are treated, if present.
7. Arterial blood gases are monitored when severe acidosis is present.
8. Sodium bicarbonate to elevate plasma pH.
9. If respiratory problems develop, ventilator measures are started.
10. Phosphate-binding agents to control elevated serum phosphate concentrations.
11. Replacement of dietary proteins is individualized to provide the maximum benefit and minimize uremic symptoms.
12. Caloric requirements are met with high-carbohydrate feedings; parenteral nutrition (PN).
13. Foods and fluids containing potassium and phosphorus are restricted.
14. Blood chemistries are evaluated to determine amount of sodium, potassium and water replacement during oliguric phase.
15. After the diuretic phase, high-protein and high-calorie diet is given with gradual resumption of activities.

Nursing Management

- Monitor for complications
- Assist in emergency treatment of fluid and electrolyte balances
- Assess progress and response for treatment; provide physical and emotional support
- Keep family informed about condition and provide support.

Monitoring Fluid and Electrolyte Balance

1. Screen parenteral fluids, all oral intake and all medications for hidden sources of potassium.
2. Monitor cardiac function and musculoskeletal status for hyperkalemia.
3. Pay careful attention to fluid intake (IV medications should be administered in the smallest volume possible), urine output,

apparent edema, distention of the jugular veins, alterations in heart sounds and breath sounds, and increasing difficulty in breathing.

4. Maintain daily weight and intake and output records.
5. Report indicators of deteriorating fluid and electrolyte status immediately. Prepare for emergency treatment of hyperkalemia. Prepare patient for dialysis as indicated to correct fluid and electrolyte imbalances.

Reducing Metabolic Rate

- Reduce exertion and metabolic rate during most acute stage with bedrest
- Prevent or treat fever and infection promptly.

Promoting Pulmonary Function

- Assist patient to turn, cough and take deep breaths frequently
- Encourage and assist patient to move and turn.

Preventing Infection

- Practice asepsis when working with invasive lines and catheters
- Avoid using an indwelling catheter, if possible.

Providing Skin Care

- Perform meticulous skin care
- Bath the patient with cool water, turn patient frequently, keep the skin clean and well-moisturized and fingernails trimmed for patient comfort and to prevent skin breakdown.

Providing Psychosocial Support

- Assist, explain and support patient and family during hemodialysis treatment; do not overlook psychological needs and concerns
- Explain rationale of treatment to patient and family, repeat explanations and clarify answers as needed
- Encourage family to touch and talk to patient during dialysis
- Continually assess patient for complications and their participating causes.

CHRONIC RENAL FAILURE

When a patient has sustained enough kidney damage to require renal replacement therapy on a permanent basis, the patient has moved into the final stage of chronic kidney disease, also referred to as chronic renal failure (CRF) or end-stage renal disease (ESRD).

The rate of decline in renal function and progression of ESRD is related to the underlying disorder, the urinary excretion of protein and the presence of hypertension. The disease tends to progress more rapidly in patients who excrete significant amount of protein or have elevated blood pressure than in those without these conditions.

Clinical Manifestations

1. Cardiovascular: Hypertension, pitting edema (feet, hands, sacrum), periorbital friction rub, engorged neck veins,

pericarditis, pericardial effusion, pericardial tamponed, hyperkalemia, hyperlipidemia.
2. Integumentary: Gray-bronze skin color, dry flaky skin, severe pruritus, ecchymosis, purpura, thin brittle nails, coarse thinning of hair.
3. Pulmonary: Crackles, thick, tenacious sputum, depressed cough reflex, pleuritic pain, shortness of breath, tachypnea, Kussmaul's respiration, uremic pneumonia.
4. Gastrointestine: Ammonia odor to breath, metallic taste, mouth ulcerations and bleeding, anorexia, nausea and vomiting, hiccups, constipation or diarrhea, bleeding from GI tract.
5. Neurological: Weakness and fatigue, confusion, inability to concentrate, disorientation, tremors, seizures, asterixis, restlessness of legs, burning of soles of feet, behavior changes.
6. Musculoskeletal: Muscle cramps, loss of muscle strength, renal osteodystrophy, bone pain, fractures, foot drop.
7. Reproductive: Amenorrhea, testicular atrophy, infertility decreased libido.
8. Hematological: Anemia, thrombocytopenia.

Diabetes, hypertension, chronic glomerulonephritis, intestinal nephritis and urinary tract obstruction are the causes of ESRD in the elderly. The symptoms of other disorders (heart failure dementia) can mask the symptoms of nephritic syndrome such as edema and proteinuria. The elderly patient may develop non-specific signs of disturbed renal function and fluid and electrolyte imbalances. Hemodialysis and peritoneal dialysis have been used effectively in elderly patients. Concomitant disorders have made transplantation a less common treatment for the elderly. Conservative management including nutritional therapy, fluid control and medications (such as phosphate binders) may be used, if dialysis or transplantation is not suitable.

Medical Management

Goals of management are to retain kidney function and maintain homeostasis for as long as possible. All factors that contribute to ESRD and those that are reversible (e.g. obstruction) are identified and treated.

Medication Therapy

Complications can be prevented or delayed by administering prescribed phosphate-binding agents, calcium supplements, antihypertensive and cardiac medications antiseizures medications, and erythropoietin (Epogen):

1. Hyperphosphatemia and hypocalcemia are treated with medications that bind dietary phosphorus in the GI tract (e.g. calcium carbonate, calcium acetate, sevelamer hydrochloride), all binding agents must be administered with food.
2. Hypertension is managed by intravascular volume control and antihypertensive medication.
3. Heart failure and pulmonary edema are treated with fluid restriction, low-sodium diet, diuretics, inotropic agents (e.g. digoxin or dobutamine) and dialysis.
4. Metabolic acidosis is treated, if necessary with sodium bicarbonate supplements or dialysis.

5. Patient is observed for early evidence of neurological abnormalities (e.g. slight twitching, headache, delirium or seizure activity); IV diazepam (Valium) or phenytoin (Dilantin) is administered to control seizures.
6. Anemia is treated with recombinant human erythropoietin (Epogen) hemoglobin and hematocrit are monitored frequently.
7. Heparin is adjusted as necessary to prevent clotting of dialysis lines during treatment.
8. Supplementary iron may be prescribed.
9. Blood pressure and serum potassium levels are monitored.

Nutritional Therapy

1. Dietary intervention is needed with careful regulation of protein intake, fluid intake to balance fluid losses and sodium intake, and with some restrictions of potassium.
2. Adequate intake of calories and vitamins is ensured. Calories are supplied with carbohydrates and fats to prevent wasting.
3. Protein restricted, allowed protein must be of high biological value (dairy products, eggs, meats).
4. Fluid allowance is 500–600 mL of fluid or more than the previous day's 24-hours urine output.
5. Vitamin supplementation.

Dialysis

The patient with increasing symptoms of renal failure is referred to a dialysis and transplantation center early in the course of progressive renal disease. Dialysis is usually initiated when the patient cannot maintain a reasonable lifestyle with conservative treatment.

Nursing Management

- Asses fluid status and identify potential sources of imbalance
- Implement a dietary program to ensure proper nutritional intake within the limits of the treatment regimen
- Promote positive feelings by encouraging increased and greater independence
- Provide explanation and information to the patient and family concerning ESRD, treatment options and potential complications
- Provide emotional support.

Promoting Family-based Care and Follow-up

- Provide ongoing explanations and information to patient and family concerning ESRD, treatment options and potential complications, monitor the patient's progress and compliance with treatment regimen
- Refer patient for dietary counseling and assist with nutritional planning
- Teach patient how to check the vascular access device for patency and appropriate precautions such as avoiding venipuncture and BP measurements on the arm with the access device
- Teach patient and family about problems to report: Signs of worsening renal failure, hyperkalemia, access problems
- Stress the importance of follow-up examinations and treatment

- Refer patient to home care nurse for continued monitoring and support
- Reinforce the dietary restrictions required including fluid sodium, potassium and protein restriction
- Remind the patient about the need for health promotion activities and health screening.

16 Chapter Reproductive Health Nursing

PELVIC INFECTION (PELVIC INFLAMMATORY DISEASE)

Pelvic inflammatory disease (PID) is an inflammatory condition of the pelvic cavity that may begin with cervicitis and may involve the uterus (endometritis), fallopian tubes (salpingitis), ovaries (oophoritis), pelvic peritoneum or pelvic vascular system. Infection, which may be acute, subacute, recurrent or chronic and localized or widespread, is usually caused by bacteria but may be attributed to a virus, fungus or parasite.

Pathophysiology

Pathogenic organisms usually enter the body through the vagina, pass through the cervical canal into the uterus may proceed to one or both fallopian tubes and ovaries, and into the pelvis. Infection most commonly occurs through sexual transmission but also may be caused by invasive procedures such as endometrial biopsy, surgical abortion, hysteroscopy or insertion of an intrauterine device (IUD). The most common organisms involved are *Neisseria gonorrhoeae* and *Chlamydia*. The infection is usually bilateral. Risk factors include early age to first intercourse, multiple sexual partners, frequent intercourse, intercourse without condoms, sex with a partner with sexually transmitted disease (STD) and a history of STDs or previous pelvic infection.

Clinical Manifestations

Symptoms may be acute and severe or low grade and subtle:

1. Vaginal discharge, dyspareunia, lower abdominal pelvic pain and tenderness that occurs after menses; pain increases during voiding or defecating.
2. Systemic symptoms include fever, general malaise, anorexia, nausea, headache and possibly vomiting.
3. Intense tenderness is noted on palpation of the uterus or movement of cervix (cervical motion tenderness) during pelvic examination.

Complications

1. Pelvic or generalized peritonitis, abscesses, strictures and fallopian tube obstruction.
2. Adhesions that eventually may require removal of the uterus, tubes and ovaries.
3. Bacteremia with septic shock and thrombophlebitis with possible embolization.

Medical Management/Therapeutic Measures

Broad-spectrum antibiotic therapy is instituted, with mild-to-moderate infections being treated on an outpatient basis. If the patient is acutely ill, hospitalization may be required. Once hospitalized, the patient is placed on a regimen of bedrest, intravenous (IV) fluids and IV antibiotic therapy. Nasogastric and suction are used if ileus is present, vital agents are monitored. Treatment of sexual partners is necessary to prevent reinfection.

Nursing Management

Nursing measures include nutritional support of the patient and administration of antibiotic therapy as prescribed. Vital signs are assessed as are characteristics of the disorder and the amount of vaginal discharge.

Comfort measures include applying heat safely to the abdomen and administering analgesics agents for pain relief. Another nursing intervention is prevention of transmission of infection to others by impeccable hand hygiene and use of barrier precautions, and hospital guidelines for disposing of biohazardous articles (e.g. pads).

Hospitalized patients must maintain bedrest. While in bed, they remain in semi-Fowler's position to facilitate dependent drainage. Before discharge, patients are taught self-care measures:

1. Inform patient of the need for precaution and encourage to take part in procedures to prevent infecting others and protect themselves from reinfection. Stress that if a partner is not well known to her or has had other sexual partners recently. Use of condoms is essential to prevent infection and sequel.
2. Explain how pelvic infections occur, how they can be controlled and avoided, and their signs and symptoms such as abdominal pain, nausea and vomiting, fever, malaise, malodorous purulent vaginal discharge and leukocytosis.
3. Evaluate any pelvic pain or abnormal discharge, particularly after sexual exposure, childbirth or pelvic surgery.
4. Inform patient that IUDs may increase the risk for infection and for that antibiotics may be prescribed.
5. Instruct the patient to use proper perineal care, wiping from front to back.
6. Instruct patient to avoid douching, which can reduce natural flora.
7. Teach patient to consult with healthcare provider if unusual vaginal discharge or odor is noted.
8. Educate patient to maintain optimal health with proper nutrition, exercise, weight control and safer sex practices (e.g. using condoms, avoiding multiple sexual partners).
9. Advise patient to have a gynecological examination at least once a year.
10. Provide information about signs and symptoms of ectopic pregnancy (pain, abnormal bleeding, faintness, dizziness and shoulder pain).

PREMENSTRUAL SYNDROME

Premenstrual syndrome (PMS) is a recurrence problem for many women. Exact cause is not understood, but ovarian hormones, aldosterone and neurotransmitters such as monoamine oxidase and serotonin may play a role in PMS.

Clinical Manifestations

- Water retention, headaches
- Discomfort of joints, muscles and breasts

- Changes in effect, concentration and coordinations
- Sensory changes
- Some experience serious enough to interfere with work or relationships.

Therapeutic Measures

1. There are a variety of drugs available to combat PMS.
2. Drugs used to affect prostaglandin production and reuptake (antidepressants) as well as diuretic.
3. Supplement calcium, magnesium, vitamin B_6, vitamin E.

Nursing Management

1. Give prescribed medications.
2. Psychological counseling if psychological impaired.
3. Provide education materials on lifestyle measures such as restriction of alcohol, caffeine, nicotine, salt, simple sugar, participation and regular exercise, and development of stress managerial skills to reduce symptoms.

DYSMENORRHEA

Dysmenorrhea or painful menstruation is common problem in women. These are of two types:

1. Primary dysmenorrhea (menstrual cramps) is not a pathological and thought to be caused mainly by the action of indigenous prostaglandins that stimulate uterine contractions, producing cramping pain.
2. Secondary dysmenorrhea is caused by a reproductive tract disorder such as endometriosis, pelvic infection and retroversion of uterus or fibroid tumor.

Diagnostic Tests

- Hormonal tests for estrogen and progesterone
- Laparoscopic examination, biopsies or cultures.

Therapeutic Measures

1. Treated with drugs that inhibit prostaglandin synthesis such as Aspirin and non-steroidal anti-inflammatory drugs (NSAIDs) for primary dysmenorrhea.
2. Hormonal adjustment with oral contraception or hormones (D&C).
3. Dilation and curettage or other surgical or medical intervention.

Nursing Management

1. Women are advised to read label and take Aspirin or NSAIDs.
2. If dysmenorrhea related to uterine retroversion ask them to assuming knee-to-chest position to relieve discomfort.
3. Suddenly occurred cases are advised to proper investigation.

CANCER OF THE VAGINA

Cancer of the vagina is rare and usually takes years to develop. Primary cancer of the vagina is usually squamous in origin. Malignant melanoma and sarcomas can occur. Risk factors include previous cervical cancer, in utero exposure to diethylstilbestrol (DES), previous vaginal or vulvar cancer, previous radiation therapy, history of human papillomavirus (HPV) infection or pessary use. Any patient with previous cervical cancer should be examined regularly for vaginal lesion.

Clinical Manifestations

1. Often asymptomatic, but slight bleeding after intercourse may be reported.
2. Spontaneous bleeding, vaginal discharge, pain, urinary or rectal symptoms.

Diagnostic Methods

1. Colposcopy for women exposed to DES in utero.
2. Pap smear of the vagina.

Medical Management/Therapeutic Measures

1. Treatment of early lesions may include local excision, topical chemotherapy or laser.
2. Surgery for more advanced lesions (depends on the size and the stage of the cancer) followed by reconstructive surgery, if needed and radiation.

Nursing Management

1. Encourage close follow-up by healthcare providers.
2. Provide emotional support.
3. Inform women who had vaginal reconstructive surgery that regular intercourse may be helpful in preventing vaginal stenosis.
4. Inform patient that water-soluble lubricants are helpful in reducing dyspareunia.

CANCER OF THE VULVA

Primary cancer of vulva is seen mostly in postmenopausal women, but this incidence in younger women is rising. Squamous cell carcinoma accounts for most primary vulvar tumors; less common are Bartholin's gland cancer, vulvar sarcoma and malignant melanoma. The median age of cancer limited to the vulva is 50 years; the median age for invasive vulvar cancer is 70 years. Possible risk factors include smoking, HPV infection, human immunodeficiency virus (HIV) infection.

Clinical Manifestations

1. Long-standing pruritus and soreness are the most common symptoms; itching occurs in half of all patients.
2. Bleeding, foul-smelling discharge and pain are signs of advanced disease.
3. Early lesions appear as chronic dermatitis; later a lump that continues to grow and becomes a hard, ulcerated, cauliflower-like growth.

Diagnostic Methods

- Regular pelvic examinations, Pap smears and vulvar self-examination are helpful in early detection

- Biopsy
- Vulvar self-examination.

Medical Management/Therapeutic Measures

1. Preinvasive (vulvar carcinoma in situ): Local excision, laser ablation, chemotherapeutic creams (fluorouracil) or cryosurgery.
2. Invasive: Wide excision or vulvectomy, external beam radiation, laser therapy or chemotherapy.
3. If a widespread area is involved or the disease is advanced, radical vulvectomy with bilateral groin dissection may be performed; antibiotic and heparin prophylaxis may be continued postoperatively; graduated compression stockings applied.

Nursing Management

Assessment

1. Perform health history; tactfully elicit the reason who delay, if occurred, in seeking health care.
2. Assess health habits and lifestyle; evaluate receptivity teaching.
3. Assess psychological factors; give preoperative preparation and psychological support.

Nursing Interventions

Preoperative

Relieving anxiety

1. Allow time for patient to talk and ask questions.
2. Advise patient that the possibility of having sexual relation is good and pregnancy is possible after a wide excision.
3. Reinforce information about surgery.
4. Skin preparation may include cleansing the lower abdomen, inguinal areas, upper thighs and vulva with a germicide for several days before the surgical procedure. Patient may be instructed to do this at home.

Postoperatively

Relieving pain and discomfort

- Administer analgesic agents preventively
- Position patient to relieve tension on incision (pillow to knees or low-Fowler's position) and give soothing back support.

Improving skin integrity

- Provide pressure-reducing mattress
- Install over-bed trapeze
- Protect intact skin from drainage and moisture
- Change dressings as needed to ensure patient comfort, perform wound care and irrigation (if prescribed) that permit after observation of the surgical site
- Always protect patient from exposure, when visitors or someone else enters the room.

Support positive sexuality and sexual function

- Establish a trusting relationship with patient
- Encourage patient to share and discuss concerns with usual partner

- Consult with surgeon to clarify expected changes
- Refer patient and partner to a sex counselor, as indicated.

Managing complications

- Monitor closely for local and systemic signs and symptoms of infection; purulent drainage, redness, increased fever, increased white blood cell (WBC) count
- Assist in obtaining tissue specimens for culture
- Administer antibiotics as prescribed
- Avoid cross-contamination; carefully handle catheter drainage and dressings; hand hygiene is crucial
- Provide a low-residue diet to prevent straining on detention and wound contamination
- Assess for signs and symptoms of deep vein thrombosis and pulmonary embolism; apply elastic compression stock encourage ankle exercise
- Encourage and assist in frequent position changes, avoiding pressure behind the knees
- Encourage fluid intake to prevent dehydration
- Monitor closely for signs of hemorrhage and hypovolemic shock.

Promoting family-based care and follow-up

- Encourage patient to share concerns as she recovers
- Encourage for participation in dressing changes and self-care
- Give complete instructions to family members or others, who will provide posthospital care regarding wound care, urinary catheterization and possible complications
- Encourage communication with home care nurse to ensure continuity of care
- Reinforce teaching with follow-up call between home visits.

ENDOMETRIOSIS

Endometriosis is a condition in which functioning endometrial tissue is located outside the uterus. The development of this condition may be due to faulty development and differentiations of cells, transport of endometrial cells via blood and lymph to other parts of the body and retrograde menstruations.

Endometriosis is a benign lesion with cells to those lining the uterus, growing aberrantly in the pelvic cavity outside the uterus. During menstruation, this ectopic tissue bleeds, mostly into area having no outlet, which causes pain and adhesions. Endometrial tissue can also be spread by lymphatic or venous channels. There is a high incidence among patients, who bear children later and have fewer children. It is usually found in nulliparous women between 25 and 35 years of age and in adolescents, particularly those with dysmenorrheal that does not respond to NSAIDs or oral contraceptives. There appears to be a familial predisposition to endometriosis. It is a major cause of chronic pelvic pain and infertility.

Clinical Manifestations

Endometrial cells grow on areas, where sufficient blood supply extending into tissues such as intestinal walls, ovaries and other abdominal structures:

1. On a cyclic basis, mediated by ovarian hormones, these cells building and slough just as they would in the uterus, but sloughing and bleeding occurs in the enclosed abdominal cavity or into the tissue that they have invaded.

2. The buildup of the blood and cells can result in pain, swelling, damage to abdominal organs and structures, scar tissues development and infertility.
3. Symptoms vary but include dysmenorrhea, dyspareunia and pelvic discomfort or pain (some patients have no pain).
4. Dyschezia (pain with bowel movements) and radiation of pain to the back or leg may occur.
5. Depression, inability to work due to pain and difficulties in personal relationship may result.
6. Infertility may occur.

Diagnostic Methods

A health history, including an account of the menstrual pattern, is necessary to elicit specific symptoms. On bimanual pelvic examination fixed tender nodules are sometimes palpated and uterine mobility may be limited, indicating adhesions. Laparoscopic examination confirms the diagnosis and enables clinicians to determine the disease's stage.

Medical Management/Therapeutic Measures

Treatment depends on symptoms, desire for pregnancy and extent of the disease. In asymptomatic cases, routine examination may be all, i.e. required. Other therapy for varying degrees of symptoms may be NSAIDs, oral contraceptives, gonadotropin-releasing hormone (GnRH) agonists or surgery. Pregnancy often alleviates symptoms because neither ovulation nor menstruation occurs.

Medication Therapy

1. Palliative measures (e.g. use of medications such as analgesic agents and prostaglandin inhibitors) for pain.
2. Oral contraceptives.
3. Synthetic androgen, danazol (Danocrine), causes atrophy of the endometrium and subsequent amenorrhea (danazol is expensive and may cause troublesome side effects such as fatigue, depression, weight gain, oily skin, decreased breast size, mild acne, hot flashes and vaginal atrophy).
4. Gonadotropin-releasing hormone agonists decreased estrogen production and cause subsequent amenorrhea. Side effects are related to low estrogen levels (e.g. hot flashes and vaginal dryness).

Surgical Management

1. Laparoscopy to fulgurate endometrial implants and to release adhesions.
2. Laser surgery to vaporize or coagulate endometrial implants, thereby destroying the tissue.
3. Other surgical procedures may include endocoagulation and electrocoagulation, laparotomy, abdominal hysterectomy, oophorectomy, bilateral salpingo-oophorectomy and appendectomy. Hysterectomy may be an option for some women.

Nursing Management

1. Obtain health history and physical examination report, concentrating on identifying when and how long-specific

symptoms have been bothersome, the effect of prescribed medications and the women's reproductive plans.
2. Explain various diagnostic supports to the woman and her partner, who wish to have children.
3. Respect and address psychological impact of realization that pregnancy in not easily possible. Discuss alternatives such as in vitro fertilization (IVF) or adoption.
4. Encourage patient to seek care of dysmenorrheal or abnormal bleeding patterns.
5. Direct patient to the Endometriosis Association for more information and support.

UTERINE PROLAPSE

Uterine prolapse occurs when the uterus sags into the vagina. The amount of sagging can vary and may increase overtime as a result of the effect of gravity, poor pelvic support:
1. First degree prolapsed, less than half the uterus sags into the vagina.
2. Second degree prolapse, the entire uterus sags into the vagina.
3. Third degree prolapse, the uterus sags outside the body.

Clinical Manifestations

Uterine prolapse can be very uncomfortable, resulting:
- Back pain, pelvic pain with intercourse or inability to have intercourse, urinary incontinence, constipation and development of hemorrhoid
- Pressure on the uterus also may compromise circulation, resulting tissue necrosis
- Vaginal vault prolapse may occur in who have had hysterectomy
- Pain with menses or sexual intercourse
- Infertility
- Spontaneous abortion or preterm labor
- Prolapsed of uterus, bladder or rectum into vagina or outside of body.

Diagnostic Measures

- Physical examination
- Ultrasound, hysteron-salpingography
- Computed tomography (CT), magnetic resonance imaging (MRI), endoscopy.

Medical Management/Therapeutic Measures

- Minor cases treated with use of a pessary
- Kegel exercises are effective for prevention of uterine prolapsed
- Surgical interventions for resuspension of uterus, hysterectomy.

Nursing Management

- Take measure to relieve pain; analgesics required
- Take measures to incontinence or constipation related to structural abnormalities
- Take measure to relieve sexual dysfunction, correct self-concept
- Counseling require to grief related to absence or loss of reproductive status.

CERVICAL POLYPS

Polyp has benign growth that grow inside the uterus or on the cervix and may bleed after intercourse or between menstrual cycles. They are generally teardrops-shaped and are attached by a stalk. The cause is unknown, but estrogen plays a role in it.

Therapeutic Measures

Polyps are removed vaginally or transcervically by separating the stalk from the uterus and stopping bleeding by use of chemical, electrical or laser cautery.

Nursing Management

- Assist in surgical procedures
- Take measures in relieve pain related to lesion or surgery
- Take measure to relieve constipation or incontinence
- Take measure to disturbed body image related to body structures abnormality
- Take measure to develop self-confidence.

CANCER OF THE CERVIX

Cancer of the cervix is predominantly squamous cell cancer and also includes adenocarcinomas. It is less common than it once was because of early detection by the Pap test, but it remains the third most common reproductive cancer in women and is estimated to affect more than 11,000 women in the United States every year. Risk factors vary from multiple sex partners to smoking to chronic cervical infection (exposure to HPV).

Clinical Manifestations

1. Cervical cancer is most often symptomatic. When discharge, irregular bleeding or pain, or bleeding after sexual intercourse occurs, the disease may be advanced.
2. Vaginal discharge gradually increases in amount, becomes watery and finally is dark and foul smelling because of necrosis and infection of the tumor.
3. Bleeding occurs at irregular intervals between periods or after menopause, may be slight (enough to spot undergarments) and is usually noted after mild trauma (intercourse, douching or defecation). As disease continues, bleeding may persist and increase.
4. Leg pain, dysuria, rectal bleeding and edema of the extremities signal advanced disease.
5. Nerve involvement, producing excreting pain in the back and legs, occurs as cancer advances and tissues outside the cervix are invaded, including the fundus and lymph glands anterior to the sacrum.
6. Extreme emaciation and anemia, often with fever due to secondary infection and abscesses in the ulceration mass, and fistula formation may occur in the final stage.

Diagnostic Findings

1. Pap smear and biopsy results show severe dysplasia, high-grade squamous intraepithelial lesions (HGSIL) or carcinoma in situ.

2. Other tests may include X-rays, laboratory tests, special examinations (e.g. punch biopsy and colposcopy), D&C, CT, MRI, IV urography, cystography, positron emission tomography (PET) and barium X-ray studies.

Medical Management

Disease may be staged (usually TNM system; T describes the size of tumor, N describes lymph nodes that are involved and M descries distant metastasis) to estimate the extent of the disease, so that treatment can be planned more specifically and prognosis:

1. Conservative treatments include monitoring, cryotherapy (freezing with nitrous oxide), laser therapy, loop electrosurgical excision procedure (LEEP) or conization (removing a cone-shaped portion of cervix).
2. Simple hysterectomy if preinvasive cervical cancer (carcinoma in situ), platinum-based agents or a combination of these approaches may be used.
3. For recurrent cancer, pelvic exenteration is considered.

Nursing Management

Assessment

- Obtain a health history
- Perform physical and pelvic examination, and laboratory studies
- Gather data about the patient's psychological supports and responses.

Nursing Diagnoses

1. Anxiety related to diagnosis of cancer, fear of pain, perceived loss of feminity or childbearing potential.
2. Disturbed body imaged related to altered fertility, fears about sexuality and relationships with patient and family.
3. Pain related to surgery and other adjuvant therapy.
4. Deficient knowledge of perioperative aspects of hysterectomy and self-care.

Potential complications are hemorrhage, deep vein thrombosis, bladder dysfunction, infection.

Planning (Goals and Objectives)

The major goals may include relief of anxiety, acceptance of loss of the uterus, absence of pain or discomfort, increased knowledge of self-care requirements and absence of complications.

Nursing Interventions (Implementations)

Relieving Anxiety

1. Determine how this experience affects the patients and allow the patient to verbalize feelings and identify strengths.
2. Explain all preoperative, postoperative and recovery period preparations and procedures.

Improving Body Image

1. Assess how patients feels about undergoing a hysterectomy related to the nature of diagnosis, significant others, religious beliefs and prognosis.
2. Acknowledge patient's concern about ability to have children, loss of feminity and impact on sexual relations.
3. Educate patient about sexual relations such as sexual satisfaction, orgasm arise from clitoris stimulation, sexual feelings or comfort related to shortened vagina.
4. Explain that depression and heightened emotional sensitivity are expected because of upset hormonal balances.
5. Exhibit interest, concern and willingness to listen the fears.

Relieving Pain

1. Assess the intensity of the patient's pain and administer analgesics.
2. Encourage patient to resume intake of food and fluids gradually, when peristalsis is auscultated (1–2 day).
3. Encourage early ambulation.
4. Apply heat to abdomen or insert rectal tube, if prescribed for abdominal distention.

Managing Complications

1. Hemorrhage: Count perineal pads used and assess extent of saturation; monitor vital signs; check abdominal dressings for drainage; give guidelines for restricting activity to promote healing and prevent bleeding.
2. Deep vein thrombosis: Apply elastic compression stockings; encourage and assist in changing positions frequently; assist with early ambulation and leg exercises; monitor leg pain; instruct patient to avoid prolonged pressures at knees (sitting) and immobility.
3. Bladder dysfunction: Monitor for urinary output and assess for abdominal distention after catheter is removed; initiate measures to encourage voiding.

Promoting Family-based Care and Follow-up

1. Tailor information according to patient's need; no menstrual cycles, need for hormones.
2. Instruct patient to check surgical incision daily and report redness, purulent drainage or discharge.
3. Stress the importance of adequate oral intake and maintaining bowel and urinary tract function.
4. Instruct patient to resume activities gradually, no sitting for long periods; postoperative fatigue should gradually decrease.
5. Teach that showers are preferable to tub baths to reduce risk for infection and injury getting in and out of tub.
6. Avoid lifting, straining, sexual intercourse or driving until advised by physician.
7. Report vaginal discharge, foul odor, excessive bleeding, leg redness or pain, or elevated temperature to healthcare professional promptly.

8. Make follow-up telephone contact with patient to address concerns and determine progress; remind patient about postoperative follow-up appointments.
9. Remind patient to discuss hormone therapy with primary physician, if ovaries are removed.

Evaluation

Evaluation is done on the basis of objectives of care/expected patient outcome:
- Experiences decreased anxiety
- Has improved body image
- Experiences minimal pain and discomfort
- Verbalizes knowledge and understanding of self-care
- Experiences no complications.

FIBROID TUMOR

Fibroid tumor or leiomyoma are benign tumors made up of endometrial cells than have implanted on or within the walls of uterus.

Clinical Manifestations

1. Fibroid can grow very large and may cause:
   a. Pain or menstrual disorder.
   b. Exert pressure on the bladder and bowel causes necrosis, and interfere with fertility.
2. Fibroids are estrogen sensitive, needs hormone suppression.
3. Surgery: Myomectomy through abdomen or vaginal incision through laparoscope or hysterectomy may be for large fibroids.

Nursing Management

For more details refer 'Cervical Polyps.'

CANCER OF OVARY

Ovarian cancer is the leading cause of gynecological cancer deaths in the United States, with peak incidence in the early 1980s. Despite care physical examination, ovarian tumors are often difficult to detect because they are usually deep in the pelvis. No definitive causative factors have been determined, but pregnancy and oral contraceptives appear to provide a protective effect. Most (90%) ovarian cancers are epithelial in origin; other tumors include germ cell tumors and stromal tumors. Risk factors include a history of breast cancer, a family history of ovarian cancer, old age, low parity and obesity.

Clinical Manifestations

1. Increased abdominal girth, pelvic pressure, bloating, back pain, constipation, abdominal pain, urinary urgency, indigestion, flatulence, increased waist size, leg pain and pelvis pain.
2. Vague gastrointestinal (GI) symptoms or a palpable ovary in a postmenopausal woman.

Diagnostic Methods

1. No screening mechanism exists; tumor markers are being explored. Biannual examination is recommended for at risk women.
2. Any enlarged ovary must be investigated; pelvic examination does not detect early ovarian cancer and pelvic imaging techniques are not always definitive.
3. Transvaginal ultrasound and CA-125 antigen testing are helpful for high-risk women.

Medical Management/Therapeutic Measures

1. Surgical removal is the treatment of choice.
2. Preoperative work-up can include a barium enema or colonoscopy under GI series, MRI, ultrasound, chest X-rays, IV urography and CT.
3. Staging of the tumor is preformed to direct treatment.
4. Likely treatment involves a total abdominal hysterectomy with removal of the fallopian tubes and ovaries and possibly, the omentum (bilateral salpingo-oophorectomy and omentectomy); tumor debulking; para-aortic and pelvic lymph node sampling; diaphragmatic biopsies; random peritoneal biopsies and cytological washings.
5. Chemotherapy including liposomal and intraperitoneal delivery is the most common form of treatment for advanced disease [e.g. cisplatin, paclitaxel (Taxol)].
6. Gene therapy is a future possibility.

Nursing Management

1. Perform nursing measures, including treatment related to surgery, radiation, chemotherapy and palliation. Refer 'Nursing Management' under 'Cancer.'
2. Monitor for complications of therapy and abdominal surgery; report manifestations of complications to physician.
3. Determine patient's emotional needs, including desire for childbearing. Provide emotional support by giving comfort, showing attentiveness and caring. Allow patient to express feelings about condition and risk for death.

CANCER OF THE ENDOMETRIUM

Cancer of the uterine endometrium (fundus or corpus) is the fourth most common cancer in women. Most uterine cancers are endometrioid (i.e. originating in the lining of the uterus) type I, which accounts for the majority of cases, is estrogen related and occurs in about 10% of cases, in high grade and usually serous cell or clear cell. It affects older women. Type III, which also occurs in about 10% of cases, is hereditary or genetic types, some of which are related to the Lynch II syndrome (this syndrome is associated with the occurrence of breast, ovarian, colon, endometrial and other cancers throughout a family). Cumulative exposure to estrogen is considered the major factor. Other risk factor includes age above 55 years, obesity, early menarche, late menopause, nulliparity, anovulation, infertility and diabetes as well as use of tamoxifen.

Clinical Manifestations

Irregular bleeding and postmenopausal bleeding raise suspicion of endometrial cancer.

Diagnostic Methods

- Annual check-up and gynecological examination
- Endometrial aspiration or biopsy is performed with perimenopausal or menopausal bleeding
- Ultrasonography.

Medical Management/Therapeutic Measures

Refer 'Medical Management/Therapeutic Measures' under 'Cancer of the Breast' discussed later in this chapter.

Nursing Management

Refer 'Nursing Management' under 'Cancer' for additional information and 'Nursing Management' of 'Cancer of the Breast'.

Implementation/Nursing Intervention

Refer 'Postoperative' and 'Preoperative' 'Nursing Intervention' of 'Cancer of the Breast' for details.

Evaluation

Refer 'Evaluation' of 'Cancer of the Breast' for more information.

EPIDIDYMITIS

Epididymitis is an infection of the epididymis, which usually spreads form an infected urethra, bladder or prostate. In prepubertal males, older men and homosexual men, the predominant causal organism is *Escherichia coli,* although in older men, the condition may also be a result of urinary obstruction. In sexually active men aged 35 years and younger, the pathogens are usually related to bacteria associated with STDs (e.g. *Chlamydia trachomatis, Neisseria gonorrhoeae*).

Clinical Manifestations

1. Often slowly develops over 1–2 days, beginning with a low-grade fever, chills and heaviness in the affected testicles.
2. Unilateral pain and soreness in the inguinal canal along the course of the vas deferens.
3. Pain and swelling in the scrotum and groin.
4. There may be discharge from the urethra, blood in the semen, pus (pyuria) and bacteria (bacteriuria) in the urine, and pain during intercourse and ejaculation.
5. Urinary frequency, urgency or dysuria and testicular pain aggravated by bowel movement.

Medical Management/Therapeutic Measures

1. If epididymitis is associated with STD, the patient's partner should also receive antimicrobial therapy.

2. If seen within first 24 hours after onset of pain, patient's spermatic cord may be infiltrated with a local anesthetic agent for relief.
3. Support interventions include reduction in physical activity, scrotal support and elevation, ice packs, anti-inflammatory agents, analgesics, including nerve blocks and sitz baths.
4. Observe for abscess formation.
5. Epididymectomy (excision of the epididymis from the testes) may be performed for patients, who have recurrent, refractory, incapacitating episodes of this infection.

Nursing Management

1. Place patient on bedrest with scrotum elevated with a scrotal bridge or folded towel to prevent traction on spermatic cord, to improve venous drainage and to relieve pain.
2. Give antimicrobial medications as prescribed.
3. Provide intermittent cold compresses to scrotum to help ease pain; later, local heat or sitz baths may hasten resolution of inflammatory process.
4. Give analgesics agents as prescribed for pain relief.
5. Instruct patient to avoid straining, lifting and sexual stimulation until infection in under control.
6. Instruct patient to continue with analgesic and antibiotic medications as prescribed and to use ice packs as necessary for discomfort.
7. Explain that it may take 4 weeks or longer for the epididymis to return to normal.

ORCHITIS

Orchitis is a rare inflammation or infection of testicles. The problem may be caused by trauma or infection from epididymitis, urinary tract injection (UTI), sexually transmitted infection (STI) or systemic diseases such as influenza, infection mononucleosis, tuberculosis, gout, pneumonia or mumps after puberty.

Clinical Manifestations

1. The patient has swollen, extremely tender testicles, red scrotal skin and fever.
2. Complications such as sterility as orchitis caused by mumps.

Therapeutic Measure and Nursing Management

1. Bedrest with scrotal support.
2. Antibiotic, analgesics, antipyretics as ordered.
3. Taking mumps vaccine at early age.

MASTITIS

Mastitis is a breast infection with inflammation. It can occur as a result of injury or introduction of bacteria into the breast. This condition more commonly occurs while breastfeeding.

Clinical Manifestation

The breast becomes swollen, hot, red and purple, and can form an abscess.

Therapeutic Measures

1. Can be treated either with antibiotics or by incision and drainage (I&D) of the abscessed area.
2. Warm packs, NSAIDs and breast support are often used to control pain and swelling.

Nursing Management

1. Assist with an I&D by setting out the equipment, i.e. a wrapped sterile sharp pointed scalpel blade, a blade handle, clean gloves and dressing materials.
2. A dressing may be applied over the I&D site to absorb drainage.
3. Teach patient to wash hand carefully to prevent spread of infection.
4. If the patient has to give breastfeeding, it is often continued and promotes drainage of the breast, mother-infant bonding and infant nutrition.

CANCER OF THE BREAST

Cancer of the breast is a pathological entity that starts with a genetic alteration in a single cell and may take several years to become palpable. The most common histological type of breast cancer is infiltrating ductal carcinoma (80% of cases), whereby tumors arise from the duct system and invade the surrounding tissues. Infiltrating lobular carcinoma accounts for 10%–15% of cases. These tumors arise from the lobular epithelium and typically occur as an area of ill-defined thickening in the breast. Infiltrating ductal and lobular carcinomas usually spread to bone, lung, liver, adrenals, pleura, skin or brain. Several less common invasive cancers such as medullary carcinoma (5% of cases), mucinous carcinoma (3% of cases) and tubular ductal carcinoma (2% of cases) have very favorable prognoses. Inflammatory carcinoma and Paget's disease are less common forms of breast cancer. Ductal carcinoma in situ is a non-invasive form of cancer (also called intraductal carcinoma), but if left untreated there is an increased likelihood that it will progress to invasive cancer. There is no specific cause of breast cancer; rather, a combination of genetic, hormonal and possibly environmental events may contribute to its development. If lymph nodes are unaffected, the prognosis is better. They key to improved cure rates is early diagnosis, before metastasis.

Risk Factors

1. Gender (female) and increasing age.
2. Previous breast cancer: The risk of developing cancer in the same or opposite breast is significantly increased.
3. Family history: Having first-degree relative with breast cancer (mother, sister, daughter) increases the risk two fold; having two first-degree relatives increases the risk five fold.
4. Genetic mutations *(BRCA1 or BRCA2)* account for majority of inherited breast cancers.
5. Hormonal factors: Early menarche (before 12 years of age), nulliparity, first birth after 30 years of age, late menopause (after 55 years of age) and hormone therapy.
6. Other factors may include exposure to ionizing radiation during adolescence and early adulthood obesity, alcohol intake (beer, wine or liquor), high-fat diet (controversial, more research needed).

Protective Factors

Protective factors may include regular vigorous exercise (decreased body fat), pregnancy before age 30 years and breastfeeding.

Prevention Strategies

Patients at high risk for breast cancer may consult with specialists regarding possible or appropriate prevention strategies such as the following:

- Long-term surveillance consisting of twice-yearly clinical breast examinations starting at age 25 years, yearly mammography and possibly MRI (in *BRCA1* and *BRCA2* carriers)
- Chemoprevention to prevent disease before it starts, using tamoxifen (Nolvadex) and possibly raloxifene (Evista)
- Prophylactic mastectomy ('risk-reducing' mastectomy) for patients with strong family history of breast cancer, a diagnosis of lobular carcinoma in situ (LCIS) or atypical hyperplasia, a *BRCA* gene mutation, an extreme fear of cancer (cancer phobia) or previous cancer in one breast.

Clinical Manifestations

- Generally, lesions are nontender, fixed and hard with irregular borders; most occur in the upper outer quadrant
- Some women have no symptoms and no palpable lump but have an abnormal mammogram
- Advanced signs may include skin dimpling, nipple restraction or skin ulceration.

Diagnostic Methods

- Biopsy (e.g. percutaneous, surgical) and histological examination of cancer cells
- Tumor staging and analysis of additional prognostic factors are used to determine the prognosis and optimal treatment regimen
- Chest X-rays, CT, MRI, PET scan, bone scans and blood tests [complete blood cell count, comprehensive metabolic panel, tumor markers, i.e. carcinoembryonic antigen (CEA/CA 15-3)].

Staging of Breast Cancer

Classifying tumors as stage 0, I or IV is fairly straightforward; stage II and III tumors represent a wide spectrum of breast cancers and are subdivided into stage IIA, IIB, IIIA, IIIB and IIIC. Factors determining stages include number and characteristic of axillary lymph nodes, status of other regional lymph nodes and involvement of the skin or underlying muscle. Refer 'Staging' under 'Cancer'.

Medical Management/Therapeutic Measures

Various management options are available. The patient and physician may decide on surgery, radiation therapy chemotherapy or hormonal therapy, or combination therapies. These are the following:

1. Modified radical mastectomy involves removal of the entire breast tissue including the nipple-areaola complex and portion of the axillary lymph nodes.

2. Total mastectomy involves removal of the breast and nipple areola complex, but does not include ALND.
3. Breast-conserving surgery: Lumpectomy, wide excision, partial or segmental mastectomy, quadrantectomy followed by lymph node removal for invasive breast cancer.
4. Sentinel lymph node biopsy: Considered a standard of care for the treatment of early-stage breast cancer.
5. External-beam radiation therapy: Typically whole breast radiation, but partial breast radiation (radiation to the lumpectomy site alone) is now being evaluated at some institution in carefully selected patients.
6. Chemotherapy to eradicate micrometastic spread of the disease: Cyclophosphamide (Cytoxan), methotrexate, fluorouracil, anthracyline-based regimens [e.g. doxorubicin (Adriamycin) epirubicin (Ellence), taxanes. (paclitaxin, Taxol), docetaxel (Taxotere)].
7. Hormonal therapy based on the index of estrogen and progestrone receptors: Tamoxifen (Soltamox) is the primary hormonal agent used to suppress hormonal dependent tumors: others are inhibitors anastrozole (Arimidex), letrozole (Femara) and exemestane (Aromasin).
8. Targeted therapy: Trastuzumab (Herceptin), bevacizumab (Avastin).
9. Breast reconstruction.

Nursing Management

Refer 'Nursing Management' under 'Cancer' for additional information.

Assessment

- Perform a health history
- Assess the patient's reaction to the diagnosis and ability to cope with it
- Ask about coping skills, support systems, knowledge deficit and presence of discomfort.

Preoperative Nursing Diagnoses/Problems

- Deficient knowledge about the planned surgical treatments
- Anxiety related to cancer diagnosis
- Fear related to specific treatments and body image changes
- Risk for ineffective coping (individual or family) related to the diagnosis of breast cancer and treatment options
- Decisional conflict related to treatment options.

Postoperative Nursing Diagnoses/Problems

- Pain and discomfort related to surgical procedure
- Disturbed sensory perception related to nerve irritation in affected arm, breast or chest wall
- Disturbed body image related to loss or alteration of the breast
- Risk for impaired adjustment relate to the diagnosis of cancer and surgical treatment
- Self-care deficit related to partial immobility of upper extremity on operative side

- Risk for sexual dysfunction related to loss of body part change in self-image and fear of partner's responses
- Deficient knowledge: Drain management after breast surgery, arm exercises to regain mobility of affected extremity, hand and arm care after an ALND.

Potential complications: Lymphedema, hematoma/seroma formation, infection.

Planning and Goals

The major goals may include increased knowledge about the disease and its treatment; reduction of preoperative and postoperative fear anxiety and emotional stress; improvement of decision-making ability; pain management; improvement in coping abilities improvement in sexual function and the absence of complications.

Preoperative Nursing Interventions

Providing Education and Preparation about Surgical Treatments

1. Review treatment options by reinforcing information provided to the patient and answer any questions.
2. Fully prepare the patient for what to expect before, during and after surgery.
3. Inform patient that she will often have decreased arm and shoulder mobility after an ALND; demonstrate range-of-motion exercises prior to discharge.
4. Reassure patient that appropriate analgesia and comfort measures will be provided.

Reducing Fear and Anxiety and Improving Coping Ability

1. Help patient cope with the physical and emotional effects of surgery.
2. Provide patient with realistic expectations about the healing process and expected recovery to help alleviate fears (e.g. fear of pain, concern about inability to care for oneself and one's family).
3. Inform patient about available resources at the treatment facility as well as in the breast cancer community (e.g. social workers psychiatrists and support groups) patient may find it helpful to talk to a breast cancer survivor who has undergone similar treatments.

Promoting Decision-making Ability

1. Help patient and family to weigh the risks and benefits of each option.
2. Ask patient questions about specific treatment options to help her focus on choosing an appropriate treatment (e.g. how would you feel about losing your breast? Are you considering breast reconstruction? If you choose to retain your breast, would you consider undergoing radiation treatments 5 days a week for 5–6 weeks?).
3. Support whatever decision the patient makes.

Postoperative Nursing Interventions

Relieving Pain and Discomfort

1. Carefully assess patient for pain; individual pain varies.
2. Encourage patient to use analgesics.
3. Prepare patient for a possible slight increase in pain after the first few days of surgery; this may occur as patients regain sensation around the surgical site and become more active.
4. Evaluate patients, who complain of excruciating pain to rule out any potential complications such as infection or a hematoma.
5. Suggest alternative methods of pain management (e.g. taking warm showers, using distraction methods such as guided imagery).

Managing Postoperative Sensations

Reassure patients that postoperative sensations (e.g. tenderness, soreness, numbness, tightness, pulling and twinges; phantom sensations after a mastectomy) are a normal part of healing and these sensations are not indicative of a problem.

Promoting Positive Body Image

1. Assess the patient's readiness to see the incision for the first time and provide gentle encouragement; ideally the patient will be with the nurse or another healthcare provider for support.
2. Maintain the patient's privacy.
3. Ask the patient what she perceives, acknowledge her feelings and allow to express her emotions; reassure patient that her feelings are normal.
4. If desired, provide patient, who has not had immediate reconstruction with a temporary breast form to place in her bra.

Promoting Positive Adjustment and Coping

1. Provide ongoing assessment of how the patient is coping with her diagnosis and treatment.
2. Assist patient in identifying and mobilizing her support systems the patient's spouse or partner may also need guidance, support and education; provide resources (e.g. reach to recovery program of the American Cancer Society, advocacy groups or a spiritual advisor).
3. Encourage the patient to discuss issues and concerns with other patients, who have had breast cancer.
4. Provide patient with information about the plan of care after treatment.
5. If patient displays ineffective coping, consultation with a mental health practitioner may be indicated.

Improving Sexual Function

1. Encourage the patient to discuss how she feels about herself and about possible reasons for a decrease in libido (e.g. fatigue, anxiety, self-consciousness).
2. Suggest that the patient vary the time of day for sexual activity (when the patient is less fired), assume positions that are more

comfortable and express affection using alternative measures (e.g. hugging, kissing, manual stimulation).

3. If sexual issues cannot be resolved, a referral for counseling (e.g. psychologist psychiatrist, psychiatric clinical nurse specialist, social worker, sex therapist) may be helpful.

Managing Potential Complications

1. Promote collateral or auxiliary lymph drainage by encouraging movement and exercise (e.g. hand pumps) through postoperative education.
2. Elevate arm above the heart.
3. Obtain referral for patient to therapist for compression sleeve and/or glove, exercises, manual lymph drainage and a discussion of ways to modify daily activities.
4. Teach patient proper incision care, signs and symptoms of infection and when to contact surgeon or nurse.
5. Monitor surgical site for gross swelling or drainage output and notify surgeon promptly.
6. If ordered, apply compression wrap to the incision.

Family and Community-based Care

Teaching patient's self-care

1. Assess patient's readiness to assume self-care; focus on teaching incision care, signs to report (infection, hematoma/seroma, arm swelling) pain management, arm exercises, hand and arm care, drainage management, activity restriction, and also include family member.
2. Provide follow-up with telephone calls to discuss concerns about incision, pain management, and patient and family adjustment.

Continuing care

1. Reinforce earlier teaching as needed.
2. Encourage patient to call with any questions or concerns.
3. Refer patient for home care as indicated or desired by patient.
4. Remind patient of the importance of participating in routine health screening.
5. Reinforce need for follow-up visits to the physician (every 3–6 months for the first several years).

Evaluation

Expected patient outcomes:

- Exhibits knowledge about diagnosis and treatment options
- Verbalizes willingness to deal with anxiety and fears
- Demonstrates ability to cope with diagnosis and treatment
- Makes decisions regarding treatment options in a timely manner
- Reports pain has decreased and states pain management strategies
- Identifies postoperative sensations and recognizes that they are a normal part of healing
- Exhibits clean, dry and intact surgical incision without signs of inflammation or infection
- Lists signs and symptoms of infection to be reported
- Verbalizes feelings regarding change in body image

- Participates actively in self-care activities
- Demonstrates knowledge of postdischarge recommendations and restrictions
- Experiences no complications.

CANCER OF THE TESTIS

Testicular cancer is the most common cancer in men aged 13–35 years and the second most common cancer in men aged 35–39 years. Testicular cancer is classified as germinal and non-germinal (stomal). Germinal tumors make up approximately 90% of all cancers of the testis and may further classified as seminomas (slow-growing, remain localized) and fast growing non-seminomas [choriocarcinomas (rare), embryonal carcinomas, teratomas and yolk sac tumors]. Non-germinal tumors (Leydig cell tumors and Sertoli cell tumors) may develop in the suppurative and hormone-producing tissues of stroma of the testicles. Risk factors for testicular cancer include undescended testicles (cryptorchidism), family history of testicular cancer and personal history testicular cancer. Other risk factors include race and ethnicity, HIV infection and occupational hazards (e.g. exposure to chemicals). Some testicular tumors tend to metastasize early, spreading from the testis to the lymph nodes in the retroperitoneum and to the lungs. Secondary testicular tumors (lymphoma) metastasize from other organs.

Clinical Manifestations

1. Symptoms appear gradually with a mass or lump on the testicle.
2. Painless enlargement of the testis occurs. Patient may complain of heaviness in the scrotum, inguinal area or lower abdomen.
3. Backache, pain in the abdomen, weight loss and general weakness may result from metastasis.

Diagnostic Methods

1. Testicular self-examination (TSE) is an effective early detection method.
2. Elevated alpha-fetoprotein (AFP) and beta-human chorionic gonadotropin (β-hCG) levels are used as tumor markers.
3. Tumor markers levels are used for diagnosis, staging and monitoring response to treatment.
4. Blood chemistry including lactate dehydrogenase.
5. Chest X-ray to assess for metastasis in the lungs and a transscrotal testicular ultrasound.
6. Inguinal orchiectomy, abdominal/pelvic CT and chest CT (if abdominal CT or chest X-ray is abnormal), brain MRI and bone scan.

Medical Management/Therapeutic Measures

The goals of management are to eradicate the disease and achieve a cure. Therapy is based on the cell type, the stage of the disease and risk classification tables (determined as good, intermediate and poor risks):

1. Orchiectomy and retroperitoneal lymph node dissection (RPLND); alternatives to more invasive open RPLND include nerve-sparing and laparoscopic RPLND.
2. Sperm banking before surgery is suggested.
3. Chemotherapy or radiation therapy.

4. Good results may be obtained by combining different types of treatments including surgery, radiation therapy and chemotherapy.

Nursing Management

1. Assess the patient's physical and psychological status, and monitor for response to and possible effects of surgery, chemotherapy and radiation therapy.
2. Address issues related to body image and sexuality.
3. Encourage patient to maintain a positive attitude during therapy.
4. Encourage follow-up evaluation studies and continual TSE (a patient with a history of one tumor of the testis has a greater chance of developing subsequent tumors).
5. Encourage healthy behaviors, including smoking cessation, healthy diet, minimization of alcohol intake and cancer screening activities.

Refer 'Nursing Management' under 'Cancer' for additional information.

PROSTATITIS

Prostatitis is an inflammation of the prostate gland that is often associated with lower urinary tract symptoms and symptoms of sexual discomfort and dysfunction. Prostatitis may be caused by infectious agent (bacteria, fungi, *Mycoplasma)* or other conditions (e.g. urethral stricture, benign prostatic hyperplasia). *E. coli* is the most commonly isolated organisms. There are four types of prostatitis; acute bacterial prostatitis (type I), chronic bacterial prostatitis (type II), chronic prostatitis/chronic pelvic pain syndrome (CP/CPPS) (type III) and asymptomatic inflammatory prostatitis (type IV).

Clinical Manifestations

1. Acute prostatitis is characterized by the sudden onset of fever, dysuria, perineal prostatic pain and severe lower urinary tract symptoms; dysuria, frequency, urgency, hesitancy and nocturia.
2. Approximately 5% of cases of type I prostatitis (acute prostatitis) progress to type II prostatitis (chronic bacterial prostatitis); patients with type II disease are typically asymptomatic between episodes.
3. Patients with type III prostatitis often have no bacteria in the urine in the presence of genitourinary pain.
4. Patients with type IV prostatitis are usually diagnosed incidentally during workup for infertility, an elevated prostate-specific antigen (PSA) test or other disorders.

Medical Management/Therapeutic Measures

The goal of treatment is to eradicate the casual organisms. Specific treatment is based on the type of prostatitis and on the results of culture and sensitivity testing of the urine:

1. If bacteria are cultured from the urine, antibiotics including trimethoprim-sulfamethoxazole (TMP-SMZ) or fluoroquinolone [e.g. ciprofloxacin (Cipro)], may be prescribed,

and continues therapy with low-dose antibiotics may be used to suppress the infection.
2. If the patient is afebrile and has a normal urinalysis, anti-inflammatory agents may be used; α-adrenergic blocker therapy [e.g. tamsulosin (Flomax)] may be prescribed to promote bladder and prostate relaxation.
3. Supportive, non-pharmacological therapies may be prescribed (e.g. biofeedback, pelvic floor training, physical therapy, sitz baths, stool softener).

Nursing Management

1. Administer antibiotics as prescribed.
2. Recommend comfort measures; analgesics, sitz baths for 10–20 minutes several times daily.
3. Instruct patient to complete prescribed course of antibiotics and recognize recurrent signs and symptoms of prostatitis.
4. Encourage fluids to satisfy thirst but do not 'force' them, because effective drug levels must be maintained in urine.
5. Instruct patient to avoid foods and drinks that have diuretic action or increase prostatic secretions, including alcohol, coffee, tea, chocolate, cola and spices.
6. Instruct patient to avoid sexual arousal and intercourse during periods of acute inflammation.
7. Advise patient to avoid sitting for long periods to minimize discomfort.
8. Emphasize that medical follow-up is necessary for at least 6 months to 1 year.
9. Advise patient that the UTI may recur and is taught to recognize its symptoms.

BENIGN PROSTATIC HYPERPLASIA AND PROSTATECTOMY

Benign prostatic hyperplasia (BPH) is enlargement or hypertrophy of the prostate gland. The prostate gland enlarges, extending upward into the bladder and obstructing the outflow of urine. Incomplete emptying of the bladder and urinary retention leading to urinary stasis may result in hydronephrosis, hydroureter and UTIs. The cause is not well understood, but evidence suggests hormonal involvement. BPH is common in men older than 40 years.

Clinical Manifestations

1. The prostate is large, rubbery and nontender. Prostatism (obstructive and irritative symptom complex) is noted.
2. Hesitancy is starting urination, increased frequency of urination, nocturia, urgency, abdominal straining.
3. Decrease in volume and force of urinary stream, interruption of urinary stream, dribbling.
4. Sensation of incomplete emptying of the bladder, acute urinary retention (more than 60 mL) and recurrent UTIs.
5. Fatigue, anorexia, nausea and vomiting, and pelvic discomfort are also reported, and ultimately azotemia and renal failure result with chronic urinary retention and large residual volumes.

Diagnostic Methods

1. Physical examination including digital rectal examination (DRE) and health history.

2. Urinalysis to screen for hematuria and UTI.
3. Prostate-specific antigen level is obtained if the patient has at least 10 years life expectancy and for whom knowledge of the presence of prostate cancer would change management.
4. Urinary flow-rate recording and the measurement of postvoid residual (PVR) urine.
5. Urodynamic studies, urethrocystoscopy and ultrasound may be performed.
6. Complete blood studies including clotting studies.

Medical Management/Therapeutic Measures

The treatment plan depends on the causes, severity of obstruction and condition of the patient. Treatment measures include the following:

1. Immediate catheterization if patient cannot void (an urologists may be consulted if an ordinary catheter cannot be inserted). A suprapubic cystostomy is sometimes necessary.
2. Watchful waiting to monitor disease progression.

Medications Used

1. Alpha-adrenergic blockers (e.g. alfuzosin, terazosin), which relax the smooth muscle of the bladder neck and prostate and 5α-reductase inhibitors.
2. Hormonal manipulation with antiandrogen agents [finasteride (Proscar)] decreases the size of the prostate and prevents the conversion of testosterone to dihydrotestosterone (DHT).
3. Use of phytotherapeutic agents and other dietary supplements [*Serenoa repens* (saw palmetto berry) and pygeum africanum (African plum)] are not recommended, although they are commonly used.

Surgical Management

1. Minimally invasive therapy: Transurethral microwave thermotherapy (TUMT; application of heat to prostatic tissue); transurethral needle ablation (TUNA; via thin needles placed in prostate gland); prostatic stents (but only for patients with urinary retention and in patients, who are poor surgical risks).
2. Surgical resection: Transurethral resection of the prostate, benchmark for surgical treatment; transurethral incision of the prostate (TUIP); transurethral electrovaporization laser therapy; and open prostatectomy.

Nursing Management

Refer 'Nursing Management of Prostatectomy' under 'Cancer of the Prostate' for additional information.

CANCER OF THE PROSTATE

Cancer of the prostate is the most common cancer in men (other than non-melanoma skin cancer) and is the second most common cause of cancer deaths in American men. African American men are twice likely than men of any other racial or ethnic group to die of prostate cancer.

Risk factors include increasing age, family history and possibly high-fat diet. Endogenous hormones, such as androgens and estrogens, also may be associated with the development of prostate cancer.

Clinical Manifestations

- Usually asymptomatic in early stage
- Nodule felt within the substance of the gland or extensive hardening in the posterior lobe.

In Advanced Stage

1. Lesion is stony hard and fixed.
2. Obstructive symptoms occur late in the disease; difficulty and frequency of urination, urinary retention, decreased size and force of urinary stream.
3. Blood in urine or semen; painful ejaculation.
4. Cancer can spread to lymph nodes and bone.
5. Symptoms of metastasis include backache, hip pain, personal and rectal discomfort, anemia, weight loss, weakness, nausea, oliguria and spontaneous pathological fractures; hematuria may result from urethral or bladder invasion.
6. Sexual dysfunction.

Diagnostic Methods

1. Digital rectal examination (preferably by the same examiner).
2. The diagnosis is confirmed by a histological examination of tissue removed surgically by transurethral resection of the prostate (TURP) open prostatectomy, ultrasound-guided transrectal needle biopsy or fine-needle aspiration.
3. Prostate-specific antigen level; transrectal ultrasound; bone scans, skeletal X-rays and MRI; pelvic CT or monoclonal antibody-based imaging may also be used.

Medical Management/Therapeutic Measures

Treatment is based on the patient's life expectancy, symptoms, risk of recurrence after definitive treatment, size of the tumor; Gleason score, PSA level, likelihood of complications and patient reference. Management can range from non-surgical methods that involve 'watchful waiting' to surgery (e.g. prostatectomy).

Radical Prostatectomy

1. Removal of the prostate, seminal vesicles, tips of the vas deferens, and often the surrounding fat, nerves and blood vessels through suprapubic approach (greater blood loss), perineal approach (easily contaminated, incontinence, impotence and rectal injury common) or retropubic approach (infection can readily start).
2. This procedure is used with patients, whose tumor is confined to the prostate.
3. Sexual impotency and various degrees of urinary incontinence commonly follow radical prostatectomy.

Radiation Therapy

1. Teletherapy [external beam radiation therapy (EBRT)] treatment option for patients with low-risk prostate cancer.
2. Brachytherapy (internal implants) commonly used therapy treatment option for early clinically organ-confined prostate cancer.
3. Side effects inflammation of the rectum, bowel and bladder (proctitis, enteritis and cystitis); acute urinary dysfunction; pain with urination and ejaculation; rectal urgency diarrhea and tenesmus; rectal proctitis, bleeding and rectal fistula; painless hematuria, chronic interstitial cystitis; urethral stricture erectile dysfunction and rarely, secondary cancers of the rectum and bladder.

Hormonal Treatment

1. Androgen deprivation therapy (ADT) accomplished either by surgical castration (bilateral orchiectomy, removal of the testes) or by medical castration with the administration of medications, such as luteinizing hormone-releasing hormone (LHRH) agonists.
2. Hypogonadism is responsible for the adverse effects of ADT, which include vasomotor flushing, loss of libido, decreased bone density (resulting in osteoporosis and fractures), anemia, fatigue, increased fat mass, lipid alterations, decreased muscle mass, gynecomastia (increased breast tissue) and mastodynia (breast/nipple tenderness).

Other Therapies

1. Chemotherapy.
2. Cryosurgery for those who cannot physically tolerate surgery or for recurrence.
3. Repeated TURPs to keep urethra patent; suprapubic of transurethral catheter drainage, when repeated transurethral resection (TUR) is impractical.
4. Opioid or non-opioid medications to control pain with metastasis to bone.
5. Blood transfusions to maintain adequate hemoglobin levels.
6. Various forms of complementary and alternative medicine (CAM).

Nursing Management of Prostatectomy

Assessment

1. Take a complete history with emphasis on urinary function and the effect of the underlying disorder on patient's lifestyle.
2. Note reports of urgency, frequency, nocturia, dysuria, urinary retention, hematuria or decreased ability to initiate voiding.
3. Note family history of cancer, heart disease or kidney disease, including hypertension.

Nursing Diagnoses

Preoperative

1. Anxiety related to inability to void.
2. Acute pain related to bladder distention.
3. Deficient knowledge of the problem and treatment protocol.

Postoperative

1. Acute pain related to surgical incision, catheter placement and bladder spasms.
2. Deficient knowledge about postoperative care.

Potential complications are hemorrhage and shock, infection, deep vein thrombosis, catheter obstruction, sexual dysfunction.

Planning (Goals and Objectives)

The major preoperative goals for the patient may include reduced anxiety and learning about his prostate disorder and the perioperative experience. The major postoperative goals may include maintenance of fluid volume balance, relief of pain and discomfort, ability to perform self-care activities, and absence of complications.

Nursing Interventions/Implementation

Preoperative

Reducing anxiety

1. Clarify the nature of the surgery and expected postoperative outcomes.
2. Provide privacy, and establish a trusting and professional relationship.
3. Encourage patient to discuss feelings and concerns.

Relieving discomfort

1. While patient is on bedrest, administer analgesic agents; initiate measures to relieve anxiety.
2. Monitor voiding patterns; watch for bladder distention.
3. Insert indwelling catheter if urinary retention is present or if laboratory tests results indicate azotemia.
4. Prepare patient for a cystostomy if urinary catheter is not tolerated.

Refer 'Preoperative' and 'Postoperative' under 'Nursing Management of Prostatectomy' for additional information.

Providing instruction

1. Review with the patient's anatomy of the affected structures and their function in relation to the urinary and reproductive system, using diagrams and other teaching aids if indicated.
2. Explain what will take place while the patient is prepared for diagnostic tests and then for surgery (depending on the type of prostatectomy planned).
3. Reinforce information given by the surgeon.
4. Explain procedures expected to occur during the immediate perioperative period, answer questions the patient or family may have, and provide emotional support.
5. Provide information about postoperative pain management.

Preparing patient for treatment

1. Apply graduated compression stockings.
2. Administer enema, if ordered.

Postoperative

Maintaining fluid balance

1. Closely monitor urine output and the amount of fluid used for irrigation maintain intake and output.

2. Monitor for electrolyte imbalances (e.g. hyponatremia), increasing blood pressure, confusion and respiratory distress.

Relieving pain

1. Distinguish cause and location of pain, including bladder spasms.
2. Give analgesic agents for incisional pain and smooth muscle relaxants for bladder spasms.
3. Monitor drainage tubing and irrigate drainage system to correct any obstruction.
4. Secure catheter to leg or abdomen.
5. Monitor dressings and adjust to ensure they are not too snug or not too saturated, or are improperly placed.
6. Provide stool softener, prune juice or an enema is prescribed.

Managing complications

Hemorrhage: Observe catheter drainage; note bright red bleeding with increased viscosity and clots; closely monitor vital signs, administer medications, IV fluids and blood component therapy as prescribed; maintain accurate record of intake and output; and carefully monitor drainage system. Provide explanations and reassurance to patient and family.

Infection: Use aseptic technique with dressing changes; avoid rectal thermometers, tubes and enemas; provide sitz bath and heat lamps to promote healing after sutures are removed; assess UTI and epididymitis; administer antibiotics as prescribed.

Thrombosis: Assess for deep vein thrombosis and pulmonary embolism; apply compression stockings. Assist patient to progress from dangling the day of surgery to ambulating the next morning; encourage patient to walk but not to sit for long periods of time. Monitor the patient receiving heparin for excessive bleeding.

Obstructed catheter: Observe lower abdomen for bladder distention; examine drainage bag, dressings and surgical incision for bleeding; monitor vital signs to detect hypotension; observe patient for restlessness, diaphoresis, pallor, any drop in blood pressure and an increasing pulse rate. Provide for patent drainage system; perform gentle irrigation as prescribed to remove blood clots.

Urinary incontinence: Encourage patient to take steps to prevent incontinence, improve continence, anticipate leakage and fatigue may be a concern soon or months after surgery. Medications, surgically placed implants of negative pressure devices may help restore function. Reassurance that libido usually returns and fatigue diminishes after recuperation may help. Providing privacy, confidentially and time to discuss issues of sexuality is important. Refer all to a sex therapist may be indicated. Urinary leakage around the wound may be noted after catheter removal.

Promoting family-based care and follow-up

1. Teach patient and family how to manage drainage system, monitor urinary output, perform wound care and use strategies to prevent complications.
2. Inform patient about signs and symptoms that should be reported to the physician (e.g. blood in the urine, decreased urine output, fever, change in wound drainage or calf tenderness).
3. Teach perineal exercises to help regain urinary control.
4. As indicated, discuss possible sexual dysfunction (provide a private environment) and refer for counseling.

5. Instruct patient not to perform Valsalva maneuver for 6–8 weeks because it increases venous pressure and may produce hematuria.
6. Urge patient to avoid long car trips and strenuous exercise, which increases tendency to bleed.
7. Inform patient that spicy foods, alcohol and coffee can cause bladder discomfort.
8. Encourage fluids to avoid dehydration and clot formation.
9. Refer for home care as indicated for follow-up.
10. Remind patient that return of bladder control may take time.

Evaluation

Expected Preoperative Patient Outcomes

1. Demonstrates reduced anxiety.
2. States pain and discomfort are decreased.
3. Relates understanding of surgical procedure and postoperative care (perineal muscle exercises and bladder control techniques).

Expected Postoperative Patient Outcomes

1. Relates relief of discomfort.
2. Exhibits fluid and electrolyte balance.
3. Performs self-care measures.
4. Remains free of complications.
5. Reports understanding of changes in sexual function.

PHIMOSIS

Phimosis is the term used to describe a condition in which the foreskin of an uncircumcised made becomes so tight that it is difficult or impossible to pull back away from the head of the penis. So it is impossible to clean the area underneath. Smegma, a cottage cheese-like secretion made by the glands of foreskin, becomes trapped under the foreskin leads to infection.

Therapeutic Measures

1. The physician may cut a small slit in the foreskin to relieve the pressure and treat the infection.
2. Full circumcision may be needed by surgeon.
3. Phimosis can be prevented by teaching uncircumcised male to pull the foreskin back carefully, wash with mild soap and water daily and replace the foreskin to its normal position.

PARAPHIMOSIS

Paraphimosis occurs when the uncircumcised foreskin is pulled back, during intercourse or bathing and not immediately replaced in a forward position. This causes constriction of the dorsal veins, which leads to edema and pain.

Therapeutic Measures

1. Moderate to severe paraphimosis are medical emergency require immediate intervention—longer the problem and possible gangrene.

2. Prevention through daily cleaning and replacing the foreskin in its normal place.

CANCER PENIS

Cancer penis has been found in men, who were not circumcised as infants or have acquired human papillomavirus (HPV).

Clinical Manifestations

Tumor is typically squamous cell carcinoma and look like a small, round, raised wart, induration or red area. It may spread the sexual partner.

Therapeutic Measures

1. Treated with minor surgery such as circumcision or laser removal of growth.
2. If the cancer is spread may require surgical removal, radiation and/or chemotherapy.
3. Penile reconstruction may be needed after and surgery.

PRIAPISM

Priapism is a painful erection that lasts longer than 4 hours. If not relieved it becomes medical emergency. The small veins in the corpora cavernosa spasm, so blood cannot drain penile tissues does not get oxygen and permanent tissue damage may result. There may be complete loss of erection ability after the priapism episode. Prolonged priapism can cause bladder and kidney problems.

Some causes of priapism are sickle cell anemia, leukemia, widespread cancer, spinal cord injury or tumors, use of medication to manage erectile dysfunction (Viagra) or recreational drugs (crack cocaine).

Therapeutic Measures

1. Medical emergency includes apply icepacks, use of sedatives, analgesics.
2. Inject medication directly into penis to relax vein systems, needle aspiration and irrigation of corpora.
3. Surgery to implant a shunt than reroutes blood flow.

ERECTILE DYSFUNCTION

Erectile dysfunction is an inability to have an erection sufficient for sexual intercourse. This condition may be caused by psychological and physical, i.e. often caused by stress, illness, fatigue or an excessive use of alcohol or drugs, which includes smell, anxiety, depression, fatigue, illness such as Peyronie's disease, kidney failure, treatment of prostate disease, low testosterone levels, diabetes mellitus, heart disease, atherosclerosis, metabolic syndrome stroke, spinal cord injury, parkinsonism disease, multiple sclerosis; tobacco use, alcohol use, drugs (marijuana) and medication such as antianxiety agents, antidepressants, antihistamine, antihypertensive, lauretis, muscle relaxation, opioids, NSAIDs, etc.

Diagnosis Measures

1. History: Medical surgical condition, medication, etc.
2. Blood tests: Glucose level, hormonal imbalances.
3. Sign of infection and other diseases.
4. Reported problem of obtain erection and key dissatisfaction with sexual performance.

Therapeutic Measures

Find out the cause and treat and nursing care accordingly:
- Oral medication
- Hormonal treatment
- Herbal remedies
- Surgical such as penile implants, vascular surgery as per cause
- Sexual devices and techniques.

Nursing Management

- Counseling
- Medication to increase blood flow to the penis
- Assist in surgical implants or repair of structural disorders
- Teach about cause and treatment of sexual dysfunction.

GONORRHEA

Sexually transmitted diseases are infection that can be transmitted through intimate contact with genitals, mouth or rectum of another individual. Some STDs can also be spread by other routes such as blood or body fluids.

Gonorrhea is caused by the bacterium *N. gonorrhoeae* and may be transmitted vaginally, rectally, orally or via contact with other mucous membranes or through contact with blood or body fluids.

Clinical Manifestations

1. In men it may be asymptomatic or may have urethritis with a yellow urethral discharge.
2. In women:
   a. Either no noticeable symptoms or have a sore throat, mucopurulent cervicitis (MPC), urethritis.
   b. Abnormal menstrual symptoms such as bleeding between periods.
   c. Pelvic inflammatory disease (PID) is caused by gonorrhea, it can also cause Fitz-Hugh-Curtis syndrome.
3. Fever, nausea, vomiting, lower abdominal pain may be present.
4. It may affect throat and rectum.
5. Inflammation of joints, skin, meninges and lining of heart.

Therapeutic Measure/Nursing Management

1. Use caution with penicillin allergies or renal or hepatic dysfunction.
2. Avoid excess sun exposure.
3. Administer cephalosporin per os (PO), intramuscular (IM) or IV as ordered.

4. Monitor side effects: GI upset, central nervous system (CNS) disturbance, rash, pruritus, elevated liver enzyme, pain at injection site.
5. Nurse's best protection against catching disease from blood and body fluids of infected patients is the strict precautions and maintaining his/her own healthy intact skin.

SYPHILIS

Syphilis is an ancient disease that has not disappeared, although it is overshadow by commonly occurring disease such as chlamydia. It occurs in three stages (refer Clinical Manifestations). It is caused by *Treponema pallidum,* a spirochete.

Clinical Manifestations

Primary Stage

Primary stage develops with an entry of organisms through the skin or mucous membrane. Between 3 and 90 days later a papula develops at the site of entry then slough off, leaving a painless red, ulcer are called chancre. Same time chancer may also develop in other areas of the body. It is only a typical symptom of syphilis. It may eventually heal, but organisms remain active in the infected person and can be passed on to them.

Secondary Stage

Secondary stage syphilis begin 2–8 weeks later and affects the body more generally, causing problems such as flu-like symptoms, joint pain, hair loss, skin rashes on soles of hand and feet, mouth sores and condylomatous growth in moist area of body.

Tertiary Stage

Tertiary stage, if untreated serious damage can occur. It can involve any organ system of the body. Spirochete may form gummas [tumor, of a rubbery consistency than can breakdown and ulcerate leaving holes in the body tissues. Common can damage the heart, circulatory system and nervous system. Ulceration can destroy area of vital tissue lead to mental and physical disability [general paralysis of insane (GPI), syphilitic heart disease (SHD)].

Syphilis can pass on to unborn child resulting hepatosplenomegaly, increased bilirubin, destruction of RBCs, birth defects (face), lymphadenopathy.

Diagnostic Measures

- Serological test for syphilis (STS)
- Venereal Disease Research Laboratory (VDRL) test
- Rapid plasma region (RPR)
- Automated reagin test (ART)
- Enzyme-linked immunosorbent assay (ELISA)
- Fluorescent treponemal antibody-absorption (FTA-ABS)
- Polymerase chain reaction (PCR).

Therapeutic Measures/Nursing Management

1. Administer antibiotics (penicillin, tetracycline, doxycycline)—give deep IM or slow IV.
2. Apply icepacks to injection site as needed.
3. Administer PO on empty stomach.
4. Monitor GI upset, CNS disturbance, rash, itching, fever, pain.
5. Instruct patient to report fever/rash.
6. Avoid tetracycline in children and pregnant women.

HERPES GENITALIS

Herpes infection is caused by the herpes simplex virus (HSV) types 1 and 2. These viruses have an affinity for tissues of the skin and nervous system and can lie dormant in nervous system tissues and then reactivate periodically when the body undergoes stress, fever or immune system compromise.

Clinical Manifestations

1. Herpes simplex virus can cause fever, blisters of the mouth as well as genital lesion.
2. Mostly associated with oral lesion (HIV-1), genital lesion (HIV-2).
3. After infection vesicles develop, spontaneously rupture and produce painful ulceration of the underlying skin tissues.
4. Asymptomatic latent periods are usually interrupted between the vesicular outbreaks.
5. Initial outbreak occurs from 2 days to 2 weeks after exposure may produce flu-like symptoms, urethritis cystitis, and MPC with vaginal discharge.
6. Infection of spinal nerve roots results sacral radiculopathy causing retention of urine and feces.
7. Later urethral stricture and risk for cervical cancer.

Diagnostic Measures

1. Testing for HSV: Collected swabs and scrapped specimen from lesions.
2. Blood-test: Western blot assay.

Therapeutic Measure/Nursing Management

1. Administer antiviral medication (acyclovir) inhibits deoxyribonucleic acid (DNA) synthesis.
2. Use systematic preparations cautiously with CNS, hepatic or renal disorder.
3. Infuse IV slowly.
4. Maintain hydration.
5. Caution patient that viral transmission can still occur during treatment.
6. Monitor GI upset, CNS disturbance, rash, urticaria elevated liver enzyme/blood urea nitrogen (BUN) levels.

GENITAL WARTS

Genital warts or condylomata acuminate common STD infection with HPV produces condylomata.

Clinical Manifestations

1. A soft, raised and verrucous fleshy tumor, which may also have finger-like projections and resemble cauliflower.
2. Lesions most commonly develop on external genitalia and perineum as well as internal vaginal walls and cervix in women.
3. Lesions may also develop on the other area of the body.
4. Some people remain asymptomatic, but still can transmit infection.
5. The HPV can passed on from pregnant woman to baby.

Diagnosis (Identifying HPV)

1. Apply dilute acetic acid to skin of the external genital area and anus. Examining with colposcope the area that turns a higher colon.
2. Biopsy for suspected soul turn and dot blot tests.

Therapeutic Measures

1. Administer antimitotics and acidic agents [trichloroacetic acid (TCA)/bichloroacetic acid (BCA) typically].
2. Instruct patient to return for repeated applications as needed.
3. Avoid medication contact with eyes or tissue surrounding lesion.
4. Apply antimitotic agents (podofilox solution) that can be applied by patient at home with cotton tipped applicator.
5. Instruct patient to apply warts only and allow to dry completely or as ordered by provider.
6. Apply antiviral/immune response modifier cream, which can be applied by patient at home.
7. Instruct patient to apply thin film to clean dry skin at bedtime as ordered by provider.
8. May take up to 16 weeks to complete clean warts.
9. Monitor side effects such as local pain, burning, inflammation, erosion, itching or local irritation and report.
10. The warts may be treated by freezing, burning or chemical destroying.
11. Cryotherapy (freezing).
12. Electrocoagulated with a electrocautery (burning) or laser.
13. No cytotoxic drugs during pregnancy.

TRICHOMONIASIS

Trichomoniasis caused by carriers of *Trichomonas vaginalis.* A decrease in resident bacteria, injuries to the vaginal tissue and development of lesions from other STDs or from some form of cancer can activate the organism.

Clinical Manifestation

1. Asymptomatic for several years until changes in vaginal or urethral condition, encourage an outbreak of disease.
2. Symptoms include redness, swelling, itching and burning of the genital area; pain with intercourse and voiding and frothy, foul-smelling discharge.

3. Men with trichomonal infection can develop prostatitis and infertility.
4. Pregnant women with infection, are in risk preterm delivery or low-birth-weight baby.

Diagnostic Measures

1. Visualization of cervix shows strawberry cervix.
2. Pap smear readings.

Therapeutic Measures

1. Treat with amebicides/antiprotozoals, e.g. metronidazole.
2. Bind to DNA to inhibit synthesis and cause cell death.
3. Administer with food (PO or IV).
4. Avoid alcohol; abstain for minimum of 48 hours following treatment to prevent severe flu-like reaction.
5. Treat partner as well as patient.
6. Monitor side effects like GI upset, anorexia, headache, metallic taste or dry mouth, dysuria.
7. Monitor, rare but serious, seizures and peripheral neuropathy, and ECG changes.

BACTERIAL VAGINOSIS

The normal vaginal environment is a balanced ecosystem with pH of less than 4.2 as a result of lactic acid and hydrogen peroxide production by cells in the vagina. This protects against many pathogenic microorganism.

Various causative agents can irritate the vulva and the vagina. Signs and symptoms are often similar, but there as some deficiency. Bacterial vaginosis caused by *Gardnerella vaginalis, Mycoplasma* or anaerobic over growth.

Several conditions can predispose to an overgrowth of resident microbes such as poor nutrition (higher single sugars), inconsistent control of blood glucose (DM, stress, pregnancy), hormonal fluctuations, pH changes, prolonged overheating of genital area, changes on vaginal flora by antibiotic and douchers.

Clinical Manifestations

1. None and vulvar or vaginal irritation or asymptomatic.
2. Involve redness, itching, burning, excoriation, pain, swelling of the vagina and labia and discharge.
3. White or gray, homogenous, foul-smelling discharge.
4. pH more than 4.5.

Diagnostic Test

Wet mount slides show 'clue cells' or release fishy odor, when potassium hydroxide applied.

Therapeutic Measure

Administer antibiotic as prescribed.

CHLAMYDIA

Chlamydia is commonly diagnosed STD. It can be transmitted sexually and by the blood and body fluids contact. It is caused *Chlamydia trachomatis (C. trachomatis).*

Clinical Manifestations

1. Chlamydia is asymptomatic in women (a salient STD), but can cause urethritis, MPC and conjunctivitis.
2. In men urethritis, epididymitis, prostatitis.
3. Complications: Fitz-Hugh-Curtis syndrome.
4. Increased susceptibility to HIV infection.
5. Infertility, PID.
6. Transmission to baby at birth.
7. Coinfection with gonorrhea.

Diagnosed Measures

Nucleic acid amplification testing (NAAT) by collecting collections of specimens.

Therapeutic Measures

Treat with antibiotic such as:

1. Macrolides (erythromycin, azithromycin), which inhibits bacterial protein synthesis (IV or PO). Administer on empty stomach, but do not administer with antacids, use caution with hepatic disorders.
2. Tetracycline (doxycycline) inhibits protein synthesis by binding ribosomes. Do not give during pregnancy and do not give with antacids or diary product.
3. Amoxicillin binds to bacterial cells walls, causing cell death. Administer on empty stomach, avoid unnecessary exposure to sunlight.
4. Fluoroquinolones inhibits cell wall synthesis. Safety under age 18 not established, do not give the antacids. Use caution with other medications and with renal, hepatic and cardiovascular system (CVS) disorder.
5. Monitor side effects like abdominal pain, cramping, GI upset, rash are growth of non-susceptible bacteria, anorexia, dysphagia, photosensitivity urticaria, increased pigmentation, may increase anticoagulation/dizziness, headache, CVS disturbance, flatulence/pruritus, etc.

HEPATITIS B (STD CATEGORY)

Hepatitis B (HB) is an infection of the liver caused by Hepatitis B virus (HBV). It can be transmitted through sexual contact with blood and body fluids. During pregnancy HBV may be transmitted to the fetus, which can result in acute hepatitis.

Clinical Manifestations

1. Early signs are loss of appetite, rashes, malaise muscle and joint pain, headache, nausea and vomiting.

2. Since not affects livers, urine may darken and stool color may lighten due to therapy on bile excretion.
3. Liver enzymes may raise and jaundice may appear.
4. Enlargement of spleen, tenderness of liver, necrosis of liver cells, cirrhosis, coma and death may occur.
5. Chronicity may lead to liver cancer.

Diagnostic Test

Blood test based on antigen and antibodies, liver enzyme, liver biopsy.

Therapeutic Measures

1. If person exposed to HBV, hepatitis B immunoglobulin should be injected within 24 hours.
2. Supportive medical care with avoidance drugs that require liver metabolism.
3. Interferon-alpha therapy and antiviral agents as prescribed.
4. The HBV vaccine for healthcare worker for prevention of HB.
5. Use standard precaution, when contact with body fluids.
6. The HBV vaccine at birth before discharge from hospital can be repeated after 1–2 months and final close at age of 24 weeks or older.
7. Infant whose mother HBV+ve will receive HBV immunoglobulin and HBV vaccine within 12 hours.

17

Chapter Dermatological Nursing

PEDICULOSIS

Pediculosis is an infestation by lice. There are three basic types:

- Pediculosis capitis (head lice)
- Pediculosis corporis (body lice)
- Pediculosis pubis (pubic and crab like).

Generally, the lice bite the skin and feed on human blood, leaving their eggs and excrement, which can cause intense itching.

Clinical Manifestation

1. Pediculosis capitis: No itching or intense itching and scratching, especially at the back of the head and it may be attached to hair (a papular rash).
2. Pediculosis corporis: May appear as tiny hemorrhage paints. Excoriations may be noted on the back, shoulders, abdomen and extremities or may cause itching.
3. Pediculosis pubis—mild to severe itching especially at night:
   a. Black or reddish brown dots (like excreta) may be noted on the base of the hairs or in underclothing.
   b. Gray-blue macules may be noted on the trunk, thighs and axilla, this is the result of insects saliva mixing bilirubin.

Complications

Bacterial infections, impetigo, furundes, pustules, crusts matted hairs (for Pediculosis capitis), secondary infections, hyperpigmentation (for Pediculosis corporis), dermatitis and coexistence, and sexually transmitted diseases (STDs) (for Pediculosis pubic).

Diagnostic Test

- History
- Physical examination
- Sexually transmitted disease (STD) tests.

Therapeutic Measures

1. Treatment aimed at killing the parasite and mechanic removal.
2. Permethrin (Nix) application or over-the-counter (OTC) medication and preparing.
3. Lindanne if OTC not affecting.
4. Complications are treated with antipruritic, topical steroids and systemic antibiotics.
5. Ophthalmic ointment if eye or eyelash affecting with precaution.
6. Prevention involves avoidance of contact with infected person to objects.
7. Brushes, combs, hats other personal items should not be shared.
8. Good personal hygiene, routine clothes washing and wearing.
9. Reassurance the patient and family.

10. Instruct patient to bathe with soap and water, disinfect comb, and brushes in hot medicated soapy water.
11. Nits can removed from eyebrows and eyelashes.
12. Linen, clothing should be laundered in hot water using detergent and hygiene measure followed.
13. Use shampoos and lotion to kill nits.

SCABIES

Scabies is a contagious skin diseases caused by the mite *Sarcoptes scabiei.* It results from intimate or prolonged skin contact or prolonged contact with infected clothing, bedding or animals (e.g. dogs, cats). These burrows appear as short, wavy brownish and black lines.

Clinical Manifestation

1. The patient is asymptomatic while organism multiple lice, but not it is contagious at this time. Symptoms do not occur until 4 weeks after contact.
2. The major complains are itching and rash.
3. Itching intense at night, occurs after 1 month after infestation and may persists for days to weeks after treatment.
4. Rash appears as small, scattered erythematous papules, concentrated in finger webs, axillae, wrist folds, umbilicus, groin and genitals.
5. Crusts and scales may be present.
6. Male patient may have excoriated papules on the penis and groin area.
7. Complication: Crusted lesions, vesicles, pustules, excoriates and heat infection (hypersensitive reaction).

Diagnosis

Diagnosis includes superficial sharing of lesion and microscopic examination for adult mites, eggs, feces.

Therapeutic Measures

1. Application of scabicides (permethrin, crotamiton) are used for chemical disinfection.
2. Usually cream or lotion applied in a thin layer to the entire body from neck to feet (including genitals, umbilicus and skin fold areas) is left on overnight 8–12 hours, and washed off in morning.
3. Package instruction should be observed.
4. This application usually curative, depending upon agents prescribing.
5. Antipruritic may be used for itching.
6. All patient and animals in intimate contact with infected patients should be treated and evaluation for mites.
7. Bed linen, clothes, towels should be washed properly.
8. Educate patient to have a warm soapy bath or shower, remove seals and skin debris.
9. Advise the patient to apply topical medication as ordered.
10. Treat family members with close contacts to eliminate mites.
11. To wear clean clothing and to use clean linen.
12. Remind the patient that itching may continue up to 2 weeks after treatment.

CANDIDIASIS

Infection of skin or mucous membranes with *candida* called candidiasis. It grows in warm moist areas such as under breasts, in groin, vagina or oral mucous membranes. Oral candidiasis are called thrush.

Clinical Manifestation

1. Appears as white patches in mouth, white vaginal discharge or red irritates areas in skin folds.
2. May occur as a result of antibiotic therapy, because normal flora than usually keep *candida* in check are destroyed or with corticosteroid therapy.

Therapeutic Measures/Nursing

1. Oral or topical antifungal agents are used. For example, 'nystatin swish and swallow' or Lozenges for oral thrush, nystatin powder or ointment for skin infections or vaginal suppositories or creams.
2. Teach the patient to keep skin clean and dry, especially in skinfold area. Treatment is important to prevent systemic infections.

IMPETIGO

Impetigo is a superficial infection of the skin caused by staphylococci, streptococci or multiple bacteria. Exposed area of the body, face, hands, neck and extremities are most frequently involved. Impetigo is contagious and may spread to other parts of the skin or to other members of the family, who touch the patient or who use towels or combs that are soiled with exudates of the lesion. Impetigo is seen in people of all ages. It is particularly common among children living in poor hygiene conditions. Chronic health problems, poor hygiene and malnutrition may predispose adults to impetigo.

Clinical Manifestations

1. Lesions begin in small, red macules that become discrete, thin-walled vesicles that rupture and become covered with a honey-yellow crust.
2. These crusts, when removed reveal smooth, red, moist surfaces on which new crusts develop.
3. If the scalp is involved, the hair is matted, distinguishing the condition from ringworms.
4. Bullous impetigo, a deep-seated infection of the skin caused by *Staphylococcus aureus,* is characterized by the formation of bullae from original vesicles. The bullae rupture leaving a raw and red area.

Medical Management/Therapeutic Measures

Systemic antibiotic therapy is usual treatment for impetigo. It reduces contagious spread, treats deep infection and prevents acute glomerulonephritis (kidney infection):

1. Agents for non-bullous impetigo: Benzathine penicillin, oral penicillin or erythromycin.
2. Topical antibacterial therapy is the usual treatment for disease that is limited to a small area. The topical preparation is applied

to the lesions several times a day for 1 week. Lesions are soaked or washed with soap solution to remove central site of bacterial growth and to give the topical antibiotic an opportunity to reach the infected site.

Nursing Management

1. Use antiseptic solutions chlorhexidine (Hibiclens) to cleanse the skin and reduce bacterial content and prevent spread.
2. Wear gloves when giving care to patients with impetigo.
3. Instruct patient and family to bathe at least once daily with bacterial soap.
4. Encourage cleanliness and good hygiene practices to prevent spread of lesion from one skin area to another and from one person to another.
5. Instruct patient and family not to share bath towels and washcloths and to avoid physical contact between the infected person and other people until lesion heals.

FURUNCLES AND CARBUNCLES

Furuncle is a small, tender boil that occurs deep in one or more hair follicles and spreads to surrounding dermis may be single or multiple; usually caused by *Staphylococcus;* usually occurs on body areas prone to excessive perspiration, friction and irritation (i.e. buttocks, axillae) can recur. The boil eventually becomes to a soft yellow, black or white head; there is localized pain, tenderness and surrounding cellulitis lymphadenopathy may be present. Furuncles may progress to more several carbuncles.

A carbuncles is an abscess of skin and subcutaneous tissue, deeper than a furuncle; usually caused by *Staphylococcus;* usually appears where skin in thick, fibrous and elastic (i.e. back of the neck, upper back and buttock); associated symptoms may include fever, pain, leukocytosis, prostration. Carbuncle may progress to infection of bloodstream. Further spread of infection can occur to self and others.

Treatment/Nursing Management

1. Assist physician with draining lesion.
2. Administer antibiotics as prescribed.
3. Prevent trauma, avoid squeezing or irritations.
4. Cleanse surrounding skin with antibacterial soaps followed by application of antibacterial ointment.
5. Surgical incision and drainage maybe performed.
6. Cover draining lesion with dressings.
7. Follow universal standard precautions. Double soiled dressings and dispose of them properly.

FUNGAL INFECTIONS (DERMOTOMYCOSIS)

Dermatomycosis or fungal infection of the skin occurs when there is an impairment of the skin integrity in a warm moist environment. This infection occurs through direct contact with infected humans, animals or objects. Tinea is the term used to describe fungal infection, tenea indication the body area affected.

HERPES SIMPLEX

Herpes simplex virus (HSV) infection is common viral infection that tends to recur repeated. There are two types: HSV-1, which occurs above the waist and causes fever and blister or cold sore and HSV-2 occurs below the waist cause of genital herpes. Primary HSV infection occurs through direct contact, respiratory droplet or fluid exposure from another infected person.

Clinical Manifestations

1. Following initial infection, the virus lives dormant in nerve ganglia near the spinal column, where the immune system cannot destroy it. So passive in asymptomatic.
2. Recurrence of symptomatic infection happens, simultaneously or may triggered by stress such as fever, sunburn, illness, menses, fatigue or injury.
3. The secondary lesion may appear isolated or a groups of small vesicles or pustules on erythematous base.
4. Crusts eventually forms and lesion heals, almost 1 week the lesion are contagious.
5. Some patients may have prodromal phase of burning and tingling at the site for a few hours before eruption.
6. They become erythematous, swollen, there may be redness with no blistering.
7. Lesions can burn itch and be painful.

Complications

- Herpes simplex virus in vagina at childbirth, newborn are also infected
- Touched organs may be infected.

Diagnosis

- Culture of lesion
- History
- Signs and symptoms.

Therapeutic Measures

1. Topical acyclovir ointment for primary lesions.
2. Oral antiviral medications as ordered.
3. Various lotions, creams and ointments may be prescribed to accelerate drying healing of lesions, e.g. camphor, phenol, alcohol.
4. Antibiotic secondary infection.

HERPES ZOSTER (SHINGLES)

Herpes zoster or shingles is an acute inflammation and infectious disorder that produces a painful vascular eruption on bright red edematous plaques along with distribution of nerve from one or more posterior ganglia. This eruption follow the course of the cutaneous sensory nerve and are almost always unilateral. It is caused by the varicella zoster virus (which causes chickenpox). It may occur in those who have diminished resistance except elderly or acquired immunodeficiency syndrome (AIDS).

Clinical Manifestations

1. The incubation period of herpes zoster is 7–21 days.
2. Vesicles appear over the course of 3–4 days.
3. Eruption occurs posteriorly and progress anteriorly and peripherally along dermatome.
4. Total duration of outbreak can vary from 10 to 5 weeks.
5. In addition to vesicles and plague, there may be irritation, fever, malaise and depending on locations of lesions, and visceral involvement.
6. Lesions maybe very painful; incidence of pain increase with age.

Complications

- Postherpetic neuralgia
- Cranial nerve involvement leads to hearing loss
- Tinnitus
- Facial paralysis
- Vertigo.

Diagnostic

- History
- Physical examination
- Culture test for secondary infections.

Therapeutic Measures

The objective is to control outbreak, reducing pain, discomfort and complication:

1. Mild cases may heal without medication.
2. Antiviral agents for severe infections, e.g. acyclovir.
3. Analgesic on prescribed.
4. Anticonvulsant or antidepressants for neuropathic pain.
5. Antihistamine to control itching.
6. Antibiotics for secondary bacterial infection.
7. In addition to medications, cold compresses or both may help with pain and itching.
8. Topical agents containing calamine or lidocaine are helpful, but not in steroid preparations.
9. The disease can be prevented by avoidance of person with herpes zoster, during contagious phase:
   - Varicella vaccine for children and adult who has not had chickenpox (Zostavax vaccine for patient aged 60 year).

ACNE VULGARIS/VERRUCA VULGARIS

Acne vulgaris is common skin disorder of the sebaceous gland and their hair follicles that usually occurs on the face, chest, upper back and shoulder. The most common cause is hormonal changes during puberty. The sebaceous of androgens (in adolescence or menstrual cycle) in turn stimulates the sebaceous glands to increase sebum production. This along with gradual obstruction of the pilosebaceous ducts with accumulation debris, rupture of sebaceous glands, which causes inflammation. It may be due to hereditary, stress, external irritation (soaps and cosmetics).

Clinical Manifestations

1. The initial lesions are called comedone, closed comedones or white heads are small white papules with tiny follicular openings.
2. These may eventually become open comedones or blackheads.
3. The color is not caused by dirt, but by lipids and melanin pigment.
4. Scarring occurs, picking can lead to inflammation and further scarring.
5. Inflammatory reactions that may lead to papules, pustules, nodules and cysts.

Therapeutic Measures

1. Need to prevent new lesions and control current lesion.
2. Effective topical agent (benzoyl peroxide), which is antibacterial prevents pore plugging.
3. Antibiotic (erythromycin, tetracycline) to kill bacteria in follicles.
4. Topical agent may be used alone or in combination as prescribed.
5. Medication should not be applied near eyes, nasolabial folds or corners of the mouth.
6. Estrogen therapy for young women with precautions.
7. Other medical treatments include:
   - Comedone extraction, cryosurgery (freezing with liquid nitrogen)
   - Mild peeling [ultraviolet (UV) light, CO_2 liquid nitrogen, mild]
   - Dermabrasion (deep chemical peel)
   - Excision of scars and infection of fibrin or collagen below the scars. The treatment depends on severity, age, condition, physique and patient preference.

WARTS

Warts are small, common, benign growth of skin resulting from the hypertrophy of the papillae and epidermis, caused by virus. Common warts often seen on hands and fingers, appears as raised, flesh-colored papules that have rough surface. These warts only crack, fissure, bleed are painful to lateral pinching and direct firm pressure.

Plantar warts occur on the sole of the foot. They may appear granular, pitted or protuberant, with a callous surrounding the normal skin. Incubation period can be several weeks to months. Virus spread by direct contact into areas broken skin or other nails cuticle biting.

Therapeutic Measures/Nursing

1. If there is no pain or discomfort, no treatment may be indicated.
2. Patient should be cautioned not to spread lesions by picking or biting them.
3. Treatment is indicated, for symptomatic warts and for cosmetic purpose, which include:
   - Keratolytic agents (a salicylic acid plasters to soften and reduce keratin)
   - Cryotherapy (liquid nitrogen) and light electrodescication and curettage (require local anesthesia).

4. Treatment choice usually cryotherapy because local anesthesia not required and it leaves with scarring.

DERMATITIS

Dermatitis is inflammation of the skin and is characterized by itching, redness and skin lesions with varying borders, and disturbances patterns. There are three common types of dermatitis—contact dermatitis, atopic dermatitis and seborrheic dermatitis:

1. Contact dermatitis caused by exposure to an allergen or irritant such as soaps, perfumes or poison ivy.
2. Atoptic dermatitis tends to be hereditary and is associated with allergies, asthma, and hay fever.
3. Seborrheic dermatitis occurs most often on the scalp, usually on individuals with oily skin.

All types tend to the chronic and respond well to treatment.

Clinical Manifestations

- Itching, rashes
- Lesions vary depending on the type and location of dermation
- Rashes and lesions may present as dry, flaky scales, yellow crusts, redness, fissures, macules, papules and vesicles
- Scratching can make any of these lesions worse.

Complication

Infections of the skin.

Diagnosis

- History
- Symptoms
- Clinical findings.

Therapeutic Measures

1. Treatment varies according to symptoms, the goals of it is to control itching, alleviate discomfort and pain decrease inflammation, control or prevent crust formation and oozing prevent infection, prevent further damage and heal as early as possible.
2. Antihistamine, analgesic, antipruritic to relieve itching or discomfort.
3. Colloidal oatmeal preparations added to baths may help.
4. Steroids with an hydrocortisone to suppress inflammation.
5. Topical, intralesional, system agent for applications as prescribed.
6. Tub bath and wet dressings help control oozing and prevent crust form.
7. Clean area and apply topical medications.
8. Skin is protected by lightly patting dry, avoiding friction, avoiding hot water and using sun screen agents when outside.
9. It can be prevented by avoiding irritants, allergens, excessive heat and dryness and by control perspiration:
   - Baths should be short, tepid water deodorant soap should be avoided

- Dry skin can be lubricated with creams, oil and ointment asymptomatic.

Contact Dermatitis

Contact dermatitis is an inflammatory reaction of the skin to physical, chemical or biological agents. It may be of the primary irritant type or it may be allergic. The epidermis is damaged repeated physical and chemical irritation. Common causes of irritant dermatitis are soaps, detergents, scouring compounds and industrial chemicals. Predisposing factor includes extremes of heat, cold, frequent use of soap and water, and pre-existing skin disease.

Clinical Manifestations

1. Eruptions when the causative agent contacts the skin.
2. Itching, burning and erythema are followed by edema, papules, vesicles, and oozing or weeping as first reactions.
3. In the subacute phase, the vesicular changes are less marked and alternate with crusting, drying, fissuring, and peeling.
4. If repeated reactions occur or the patient continually scratches the skin, lichenification and pigmentation occur, and secondary bacterial invasion may follow.

Medical Management/Therapeutic Measures

1. Soothe and heal the involved skin and protect it from further damage.
2. Determine the distribution pattern of the reaction to differentiate between allergic type and irritant type.
3. Identify and remove the offending irritant; soap is generally not used on site until healed.
4. Use bland, unmedicated lotions for small patches of erythema; apply cool wet dressings over small areas of vesicular dermatitis; a corticosteroid ointment may be used.
5. Medicated bath at room temperature are prescribed for larger areas of dermatitis.
6. In severe, widespread conditions, a short course of systemic steroids may be prescribed.

Nursing Management

Instruct patient to adhere to the following instructions for at least 4 months, until the skin appears completely healed:

1. Think about what may have caused the problem.
2. Avoid contact with the irritants or wash skin thoroughly immediately after exposure to irritants.
3. Avoid heat, soap and rubbing the skin.
4. Choose bath soaps, detergents and cosmetics that do not contain fragrance; avoid using a fabric softener dryer sheet.
5. Avoid topical medications, lotions or ointments, except when prescribed.
6. When wearing gloves (e.g. for washing dishes, cleaning), make sure that they are cottonlined; do not wear for more than 15–20 minutes.

Exfoliative Dermatitis

Exfoliative dermatitis is a serious condition characterized by progressive inflammation in which erythema and scaling occur. The condition starts acutely either a patchy or a generalized erythematous eruption. Exfoliative dermatitis has a variety of causes. It is considered to be a secondary or reactive process to an underlying skin or systemic disease. It may appear as part of the lymphoma group of diseases and may precede the appearance of lymphoma. Pre-existing skin disorders implicated as a cause including psoriasis, atopic dermatitis and correct dermatitis. It also appears as a severe medication reaction to penicillin and phenylbutazone. The cause is unknown in about 25% of cases.

Clinical Manifestations

1. Chills, fever, malaise, prostration, severe toxicity, a pruritic scaling of the skin and occasionally gastrointestinal symptoms.
2. Profound loss of stratum corneum (outermost layer of the skin), causing capillary leakage, hypoproteinemia and negative nitrogen balance.
3. Widespread dilation of cutaneous vessels, resulting in large amount of body heat loss.
4. Skin color changes from pink to dark red after a week, exfoliation (scaling) begins in the form of thin flakes that leave the underlying skin smooth and red, with new scales forming as the older ones come off.
5. Possible hair loss.
6. Relapse common.
7. Systemic effects: High-output heart failure, other gastrointestinal disturbances, breast enlargement, hyperuricemia and temperature disturbances.

Medical Management/Therapeutic Measures

Goals of management are to maintain fluid and electrolyte balance and to prevent infection. Treatment is individualized and supportive, and is started as soon as condition is diagnosed:

1. Hospitalize patient and place on bedrest.
2. Discontinue all medications that may be implicated.
3. Maintain comfortable room temperature because of patient's abnormal thermoregulatory control.
4. Maintain fluid and electrolyte balance because of considerable water and protein loss from skin surface.
5. Give plasma expanders as indicated.
6. Observe for signs and symptoms of high-output heart failure due to hyperemia and increased blood flow.

Nursing Management

1. Carry out continual nursing assessment to detect infection.
2. Administer prescribed antibiotics on the basis of culture and sensitivity test results.
3. Assess for hypothermia because of increased skin blood flow coupled with increased heat and water loss through the skin.
4. Closely monitor and report changes in vital signs.
5. Use topical therapy for symptomatic relief.

6. Recommend soothing baths, compresses and lubricating with emollients to treat extensive dermatitis.
7. Administer prescribed oral or parenteral corticosteroids when disease is not controlled by more conservative therapy.
8. Advise patient to avoid all irritants, particularly medications.

Seborrheic Dermatitis

Seborrhea is an excessive production of sebum (secretion of sebaceous glands). Seborrheic dermatitis is a chronic inflammatory disease of the skin with a predilection for areas that are well supplied with sebaceous glands or that lie between folds of the skin, where the bacterial count is high. Seborrheic dermatitis has a genetic predisposition, hormones, nutritional status, infection and emotional stress influence its course. There are remissions and exacerbations of this condition. Areas most often affected are the face, scalp, cheeks, ears, axillae and various skin folds.

Clinical Manifestations

Two forms can occur: An oily form and a dry form. Either form may start in childhood with fine scaling of the scalp or other areas.

Oily form: Moist or greasy patches of swallow, greasy-appearing skin, with or without scaling and slight erythema (redness); small pustules of papulopustules on trunk resembling acne.

Dry form: Flaky desquamation of the scalp (dandruff) and asymptomatic mild forms or scaling often accompanied by pruritus leading to scratching and secondary infections and excoriation.

Medical Management/Therapeutic Measures

Because there is no known cure for seborrhea, the objectives of therapy are to control the disorder and allow the skin to repair itself. Treatment measures include the following:

1. Administering topical corticosteroid cream to body and face (use with caution near eyes).
2. Aerating skin and careful cleansing of creases or folds to prevent candidal yeast infection (evaluate patients with persistent candidiasis for diabetes).
3. Shampooing hair daily or at least three times weekly with medicated shampoos. Two or three different types of shampoos are used in rotation to prevent the seborrhea from becoming resistant to a particular shampoo.

Nursing Management

1. Advise patient to avoid external irritants, excess heat and perspiration; rubbing and scratching prolong the disorder.
2. Instruct patient to avoid secondary infections by airing the skin and keeping skin folds clean and dry.
3. Reinforce instructions for using medicated shampoos; frequent shampooing is contrary to some cultural practices, be sensitive to these differences, when teaching the patient about home care.
4. Caution patient that seborrheic dermatitis is a chronic problem that tends to reappear. The goal is to keep it under control.
5. Encourage patient to adhere to treatment program.

6. Treat patients with sensitivity and an awareness of their need to express their feelings when they become discouraged by the disorder effect on body image.

PRURITUS

Pruritus (itching) is one of the most common dermatological complaints. Scratching the itchy area causes the inflamed cells and nerve endings to release histamine, which produces more pruritus and in turn, a vicious itch-scratch cycle. Scratching can result in altered skin integrity with excoriation, redness, raised areas (wheals), infection or changes in pigmentation. Although pruritus usually due to primary skin disease, it may also reflect systemic internal disease, such as diabetes mellitus, renal, hepatic, thyroid or blood disorders, or cancer. Pruritus may be caused by certain oral medications (Aspirin, antibiotics, hormones, opioid), contact with irritating agents (soaps, chemicals) or prickly heat (miliaria). It may also be a side effect of radiation therapy, a reaction to chemotherapy or a symptom of infection. It may occur in elderly patients' as a result of dry skin. It may also be caused by psychological factors (emotional stress).

Clinical Manifestations

1. Itching and scratching, often more severe at night (itch-scratch-itch cycle).
2. Excoriations, redness, raised areas on the skin (wheals) are result of scratching.
3. Infectious or changes in pigmentation.
4. Debilitating itching in severe cases.

Medical Management/Therapeutic Measures

The cause of pruritus needs to be identified and treated. The patient is advised to avoid washing with soap and hot water. Cold compresses, ice cubes or cool agents that contain soothing menthol and camphor may be applied:

1. Bath oils (Lubath or Alpha Keri) are prescribed, except for elderly patients or those with impaired balance, who should not add oil to the bath because of the danger of slipping.
2. Topical corticosteroids are prescribed to decrease itching.
3. Oral antihistamines [diphenhydramine (Benadryl)] may be used.
4. Tricyclic antidepressants [doxepin (Sinequan)] may be prescribed when pruritus is of neuropsychogenic origin.

Nursing Management

1. Reinforce reasons for the prescribed therapeutic regimen.
2. Remind patient to use tepid (not hot) water and to shake off excess water and blot between intertriginous areas (body folds) with a towel.
3. Advise patient to avoid rubbing vigorously with towel, which over stimulates skin, causing more itching.
4. Lubricate skin with an emollient that traps moisture (specifically after bathing).
5. Advise patient to avoid situations that cause vasodilation (warm environment, ingestion of alcohol or hot foods and liquids).
6. Keep room cool and humidified.

7. Advise patient to wear soft cotton clothing next to skin and avoid activities that result in perspiration.
8. Instruct patient to avoid scratching and to trim nails short to prevent skin damage and infection.
9. When the underlying cause of pruritus in unknown and further testing is required, explain each test and the expected outcomes.

TOXIC EPIDERMAL NECROLYSIS AND STEVENS-JOHNSON SYNDROME

Toxic epidermal necrolysis and Stevens-Johnson syndrome are potentially fatal skin disorders and the most severe forms of erythema multiforme. Both conditions are triggered by medications. Antibiotics, antiseizures agents, non-steroidal anti-inflammatory drugs (NSAIDs), and sulfonamides are the medications most commonly implicated. The complete body surface may be involved, with widespread areas of erythema and blisters. Sepsis and keratonconjunctivitis are possible complications.

Clinical Manifestations

1. Initial signs are conjunctival burning or itching, cutaneous tenderness, fever, headache, cough, sore throat, extreme malaise and myalgias (aches and pains).
2. Rapid onset of erythema follows, involving much of the skin surface and mucous membranes, large flaccid bullae in some areas; in other areas, large sheets of epidermis are shed, exposing underlying dermis; fingernails, toenails, eyebrows and eyelashes may all be shed, along with surrounding epidermis.
3. Excruciatingly tender skin and loss of skin lead to a weeping surface similar to that of a total body partial thickness burn; this condition may be referred to as scalded skin syndrome.
4. In severe case of mucous involvement, there may be danger of damage to the larynx, bronchi and esophagus from ulcerations.

Diagnostic Measures

- Histological studies of frozen skin cells
- Cytodiagnosis of cells from a freshly denuded area
- Immunofluorescent studies for atypical epidermal autoantibodies.

Medical Management

Treatment goals include control of fluid and electrolyte balance, prevention of sepsis, and prevention of ophthalmic complications. The mainstay of treatment is supportive care:

1. All non-essential medications are discontinued immediately.
2. If possible, patient is treated in a regional burn center.
3. Surgical debridement or hydrotherapy is used initially to remove involved skin.
4. Tissues samples form nasopharynx, eyes, ears, blood, urine, skin and unruptured blisters are used to identify pathogens.
5. Intravenous fluids are prescribed to maintain fluid and electrolyte balance.
6. Fluid replacement is accomplished by nasogastric tube and orally as soon as possible.
7. Systemic corticosteroids are given early in the disease process (controversial).

8. Administration of intravenous immunoglobulin (IVIG) may provide rapid improvement and skin healing.
9. Skin is protected with topical agents; topical antibacterial and anesthetic agents are used to prevent wound sepsis.
10. Temporary biological dressings (pigskin, amniotic membranes or plastic semipermeable dressings (Vigilon) are applied.
11. Meticulous oropharyngeal and eye care is essential when there is severe involvement of mucous membranes and eyes.

Nursing Management

Assessment

1. Inspect appearance and extent of involvement of skin.
2. Monitor blister drainage for amount, color and odor.
3. Inspect oral cavity for blistering and erosive lesions daily.
4. Determine patient's ability to swallow and drink fluids, as well as speak normally.
5. Assess eye daily for itching, burning and dryness.
6. Monitor vital signs, paying special attention to fever, respiratory status and secretions.
7. Assess high fever, tachycardia, extreme weakness and fatigue (indicate the process of epidermal necrosis, increased metabolic needs, possible gastrointestinal and respiratory mucosal sloughing).
8. Monitor urine volume, specific gravity and color.
9. Inspect intravenous insertion sites for local signs of infection.
10. Record daily weight.
11. Question patient about fatigue and pain levels.
12. Assess level of anxiety and coping mechanisms, identify new effective coping skills.

Nursing Diagnoses/Problems

1. Impaired tissue integrity (oral, eye and skin) related to epidermal shedding.
2. Deficient fluid volume and electrolyte losses related to loss of fluids from denuded skin.
3. Risk for imbalanced body temperature (hypothermia) related to heat loss, secondary to skin loss.
4. Acute pain related to denuded skin, oral lesions and possible infection.
5. Anxiety related to the physical appearance and prognosis.

Potential complications: They are:

- Sepsis
- Conjunctival retraction
- Scars
- Corneal lesions.

Planning (Goals and Objectives)

Major goals may include skin and oral tissue healing, fluid balance, prevention of heat loss, relief of pain, reduced anxiety and absence of complications.

Nursing Intervention/Implementation

Maintaining Skin and Mucous Membranes Integrity

1. Take special care to avoid friction involving the skin when moving the patient in bed; check skin after each position change to ensure that no new denuded areas have appeared.
2. Apply prescribed topical agents to reduce wound bacteria.
3. Apply warm compresses gently, if prescribed, to denuded areas.
4. Use topical antibacterial agent in conjunction with hydrotherapy; monitor treatment and encourage patient to exercise extremities during hydrotherapy.
5. Perform oral hygiene carefully. Use prescribed mouthwashes, anesthetics or coating agents frequently to rid mouth of debris, soothe ulcerative areas and control odor. Inspect oral cavity frequently, note changes and report. Apply petrolatum to lips.

Fluid Balance Maintenance

1. Observe vital signs, urine output and sensorium for signs of hypovolemia.
2. Evaluate laboratory tests and report abnormal results.
3. Check weight of patient daily.
4. Provide enteral nourishment or if necessary, parenteral nutrition.
5. Record of intake and output, and daily calorie count.

Preventing Hypothermia

1. Maintain patient's comfort and body temperature with cotton blankets, ceiling-mounted heat lamps or heat shields.
2. Work rapidly and efficiently when large wounds are exposed for wound care to minimize shivering and heat loss.
3. Monitor patient's temperature carefully and frequently.

Relieving Pain

1. Assess the patient's pain, its characteristics, factors that influence the pain, and the patient's behavioral responses.
2. Administer prescribed analgesic agents and observe for pain relief, and side effects.
3. Administer analgesic agents before painful treatment.
4. Provide explanations and speak calmly to patient during treatments to allay anxiety, which may intensify pain.
5. Provide measures to promote rest and sleep; provide emotional support, and reassurance to achieve pain control.
6. Teach self-management techniques for pain relief, such as progressive muscle relaxation and imagery.

Reducing Anxiety

1. Assess emotional state (anxiety, fear of dying and depression); reassure patient that these reactions are normal.
2. Give support, be honest and offer hope that the situation will improve.
3. Encourage patient to express feelings to someone he/she trusts.
4. Listen to patient's concerns; provide skillful, compassionate care.
5. Provide emotional support during the long recovery period with psychiatric nurse, chaplain, psychologist or psychiatrist.

Managing Potential Complications

Sepsis: Monitor vital signs and note changes to allow early detection of infection. Maintain strict asepsis. If a large portion of the body is involved, place the patient in a private room with protective isolation.

Conjunctival retraction, scars and corneal lesion: Inspect eyes for progression of disease to keratoconjunctivitis (itching, burning and dryness). Administer eye lubricant. Use eye patches. Encourage patient to avoid rubbing eyes. Document and report the progression of symptoms.

Evaluation

Evaluations are done according to the objectives of care/expected patient outcomes:
- Achieves increasing skin and oral tissue healing
- Attains fluid balance
- Attains thermoregulation
- Achieves pain relief
- Appears less anxious
- Experiences no complication, such as asepsis and impaired vision.

PEMPHIGUS

Pemphigus is a group of serious disease of the skin characterized by the appearance of bullae (blisters) on apparently normal skin and mucous membranes (mouth, vagina). Evidence indicates that pemphigus is an autoimmune disease involving immunoglobulin G (IgG).

Pathophysiology

A blister forms from the antigen-antibody reaction. The level of serum antibody is predictive of disease severity. The condition may be associated with ingestion of penicillin, captopril and with myasthenia gravis. Genetic factors may also play a role, with the highest incidence in those of Jewish or Mediterranean descent. It occurs with equal frequency in men and women in middle, and late adulthood.

Clinical Manifestations

1. Most cases present with oral lesion appearing as irregularly shaped erosions that are painful, bleed easily and heal slowly.
2. Skin bullae enlarge, rupture and leave large painful eroded areas with crusting and oozing.
3. A characteristic odor emanates from the bullae and the exuding serum.
4. Blistering or sloughing of uninvolved skin occurs when minimal pressure is applied (Nikolsky's sign).
5. Eroded skin heals slowly and eventually huge areas of the body involved. Fluid and electrolyte imbalances and hypoalbuminemia may result from loss of fluid and protein.
6. Bacterial superinfection is common.

Diagnostic Findings

Diagnosis is confirmed by histological examination of a biopsy specimen and immunofluorescent examination of the serum, which show circulating pemphigus antibodies.

Medical Management/Therapeutic Measures

Goals of therapy are to bring the disease under control as secondary infection and promote re-epithelialization of the skin:

1. Corticosteroids are administered in high doses to control the disease and keep the skin free of blisters. The high dosage level is maintained until remission is apparent (monitor for serious toxic effects from high dose corticosteroid therapy).
2. Immunosuppressive agents (e.g. azathioprine, cyclophosphamide, gold) may be prescribed to help control the disease and reduce the corticosteroids dose.
3. Plasmapheresis is usually reserved for life-threatening cases.

Nursing Diagnoses/Problems

- Acute pain of oral cavity and skin related to blistering, and erosions
- Impaired skin integrity related to ruptured bullae and denuded areas of skin
- Anxiety and ineffective coping related to appearance of skin and no hope of cure
- Deficient knowledge about medications and side effects.

Potential complications: They are:

- Infection and sepsis related to loss of protective barrier of skin and mucous membranes
- Fluid volume deficit and electrolyte imbalance related to loss of tissue fluids.

Planning (Goals and Objectives)

The major goals may include relief of discomfort from lesions, skin healing, reduced anxiety and improved coping capacity, and absence of complications. The objective of care will be that the patient:

- Achieves relief from pain of oral lesions
- Achieves skin healing
- Experiences decreased anxiety and increased ability to cope
- Experiences no complications
- Disease activity is monitored by examining the skin for the appearance of new blisters as well as sign and symptoms of infection.

Nursing Interventions/Implementation

Relieving Oral Discomfort

1. Provide meticulous oral hygiene for cleanliness and regeneration of epithelium.
2. Provide frequent prescribed mouthwashes to rinse mouth of debris. Avoid commercial mouthwashes.
3. Keep lips moist with lanolin, petrolatum or lip balm.
4. Humidify environmental air.

Enhancing Skin Integrity and Relieving Discomfort

- Provide cool, wet dressings or baths (protective and soothing)
- Premedicate with analgesic agents before skin care is initiated
- Dry skin carefully and dust with non-irritating powder
- Avoid use of tape, which may produce more blisters
- Keep patient warm to avoid hypothermia.

Refer 'Nursing Management' under 'Burn Injury' for additional information.

Reducing Anxiety

- Demonstrate a warm and caring attitude: Allow patient to express anxieties, discomfort and feelings of hopelessness
- Educate patient and family regarding the disease
- Refer to psychological counseling as needed.

Managing Potential Complications

1. Keep skin clean to eliminate debris, dead skin and prevent infection.
2. Inspect oral cavity for secondary infections and *Candida albicans* infection from high-dose steroid therapy; report if noted.
3. Investigate all 'trivial' complaints or minimal changes because corticosteroids mask typical symptoms of infection.
4. Monitor for temperature fluctuations and chills; monitor secretions and excretions for changes suggestive of infection.
5. Administer antimicrobial agents as prescribed and note response to treatment.
6. Employ effective hand drying techniques; use protective isolation measures and standard precautions.
7. Avoid environmental contamination (have housekeeping department dust with a damp cloth and wash floor with a wet mop).

Achieving Fluid and Electrolyte Balance

- Administer saline infusion for sodium (Na) and depletion
- Administer blood component therapy
- Monitor serum albumin, Hb%, hematocrit of protein level
- Encourage adequate oral intake
- Provide cool, non-irritating fluids
- Provide parenteral nutrition, if patient cannot eat.

PSORIASIS

Psoriasis is a chronic, noninfectious, inflammatory disease of the skin in which the production of epidermal cells occurs faster than normal. Onset may occur at any age, but is most common between ages of 15 and 35 years. Main sites of the body affected are the scalp, areas over the elbows, knees, lower part of the back and genitalia, as well as the nails. Bilateral symmetry often exists. Psoriasis may be associated with asymmetric rheumatoid factor—negative arthritis of multiple joints. An exfoliative psoriatic state may develop in which the disease progresses to involve the total body surface (erythrodermic psoriatic state).

Pathophysiology

The basal skin cells divide too quickly and the newly formed cells become evident as profuse scales or plaques of epidermal tissue. As a result of the increased number of basal cells and rapid cell passage, the normal events of cell maturation and growth cannot occur, which prevents the normal protective layers of the skin to form. Current evidence supports an immunological basis for psoriasis. The primary defect is unknown. Periods of emotional stress and anxiety aggravate the condition and trauma, infections, seasonal and hormonal changes are also trigger factors.

Clinical Manifestations

Symptoms range from a cosmetic annoyance to a physically disabling and disfiguring affliction:

1. Lesions appear as red, raised patches of skin covered with silvery scales.
2. If scales are scraped away, the dark red base of lesion in exposed, with multiple bleeding point.
3. Patches are dry and may or may not itch.
4. The condition may involve nail pitting, discoloration, crumbling beneath the free edges and separation of the nail plate.
5. In erythrodermic psoriasis, the patient is acutely ill, with fevers, chills and electrolyte imbalance.
6. Psoriasis may cause despair and frustration. Observer may state, comment and ask embarrassing questions or even avoid the person.
7. The condition can eventually exhaust resources, interfere with work and negatively affect many aspects of life.
8. Teenagers are especially vulnerable to its psychological effects.

Diagnostic Findings

- Presence of classic plaque-type lesions (change histologically progressing from early to chronic plaques)
- Signs of nail and scalp involvement and positive family history.

Medical Management/Therapeutic Measures

Goals of management are to slow the rapid turnover of epidermis, to promote resolution of the psoriasis lesions and dermis, to control the natural cycles of the disease. There is no known cure. The therapeutic approach should be understandable, cosmetically acceptable and not too disruptive of lifestyle.

First, any precipitating or aggravating factors are addressed. An assessment is made of lifestyle, because psoriasis is significantly affected by stress. The most important principle of psoriasis treatment is gentle removal of scales (bath oils, coal tar preparations and a soft brush used to scrub the psoriasis plaques). After bathing, the application of emollient creams containing α-hydroxy acids (Lac-Hydrin, Penederm) of salicylic acid will continue to soften thick scales. Three types of therapy are standard: topical, systemic and phototherapy.

Topical Therapy

1. Topical therapy is used to slow the overactive epidermis.
2. Topical corticosteroids therapy acts to reduce inflammation.
3. Medications include tar preparations [e.g. coal tar topical (Balnetar)], α-hydroxy acids or salicylic acid and corticosteroids. Calcipotriene (Dovonex, not recommended for use by elderly patients because of their more fragile skin or in pregnant, or lactating women) and tazarotene (Tazorac) as well as vitamin D are additional non-steroidal agents. Occlusive (plastic) dressing may improve effectiveness. Medications may be in the form of lotions, ointments, pastes, creams and shampoos.

4. Assess the flammability of any plastic substances used; caution patients not to smoke or go near open flame.

Systemic Therapy

1. Biological agents act by inhibiting activation and migration, eliminating the T cells completely, slowing postsecretory cytokines or inducing immune deviation: Infliximab (Remicade), etanercept (Enbrel), efalizumab (Raptiva), alefacept (Amevive), and adalimumab (Humira). Biological agents have significant side effects, making close monitoring essential.
2. Oral agents: Methotrexate (patients should avoid drinking alcohol, should not be administered to pregnant women), cyclosporine A, oral retinoids (i.e. synthetic derivatives of vitamin A and its metabolite, vitamin A acid), etretinate; laboratory studies are monitored to ensure that hepatic, hematopoietic and renal system are functioning adequately.

Photochemotherapy

1. Psoralens and ultraviolet A (PUVA) therapy may be used for severely debilitating psoriasis.
2. Photochemotherapy is associated with long-term risks of skin cancer, cataracts and premature aging of the skin.
3. Ultraviolet B (UVB) light therapy may be used to treat generalized plaque and may be combined with the topical cream, calcipotriene (Dovonex). Excimer laser therapy may be another treatment.

Nursing Management

Assessment

Assessment focuses on how the patient is coping with the skin condition, the appearance of 'normal' skin and the appearance of skin lesions:

- Examine areas especially affected: Elbows, knees, scalp, gluteal cleft and all nails for small pits
- Assess the impact of the disease on the patient and the coping strategies used for conducting normal activities and interactions with family and friends
- Instruct the patient that the condition is not infectious, it is not a reflection of poor personal hygiene and is not skin cancer
- Create an environment in which the patient feels comfortable discussing important quality of life, issues related to his/her psychological and physical response to this chronic illness.

Planning

The goals of management include understanding the disease, promote skin integrity, improving self-concept and body image, management of complications, etc.

Nursing Interventions/Implementation

Promoting Understanding

1. Explain with sensitivity that there is no cure and that lifetime management is necessary; the disease process can usually be controlled.

2. Review pathophysiology of psoriasis and factors that provoke it. Any irritation or injury to the skin (cut, abrasion, sun burn), any current illness, emotional stress, unfavorable environment (cold) and drug (caution patient about non-prescription medication).
3. Review and explain treatment regimen to ensure compliance; provide patient education materials in addition to face-to-face discussions.

Increase Skin Integrity

- Advise patient not to pick the scratch areas
- Encourage patient to prevent the skin from drying out; dry skin causes psoriasis to worsen
- Inform patient that water should not be too hot and skin should be dried by patting with a towel
- Teach patient to use bath oil or emollient cleansing agent for sore and scaling skin.

Improving Self-concept and Body Image

Introduce coping strategies and suggestions for reducing or coping stressful situations to facilitate a more positive outlook and acceptance of the diseases.

Managing Complications

- Psoriatic arthritis: Note joint discomfort and evaluate further
- Educate patient about care and treatment and need for compliance
- Consult a rheumatologist to assist in the diagnosis and treatment of the arthropathy.

Promoting Family-based Care

1. Advise patient that topical corticosteroid preparations on face and around eyes predispose to cataract development.
2. Follow strict guidelines to avoid overuse.
3. Teach patient to avoid exposure to sun when undergoing PUVA treatments; if exposure is unavoidable, the skin must be protected with sunscreen and clothing, and sunglasses should be worn.
4. Remind patient to schedule ophthalmic examinations on a regular basis.
5. Advise female patient of childbearing age that PUVA therapy is teratogenic (can cause fetal defects); they may consider using contraceptives during therapy.
6. If indicated, refer to mental health professional, who can help ease emotional strain and give support.
7. Encourage patient to join a support group and to contact.

CANCER OF THE SKIN (MALIGNANT MELANOMA)

A malignant melanoma is a malignant neoplasm in which atypical melanocytes (pigment cells) are present in both the epidermis and the dermis (and sometimes the subcutaneous cells). It is the most lethal of all skin cancers. It can occur in one of several forms; superficial spreading melanoma, lentigo maligna melanoma, nodular melanoma and acral lentiginous melanoma.

Most melanomas are derived from cutaneous epidermal melanocytes; some appear in pre-existing nevi (moles) in the skin or develop in the uveal tract of the eye. Melanomas occasionally appear simultaneously with cancer of other organs. The incidence and mortality rates of malignant melanoma are increasing, probably related to increased recreational of exposure and better early detection. Prognosis is related body depth of dermal invasion and the thickness of the lesions. Malignant melanoma can spread through both the bloodstream and lymphatic system and can metastasize to the bones, lungs, liver, spleen, central nervous system (CNS) and lymph nodes.

The cause of malignant melanoma is unknown, but UV rays are strongly suspected. Risk factors include the following:

- Fair complexion, blue eyes, red or blonde hair and freckle
- Celtic or Scandinavian origin
- Tendency to burn and not tan; significant history of severe sunburn
- Older age; residence in the Southwestern United States
- Family or personal history of melanoma, the absence of a gene or chromosome 9P, presence of giant congenital nerve
- Dysplastic nevus syndrome.

Clinical Manifestations

Superficial Spreading Melanoma

1. Most common form usually affects middle-aged people, occurs most frequently on trunk and lower extremities.
2. Circular lesions with irregular outer portions.
3. Margins of lesion flat or elevated and palpable.
4. May appear in combination of colors, with hues of tan, brown, and black mixed with gray, bluish black or white. Sometimes a dull, pink-rose color is noted in a small area within the lesion.

Lentigo Maligna Melanoma

1. Slowly evolving pigmented lesion.
2. Occurs on exposed skin areas: Hand, head and neck in elderly patient.
3. First appears as tan, flat lesion, which in time undergoes changes in size and color.

Nodular Melanoma

- Spherical, blueberry-like nodule with relatively smooth surface and uniform blue-black color
- May be dome-shaped with a smooth surface or have other shadings of red, gray or purple
- May appear as irregularly shaped plaques
- May be described as a blood blister that fails to resolve
- Invades directly into adjacent dermis (vertical growth); poor prognosis.

Acral Lentiginous Melanoma

- Occurs in areas not excessively exposed to sunlight and where hair follicles are absent

- Found on the palms of the hand, soles, in nail beds and mucous membranes in dark-skinned people
- Appears as irregular pigmented macule that develops nodules
- Becomes invasive early.

Diagnostic Methods

1. Excisional biopsy specimen; incisional biopsy when the suspicious lesion is too large to be removed safely without extensive scarring.
2. Chest X-ray, complete blood cell count, liver function tests and radionuclide or CT are ordered for staging once melanoma is confirmed.

Medical Management/Therapeutic Measures

The therapeutic approach to malignant melanoma depends on the level of invasion and the depth of the lesion. In addition to surgery, chemotherapy and induced hyperthermia may be used to enhance treatment. Investigations are exploring the potential for the use of lipid-lowering medications and vaccine therapy to prevent melanoma.

Surgical Management

- Surgical excision is the treatment of choice for small superficial lesions
- Deeper lesions require wide local excision and skin graft
- A regional lymph node dissection may be performed to rule out metastasis, although newer approaches call for sentinel node biopsy to avoid problems from extensive lymph node removal
- Debulking the tumor or other palliative procedures may be performed.

Nursing Management

Assessment

1. Question patient with a lesion specifically about pruritus tenderness and pain, which are not features of a benign nevus. Also investigate changes in pre-existing moles of development of new pigmented lesions. Assess people at risk carefully, focusing on the skin.
2. Use a magnifying lens to examine for irregularity and changes in the moles.
3. Signs that suggest malignant changes include asymmetry (irregular surface), irregular border, variegated color and large diameter; referred to as the ABCDs of moles.
4. Pay attention to common sites of melanoma (e.g. back, legs, between toes, face, feet, scalp, fingernails and backs of hands).

Nursing Diagnoses/Problems

- Acute pain related to surgical incision and grafting
- Anxiety and depression related to possible life-threatening consequences of melanoma and disfigurement
- Deficient knowledge about early signs of melanoma.

Potential complications: They are:
- Metastasis
- Infection of surgical site.

Planning (Goals and Objectives)

The major goals for the patient may include relief of pain, discomfort, reduced anxiety and depression, increased knowledge of early signs of melanoma, and absence of complications. The objective will be that patient:
- Experiences relief of pain and discomfort
- Achieves reduced anxiety
- Demonstrates understanding of the means for detecting and preventing melanoma
- Experiences absence of complications.

Nursing Intervention/Implementation

Relieving Pain and Discomfort

Promote comfort and anticipate need for administer appropriate analgesic agents.

Reducing Anxiety

- Give support and allow patient to express feelings (e.g. anxiety, depression)
- Convey understanding of feelings
- Answer questions and clarify information during the diagnostic workup and staging of the tumor
- Print out resources, past effective coping mechanisms and support systems to help the patient cope with diagnosis and treatment
- Include family in all discussion to clarify information and provide emotional support.

Managing Potential Complications: Metastasis

1. Educate patient about treatment, deliver supportive care and clarify information about the therapy, and the rationale for its use. Identify potential side effects of therapy and ways to manage them, instruct the patient and family about the expected outcomes of treatment.
2. Monitor and document symptoms that may indicate metastasis: Lung (e.g. difficulty breathing, shortness of breath, increasing cough), bone (e.g. pain, decreased mobility and function, pathological fractures), and liver (e.g. change in liver enzyme levels, pain, jaundice).
3. Encourage patient to have to cope in the therapy while being realistic.
4. Provide time for patient to express fears and concerns about the future.
5. Offer information about support groups and contact people.
6. Arrange for hospice and palliative care services.
7. Refer 'Cancer' overview for additional nursing care measures.

PRESSURE ULCERS

Pressure ulcers are often referred to by patient with old terms such as bedsores, decubitus ulcer or pressure sores. Essentially, a pressure ulcer is a lesion caused by prolonged pressure against the skin:

- This is may result from spending prolonged pressure in one position causing weight of the body to compress the capillaries against bed or chair especially over bony prominence
- Pressure ulcers are the result of tissue anoxia and begin to develop within 20–40 minutes of unrelieved pressure on the skin
- Other causes, pressure from splinter cast, traction or other devices
- Those at risk are immobile patients, those with decreased circulation and those with impaired sensory perceptional or neurological function
- Mechanical factors (pressures, friction and shear) lead to formation of ulcer.

Preventive Measures

- Examine and document the condition daily, so all are aware of developing problems
- Gently cleanse the skin daily with tepid water and mild soaps to prevent drying
- To reduce friction, pat the skin dry rather than rubbing dry
- After bathing daily lubricating with moisturizer to prevent dryness on skin
- Thoroughly dry skin-to-skin surfaces, such as breasts, skinfolds (groin, abdomen) and between toes to prevent prolonged exposure to moisture
- If incontinence clean the skin promptly with tepid water and mild soap
- Pat dry and apply moisture barriers to prevent breakdown
- Avoid massaging bony prominences or reddened skin areas to prevent damaging blood vessels.

Nursing Management

1. Teach the patient to weight shift for every 15 minutes if possible.
2. When the patient immobile, the higher possible mobility should be maintained.
3. Frequent active or passive range of motion exercise should be performed as changing the position, turning as scheduled accordingly.
4. Avoid elevating the head of the bed more than 30° to reduce pressure on coccyx and to reduce friction, and shear damage from sliding down.
5. Elevate the heels off the bed with pillows placed lengthwise under the calf or with heel elevators.
6. Be sure to also protect the patients elbow, sacrum, scapular, ears, occipital from pressure ulcers.
7. Avoid the use of donut-shaped cushions. They create a circle of pressure that cut circulation.
8. Provide pressure reducing or relieving mattress.
9. Take measures to prevent malnutrition, dehydration by ensuring adequate intake of protein and fluids.

BURNS

Burns are wounds caused by an energy transfer from a heat source to the body, heating the tissue enough to cause damage. Locally the heat denatures cellular protein and interrupts the blood supply. The three zones of tissue damage that occurs with burns are partial-thickness (superficial), partial thickness (deep) and full-thickness (protein layers including 1°, 2°, 3°). The amount of skin damage is related to the temperature of burning agent, the burning agent itself, duration of exposure, the conductivity of the tissue and thickness of the involved dermal structure.

Alteration of normal skin functioning resulting from major burns injury includes loss of protective functions, impaired ability to regulate temperature, increased risk of infection, changes in sensory function, loss of fluids, impaired skin regeneration, impaired secretory and excretory function.

Burns may be caused by flame, contact, scalp, chemical, clin or radiation.

Clinical Manifestations

- Pain
- Superficial partial thickness: Pink to red skin and blisters
- Deep partial thickness: Pink to light red or white skin, blisters and blanching
- Full thickness: White, gray or brown color, firm and leathery
- Complete: Shock and wound infection.

Diagnostic Tests

- Wound culture
- Complete blood count, blood urea nitrogen (BUN), glucose, electrolyte, urine studies.

Therapeutic Measures

- Intravenous (IV) fluids replacement
- Antibiotic/Antimicrobial agents
- Analgesics.

Nursing Management

Managing the:
- Impaired gas exchange
- Impaired skin integrity
- Deficient fluid volume
- Pain-related burns
- Ineffective peripheral tissue perfusion
- Risk for infection.

Burn Injury

Burns are caused by a transfer of energy from a heat source to the body. The depth of the injury depends on the temperature of the burning agent and the duration of contact with it. Burns disrupt the skin, which leads to increased fluid loss, infection, hypothermia, scarring, compound immunity and changes in function, appearance, and body image. Young children and the elderly continue to have increased morbidity, and mortality when compared to other age groups with similar injuries. Inhalation injuries in addition to cutaneous burns worsen the prognosis.

Depth of Burn

The depth of a burn injury depends on the type of injury, causative agent, temperature of the burn agent, duration of contact with the agent and the skin thickness.

Burns are classified according to the depth of tissue destruction:

1. Superficial partial-thickness burns (similar to 1°) such as sunburn: The epidermis and possibly a portion of the dermis are destroyed.
2. Deep partial-thickness burns (similar to 2°) such as scald: The epidermis and upper to deeper portions of the dermis are injured.
3. Full-thickness burns (3°) such as burn from a flame or electric current: The epidermis, entire dermis and sometimes the underlying tissues, muscle, and bone are destroyed.

Extent of Body Surface Area Burned

How much total body surface area burned is determined by one of the following methods:

1. Rules of nine: An estimation of the total body surface area burned by assigning percentages in multiple of nine to major body surfaces.
2. Lund and Browder method: A more precise method of estimating the extent of the burn; takes into account that the percentage of the surface area is represented by various anatomic parts (head and legs) changes with growth.
3. Palm method: Used to estimate percentage of scattered burns, using the size of the patient's palm (about 1% of body surface area) to assess the extent of burn injury.

Elderly people are at higher risk for burn injury because of reduced coordination, strength, sensation and changes in vision. Predisposing factors and the health history, in the older adult, influence the complexity of the care for the patient. Pulmonary function is limited in the older adult and therefore airway exchange, lung elasticity, and ventilation can be affected. This can be further affected by a history of smoking. Decreased cardiac function and coronary artery disease increase the risk of complications in elderly patients with burn injuries. Malnutrition and presence of diabetes mellitus or other endocrine disorders present nutritional challenges and require close monitoring. Varying degrees of orientation may present themselves on admission or through the course of care making assessment of pain and anxiety a challenge for the burn team. The skin of the elderly is thinner and less elastic, which affects the depth of injury and its ability to heal.

Education on the prevention of burn injury is especially important among the elderly. Assess an elderly patient's ability to safely perform activities of daily living (ADLs), assist elderly patient and families to modify their environment to ensure safety, and make referrals as needed.

Medical Management/Therapeutic Measures

Four major goals relating to burn management are prevention, institution of life-saving measures for the severely burned person, prevention of disability, disfigurement and rehabilitation.

Emergent/Resuscitative Phase

Nursing Management

1. Focus on the major priorities of any trauma patient.
2. The burn wound is a secondary consideration, although aseptic management of the burn wounds and invasive lines continues.
3. Assess circumstances surrounding the injury, time of injury, mechanism of burn, whether the burn occurred in a closed space, the possibility of inhalation of noxious chemicals and any related to trauma.
4. Monitor vital signs frequently, monitor respiratory status closely, evaluate apical, carotid and femoral pulses particularly in areas of circumferential burn injury to an extremity.
5. Start cardiac monitoring if indicated (e.g. history of cardiac or respiratory problems, electrical injury).
6. Check peripheral pulses on burned extremities hourly; use Doppler as needed.
7. Monitor fluid intake (IV fluids) and output (urinary catheter), and measure hourly. Note the amount of urine obtained when catheter is inserted (indicates preburn renal function and fluids status).
8. Assess body temperatures, body weight, history of preburn weight, allergies, tetanus immunization, past medical-surgical problems, current illness and use of medications.
9. Arrange for patients with facial burns to be assessed for corneal injury.
10. Continue to assess the extent of the burns; assess depth or wound and identify areas of full, and partial thickness injury.
11. Assess neurological status: Consciousness, psychological status pain, anxiety levels and behavior.
12. Assess patient and family understanding of injury, and treatment. Assess patients support system and coping skills.

Nursing Interventions/Implementation

Promoting gas exchange and airway clearance

1. Provide humidified oxygen, monitor arterial blood gases (ABGs), pulse oximetry and carboxyhemoglobin levels.
2. Assess breath sounds, respiratory rate, rhythm, depth and symmetry; monitor for hypoxia.
3. Observe for signs of inhalation injury, blistering of lips and buccal mucosa; signed nostrils; burns of face, neck or chest increasing hoarseness; or soot in sputum or respiratory secretions.
4. Report labored respirations, decreased depth of respirations, signs of hypoxia to physician immediately. Prepare to assist with intubation and escharotomies.
5. Monitor mechanically ventilated patient closely.
6. Institute aggressive pulmonary care measures; turning, coughing, deep breathing; periodic forceful inspiration using spirometry and tracheal suctioning.
7. Maintaining proper positioning to promote removal of secretions, patient airway and to promote optimal chest expansion; use artificial airway as needed.

Restoring fluid and electrolyte balance

1. Monitor vital signs and urinary output (hourly), central venous pressure (CVP), pulmonary artery pressure, and cardiac output.

2. Note and report signs of hypovolemia or fluid overload.
3. Maintain IV lines and regular fluids at appropriate rates, as prescribed. Document intake, output and daily weight.
4. Elevate the head of bed and burned extremities.
5. Monitor serum electrolyte levels (e.g. sodium, potassium, calcium, phosphorus, bicarbonate); recognize developing electrolyte imbalances.
6. Notify physician immediately of decreased urine output; blood pressure; central venous, pulmonary artery or pulmonary artery wedge pressures, or increased pulse rate.

Monitoring normal body temperature

1. Provide warm environment: Use heat shield, space blanket, heat lights or blankets.
2. Assess core body temperature frequently.
3. Work quickly when wounds are exposed to minimize heat loss from the wound.

Minimizing pain and anxiety

1. Use a pain scale to assess pain level (i.e. 1–10); differentiate between restlessness due to pain and restlessness due to hypoxia.
2. Administer IV opioid analgesics as prescribed and assess response to medication. Observe for respiratory depression in patient who is not mechanically ventilated.
3. Provide emotional support, reassurance and simple explanations about procedures.
4. Assess patient and family understanding of burn injury, coping strategies, family dynamics, and anxiety levels. Provide individualized responses to support patient and family coping. Explain all procedures in clear, simple terms.
5. Provide pain relief and give antianxiety medications, if patient remains highly anxious, and agitated after psychological interventions.

Managing potential complications

1. Acute respiratory failure: Assess for increasing dyspnea, stridor and changes in respiratory patterns; monitor pulse oximetry and ABG values to detect problematic oxygen saturation and increasing CO_2; monitor chest X-rays; assess for cerebral hypoxia (e.g. restlessness, confusion); report deteriorating respiratory status immediately to physician; and assist as needed with intubation or escharotomy.
2. Distributive shock: Monitor for early signs of shock (decreased pulmonary capillary wedge pressure, blood pressure or increasing pulse) or progressive edema. Administer fluid resuscitation as ordered in response to physical findings; continue monitoring fluid status.
3. Acute renal failure: Monitor and report abnormal urine output and quality, BUN and creatinine levels; assess for urine hemoglobin or myoglobin; administer increased fluids as prescribed.
4. Compartment syndrome: Assess peripheral pulse hourly with Doppler; assess neurovascular status of extremities hourly (warmth, capillary refill, sensation and movement); remove blood pressure cuff after each reading; elevate burned extremities; report any extremity pain, loss or peripheral pulses or sensation; prepare to assist with escharotomies.

5. Paralytic ileus: Maintain nasogastric tube on low intermittent suction until bowel sounds resume; auscultate abdomen regularly for distention and bowel sounds.
6. Curling's ulcer: Assess gastric aspirate for blood and pH assess stools for occult blood; administer antacids and histamine blockers [e.g. ranitidine (Zantac)] as prescribed.

Acute/Intermediate Phase

Nursing Management

The acute or intermediate phase begins 48–72 hours after the burn injury. Burn wound care and pain control are priorities at this stage:

1. Focus on hemodynamic alterations, wound healing, pain and psychological responses, and early detection of complications.
2. Measure vital signs frequently; respiratory and fluid status remains highest priority.
3. Assess peripheral pulses frequently for first few days after the burn for restricted blood flow.
4. Closely observe hourly fluid intake and urinary output, as well as blood pressure and cardiac rhythm. Changes should be reported to the burn surgeon promptly.
5. For patient with inhalation injury, regularly monitor level of consciousness, pulmonary function and ability to ventilate. If patient is intubated and placed on a ventilator, frequent suctioning and assessment of the airway are priorities.

Nursing Interventions/Implementation

Restoring normal fluid balance

- Monitor IV and oral fluid intake; use IV infusion pumps
- Measure intake, output and daily weight
- Report changes (e.g. blood pressures, pulse rate) to physician.

Preventing infection

1. Provide a clean and safe environment; protect patient from sources of cross-contamination (e.g. visitors, other patients, staff, equipment).
2. Closely scrutinize wound to detect early signs of infection.
3. Monitor culture results and white blood cell counts.
4. Practice clean technique for wound care procedures and aseptic technique for any invasive procedures. Use meticulous hand hygiene before and after contact with patient.
5. Caution patient to avoid touching wounds or dressings; wash unburned areas and change linens regularly.

Maintaining adequate nutrition

1. Initiate oral fluids slowly when bowel sounds resume; record tolerance if vomiting and distention do not occur, fluids maybe increased gradually and the patient maybe advanced to a normal diet or to tube feedings.
2. Collaborate with dietitian to plan a protein and calorie-rich diet acceptable to patient. Encourage family to bring nutritious and patient's favorite foods. Provide nutritional, vitamin and mineral supplements if prescribed.
3. Document caloric intake. Insert feeding tube, if caloric goals cannot be met by oral feeding (for continuous or bolus feedings); note residual volumes.
4. Check patient weight daily and graph the weights.

Promoting skin integrity

1. Assess wound status.
2. Support patient during distress and painful wound care.
3. Coordinate complex aspects of wound care and dressing changes.
4. Assess burn for size, color, odor, eschar, exudates, epithelial buds (small pearl-like clusters on cells on the wound surface), bleeding, granulation tissues, the status of graft take, healing of the donor site and the condition of the surrounding skin; report any significant changes to physician.
5. Inform all members of healthcare team to latest wound care procedures in use for the patient.
6. Assist, instruct, support, encourage patient and family to take part in dressing changes, and wound care.
7. Assess strengths (as early) of patient and family in preparing for discharge and home care.

Relieving pain and discomfort

1. Frequently assess pain and discomfort; administer analgesic agents and anxiolytic medications, as prescribed, before the pain becomes severe. Assess document the patient's response to medication and any other interventions.
2. Teach patient relaxation techniques. Give some control over wound care and analgesia. Provide frequent assurance.
3. By using guided imagery, distract to alter patient's perceptions and responses to pain. Hypnosis, music therapy and virtual reality are also useful.
4. Assess the patient's sleep pattern daily; administer sedatives if prescribed.
5. Work quickly to complete treatment and dressing changes.
6. Encourage patient to use analgesic medications before painful procedures.
7. Promote comfort during healing phase with oral antipruritic agents, a cool environment, frequent lubrication of the skin with water- or silica-based lotion, exercise and splinting to prevent skin contracture, and diversional activities.

Promoting physical mobility

1. Prevent complications of immobility (atelectasis, pneumonia, edema, pressure ulcers and contractures) by deep breathing, turning and proper repositioning.
2. Modify interventions to meet patient's needs. Encourage early sitting and ambulation. When legs are involved, apply elastic pressure bandages before assisting patient to upright position.
3. Make aggressive efforts to prevent contractures and hypertrophic scarring of the wound closure for a year or more.
4. Initiate passive and active range of motion exercises from admission until after grafting, within prescribed limitations.
5. Apply splints or functional devices to extremities for contracture control. Monitor for signs of vascular insufficiency, nerve compression and skin breakdown.

Strengthening coping strategies

1. Assist patient to develop effective coping strategies: Set specific expectations for behavior, promote truthful communication to build trust, help patient practice coping strategies and give positive reinforcement when appropriate.
2. Demonstrate acceptance of patient. Enlist a non-involved person for patient to vent feelings without fear of retaliation.

3. Include patient in decisions regarding care. Encourage patient to assert individually and preferences. Set realistic expectation for self-care.

Support patient and family processes

Support and address the verbal, and non-verbal concerns of the patient and family, i.e.:

1. Instruct family in ways to support patient.
2. Make psychological or social work referrals as needed.
3. Provide information about burn care and expected course of treatment.
4. Initiate patient and family education during burn management. Assess and consider preferred learning styles; assess ability to grasp and cope with information. Determine barriers to learning when planning and executing teaching.
5. Remain sensitive to the possibility of changing family dynamics.

Managing potential complications

1. Heart failure: Assess for fluid overload, decreased cardiac output, oliguria, jugular veins distention, edema or onset of S3, S4 heart sounds.
2. Pulmonary edema: Assess for increasing CVP, pulmonary artery, wedge pressures and crackles; report promptly. Position comfortably with head elevated unless contraindicated. Administer medications and oxygen as prescribed to assess response.
3. Sepsis: Assess for increased temperature, increased pulse, widened pulse pressure, flushed, dry skin in unburned areas (early signs) and note trends in the data. Perform wound and blood cultures as prescribed. Give scheduled antibiotics on time.
4. Acute respiratory failure and acute respiratory distress syndrome (ARDS): Monitor respiratory status for dyspnea, change in respiratory pattern and onset of adventitious sounds. Assess for decrease in tidal volume and lung compliance in patients on mechanical ventilation. The hallmark of onset of ARDS is hypoxemia on 100% oxygen, decreased lung compliance and significant shunting; notify physician of deteriorating respiratory status.
5. Visceral damage (from electrical burns): Monitor electrocardiogram (ECG) and report dysrhythmias; pay attention to pain related to deep muscle ischemia and report. Early detection may minimize severity of this complication. Fasciotomies may be necessary to relieve swelling, ischemia in the muscles and fascia; monitor patient for excessive blood loss, and hypovolemia after fasciotomy.

Rehabilitation Phase

Nursing Management

Rehabilitation should begin immediately after the burn has occurred. Wound healing, psychosocial support and restoring maximum functional activity remain priorities. Maintaining fluid and electrolyte balance, and improving nutrition status continue to be important.

Assessment

1. In early assessment, obtain information about patient's educational level, occupation, leisure activities, cultural background, religion and family interactions.

2. Assess self-concept, mental status, emotional response to the injury and hospitalization, level of intellectual functioning, previous hospitalization, response to pain relief measures, and sleep pattern.
3. Perform ongoing assessments relative to rehabilitation including range of motion affected joints.
4. Functional abilities in ADLs, early signs of skin breakdown from splints or positioning devices, evidence of neuropathies (neurological damage), activity tolerance, quality and condition of healing skin.
5. Document participation and self-care abilities in ambulation, eating, wound cleaning and applying pressure wraps.
6. Maintain comprehensive and continuous assessment for early detection of complications, with specific assessment as needed for specific treatment. Such as postoperative assessment of patient undergoing primary excision.

Nursing Diagnoses/Problems

- Activity intolerance related to pain on exercise, limited joint mobility, muscle wasting and limited endurance
- Disturbed body image related to altered appearance and self-concept
- Knowledge of postdischarge home care and recovery needs.

Potential complications: They are:
- Contractures
- Inadequate psychological adaptation to burn injury.

Planning (goals and objectives)

Goals include increased participation in ADLs; increased understanding of the injury, treatment and planned follow-up care. Adaption and adjustment to alterations in body image, self-concept, lifestyle, and absence of complications:
- Demonstrates activity tolerance required for desired daily activities
- Adapts to altered body image
- Demonstrates knowledge of required self-care and follow-up care
- Exhibits no complications.

Nursing Interventions/Implementation

Promoting activity tolerance

1. Schedule care to allow periods of uninterrupted sleep. Administer hypnotic agents as prescribed to promote sleep.
2. Communicate plan to care family and other caregivers.
3. Reduce metabolic stress by relieving pain, preventing chilling or fever and promoting integrity of all body system to help conserve energy. Monitor fatigue, pain and fever to determine amount of activity to be encouraged daily.
4. Incorporate physical therapy exercises to prevent muscular atrophy and maintain mobility required for daily activities.
5. Support positive outlook and increase tolerance for activity by scheduling diversion activities in periods of increasing duration.

Improving body image and self-concept

1. Take time to listen to patient's concerns and provide realistic support; refer patient to support group to develop coping strategies to deal with losses.

2. Assess patient's psychological reactions; provide support and develop a plan that help the patient to handle feelings. Promote a healthy body image and self-concept by helping patient practice responses to people who stare or ask about the injury.
3. Support patient through small gestures such as providing a birthday cake, combing patient's hair before visitors and sharing information on cosmetic resources to enhance appearance.
4. Teach patient ways to direct attention away from a disfigured body to the self within.
5. Coordinate communications of consultants, such as psychologists, social workers, vocational counselors and teachers during rehabilitation.

Managing potential complications

1. Contractures: Provide early, aggressive physical and occupational therapy; support patient if surgery is needed to achieve full range of motion.
2. Impaired psychological adaption to the burn injury. Obtain psychological or psychiatric referral as soon as evidence of major coping problems appears.

Promoting family-based care

1. Throughout the phases of burn care, make efforts to prepare patient and family for the care they will perform at home. Instruct them about measures and procedures.
2. Provide verbal and written instructions about wound care, prevention of complications, pain management, and nutrition.
3. Inform and review with patient specific exercises, use of elastic pressure garments and splints; provide written instructions.
4. Teach patient and family to recognize abnormal signs, and report them to the physician.
5. Assist the patient and family in planning for the patient's continued care by identifying, acquiring supplies and equipment that are needed at home.
6. Encourage and support follow-up wound care.
7. Refer patient with inadequate support system to home care resources for assistance with wound care and exercises.
8. Evaluate patient status periodically for modification of home care instructions and/or planning for reconstructive surgery.

18

Chapter Ophthalmo-otic Nursing

VISUAL IMPAIRMENT

Visual impairment (blindness) is the complete or almost complete absence of the sense of sight. Few people are born visually impaired (blind). It is caused by variety of factors including trauma, complications from various diseases such as hypotension and diabetes and condition such as cataract and glaucoma.

Visual impairment is produced when the rays of light on the way to optic nerve are obstructed or by disease of optic nerve or tract of the part of the brain connected with vision. It may be permanent or transient, complete or partial, or may occur only in darkness (night blindness).

Clinical Manifestations

- General loss of vision in which visual images are blurred, distorted or absent as specific areas of the visual field
- Objects may appear dark or absent around the peripheral field in glaucoma or retinitis pigmentosa (degeneration of pigment layer of retina)
- The center of the visual field may appear dark for a person with diabetic retinopathy or macular degenerations
- Half of the visual field may be impaired in patient with hemianopia
- Patient may reports that visual field appears blurry or hazy in corneal problems, in cataracts, diabetes retinopathy, as a refractive errors.

Diagnostic Measures

- Visual field examination, tonometry, slit lamp microscopic beam
- Retinal angiography to detect vascular changes
- Ultrasonography to visualize changes in posterior eye.

Therapeutic Measures

Depending on the cause of visual impairment, treatment includes medication prescription, surgical interventions, and corrective eye wear prescriptions and referred to supportive services.

Nursing Management

- Administration of medication as prescribed
- Assist in surgical intervention as indicated
- Advice to have corrective eyewears device as ordered
- Take measures to correct disturbed sensory perception vision
- Take measures to anxiety related to visual sensory deficit
- Take measure to prevent risk for injury to eyes
- Educate patient and family regarding visual impairment and suitable measure for prevention and treatment.

MACULAR DEGENERATION

Age-related macular degeneration (ARMD) is the leading cause of area on the retina where light rays converge into the sharp, central vision needed for reading and seeing small objects. The macula is also responsible for color vision. There are two types, i.e. dry (atrophic), and wet (exudative). In dry form, photoreceptors in the macula fail to function and not replaced due to advancing age. In wet form, retinal tissue degenerate, allowing vitreous fluid to block into the subretinal space. New blood vessels formed and compromise the macular tissue causing subretinal edema, fibrous scar and limit the central vision.

Clinical Manifestations

1. Dry form macula is characterized by slow, progressive loss of central or near vision. Although, usually have the condition in both eyes, but each eye may be affected in varying degree.
2. Wet form of macula also has the same loss of central or near vision, but the onset is sudden. The loss can occur in anyone or both eyes.
3. The vision loss described as blurred vision, distortion of straight lines, and dark or empty spots in the central area of vision.
4. Some may report decreased ability to distinguish colors.

Diagnostic Measures

- Visual acuity, ophthalmoscopy, examiner uses Amsler grid for visual changes
- Intravenous fluorescein (dye) angiography, digital imaging
- Optical coherence tomography for vessels leakage.

Therapeutic Measures

- No treatment for dry form ARMD, special low-vision lens can enhance remaining vision as it will not lose peripheral vision
- If wet form is diagnosed early, laser photocoagulation can seal the leaking blood vessels, slowing the rate of vision loss
- Photodynamic therapy is also available to stop bleeding vessels.

Nursing Management

Take measures to treat patient with visual impairment—spectrum, contact lens, refractive surgeries, etc.

CATARACT

Cataract is opacity in the lens of the eye than may cause a loss of visual activity. Vision is diminished because the light rays are unable to get the retina through the clouded lens. The factors contribute to cataract development may include age, ultraviolet radiation (sunlight), diabetes, smoking, steroids, nutritional deficiencies, alcohol consumption, intraocular infections, trauma, and congenital defect.

A cataract is a lens opacity or cloudiness. Cataracts can develop in one or both eyes and at any age. Cigarette smoking, long-term use of corticosteroid, especially at high doses, sunlight and ionizing radiation, diabetes, obesity, and eye injuries can increase the risk of cataracts. The three most common types of senile (age related) cataracts are defined by their location in the lens such as nuclear, cortical and posterior subcapsular. Visual impairment depends on the size, density and location in the lens. More than one type can be present in the eye.

Therapeutic Measures

- Surgical removal of the cloudy lens, it should perform one eye treatment at a time
- Implant lenses after lens removal or eyeglasses
- Complications are rare, but take measures to prevent complication after surgery, which includes inflammations, increased intraocular pressure (IOP), macular edema, retinal detachment, vitreous loss, hyphema, endophthalmitis are expulsion hemorrhage.

Clinical Manifestations

Cataracts are painless, symptoms of cataract formation includes halos around light, difficulty in reading fine print or seeing in bright light, increased sensitivity to flare such as when driving at night, double or hazy vision, or decreased color vision:

- Painless, blurry vision
- Perception that surrounding are dimmer (as if glasses need cleaning)
- Light scattering: Reduced contrast sensitivity, sensitivity to glare and reduced visual acuity.

Other effects include myopic shift [return of ability to do close work (e.g. reading fine print) without eyeglasses], astigmatism, monocular diplopia (double vision), color shift (the aging lens becomes progressively more absorbent at the blue end of the spectrum), brunescens (color values shift to yellow-brown) and reduced light transmission.

Diagnostic Methods

- Eye examination
- Degrees of visual acuity is directly proportional to density of the cataract
- Snellen's visual acuity test
- Ophthalmoscopy
- Slit lamp biomicroscopic examination.

Medical Management

Non-surgical (medications, eyedrops, eyeglasses) treatment cures cataract or prevent age-related cataracts. Studies have found no benefit from antioxidant supplements, vitamins C and E, beta carotene, and selenium. Glasses or contact lens, bifocal, or magnifying lenses may improve vision. Mydriatics can be used for short term, but glare will increase.

Surgical Management

In general, if reduced vision from cataract does not interfere with normal activities, surgery may not be needed. In dividing technique when cataract surgery has to be performed, the primary consideration is the methanol and visual status of patient. Surgical option includes phacoemulsification (method of extracapsular cataract surgery) and lens replacement (aphakic eyeglasses, contact lenses and intraocular lens implants). Cataracts are removed under local anesthesia in an outpatient basis. When both lenses have cataracts, one eye is treated first with least reversal weeks, preferably months, separating the two procedures.

Nursing Management

1. Prepare patient for surgery.
2. Explain that depth of perception may be affected by eye surgery, which can result on falls. So, help prevent injury.
3. Ambulate with assistance and use clearly marked stairs to prevent injury.
4. At home, beverages can be poured and stored in the refrigerator in single serving glasses to prevent spills and slippery floors.
5. Teach disease process, surgical intervention, pre- and post-operative activity restrictions, use of dark glasses to decrease the discomfort of pathophobia, use of correct technique for applying eye medication, need to repair, medical follow-up as instructed.
6. Withhold any anticoagulants that the patient is receiving, which is medically appropriate. In some cases, anticoagulant therapy may continue.
7. Administer dilating drops every 10 minutes for four doses at least 1 hour before surgery. Antibiotic, corticosteroids and anti-inflammatory drops may be administered prophylactically to prevent postoperative infection and inflammation.
8. Provide patient verbal and written instructions about the protection of the eye, administer medications, recognize of complications, and obtain emergency care.
9. Explains that there should be minimal discomfort after surgery and instruct the patient to take a mild analgesic agent such as acetaminophen, as needed.
10. Antibiotic, anti-inflammatory and corticosteroid eyedrop or ointment are prescribed postoperatively.

GLAUCOMA

Glaucoma is a group of disease characterized by abnormal pressure within the eyeball. The pressure causes damage to the cells of the optic nerves, the structure responsible for transmitting visual information form the eye to the brain. The damage is silent, progressive and irreversible until the end stages, when the peripheral vision occurs followed by reduction in central vision and eventual blindness. The three type of glaucoma are:

1. Primary glaucoma, i.e. primary open-angle glaucoma (POAG) and acute angle-closure glaucoma (AACG).
2. Secondary glaucoma caused by infection of tumors or injuries.
3. Congenital glaucoma, primary due to developmental abnormalities.

The term 'glaucoma' is used to refer a group of ocular conditions characterized by optic nerve damage. In the past, glaucoma was seen more as a condition of elevated IOP than of optic neuropathy. Increasingly that is no longer the case. There is no doubt that increased IOP damages the optic nerve and nerve fiber layer, but the degree of harm is highly variable. The optic nerve damage is related to the IOP caused by congestion of aqueous humor in the eye.

Glaucoma is the second leading causes of blindness among adults in the United States of America. Most cases are asymptomatic until extensive and irreversible damage has occurred. Glaucoma affects people of all ages, but is more prevalent with increasing age (above 40 year). Others at risk are patients with diabetes, African Americans, those individuals with a family history of glaucoma and people with previous eye trauma or surgery, or those who have had long-term steroid treatment. There is no cure for glaucoma, but the disease can be controlled.

Classification of Glaucoma

In glaucoma there are several types. Current clinical forms of glaucoma are identified as open-angle glaucoma, angle-closure glaucoma (also called papillary block), congenital glaucoma and glaucoma associated with other conditions. Glaucoma can be primary or secondary, depending on whether associated factors contribute to the rise of IOP. The two common clinical forms of glaucoma, i.e. POAG and AACG, which are differentiated by the mechanism that cause impaired aqueous outflow.

Clinical Manifestations

1. Acute angle-closure glaucoma is typically unilateral, rapid onset. In ophthalmic emergency:
   a. Patient report severe pain over the affected eye, blurred vision, rainbows around lights, photophobia, have eye redness, a steamy appearing cornea, and tearing. Increase IOP causing nausea and vomiting (excess 50 mm Hg).
2. Primary open-angle glaucoma (POAG) develops bilaterally, onset is gradual and painless. So the patient may have no noticeable symptoms or after time, may experiences mild itching in eyes, headache, halos around light, or frequently visual changes that are not corrected with eyeglasses.
3. Most patients are unaware that they have the disease until they have experienced visual changes and vision loss.
4. Symptoms may include blurred vision or 'halos' around lights, difficulty in focusing, difficult of adjusting eyes in low lightning, loss of peripheral vision, aching or discomfort around the eyes and headache.
5. Pallor and cupping of the optic nerve disk, as the optic nerve damage increases, visual perception in the area is lost.

Diagnostic Methods

- Ocular and medical history (to investigate predisposing factors)
- Diagnostic tests include tonometry (measures IOP), ophthalmoscopy (to inspect the optic nerve), gonioscopy (to examine the filtration angle of the anterior chamber), and perimetry (visual fields assessment) are major diagnostic tests.

Medical Management/Therapeutic Measures

The aim of all glaucoma treatment is prevention of optic nerve damage. Lifelong therapy is almost always necessary because glaucoma cannot be cured. Treatment focuses on pharmacological therapy, laser procedures, surgery or a combination of these approaches, all of which have potential complications and side effects. The objective is to achieve the greatest benefit at the least risk, cost and inconvenience to the patient. Although treatment cannot reverse optic nerve damage, further damage can be controlled. The goal is to maintain an IOP within a range, unlikely to cause further damage. The management includes:

- First treatment is to focus on an opening the aqueous flow by administering cholinergic agents (miotics) to constrict pupil (for free flow)
- Medication (Diamox, propane or Timoptic) may be given to slow the production of aqueous fluid, which help to decrease IOP
- Steroids eyedrops may be given as prescribed
- Analgesic may be seen on prescription
- Lifelong use of eyedrops medication once or twice daily as prescribed
- Surgical interventions such as creating an area where the aqueous humor can flow freely to prevent increased IOP:
  - Laser iridotomy/Prophylactic iridotomy to prevent AACG or POAG
  - Assess the condition, assist in surgical intervention. A drain medication as ordered.

Pharmacological Therapy

Medical management of glaucoma relies on systemic and topical ocular medications that lower IOP. Periodic follow-up examinations are essential to monitor IOP, the appearance of the optic nerve, the visual fields and side effects of medications. Therapy takes into account, the patient's health and stage of glaucoma. It includes:

1. Patient is usually started on the lowest dose of topical medication, ocular medication and then advanced to increased concentrations until the desired IOP level is reached and maintained.
2. One eye is treated first with the other eye used as a control in determining the efficacy of the medication.
3. Several types of ocular medications are used to treat glaucoma, including miotics (medications that cause papillary constriction), adrenergic agonists (i.e. sympathomimetic agents), beta blockers, α-agonist (i.e. adrenergic agents), carbonic anhydrase inhibitors and prostaglandins.

Surgical Management

- Laser trabeculoplasty or iridotomy indicated when IOP is inadequately controlled by medications
- Filtering procedures: An opening or a fistula in the trabecular meshwork; trabeculectomy is a standard technique
- Drainage implant or shunt surgery may be performed
- Trabectome surgery is reserved for patients in whom pharmacological treatment and/or laser trabeculoplasty do not control the IOP sufficiently.

Nursing Management

- Create a teaching plan regarding the nature of the disease and the importance of strict adherence to the medication regimen to help ensure compliance

- Review the patient's medication program, particularly the interactions of glaucoma-control medication with other medications
- Explain effects of glaucoma-control medications on vision (e.g. miotics and sympathomimetics result in altered focus; therefore, patients need to be cautions in navigating their surroundings)
- Refer patients with impaired mobility for low vision and rehabilitation services; patients who meet the criteria for legal blindness should be offered referrals to agencies that can assist them in obtaining federal assistance
- Provide reassurance and emotional support
- Integrate patient's family into the plan of care and because the disease has a familial tendency, encourage family members to undergo examinations at least once every 2 years to detect glaucoma early.

EYE INFECTIONS/INFLAMMATIONS

The eye may become aggravated by allergens, chemical substance or mechanical irritation leading to infection by microorganisms. Mechanical irritation may be caused by sunburn or bacterial infection. Inflammation results from allergies to environmental substances or by irritants found in perfumes, makeup, sprays or plants, viral agents includes herpes simplex, Cytomegalovirus and human adenovirus. Bacterial agents include *Staphylococcus, Streptococcus*. Eye infections are as follows:

1. Conjunctivitis is the inflammation of the conjunctiva caused by either virus or bacteria. It is contagious. The symptoms include redness and crusting exudates on the lids and in the cornea of the eyes. Patient reports of itching and pain, may tear excessively in response to the irritations. Treat with symptomatic measures by eye washes or eye irrigation and antibiotic eyedrops or ointments.
2. Blepharitis is an inflammation of eyelid margin in a chronic inflammation process dry eyes or abnormalities of the meibomian glands and then lipid secretions. Blepharitis includes:
   a. Seborrheic blepharitis: Redness of eyelids with scales and flaking at the base of the lashes.
   b. Ulcerative blepharitis produces crusts, at eyelids, reddened eyes and inflamed cornea. Eyelids infection by *Staphylococcus* become thick and may lose eyelash. Clean the eye with cotton-tipped swabs dipped in diluted baby shampoo or with sterile eye cleaner solution. Treat infection with antibiotics ointments.
3. Hordeolum (stye) and chalazion (internal hordeolum):
   a. Styes are small, raised, reddened areas, use of cosmetics on the eye may contribute to its hordeolum formats.
   b. Chalazion may form in the connective tissue of eyelids (meibomian gland).
   c. Styes may be tender, however a chalazion often puts pressure on the cornea causes more discomfort:
      - Hordeolum usually forms and heals spontaneously within few days and requires no treatment
      - Chalazion may require surgical incisions and drainage of abscess persists in prescribed antibiotics.

Clinical Manifestations

Common clinical manifestations of eye disorders are visual disturbances, pain, redness, secretions, itchiness and sensation of pressure in eyes.

Complications

Worsening vision or loss of vision and acute pain.

Diagnosis

Visual acuity, ophthalmoscopy, Amsler grid, slit lamp examination and tonometry (identify IOP).

Therapeutic Measures

- Medications: Reduce IOP; treat infections, anesthesia of the eye
- Surgery in certain conditions.

KERATITIS

Keratitis is the inflammation of the cornea and may be acute or chronic and superficial or deep. The depth may be determined by the layers of the cornea than may be affected. It may be associated with conjunctivitis. People, who have dry eyes, wear contact lenses, practice of poor contact lens hygiene, have decreased corneal sensation and are increased risk of keratitis.

Clinical Manifestations

- Cornea has many pain receptors, so inflammation is very painful
- Pain increases with movements of the lid over the cornea
- Decreased vision, photophobia, tearing and blepharospasm
- Conjunctive appears reddened, in advanced case cornea may appear opaque.

Diagnosis

- Assess ulcer is made by slit lamps or a handled lights
- Fluorescence strain may also be used to outline the area of involvement.

Therapeutic Measures

- Topical antibiotics, typical corticosteroids, topical interferons, antivirus as prescribed
- Assess the patient for pain
- Administer eye medications as ordered
- Apply warm or cool packs as ordered for soothing eyes
- Patching of the affected eye may help to reduce pain
- Reading and television should be discouraged for the rest of eyes
- Encouraging to quiet activity such as listening to music, radio or recorded book
- Assess and plan for visual impairment that may persist to promote safety
- Advice patient with one eye patched, not to drive
- Teach patient and family—how to prevent spreading of infection.

EYE TRAUMA

Injuries to the eye include foreign bodies, burns, abrasions, lacerations, and penetrating wounds:

- Foreign bodies such as dust particles or propellants may lodge in conjunctive or cornea, patient may rub the eyes to dislodge object, cause further irritations
- Burns may occur from chemical, ultraviolet or direct heat sources
- Abrasion and laceration occur as a result of something dragging across the eye such as fingernail or clothing
- Penetrating wounds are most serious, damage to the eye resulting blindness.

Clinical Manifestations

- Foreign bodies produce pain when eyeball or eyelid moves foreign body to opposing surface, causing ocular dryness eye tears excessively to an attempt to irrigate the noxious substance
- Injuries that irritate or penetrate layers of the cornea range from mild to severe pain; in abrasion sensation of pain delayed for hours
- Conjunctival redness, photo sensitivity, decreased visual acuity, erythema pruritus
- Acute pain and burning characteristic oozing for burns
- Penetrating wound results varieties of symptoms depending on the area if nerve dryness then no pain.

Diagnostic Test

Visual acuity, slit lamp microscopy, direct ophthalmoscopy and fluorescence stain.

Therapeutic Measures/Management

1. Foreign body: Treatment with normal saline flush to irrigate the object out:
   - To a patient where it can be removed with a swab
   - Topical antibiotic ointment to prevent infection as prescribed.
2. Most chemical burns are treated immediately with 15–20 minutes irrigation of either tap water at site or sterile solution in hospital:
   - Topical antibiotics
   - Burns from ultraviolet radiation are should not be irrigated.
3. Abrasion and laceration treated with anti-infective ointment or drops.
4. An eye specialist is needed to treat penetrating wounds.

Nursing Management

Take nursing measures according to therapeutic measures and routine nursing measures in eye disorder.

HEARING IMPAIRMENT

Hearing impairment may be congenital or acquired. Hearing impairment ranges from difficulty in understanding words or hearing certain sounds to total deafness. This can affect communication, social activities and work activities and can diminish quality of life:

1. Conductive hearing loss is an interference with conduction of sound impulses through the external auditory canal, the eardrum or the middle ear, but inner ear not involved. It is caused by cerumen, foreign bodies, infection, perforation of tympanic membrane, trauma, fluid in the middle ear, cysts, tumor and otosclerosis.
2. Sensorineural hearing loss originates in the cochlea and involves hair cells and nerve endings. Neural hearing loss originates in the nerve or brain. It results from disease or trauma to sensorium components of the inner ear may be due to nerve deafness complication of infection (measles, mumps, meningitis), ototoxic drugs, trauma, noise, neuromas, arteriosclerosis and the aging process. Presbycusis in hearing loss caused by aging process.
3. There may be mixed hearing loss when individual has both of the above losses.

Clinical Manifestations

- Difficulty in understanding words or certain sounds
- Total deafness
- Change in social and work activities, turns up volume on television ask, what did you say?
- Reports people are talking softly, speaks in a quiet or loud voice, anterior questions in appropriately
- Avoids activities, loss of sense of humor, appears aloof
- Reports ringing, buzzing or roaring noise in ears.

Diagnostic Tests

- Abnormal Rinne and Weber tests
- Audiometric testing indicates hearing loss.

Therapeutic Measures

- Cerumenolytics
- Anti-infective
- Anti-inflammators
- Assist devices (hearing aids, implantable middle ear hearing device, cochlear implants).

Nursing Management

Take measures for:

- Disturbed sensory perception: Hearing related to altered sensory perception and transmissions
- Impaired verbal communication related to impaired hearing
- Impaired social interactions/disturbed body image/ineffective coping of/degree.

EXTERNAL EAR DISORDER

External otitis are most common infections, due exposure to moisture, contamination or local trauma, provides an ideal environment for pathological growth of the external ear. It may be caused by *Staphylococcus*. Pneumocystis infection is seen with human immunodeficiency syndrome (HIV) cases. Bacterial or fungal external otitis occurs when water is left in the ear. A localized infection results in abscess.

Clinical Manifestations

- Pain, pruritus, swelling, redness
- Drainage, laceration, contusion, hematoma, abrasion
- Erythema, blistering, hearing loss, foreign body
- Complications such as spread of infection to other parts of ear, disfigurement, loss of hearing, scarring.

Diagnostic Test

- Complete blood count (CBC) with elevated white blood cells (WBCs) with infections
- Audiometric, Rinne, Weber and whisper voice testing
- Imaging studies to indicate extent of trauma.

Therapeutic Measures/Management

- Cerumenolytics to remove ear wax
- Anti-infectives and anti-inflammatory medications (to treat infection)
- Debridement, surgical repair
- Application of protective covering with trauma to external ear.

Nursing Management

In addition routine nursing care, measures are:
- Acute pain related to inflammation or trauma
- Disturbed sensory perception: Auditory related to altered sensory perception
- Risk for injury related to self-cleaning of external ear
- Deficient knowledge related to care of hearing aid due to lack of prior experience
- Instruct patient, how to care for ear to prevent injury
- Instruct patient, how to complete prescribed treatment to ensure complication of treatment.

OTITIS MEDIA

Otitis media is a general term for inflammation of the middle ear, mastoid and eustachian tube. Inflammation of the nasopharynx causes most cases of otitis media. As inflammation occurs, the nasopharyngeal mucosa becomes edematous and discharge is produced. When fluid, pus or air buildup in the middle ear, the eustachian tube blocked and this impair middle ear ventilation.

Clinical Manifestations

- Fever, earache and feeling of fullness in affected ear following upper respiratory infections
- Nausea and vomiting
- Mastoid tenderness
- Reddened, bulging tympanic membrane

- Progressive hearing loss
- Vertigo, disorientation.

Complications

- Perforated tympanic membrane
- Cholesteatoma
- Tympanosclerosis
- Mastoiditis
- Permanent hearing loss.

Therapeutic Measures/Management

- Antibodies, analgesics
- Myringotomy, myringoplasty
- Stapedectomy.

Nursing Management

- In addition to routine nursing measure, take care of acute pain, deficient knowledge and risk for infections
- Nursing care of the surgical interventions—preoperations and postoperations.

ACUTE OTITIS MEDIA

Otitis media is an acute infection of the middle ear usually lasting less than 6 weeks. The pathogens that cause acute otitis media are usually *Streptococcus pneumoniae, Haemophilus influenzae* and *Moraxella catarrhalis*, which enter the middle ear after eustachian tube dysfunction caused by obstruction related to upper respiratory infections, inflammation of surrounding structures (e.g. rhinosinusitis, adenoid hypertrophy) or allergic reactions (e.g. allergic rhinitis). Bacteria can enter the eustachian tube from contaminated secretions in the nasopharynx and the middle ear from a tympanic membrane perforation. The disorder is most common in children.

Clinical Manifestations

- Symptoms are vary with severity of the infection usually unilateral in adults
- Pain in and about the ear (otalgia) may be intense and relieved only after spontaneous perforation of the eardrum or after myringotomy
- Fever, drainage from the ear and hearing loss
- Tympanic membrane (TM) is erythematous and often bulging
- Conductive hearing loss due to exudates in the middle ear
- Even if the condition becomes subacute (3 week to 3 month) with purulent discharge, permanent hearing loss is rare.

Complications

- Perforation of the tympanic membrane may persist and develop into chronic otitis media
- Secondary complications involve the mastoid (mastoiditis), meningitis, or brain abscess (rare).

Management

1. With early and appropriate broad-spectrum antibiotic therapy, otitis media may clear with no serious sequelae. If drainage occurs, an antibiotic otic preparation may be prescribed.
2. Outcome depends on efficiency of therapy (prescribed dose of an oral antibiotic and the duration of therapy), the virulence of the bacteria and the physical status of the patient.

Myringotomy (Tympanotomy)

If mild cases of otitis media are treated effectively, myringotomy may not be necessary. An incision is made into the tympanic membrane to relieve pressure and to drain serous or purulent fluid in the middle ear. This painless procedure usually takes less than 15 minutes. If episodes of acute otitis media recur and there is no contraindication, a ventilating or pressure-equalizing tube may be inserted.

CHRONIC OTITIS MEDIA

Chronic otitis media results from repeated episodes of acute otitis media causing irreversible tissue pathology and persistent perforation of the tympanic membrane. Chronic infections of the middle ear cause damage the tympanic membrane, can destroy the ossicles and involve the mastoid.

Clinical Manifestations

1. Symptoms may be minimal with varying degrees of hearing loss and a persistent or intermittent foul-smelling otorrhea (discharge).
2. Pain may be present, in case of acute mastoiditis, when mastoiditis is present, postauricular area is tender; erythema and edema may be present.
3. Cholesteatoma (sac filled with degenerated skin and sebaceous material) may be present as a white mass behind the tympanic membrane visible through an otoscope. If untreated, the cholesteatoma continues to grow and destroys structures of the temporal bone possibly causing damage to the facial nerve and horizontal canal and destruction of other surrounding structures. Auditory tests often show a conductive or mixed hearing loss.

Medical Management

1. Careful suctioning and cleaning of the ear are done under microscopic guidance.
2. Antibiotic drops are instilled or antibiotic powder is applied to treat purulent discharge.
3. Tympanoplasty procedures (myringoplasty and more extensive types) may be performed to prevent recurrent infection, re-establish middle ear function, close the perforation and improve hearing.
4. Ossiculoplasty may be done to reconstruct the middle ear bones to restore hearing.
5. Mastoidectomy may be done to remove cholesteatoma, gain access to diseased structures and create a dry (noninfected) and healthy ear.

Nursing Management

Refer 'Nursing Management' under heading 'Mastoiditis' for additional information.

MASTOIDITIS

Otitis is an inflammation of the mastoid resulting from infection of the middle ear (otitis media). Since, the discovery of antibiotics, acute mastoids have been rare. Chronic otitis may cause chronic mastoiditis. Chronic mastoids can lead to the formation of cholesteatoma (ingrown of skin of the external layer of the eardrum into the middle ear). If mastoiditis is untreated, osteomyelitis may occur.

Clinical Manifestations

- Pain and tenderness behind the ear (postauricular)
- Discharge from the middle ear (otorrhea)
- Mastoid area that becomes erythematous and edematous.

Medical Management

General symptoms are usually successfully treated with antibiotics; occasionally, myringotomy is required.

Surgical Management

If recurrent or persistent tenderness, fever, headache and discharge from the ear are evident, mastiodectomy may be necessary to remove the cholesteatoma and gain access to diseased structures.

Nursing Management

Assessment

1. During the health history, collect data about the ear problem including infection, otalgia, otorrhea, hearing loss and vertigo, duration and intensity, causation, prior treatments, health problems, current medications, family history.
2. During the physical assessment, observe for erythema, edema, otorrhea, lesions and odor and color of discharge. Review results of audiogram.

Nursing Diagnoses/Problems

1. Anxiety related to surgical procedure, potential loss of hearing, potential taste disturbance and potential loss of facial movement.
2. Acute pain related to mastoid surgery.
3. Risk for infection related to mastoidectomy, placement of grafts, prostheses or electrodes; surgical trauma to surrounding tissues and structures.
4. Disturbed auditory sensory perception related to ear disorder, surgery or packing.
5. Risk for trauma related to impaired balance of vertigo during the immediate postoperative period or from dislodgement of the graft or prosthesis.
6. Disturbed sensory perception related to potential damage to facial nerve (cranial nerve VII) and chorda tympani nerve.

7. Deficient knowledge about mastoid disease, surgical procedure and postoperative care and expectations.
8. Major goals for mastoidectomy include reduced of anxiety; freedom from pain and comfort; prevention of infection; stable or improved hearing and communication; absence of vertigo and related injury; absence of or adjustment to sensory perceptual alterations and increased knowledge regarding the disease, surgical procedure and postoperative care.

Nursing Interventions (Implementation)

Reducing Anxiety

1. Reinforce information the otological surgeon has discussed: Anesthesia, the location of the incision (postauricular) and expected surgical results (hearing, balance, taste and facial movement).
2. Encourage patient to discuss any anxiety or concerns.

Relieving Pain

1. Administer prescribed analgesic agent for the first 24-hours postoperatively and then only as needed.
2. If a tympanoplasty is also performed, inform patient that he/she may have packing or a wick in the external auditory canal and may experience sharp shooting pains in the ear for 2–3 weeks postoperatively.
3. Inform patient that throbbing pain accompanied by fever may indicate infection and should be reported to the physician.

Preventing Infection

1. Explain prescribed prophylactic antibiotic regimen.
2. Instruct patient to keep water from entering the ear for 6 weeks and to keep postauricular incision dry for 2 days; a cotton ball or lambswool covered with water-insoluble substance (e.g. petroleum jelly) and placed loosely in the ear canal usually prevents water contamination.
3. Observe for and report signs of infection (fever, purulent drainage).
4. Inform patient that some serous drainage is normal postoperatively.

Improving Hearing and Communication

1. Initiate measures to improve hearing and communication. Reduce environmental noise, face patient when speaking, speak clearly and distinctly without shouting. Provide good lighting if patient must speech read and use non-verbal clues.
2. Instruct family that patient will have temporarily reduced hearing from surgery as a result of edema, packing and fluid in the middle ear; instruct family in ways to improve communication with patient.

Preventing Injury

- Administer antiemetics or antivertiginous medications (e.g. antihistamines) as prescribed, if a balance disturbance or vertigo occurs
- Assist patient with ambulation to prevent falls and injury

- Instruct patient to avoid heavy lifting, straining, exertion and nose blowing for 2–3 weeks after surgery to prevent dislodging tympanic membrane graft or ossicular prosthesis.

Preventing Altered Sensory Perception

- Reinforce to patient that a taste disturbance and dry mouth may be experienced on the operated side for several months until the nerve regenerates
- Instruct patient to report immediately any evidence of facial nerve (cranial nerve VII) weakness such as drooping in the mouth on the operated side.

Promoting Family-based Care

- Provide instructions about prescribed medications: Analgesics, antivertiginous agents, and antihistamines for balance disturbance
- Inform patient about the expected effects and potential side effects of the medications
- Instruct patient about any activity restrictions
- Teach patient to monitor for possible complications such as infection, facial nerve weakness or taste disturbances including signs and symptoms to report immediately
- Refer patients, particularly elderly patients for home care nursing
- Caution caregiver and patient that patient may experience some vertigo and will therefore require help with ambulation to avoid falling
- Instruct patient to report promptly any symptoms of complications to the surgeon
- Stress the importance of scheduling and keeping follow-up appointments.

Evaluations

Evaluation is based on the objectives of care/expected patient outcomes:

- Demonstrates reduced anxiety about surgical procedure
- Remains free of discomfort or pain
- Demonstrates no signs or symptoms of infection
- Exhibits signs that hearing has stabilized or improved
- Remains free of injury and trauma
- Adjusts to or remains free of altered sensory perception
- Verbalizes the reasons for and methods of care and treatment.

LABYRINTHITIS

Labyrinthitis is an inflammation or infections of the inner ear and can be caused by either viral or a bacterial pathogens. Pathogen enters the inner ear from middle ear, meanings or bloodstream. Serous labyrinthitis, sometimes follows drug intoxication or over indulge in alcohol. It can also be caused by allergy. Diffuse labyrinthitis occurs when acute or chronic otitis media spreads into the inner ear or after middle ear in mastoid surgery.

Clinical Manifestations

- Vertigo, tinnitus and sensorineural hearing loss
- Vertigo or dizziness occurs when the vestibular structure involved

- Tinnitus or ringing in the ear occurs when infection located in cochlea
- Sensorineural loss causes by infections in the cochlea and vestibular structure
- Nystagmus on the affected side
- Other sign and symptoms: Pain, fever, ataxia, nausea, vomiting, begining nerve deafness.

Diagnostic Test

Complete blood count, Rinne and Weber tests.

Therapeutic Measures

- Antibiotics for bacterial inner infection
- Viral infection runs about a week
- Mild sedation help patient to relax
- No specific medicine for dizziness, an antihistamine may be helpful.

Nursing Management

- Patient may be placed on bedrest
- Helping the patient manage symptoms and self-care
- Educating the patient about safety issue, while on bedrest
- Sedatives to prevent falls and injury
- Patient is advised to avoid turning head quickly to help alleviate vertigo
- Patient should be assisted to cope with anxiety.

ACOUSTIC NEUROMA

Acoustic neuroma, a tumor of VIII cranial nerve, is a benign tumor. It is slow growing, occurs at any age and occurs usually unilaterally. As it spreads, it compresses the nerve and adjacent structures.

Clinical Manifestations

- Early symptoms: Progressive unilateral sensorineural hearing loss of high-pitched sounds, unilateral tinnitus and intermittent vertigo
- Headache, pain and balance disorders may be also present
- Symptoms progresses as the tumor spreads to other structures.

Diagnostic Tests

- Neurologic, audiometric and vestibular testing are used
- Auditory brainstem evoked response (ABR)
- Electronystagmography (ENG)
- Cerebrospinal fluid (CSF) examination shows increased proteins
- Computed tomography (CT), MRI used to detect size and location of tumor.

Therapeutic Measures

- Surgical removal of tumor
- Steroids and radiation may be used to decrease size of tumor inoperable ones.

Nursing Management

Preoperative Care

- Collecting data relevant to surgery, determine if the patient understands event more the patient mental readiness, obtains baseline physiology day
- Ask understanding of surgery whether local or general anesthesia
- Help alleviate patients fear by encouraging the patient to ask questions and clarify properly
- Explain the type of pain or any packing, or dressings, etc.
- Establish baseline vital signs and document findings
- Ensure the consent taken, determine current medication in taking and document
- Leave hearing devices, if any before surgery.

Postoperative Care

- Assess the patient physiological conditions act accordingly
- Explain when to take pain medications or give analgesic as prescribed
- Monitor postoperative vital signs and return to presurgical baseline
- Tell the patient that dressing in place, hearing may be decreased
- Instruct patient with tubes to avoid getting water in the ear
- Instruct him/her to seek medical attention, if excessive bleeding or drainage
- Avoid airoplane/flights for 1 week after surgery
- Avoid strenuous work for several weeks
- Tell the patient to take prescribed medications as prescribed.

MÉNIÉRE'S DISEASE

Méniére's disease is a balance disorder. Its cause is unknown with the disease; there is dilation of the membranous labyrinth resulting from a disturbance in the fluid physiology of the endolymphatic system.

Exact cause is unknown, but it is thought to stem from hypersecretion, hypoabsorption, deficit membranes permeability, allergy, viral infections, hormonal imbalance or mental stress.

Méniére's disease in an abnormal inner ear fluid balance (too much circulatory fluid) caused by malabsorption in the sac or blockage in the duct. Endolymphatic hydrops, a dilation in the endolymphatic space, develops. Either increased pressure in the system or rupture of the inner ear membranes occurs, producing symptoms. Although it has been reported in children, Méniére's disease is more common in adults with average age of onset in the 40s. There is no cure. There are two possible subsets of the disease, cochlear and vestibular:

1. Cochlear disease is recognized as a fluctuating, progressive sensorineural hearing loss associated with tinnitus and aural pressure, in the absence of vestibular symptoms or findings.
2. Vestibular disease is characterized as the occurrence of episodic vertigo associated with aural pressure but no cochlear symptoms.

Clinical Manifestations

Symptoms of Méniére's disease include fluctuating, progressive sensorineural hearing loss; tinnitus or a roaring sound; a feeling of pressure or fullness in the ear and episodic, incapacitating vertigo often accompanied by nausea and vomiting. At the onset, only one or two symptoms may be manifested. Attacks occur with increasing frequency until eventually all of the symptoms develop:

1. A triad symptoms of vertigo, hearing loss and tinnitus.
2. Recurrent episode bouts of incapacitating triad of symptoms and nausea and vomiting.
3. The attack may occur suddenly or patient may experiences warning signs such as headache or fullness in the ears:
   - Acute episode patient experiences vertigo then lasts 2–4 hours
   - Vertigo usually accompanied by nausea, vomiting followed by dizziness an unsteadiness
   - Uncoordinated movements, while walking gait changes
   - Hearing loss-fluctuating fullness in the ear
   - Tinnitus, irritability, depression, withdrawal is common
   - It takes several weeks for symptoms to resolve.

Diagnostic Measures and Methods

Diagnostic measures are audiometry studies, neurological testing and radiographic studies. The diagnostic methods are:

- Disease is not diagnosed until the four major symptoms are present; careful history of vertigo and nausea and vomiting contributes to diagnosis
- There is no absolute diagnostic test for this disease
- Audiovestibular diagnostic procedures including Weber test are used with finding of sensorineural hearing loss in the affected ear
- Electronystagmogram may be normal or may show reduced vestibular response.

Therapeutic Measures

The goals are to preserve hearing and reduce symptoms:

- Symptomatic treated and prophylactic treatment between attacks
- Tranquilizers and vagal blockers during acute attack
- Salt-restricted diet, diuretics, antihistamine or vasodilators may be used on prophylactic treatment
- The patient should avoid alcohol, caffeine and tobacco use
- When medical measures fail, surgical interventions include labyrinthectomy (unilateral).

Nursing Management

- Management of symptoms of patient
- Provide safety during attacks
- Emotional support for patient during periods of remission, which helps to patient to cope with unpredictable nature of disease and the physical impairment associated with disease.

Medical Management

Goals of treatment include recommendations for changes in lifestyle and habits or surgical treatment. The treatment is designed to eliminate vertigo or to stop the progression of or stabilize the disease.

Psychological evaluation may be indicated if patient is anxious, uncertain, fearful or depressed.

Dietary Management

- Low sodium (1,000–1,500 mg/day or less)
- Avoidance of alcohol, monosodium glutamate (MSG), Aspirin contain medications.

Drug Therapy

1. Antihistamines such as meclizine (Antivert) to suppress the vestibular system; tranquilizers such as diazepam (Valium) help to control vertigo; antiemetics such as promethazine (Phenergan) suppositories to control the nausea, vomiting and vertigo.
2. Diuretics to lower pressure in the endolymphatic system.
3. Vasodilators are often used in conjunction with other therapies.

Surgical Management

Surgical procedures include endolymphatic sac decompression and vestibular nerve section. However, hearing loss, tinnitus and aural fullness may continue because the surgical treatment of Méniére's disease is aimed at eliminating the attacks of vertigo.

Nursing Management of the Patient with Vertigo

Preventing Injury

- Assess for vertigo
- Reinforce vestibular
- Administer and teach about antivertiginous medications and vestibular sedation; instruct in side effects
- Encourage patient to sit down when dizzy
- Recommend that patient keep eyes open and stare straight ahead when lying down and experiencing vertigo; place pillows on side of head to restrict movement
- Assist the patient in identifying the aura, which suggests an impending attacks

Adjusting to Disability

- Encourage patient to identify personal strengths and roles that can be fulfilled
- Provide information about vertigo and what to expect
- Include family and significant others in rehabilitation process
- Encourage patient in making decisions and assuming more responsibility for care.

Maintaining Fluid Volume

- Assess intake and output; monitor laboratory values
- Assess indicators of dehydration
- Encourage oral fluids as tolerated; avoid caffeine (a vestibular stimulant)
- Teach about antiemetics and antidiarrheal medications.

Relieving Anxiety

- Assess level of anxiety; help to identify successful coping skills
- Provide information about vertigo and its treatment
- Encourage patient to discuss anxieties and explore concerns about vertigo attacks
- Teach stress management; provide comfort measures.

Teaching Patients Self-care

- Teach patient to administer antiemetic and other prescribed medications to relieve nausea and vomiting
- Encourage patient to cure for bodily needs when free of vertigo
- Review diet with patient and caregivers; offer fluids as necessary.

19

Chapter Nursing the Poisoned Client

INTRODUCTION

Any substance, which produces adverse reactions/effects in the living organisms, is called 'poison'. Acute poisoning is the common cause of morbidity and mortality throughout the world and is the most common cause of non-traumatic coma in young persons (< 15 year of age). Hospital-based data suggest that about 10% of all medical admissions are due to poisoning.

TYPES OF POISONING

Poisoning can be classified into three types, which are as follows:

- **Self-poisoning** refers to the deliberate ingestion of an overdose of a substance/drug, which is not meant for consumption, it is also called suicidal or intentional poisoning, e.g. aluminum phosphide, organophosphate (OP) compound poisonings
- **Accidental poisoning** occurs in children below 5 years of age, but can occur in adults, is either due to accidental exposure (inhalation of gas) or ingestion of fluid or substance from a wrong labeled bottle and also includes strings, bites, or eating poisoned foods/plants, e.g. mushroom poisoning
- **Homicidal poisoning** means intension to kill someone by poisoning.

ASSESSMENT

History Taking

Important points on history taking will include:

- Time, route of administration, duration
- Name and amount of poison, chemical ingredients involved (summon the bottle/container/wrapper of poison to verify it)
- The print code on the pills or label may be used to identify the ingredients
- Family, friends police, pharmacists, physician and employees should be asked regarding the habits, hobbies, behavior, available medication, and clinical ground for suspicion of poisoning
- Circumstances of exposure(location, surroundings and intent)
- Symptomatology, e.g. time of onset, nature and severity of symptoms
- Time and type of first aid given
- Medical history for any acute illness
- Psychiatric illness
- History of alcohol or drug overdose.

Physical Examination

A search for clothes, belongings and place of discovery may help to recover a suicidal note or a container, which may have the remaining tablets or chemical.

The physical examination should initially focus on the vital signs and cardiopulmonary and neurological status. Before proceeding for detailed clinical examination, first ensure A, B and C of cardiopulmonary resuscitation:

- The airway (A) is clear
- The patient is breathing (B) properly and adequately
- The circulation (C) is adequate and is not compromised.

If patient is alert and hemodynamically stable, proceed to examine in the following way:

- Level of consciousness: The Glasgow coma scale may be employed to assess the degree of unconsciousness, though it has never been validated for use in poisoned patients
- Look for respiratory effort, cyanosis, and presence or absence of cough, and gag reflex
- Record pulse rate and blood pressure (BP)
- Examination of eyes (nystagmus, size of the pupil and its reaction), abdomen (for bowel activity and bladder size) and skin (for burns, bullae, color, warmth, moisture, pressure sores, puncture marks) to narrow down the diagnosis to a particular poison
- Temperature: Measure with a low reading rectal thermometer
- When history is unclear, all orifices should be examined for the presence of chemical burns and drug packets
- The odor of breath or vomitus and the color of the skin, nail or urine may give valuable information for diagnosis.

MANAGEMENT

The aims of management are:

- To support the vital functions (circulatory and respiratory)
- To delay or prevent further absorption of poison
- To enhance the excretion of poison (through feces or urine)
- To administer specific antidote, where applicable and to prevent re-exposure.

General Management

Support of Vital Functions

Supportive therapy may be needed to maintain vital function and to prevent and treat the secondary complication such as aspiration, bedsores, and generalized organ dysfunction due to prolonged hypoxia or shock.

Specific Management/Measures

Specific management depends on the route of exposure, i.e. direct contact (eye, skin), ingestion (gastrointestinal tract), inhalation (lungs) and inoculation (blood).

Steps to Delay or Prevent Further Absorption of Poison

1. Decontamination of gastrointestinal tract, the steps are:
    - **Gastric lavage** only to be done if a potentially life-threatening amount of toxic substance has been ingested within the last hour; not to be done for acids, alkalis or petroleum distillators
    - **Induced emesis** by syrup of ipecac
    - **Activated charcoal** about 50 g can be given to an adult orally if potentially toxic amount poison has been ingested during

the last hour, but only if the toxin can be bound or absorbed to charcoal; multiple doses of charcoal are given (50 g at q4h) in poisoning by carbamazepine, dapsone, quinine and theophylline

- **Catharsis** is induced by cathartic salts (disodium sulfate, magnesium, sulfate, sodium sulfate)or saccharide (mannitol or sorbitol) to promote fecal excretion of poison; it is contraindicated in corrosive poisoning and diarrhea
- **Whole bowel irrigation** is by polyethylene glycol solution is given for potentially toxic ingestion of iron, lithium theophylline and to clear packets of drugs from body packers.

2. Decontamination of other sites:
   - **Removal of clothing or skin washing** if still required by washing the skin with copious amounts of soap and water for chemical or pesticide exposure
   - **Irrigation of eyes:**
     - Wash the eyes thoroughly for at least 15 minutes with normal saline or water
     - Remove particle from palpebral fissure, if pain persists fluorescence drops and slit lamp examination for corneal damage are essential.
3. Exhalation of poison:
   - **Oxygen and bronchodilators:** Give high-flow of oxygen, e.g. 12 L/min, nebulized by β_2-adrenoceptor agonists if the patient has wheezing.

Steps to Enhance Poison Excretion

1. **Urinary alkalization:** It enhances elimination of salicylates and some pesticides. Give 1.26% of 1 liter sodium bicarbonate intravenously over 3 hours. Check urine P^H, maintain between 7.5 and 8.5. Avoid use of large volumes, i.e. forced diuresis and watch for hypokalemia.
2. **Extracorporeal methods of elimination:** For serious poisoning with salicylate, theophylline, ethylene glycol, methanol carbamazepine, the methods such as hemodialysis or hemoperfusion may be used.

Neutralization of Poison by a Specific Antidote

Antidote counteracts the effects of poisons by neutralizing them (e.g. antigen-antibody reaction), by chelating (chemical bonding) or by antagonizing their physiological effects (opposing nervous system activity, competitive inhibition). Antidote can reduce both morbidity and mortality, but more antidotes are toxic too. The antidotes to various poisons are listed in the Table 19.1.

Nursing Management of Specific Poisoning

Poisoning may be caused by chemicals (acids and alkalies), gases (carbon monoxide), plants (*Datura,* oleander and mushroom), pesticides (organochlorine) and drugs (sedatives and hypnotics). These are common medicolegal cases; therefore nurses must follow the instructions of the doctor and maintain proper record. The common poisoning encountered their symptoms and signs in nursing management as given below.

Table 19.1: Commonly employed antidotes

Sl No	Poison	Antidote
1.	Paracetamol	N-acetylcysteine, methionine
2.	Organophosphorus	Atropine (muscarine effects, pralidoxime (nicotinic effects)
3.	Carbamate	Atropine
4.	Amnita phylloides	Benzylpenicillin
5.	Calcium channel blocker	Calcium chloride/Gluconate
6.	Methanol and ethylene glycol	Ethanol
7.	Benzodiazepine	Flumazenil
8.	Iron	Deferoxamine
9.	Opiates	Naloxone
10.	Cyanide	Sodium nitrate, sodium thiosulfate
11.	Antcholinergics	Physostigmine
12.	Isoniazid	Pyridoxine
13.	Mercury, lead, copper	Calcium ethylenediaminetetraacetate (EDTA), British anti-Lewisite (BAL), D-penicillamine
14.	Anticoagulants	Vitamin K
15.	Beta blockers	Glucagon, adrenaline
16.	Digitalis	Digoxin-specific fragment antigen-binding (Fab) antibody

Corrosives (Acids)

Corrosives are the common household poisoning as acids (sulfuric acid, nitric acid and hydrochloric acid) are present in household use.

Signs and symptoms

- Pain, burn, ulcers and discoloration of mouth and throat
- Drooling of saliva, chocking
- Painful swallowing, retrosternal pain, hematemesis
- Epigastric pain, vomiting, tender abdomen.

Nursing management

Immediate Do's and Don'ts, which nurse should follow in care plan of acid poisoning are listed as follows.

Don'ts

- Do not panic
- Make arrangement to transfer the patient to a hospital; look at the oral cavity and remove any caustic granules and flakes gently
- Do not induce vomiting
- Do not put Ryle's tube as it may cause perforation of thinned mucosa of esophagus or stomach, if still required, a thin can be put only under endoscopic guidance.

Do's

- Immediate liberal use of water or milk mixed with milk of magnesia, aluminum hydroxide and magnesium oxide to neutralize the acid

- Correct hypotension with isotonic fluids and blood products; suction of ice may reduce thirst
- If the patient has respiratory distress perform immediate tracheal intubation or tracheostomy
- Give oxygen
- Intravenous hydrogen receptor blockers may be used for symptomatic relief and may help in early healing of gastric erosion
- Use antibiotics if infection supervenes
- Relief of pain by morphine or pethidine
- Skin, oral and eye lesions may irrigated with plenty of water.

Methanol

Methanol (methyl alcohol) is used as a detergent, is a component varnishes, paint removers, antifreeze solution and spirits. The poisoning commonly occurs as 'hooch tragedy' due to ingestion of cheap illicit liquor called hooch.

Signs and symptoms

- Nausea, vomiting, headache, vertigo
- Alteration in consciousness, convulsion, coma
- Metabolic acidosis leading to acidotic breathing
- Visual disturbance, e.g. clouding, dimness of vision, flashing spots before eye blindness.

Nursing management

- Removal of unabsorbed methanol by Ryle's tube aspiration and administration of 50 g activated charcoal
- Intravenous fluids to correct dehydration
- Intravenous sodium carbonate to correct acidosis
- Intravenous diazepam to control seizures
- Replacement of methanol, but medicated ethanol to saturate the enzyme alcoholic dehydrogenase; this will reduce the formation of formic acid and acetaldehyde hence reduce acidosis
- Supplement thiamine and folate
- Elimination by hemodialysis.

Carbon Monoxide

Poisoning is common after smoke inhalation (incomplete burning of wood, coal, heating system such as stoves and brick ovens) in a closed environment where the exhaust facility is not available.

Signs and symptoms

- Cherry red or pink color of skin
- Dyspnea, orthopnea and tachypnea
- Nausea, vomiting, headache, lack of concentration and fatigue
- Visual disturbance
- Confusion, collapse, seizures, flaccid paralysis
- Hypotension, slow pulse rate
- Respiratory depression, asphyxia, cyanosis
- Coma, death.

Nursing management

- Remove the patient at once in fresh air
- Supplement oxygen
- Ventilator support (e.g. endotracheal intubation and mechanical ventilation).

Organochlorine Poisoning

Organochlorine poisoning [dichlorodiphenyltrichloroethane (DDT), endosulfan, aldrin, benzene hexachloride (BHC), acute toxicity follows accidental and suicidal ingestion].

Signs and symptoms
- Nausea, vomiting
- Hyperexcitability
- Headache, parenthesis and seizure
- Paralysis and coma.

Nursing management
- Repeated skin washing with soap and water
- Gastric lavage
- Diazepam for hyperexitibility and convulsions
- Respiratory support.

Sedative and Hypnotic Poisoning

Sedative (benzodiazepines, ecstasy) and hypnotic (barbiturates) poisoning are usually taken with suicidal intent. Accidental ingestion is rare.

Signs and symptoms
- Weakness, drowsiness
- Hypotonia, hypotension
- Ataxia, dysarthria
- Constricted pupils
- Respiratory depression and coma.

Nursing management
- Gastric lavage
- Intravenous fluids to support circulation and treat dehydration
- Supplement oxygen and patient airway (endotracheal intubation, suction) if there is a cyanosis and respiratory depression
- Use the antidote, e.g. flumazenil for benzodiazepine
- Enhance excretion of barbiturates by forced alkaline diuretics
- Monitor vital sign.

Opiate Poisoning

The opiate (codeine, morphine, pethidine, meperidine, fentanyl, tramadol, methadone, pentazocine) are potent analgesics hence person abuse them frequently. Doctors, paramedical staff (chemist, pharmacist and nurses) use them for pain as well as induce sleep in acute stress. They also abuse them frequently as they are easily available to them. Opiates are also used for local parlance and offered to guests during marriage party.

Signs and symptoms
- Nausea, vomiting, decreased appetite and constipation
- Analgesia, euphoria and sedation
- Cough suppression and slow shallow breathing
- Constricted pupils
- Bradycardia, hypotension and hypothermia
- Stupor, coma, respiratory arrest and death.

Nursing management
- Gastric lavage
- Intravenous fluids for dehydration and hypotension

- Inotropes to raise BP
- Oxygen inhalation and intubation; if respiratory depression present, mechanical ventilation used if needed
- Monitor vital signs (pulse, BP, temperature, respiration)
- Use of an antidote, e.g. naloxone
- Care of unconscious patient as usual.

Organophosphate Poisoning

Acute OP poisoning is commonest in India, occurs due to skin exposure during mixing of power with solvent with naked hands (unprotected skin) or ingestion, or inhalation.

The poisoning is common among agriculturists, industrial and domestic workers.

Signs and symptoms

1. Muscarinic effect:
   - Nausea, vomiting, excessive salvation, lacrimation, nasal discharge, dyspnea, audible wheezes and crackles.
2. Nicotinic effect:
   - Muscle twitchiness, weakness, flaccid paralysis, pallor, giddiness, nightmares, confusion, tremors, ataxia, speech disturbance and convulsion; respiratory paralysis with cyanosis may occur at the end.

Nursing management

- Meticulous washing of skin with soap and water and washing of eyes with water
- Elimination of poison by induced vomiting or gastric lavage
- Maintain airway (endotracheal intubation, suction), mechanical ventilation by Ambu bag, if necessary
- Give oxygen, maintain blood gas analysis
- Control convulsion by diazepam or phenytoin
- Administer antidote, i.e. atropine for muscarinic effects and pralidoxime for nicotinic effects (for dosage, consult the doctor)
- Monitor pulse, BP, urine output and electrocardiogram (ECG) at every 1–2 hours for 24 hours.

Metal Phosphide (Aluminum and Zinc) Poisoning

Aluminum phosphide (AlP) is used as grain preservative to protect grain from pests. Zinc phosphide is used as rat poison. Both produce toxicity due to phosphine gas. Toxicity occurs due to ingestion as well as inhalation of liberated phosphine gas.

Signs and symptoms

Signs and symptoms are similar in both poisoning:

- Nausea, vomiting, thirst, pain in epigastrium
- Hypotension, shock, arrhythmias
- Cough and dyspnea
- Anxiety, fear, apprehension, restlessness, undue crying and occasional convulsion
- Organ system failure, e.g. cardiac, renal, respiratory, hepatic system.

Nursing management

- No antidote, hence, treatment is supportive
- Meticulous gastric lavage with water or potassium permanganate
- For gastric upset, use antacids and hydrogen blockers

- Intravenous fluids for fluid depict
- Resuscitate shock with fluids, saline and vasopressor (dopamine and dobutamine)
- Sodium bicarbonate for metabolic acidosis
- Intravenous magnesium sulfate therapy as membrane stabilizer to reduce the hypoxic toxicity and arrhythmias.

Household Products Poisoning

Poisoning by household products (phenol, dyes, paints and solvents) is common as they are kept in the house for use such as kerosene, turpentine and bleaching solution. Some poisonous nuts, flowers and leaves may be ingested.

Signs and symptoms

Signs and symptoms are depending on the poison ingested and duration of the poisoning. Identification of poison by questioning and observation is essential. In case of emergency with consumption of unknown poison help can be sought from the National Poison Information Centre (NPIC), All India Institutes of Medical Sciences (AIIMS), New Delhi or the state poison center.

Nursing management

These are general measure for identified or unidentified poisons:

- Identify the poison by all available means
- In case of unknown poison, observe the patient
- Send for medical help and transport the patient to the nearby hospital
- Examine the mouth and smell the breath; if anything present in mouth, remove it
- Gastric lavage, if the person is unconscious; if the patient breath smells kerosene, phenol and he/she is unconscious, induce vomiting by tickling the back of the throat
- Give fluids orally if the person is conscious and by IV if the victim is unconscious, to dilute the poison
- In hospital, the nurse must work with the doctor to keep the article ready for stomach wash, bowel wash and obtain the blood samples, vomit and aspirated fluid for chemical analysis
- Care of an unconscious victim as usual; keep the head in lower position
- Monitor vital signs
- Give cardiovascular and respiratory support, when required; keep the suction ready
- Use an antidote, if nature of the poison is known and antidote is available
- Take preventive measure to prevent further complication.

- [illegible], fatigue and [illegible]
- [illegible] hypotension, bradycardia and vasopressor (hypotensive and dysrhythmia).
- Secondary [illegible] pneumonia.
- Intravenous administration of [illegible]

Household Product Poisoning

[illegible] household products [illegible] common [illegible] as [illegible] Some poisonous [illegible] can be treated.

Signs and Symptoms

Signs and symptoms vary depending on the poison ingested and the [illegible] of the poisoning [illegible] of [illegible] [illegible] emergency [illegible] information centre [illegible]

Nursing Management

These are general [illegible]
- Identify [illegible]
- [illegible]
- [illegible] medical [illegible] and [illegible] the patient to the nearest hospital.
- [illegible]
- [illegible] breath [illegible]
- [illegible] if the person is conscious and [illegible] is [illegible] the poison.
- [illegible]
- [illegible]

Avoid vomiting
- [illegible]
- Use [illegible] the poison [illegible]
- [illegible] in the [illegible]

Index

A

B

E

F

G